A Clinical Guide to Colitis

A Clinical Guide to Colitis

Editor: Isabelle Owens

FOSTER ACADEMICS
www.fosteracademics.com

www.fosteracademics.com

FOSTER ACADEMICS

Cataloging-in-Publication Data

A clinical guide to colitis / edited by Isabelle Owens.
p. cm.
Includes bibliographical references and index.
ISBN 978-1-63242-957-5
1. Colitis. 2. Colitis--Treatment. 3. Colon (Anatomy)--Diseases. 4. Gastroenteritis. I. Owens, Isabelle.
RC862.C6 C55 2020
616.344 7--dc23

Foster Academics,
118-35 Queens Blvd., Suite 400,
Forest Hills, NY 11375, USA

ISBN 978-1-63242-957-5 (Hardback)

Contents

Preface

Colitis is an inflammatory disease of the colon. It may be an acute and self-limited condition, or a long-term condition. Colitis can be of various kinds such as ulcerative colitis, lymphocytic colitis, collagenous colitis, ischemic colitis, etc. The symptoms of colitis depend on the underlying cause of the disease, its stage and severity. These may include recurring bloody diarrhea, mild to severe abdominal pain, abdominal tenderness, flatulence, poor appetite, fatigue, etc. Severe symptoms such as irregular or fast heartbeat, fever and shortness of breath may also occur. When viewed using colonoscopy, ulcers, colonic mucosal erythema and bleeding may be observed. A review of the patient's medical history, physical examination and laboratory tests such as CBC, stool culture, stool ova, etc. are performed to diagnose colitis. Medical imaging and imaging of the rectum also help in making such diagnoses. The cause and extent of bowel damage due to colitis can be determined through a biopsy. Medications generally prescribed to treat colitis include immunosuppressant or anti-inflammatory drugs. This book contains some path-breaking studies in colitis. Also included herein is a detailed explanation of the various symptoms of colitis, and their management strategies. This book is meant for students who are looking for an elaborate reference text on colitis.

The researches compiled throughout the book are authentic and of high quality, combining several disciplines and from very diverse regions from around the world. Drawing on the contributions of many researchers from diverse countries, the book's objective is to provide the readers with the latest achievements in the area of research. This book will surely be a source of knowledge to all interested and researching the field.

In the end, I would like to express my deep sense of gratitude to all the authors for meeting the set deadlines in completing and submitting their research chapters. I would also like to thank the publisher for the support offered to us throughout the course of the book. Finally, I extend my sincere thanks to my family for being a constant source of inspiration and encouragement.

Editor

Preface

Colitis is an inflammatory disease of the colon. It may be an acute and self-limited condition, or a long-term condition. Colitis can be of various kinds such as ulcerative colitis, lymphocytic colitis, collagenous colitis, ischemic colitis, etc. The symptoms of colitis depend on the underlying cause of the disease, its stage and severity. These may include recurring bloody diarrhea, mild to severe abdominal pain, abdominal tenderness, flatulence, poor appetite, fatigue, etc. Severe symptoms such as irregular or fast heartbeat, fever and shortness of breath may also occur. When viewed using colonoscopy, ulcers, colonic mucosal erythema and bleeding may be observed. A review of the patient's medical history, physical examination and laboratory tests such as CBC, stool culture, stool ova, etc. are performed to diagnose colitis. Medical imaging and imaging of the rectum also help in making such diagnoses. The cause and extent of bowel damage due to colitis can be determined through a biopsy. Medications generally prescribed to treat colitis include immunosuppressant or anti-inflammatory drugs. This book contains some path-breaking studies in colitis. Also included herein is a detailed explanation of the various symptoms of colitis, and their management strategies. This book is meant for students who are looking for an elaborate reference text on colitis.

The researches compiled throughout the book are authentic and of high quality, combining several disciplines and from very diverse regions from around the world. Drawing on the contributions of many researchers from diverse countries, the book's objective is to provide the readers with the latest achievements in the area of research. This book will surely be a source of knowledge to all interested and researching the field.

In the end, I would like to express my deep sense of gratitude to all the authors for meeting the set deadlines in completing and submitting their research chapters. I would also like to thank the publisher for the support offered to us throughout the course of the book. Finally, I extend my sincere thanks to my family for being a constant source of inspiration and encouragement.

Editor

Expressions of Tight Junction Proteins Occludin and Claudin-1 are under the Circadian Control in the Mouse Large Intestine: Implications in Intestinal Permeability and Susceptibility to Colitis

Kyoko Oh-oka[1], Hiroshi Kono[2], Kayoko Ishimaru[1], Kunio Miyake[3], Takeo Kubota[3], Hideoki Ogawa[4], Ko Okumura[4], Shigenobu Shibata[5], Atsuhito Nakao[1,4*]

1 Department of Immunology, University of Yamanashi Faculty of Medicine, Yamanashi, Japan, **2** The First Department of Surgery, University of Yamanashi Faculty of Medicine, Yamanashi, Japan, **3** Department of Epigenetic Medicine, University of Yamanashi Faculty of Medicine, Yamanashi, Japan, **4** Atopy Research Center, Juntendo University School of Medicine, Tokyo, Japan, **5** Department of Physiology and Pharmacology, School of Advanced Science and Engineering, Waseda University, Tokyo, Japan

Abstract

Background & Aims: The circadian clock drives daily rhythms in behavior and physiology. A recent study suggests that intestinal permeability is also under control of the circadian clock. However, the precise mechanisms remain largely unknown. Because intestinal permeability depends on tight junction (TJ) that regulates the epithelial paracellular pathway, this study investigated whether the circadian clock regulates the expression levels of TJ proteins in the intestine.

Methods: The expression levels of TJ proteins in the large intestinal epithelium and colonic permeability were analyzed every 4, 6, or 12 hours between wild-type mice and mice with a mutation of a key clock gene Period2 (Per2; mPer2$^{m/m}$). In addition, the susceptibility to dextran sodium sulfate (DSS)-induced colitis was compared between wild-type mice and mPer2$^{m/m}$ mice.

Results: The mRNA and protein expression levels of Occludin and Claudin-1 exhibited daily variations in the colonic epithelium in wild-type mice, whereas they were constitutively high in mPer2$^{m/m}$ mice. Colonic permeability in wild-type mice exhibited daily variations, which was inversely associated with the expression levels of Occludin and Claudin-1 proteins, whereas it was constitutively low in mPer2$^{m/m}$ mice. mPer2$^{m/m}$ mice were more resistant to the colonic injury induced by DSS than wild-type mice.

Conclusions: Occludin and Claudin-1 expressions in the large intestine are under the circadian control, which is associated with temporal regulation of colonic permeability and also susceptibility to colitis.

Editor: Christopher R. Weber, University of Chicago, United States of America

Funding: This work was supported by grants from the Ministry of Education, Culture, Sports, Science, and Technology, Japan (H25). The funders had no role in study design, data collection and analysis, decision to publish, or preparation of the manuscript.

Competing Interests: The authors have declared that no competing interests exist.

* E-mail: anakao@yamanashi.ac.jp

Introduction

The intestinal epithelium forms the boundary between the body and external environment and provides a selective permeable barrier that limits the permeation of luminal harmful molecules, while allowing the appropriate absorption of nutrients and water. This selective permeability in the intestine depends on specialized structures composed of tight junctions (TJs) [1–3]. TJs are multiple protein complexes consisting of Occludin, Zonula occludens (Zo), Claudins, and junctional adhesion molecules (JAM), located at the apical ends of the lateral membranes of epithelial cells [2,3].

The circadian clock drives daily rhythms in physiology and behavior that enable organisms to keep track of the time of day [4–6]. Mammalian circadian clock consists of the central oscillator located in the suprachiasmatic nucleus (SCN) of the hypothalamus and peripheral oscillators present in nearly all cell types [4–6]. The central SCN clock is set by light and synchronizes the peripheral clocks via neural and endocrine pathways. At the cellular levels, the circadian clock is based on autonomous interlocking transcriptional-translational feedback loops consisting of several "clock genes". Briefly, the PAS domain helix-loop-helix proteins Clock and Bmal1 bind as heterodimers to regulatory elements of Cryptochrome (Cry) and Period (Per) genes via E-box and stimulate the transcription of these genes. Once the repressor proteins Cry and Per have reached a critical concentration, they attenuate the activity of Clock-Bmal1 heterodimers and thereby repress the transcription of their own genes. These core molecular clocks also control expression of clock-controlled genes (CCGs) via direct or indirect transcriptional activation through clock-controlled transcriptional regulators.

Previous studies suggest that the circadian clock is present in intestinal epithelial cells and plays an important role in several functions of intestinal epithelial cells, such as retaining homeostasis, cell division and lipid absorption [7–9]. A recent study suggested that intestinal permeability was also regulated by the circadian clock [10]. However, the precise mechanisms how the circadian clock affects intestinal permeability remain largely unknown. The primary aim of this study is to investigate whether the expression levels of TJ proteins that play an important role in intestinal permeability are under control of the circadian clock.

Methods

Mice

Female 5- to 6-week-old ICR mice purchased from Japan SLC (Tokyo, Japan), ICR mPer2$^{m/m}$ and Clock$^{\Delta 19/\Delta 19}$ mice were bred under specific pathogen-free conditions. All mice were housed in 12-hours light/12-hours dark conditions (L/D cycles; the light was turned on at 6:00 AM, Zeitgeber time [ZT] 0, and the light was turned off at 6:00 PM, ZT12) with ad libitum access to food and water, for at least 2 weeks. All animal experiments were approved by the institutional review board of the University of Yamanashi and the Committee for Animal Experimentation of the School of Science and Engineering at Waseda University.

Quantitative Real-time PCR (Q-PCR)

A quantitative real-time PCR analysis using cDNA from the mouse tissue specimens was performed using the AB7300 real-time PCR system (Applied Biosystems, Foster City, CA, USA) according to the manufacturer's instructions, using primers and probes for mouse Occludin, Zonula occludens (Zo)-1, Claudin-1, 2, 3, 4, 7, Junctional adhesion molecule (JAM), Myeloperoxidase (Mpo), Heme oxygenase (Ho)-1, Cyclooxygenase (Cox)-2, Prostaglandin E synthetase (Pges)-1, Per1, 2, 3, Clock, Bmal1, Cry1, IL-1β, TNF-α and Glyceraldehyde-3-phosphate dehydrogenase (GAPDH; Applied Biosystems) as previously described [11]. The ratio of each gene to that of GAPDH was calculated, and the relative expression levels are shown.

Isolation of Intestinal Epithelial Cells (IECs)

IECs were isolated as described previously [12]. Briefly, an inverted large intestine of mice was cut into four segments and the segments were transferred to a 50-ml tube containing 10 ml RPMI1640 medium/5% FCS/25mM Hepes. The tube was shaken at 37°C at 100 rpm for 45 min. After incubation, vortex the cell solution vigorously for 20s and pass through a 70 μm cell strainer. Subsequently, the cells were suspended in 30% (wt/vol) Percoll and centrifuged at 20°C at 400×g for 20 min. After centrifugation, cells at the top of the 30% Percoll were enriched with IECs.

Western Blot Analysis

IECs were lysed in buffer containing 0.1 M Tris-HCl (pH 7.5)/2% SDS/10% glycerol/5% 2-mercaptoethanol, boiled at 95°C for 5 min and centrifuged at 15000 rpm for 5 min and analyzed by reducing SDS-PAGE. Immunoblots were performed using antibodies against Claudin-1 (Abcam, Cambridge, UK, ab15098, 1:100), Occludin (Applied Biosystems, 71–1500, 1:250), Clock (Abcam, ab3517, 1:200), Bmal1 (Abcam, ab3350, 1:200) and β-actin (Santa Cruz, Texas, sc-1615, 1:200). Quantitative analysis of Western blotting was done by using the Scion Image Software package and relative intensities of the target proteins to β-actin were shown.

Chromatin Immunoprecipitation (CHiP) Assay

CHiP was performed using SimpleChIP® Enzymatic Chromatin IP Kit (Agarose Beads) (Cell signaling, Tokyo, Japan, #9002). Isolated IECs or cultured cells (HCT116 and Caco-2) were cross-linked in 1% formaldehyde, followed by the CHiP assay according to the manufacturer's protocol. Rabbit polyclonal antibodies to CLOCK (ab3517) and BMAL1 (ab3350) were from Abcam (Cambridge, UK). DNA was purified and Q-PCR was done using SYBRgreen reagent (QIAGEN, Hilden, Germany). Primers used were as follows: mouse Occludin promoter forward 5′-CTCCCATCCGAGTTTCAGGT-3′ and reverse 5′-GCTGTCGCCTAAGGAAAGAG-3′, mouse Claudin-1 promoter forward 5′-GTTTGCAGAGACCCCATCAC-3′ and reverse 5′-AGAAGCCAGGATGAAACCCA-3′, human Occludin promoter forward 5′-CTCCCATCCGAGTTTCAGGT-3′ and reverse, human Claudin-1 promoter forward 5′-CTCCCCGCCTTAACTTCCTC-3′ and reverse 5′-CAGGAAGGCGAGAATGAAGC-3′, 5′-GGAGTGTAGGTGTGGTGTGT-3′.

Isolation of Promoter Fragments and Reporter Assay

A human Occludin (–60 to +240) or Claudin-1 (–1010 to +360) promoter fragment containing E-box elements was amplified by PCR from genomic DNA of TIG120 cells and cloned into the pGL3 vector (Promega, Fitchburg, Wisconsin) upstream of firefly luciferase. Primer sequences used were as follows: human Occludin promoter forward 5′-CTCGAGAAAGTGCTGAGTGCCTGGAC-3′ and reverse 5′-AAGCTTTCGGTGACCAATTCACCTGA-3′, human Claudin-1 promoter forward 5′-CTCGAGGGAAACTACAGTCCCAGCGA-3′ and reverse 5′-AAGCTTGATGTTGTCGCCGGCATAGG-3′. These reporter constructs were transfected into HCT-116 or Caco-2 cells cultured in 96-well plates using Fugene6 (Promega) in the presence of pcDNA3, pcDNA3-Clock or pcDNA3-Bmal1 expression plasmid. pcDNA3-Clock and pcDNA3-Bmal1 expression plasmids were kindly gifted by Dr. Fuyuki Sato (Hirosaki University, Aomori, Japan). At 48 hours after transfection, the luciferase activity was measured using the luciferase reporter assay system (TOYO ink, Tokyo, Japan).

In vivo Colon Permeability Assay

Colon permeability to Evans blue was measured *in vivo*. This is a well-validated method for assessing epithelial permeability [13]. In isoflurane-N_2O anesthesia, spontaneously breathing animals were placed in a supine position on a heating pad and a laparotomy was performed. A small polyethylene tube (G22) was inserted into the proximal colon ascendens (immediately adjacent to the cecum) and secured by a ligature. Via this tube the colon was gently flushed until all stool was rinsed out, and 1 ml of Evans blue 1.5% (Sigma-Aldrich Japan, Tokyo, Japan, E2129) in PBS was instilled into the colon and left in place for 15 min. Then the colon was rinsed with PBS, until the perianal washout was clear. Animals were euthanized, and the colon was rapidly taken out. It was rinsed again with several milliliters of PBS, followed by 1 ml of 6 mM N-acetylcysteine to eliminate dye sticking in the colonic mucus. The colon was opened and rinsed once more with PBS, and its length was recorded. The whole colon was placed in 2 ml N,N-dimethylformamide for 12 h to extract the Evans blue dye. The dye concentration in the supernatant was measured spectrophotometrically at 610 nm and given as extinction per gram colonic tissue.

Ex vivo Colon Permeability Assay

Colon permeability was measured in isolated intestinal segments using FITC-dextran or Horseradish peroxidase (HRP) as described previously [14,15]. Briefly, 6-cm segments of the large intestine were removed, rinsed with ice-cold saline, everted, filled with 700 μl PBS and ligated at both ends. The filled colon segments were incubated in PBS containing 1 mM FITC-dextran (average mol wt, 4000 Sigma-Aldrich Co. Missouri, USA) or 0.4 mg/ml HRP (type IV, 300 units/mg solid, Sigma-Aldrich Co.). The colon sacs were removed after 45 minutes and the contents (~500 μL) of each sac was collected carefully using a 1-ml syringe. The amount of FITC-dextran that transverse the colon was quantified by fluorescence plate reader at 521 nm. The HRP activity in the contents of each sac was determined spectrophotometrically based on the rate of oxidation of pyrogallol.

Induction of Dextran Sodium Sulfate (DSS)-induced Colitis

Colitis was induced by feeding mice 5% DSS dissolved in drinking distilled water (mol wt 5000; Wako Pure Chemical Co., Osaka, Japan) for 7 days, as previously described [16].

Stool Scores

The stool scores were calculated based on a method by Cooper et al. with some modifications [17]. Briefly, the scoring was based on a maximum score of 4. Stool consistency was graded as: 0 = firm, 1 = loose, 2 = diarrhea. Blood in the stool was also evaluated on a 0- to 2-point scale. 0 = no blood, 1 = occult blood, 2 = gross rectal bleeding.

Enzyme-Linked Immunosorbent Assay (ELISA)

The concentrations of tumor necrosis factor-α (TNF-α) and interleukin-6 (IL-6) in the mouse colon tissue were determined using the mouse TNF-α and IL-6 enzyme-linked immunosorbent assay (ELISA) kits (R&D Inc, Minneapolis, MN), respectively, according to the manufacturer's instructions.

Generation of Bone Marrow Chimeric Mice

Recipient wild-type mice or mPer2$^{m/m}$ mice were lethally irradiated with 1050 rads using a Co irradiator and then were injected intravenously 6 hours later with 1×10^7 bone marrow cells derived from the femurs of the respective donors.

Statistical Analysis

Values represent the mean ± S.D. The statistical analysis was performed using the unpaired Studentns t-test. The statistical analysis of time-of-day-dependent variations in mRNA and protein levels was performed using a one-way analysis of variance (ANOVA). A value of $P<0.05$ was considered to be significant.

Results

Occludin and Claudin-1 Expressions Exhibit a Time of Day-dependent Variation in Colonic Epithelium, Relying on Normal Per2 Activity

The mRNA levels of Occludin, Zo-1, Claudin-1, -2, -3, -4, -7 and JAM-A, major components of TJ, were examined in the colon tissue samples obtained from wild-type mice and mice with the loss-of-function mutation of a key clock gene Period2 (Per2; mPer2$^{m/m}$) every 6 hours during the day to investigate the possible circadian variations [18]. We found that the mRNA levels of Occludin and Claudin-1, but not Claudin-2, -3, -4, -7, Zo-1, and JAM-A, in the colon showed a time of day-dependent variation in wild-type mice (**Fig. 1A**). Detailed kinetic analysis of mRNA levels of Occludin and Claudin-1 at every 4 hours during the day revealed that the mRNA levels showed a nadir at Zeitgeber time (ZT) 12 (18:00 PM) (**Fig. S1A**). We also found that Per1, Per2, Cry1, and Bmal1 mRNA levels in the colon exhibited a time of day-dependent variation (**Fig. S2**) and the kinetics of Per1 and Per2 mRNA expression were the opposite phase to Occludin and Claudin-1 mRNA kinetics (**Fig. 1A**). Consistently, the expression levels of Occludin and Claudin-1 proteins in colonic IECs showed a similar time of day-dependent variation to the mRNA expressions (**Fig. 1B and C**). Detailed kinetic analysis of protein levels of Occludin and Claudin-1 at every 4 hours during the day revealed that the protein levels showed a nadir at ZT 16 (22:00 PM) (**Fig. S1B**), suggesting that there was a time-lag between mRNA and protein expression changes of Occludin and Claudin-1. However, please note that the circadian changes of Occludin, but not Claudin-1, protein levels did not reach a statistical significance ($p = 0.053$) and showed only a trend of circadian oscillations in this analysis. In contrast to wild-type mice, mPer2$^{m/m}$ mice showed constitutively high expression levels of Occludin and Claudin-1 mRNAs and proteins without oscillations (**Fig. 1**). These results suggested that Occludin and Claudin-1 expressions in colonic epithelium showed circadian oscillations, which relied on normal Per2 activity.

Clock and Bmal1 Bind to the E-box Element in the Promoter Regions of Occludin and Claudin-1 Genes and Affect their Trancriptional Responses

The Clock-Bmal1 heterodimer binds directly to the E-box element of the clock controlled genes (CCGs) [19,20]. Occludin and Claudin-1 possess E-box elements in the promoter regions of the genes [21,22]. To examine whether Clock and Bmal1 bind to the E-box elements of Occludin and Claudin-1 promoter regions, we performed CHiP assays by using IECs isolated from the colonic tissues of wild-type and mPer2$^{m/m}$ mice every 12 hours during the day.

Clock and Bmal1 bound to the E-box elements of Occludin and Claudin-1 promoter regions in mouse colonic IECs (**Fig. 2A**). Interestingly, the ratio of binding showed a time of day-dependent variation in IECs from the colon of wild-type mice, with a high at day (ZT4: 10:00 AM) and low at night (ZT16: 10:00 PM) (**Fig. 2A**). However, such a variation was absent in mPer2$^{m/m}$ mice (**Fig. 2A**). The bindings of Clock and Bmal1 to the E-box elements of Occludin and Claudin-1 promoter regions were also confirmed in human colonic epithelial cell lines HCT-116 and Caco-2 cells (**Fig. 2B and Fig. S3A**).

To investigate whether Clock and Bmal1 regulate transcriptional responses of Occludin and Claudin-1, we performed reporter assays using luciferase-reporter plasmids containing human Occludin (–60 to +240) or Claudin-1 (–1010 to +360) promoter fragments with E-box elements. Transfection of the Occludin- or Claudin-1 promoter reporter plasmids into HCT-116 cells showed ~20-fold increases in luciferase activity compared with transfection of control pGL3-basic plasmid without containing the promoter elements (data not shown), suggesting that these plasmids were activated in HCT-116 cells. Overexpression of Clock or Bmal1 in HCT-116 cells further increased the luciferase activity of Occludin- or Claudin-1-reporter plasmids (**Fig. 2C**). Similar findings were also observed in Caco-2 cells (**Fig. S3B**). These results suggested that Clock and Bmal1 bound directly to the E-box elements of Occludin and Claudin-1 promoters and increased the transcriptional responses.

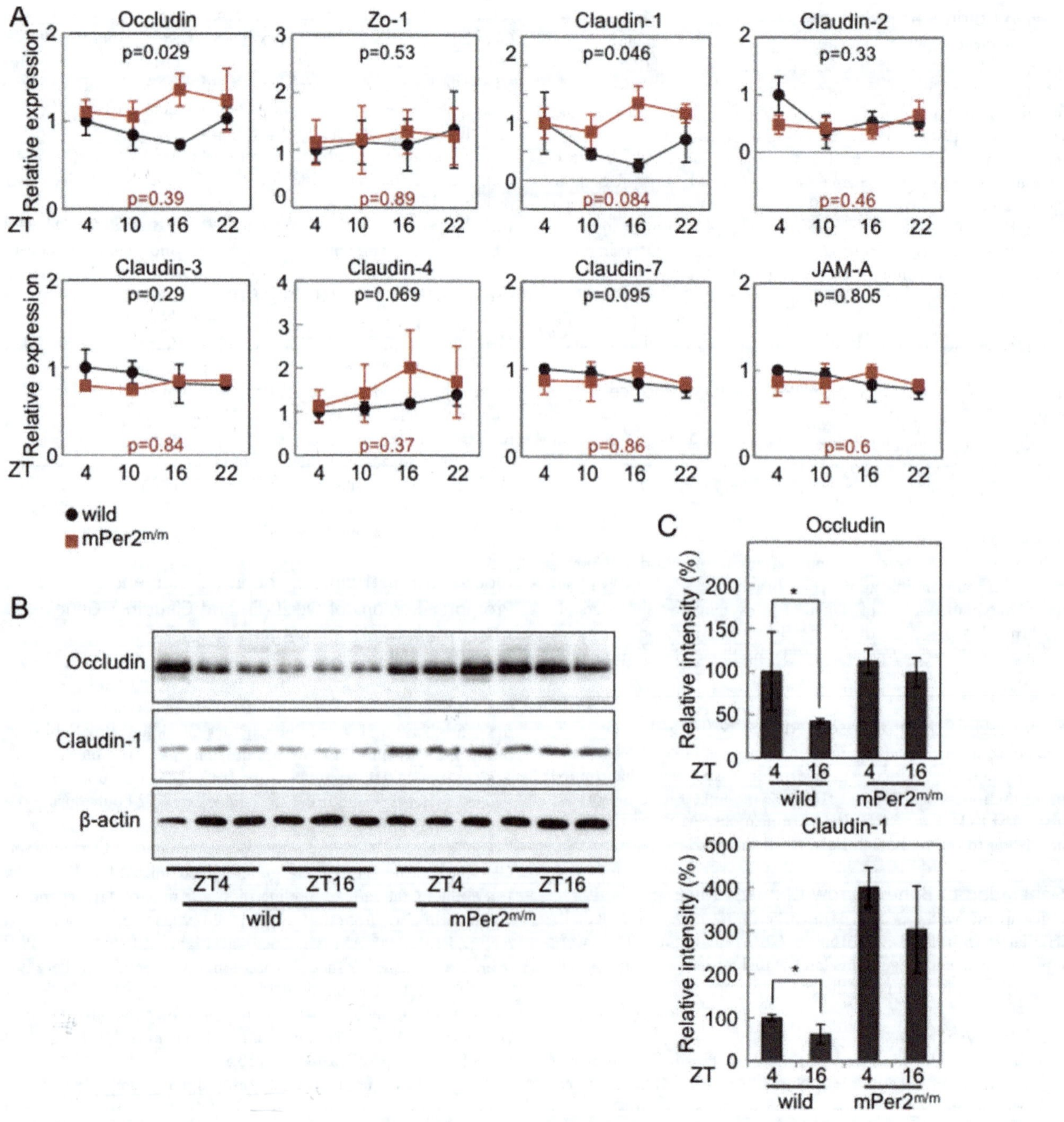

Figure 1. Occludin and Claudin-1 expressions exhibit a time of day-dependent variation in colonic epithelium, relying on normal Per2 activity. (**A**) Real-time PCR analysis for Occludin, Zo-1, Claudin-1, -2, -3, -4, -7, and JAM mRNAs expression in the colon tissue samples obtained from the wild-type mice and mPer2$^{m/m}$ mice at the indicated time points (n = 8 per group). (**B**) Representative pictures of Western blot for Occludin, Claudin-1 and β-actin expression in colonic epithelial cell samples from wild-type and mPer2$^{m/m}$ mice obtained at the indicated time points (n = 3 per group). (**C**) The quantitative analysis of (**B**) (n = 3 per group). *p<0.05.

Colonic Permeability is under the Circadian Control, which is Inversely Associated with Occludin and Claudin-1 Expression Levels

The possibility of altered epithelial permeability in wild-type and mPer2$^{m/m}$ mice was investigated since the TJ proteins play an important role in epithelial permeability through the control of the paracellular pathway for movement of intestinal fluid and macromolecules [1–3]. Colonic permeability to Evans blue *in vivo* and to FITC-dextran and HRP *ex vivo* showed a time-of-day dependent variation in wild-type mice, with a high at night (ZT16: 10:00 PM) and low at day (ZT4: 10:00 AM), which was the opposite phase to Occludin and Claudin-1 protein levels (**Fig. 2 and 3**). However, such a variation was absent in mPer2$^{m/m}$ mice and, as expected, the colonic permeability was lower in mPer2$^{m/m}$ mice than that in wild-type mice (**Fig. 3**). These results suggested that colonic permeability was under control of the circadian clock,

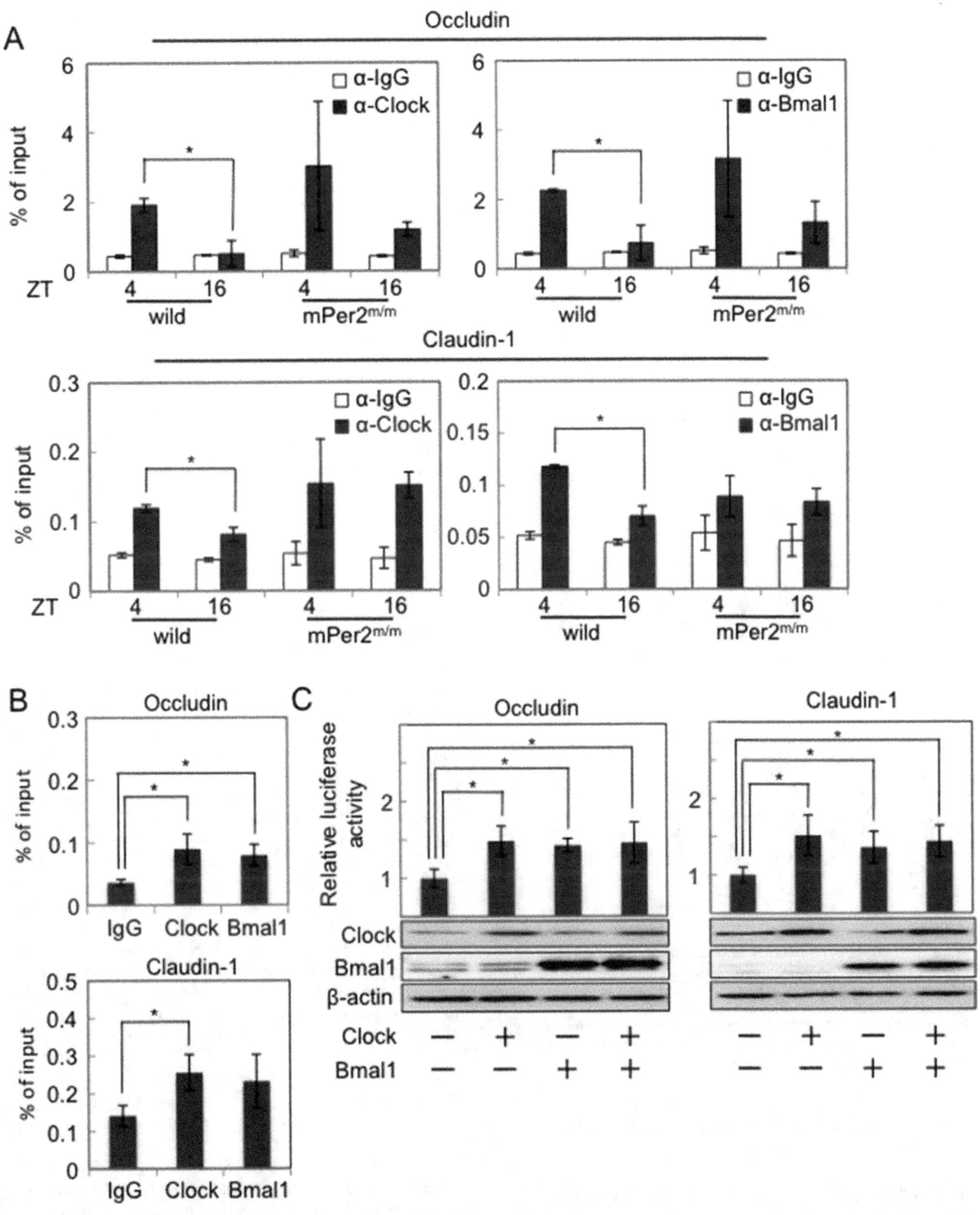

Figure 2. Clock and Bmal1 bind to the E-box element in the promoter regions of Occludin and Claudin-1 genes and affect their transcriptional responses. (**A**) CHiP assays for recruitments of Clock and Bmal1 to E-box elements in Occludin and Claudin-1 promoter region using colonic IECs obtained at the indicated time points from wild-type mice and mPer2$^{m/m}$ mice (n = 3 per group). Similar results were obtained in two independent experiments. (**B**) CHiP assays for recruitments of CLOCK and BMAL1 to E-box elements in Occludin and Claudin-1 promoter region using HCT116 cells (n = 3 per group). (**C**) Relative luciferase activity in HCT116 cells transfected with Occludin and Claudin-1 promoter reporter plasmids together with Clock and Bmal1 expression vectors or a control empty vector (n = 3 per group). *p<0.05.

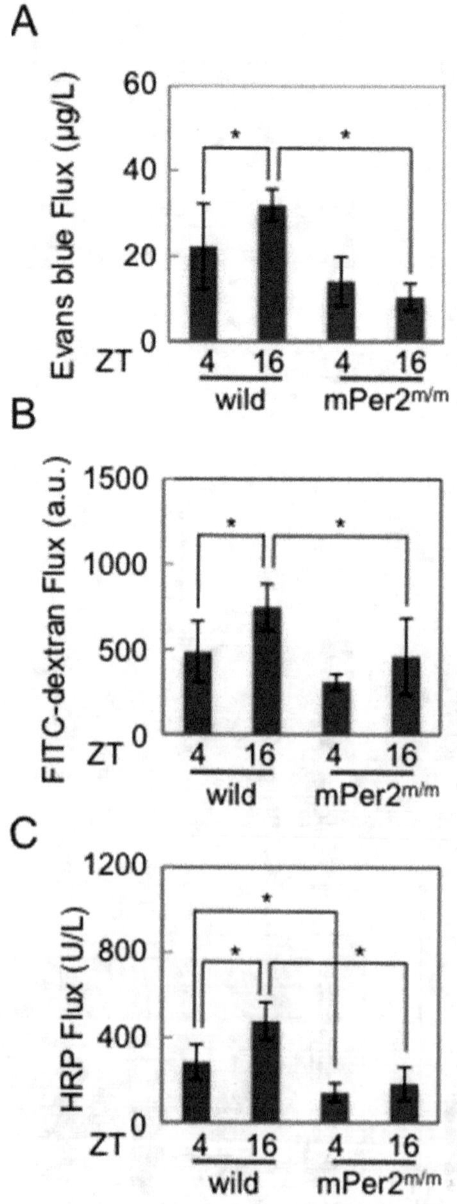

Figure 3. Colonic permeability is under the circadian control. (**A**) Permeability to evans blue *in vivo* at the indicated time points from wild-type mice and mPer2$^{m/m}$ mice (n = 5 per group). (**B**) Permeability to FITC-dextran 4000 *ex vivo* obtained at the indicated time points from wild-type mice and mPer2$^{m/m}$ mice (n = 6 per group). (**C**) Permeability to HRP *ex vivo* obtained at the indicated time points from wild-type mice and mPer2$^{m/m}$ mice (n = 8 per group). *$p<0.05$.

which was associated with temporal alterations of colonic permeability.

mPer2$^{m/m}$ Mice Show Reduced Susceptibility to DSS-induced Colitis

We then investigated whether mPer2$^{m/m}$ mice with reduced colonic permeability were more resistant to colonic injury induced by DSS, because intestinal permeability was associated with susceptibility to colitis [1–3,23].

mPer2$^{m/m}$ mice given 5% DSS in drinking water over a period of 7 days showed less body weight loss, bloody stool, and colon shrinkage than the wild-type mice. Reduced levels of TNF-α and IL-6 proteins in the colon were observed in the mPer2$^{m/m}$ mice in comparison to wild-type mice (**Fig. 4A–D**). The mRNA expression levels of pro-inflammatory molecular markers, myeloperoxidase (Mpo), heme oxygenase (Ho)-1, cyclooxygenase (Cox)-2, and prostaglandin E synthase (Pges)-1 in the colon were also less in mPer2$^{m/m}$ mice than those in wild-type mice (**Fig. S4A**). mPer2$^{m/m}$ mice drank equivalent amounts of DSS-containing water to wild-type mice per day during the period of DSS challenge (day 0–7; **Fig. S4B**). These results suggested that mPer2$^{m/m}$ mice were more resistant to DSS-induced colitis in comparison to wild-type mice.

Bone marrow chimeric mice in which the donors and/or the recipients were either wild-type or mPer2$^{m/m}$ mice were generated to further investigate whether the Per2 mutation in the tissue resident cells (most likely colonic epithelium) was important for the protection against DSS-induced colitis. DSS challenge of chimeric mice lacking the Per2 mutation in hematopoietic cells induced pro-inflammatory markers similar to those observed in wild-type mice reconstituted with wild-type bone marrow cells (**Fig. 4E–H, Fig. S5**). In contrast, chimeric mice lacking Per2 in the non-hematopoietic cells were resistant to DSS-induced colitis similar to the mPer2$^{m/m}$ mice reconstituted with mPer2$^{m/m}$ bone marrow cells, as indicated by the changes of those parameters (**Fig. 4E–H, Fig. S5**). These results suggested that the Per2 mutation conferred protection against DSS-induced colitis when it occurred in non-hematopoietic cells (presumably the cells of the colonic epithelium).

Clock$^{\Delta19/\Delta19}$ Mice Show Enhanced Susceptibility to DSS-induced Colitis

To further ascertain that the circadian clock regulated a time of day-dependent variation of Occludin and Claudin-1expression in the colon, we examined the mRNA levels of Occludin and Claudin-1 in the colon tissue samples obtained from wild-type mice and mice with the loss-of-function mutation of another key clock gene Clock (Clock$^{\Delta19/\Delta19}$ mice) every 6 hours during the day. The mRNA levels of Occludin and Claudin-1 in the colon showed a time of day-dependent variation in wild-type mice whereas the variation was absent in Clock$^{\Delta19/\Delta19}$ mice (**Fig. S6A**). Interestingly, the mRNA levels of Occludin and Claudin-1 in the colon were relative low in Clock$^{\Delta19/\Delta19}$ mice compared with those in wild-type mice. Consistently, Clock$^{\Delta19/\Delta19}$ mice were more sensitive to the colonic injury induced by DSS than wild-type mice as judged by body weight changes, stool property, and Ho-1 and Pges-1 expression (**Fig. S6B–D**). These results also suggested that disruption of the circadian clock affected TJ protein expression and barrier function. The opposite phenotypes observed in Clock$^{\Delta19/\Delta19}$ mice to those in mPer2$^{m/m}$ mice may be attributed to the opposite function of Clock and Per2 in the circadian clockwork; Clock acts as a positive limb whereas Per2 acts as a negative limb in the transcriptional-translational feedback loop in the molecular clock machinery.

IL-1β and TNF-α mRNAs Expression does not Exhibit a Time of Day-dependent Variation in the Mouse Colon

Major proinflammatory cytokines IL-1β and TNF-α have been shown to regulate epithelial barrier function [2]. To investigate whether the circadian clock also affects IL-1β and TNF-α expression, we examined mRNA levels of IL-1β and TNF-α in the colon tissue samples obtained from wild-type mice and mPer2$^{m/m}$ mice every 6 hours during the day. We found that IL-1β and TNF-α mRNA levels did not show circadian oscillations in

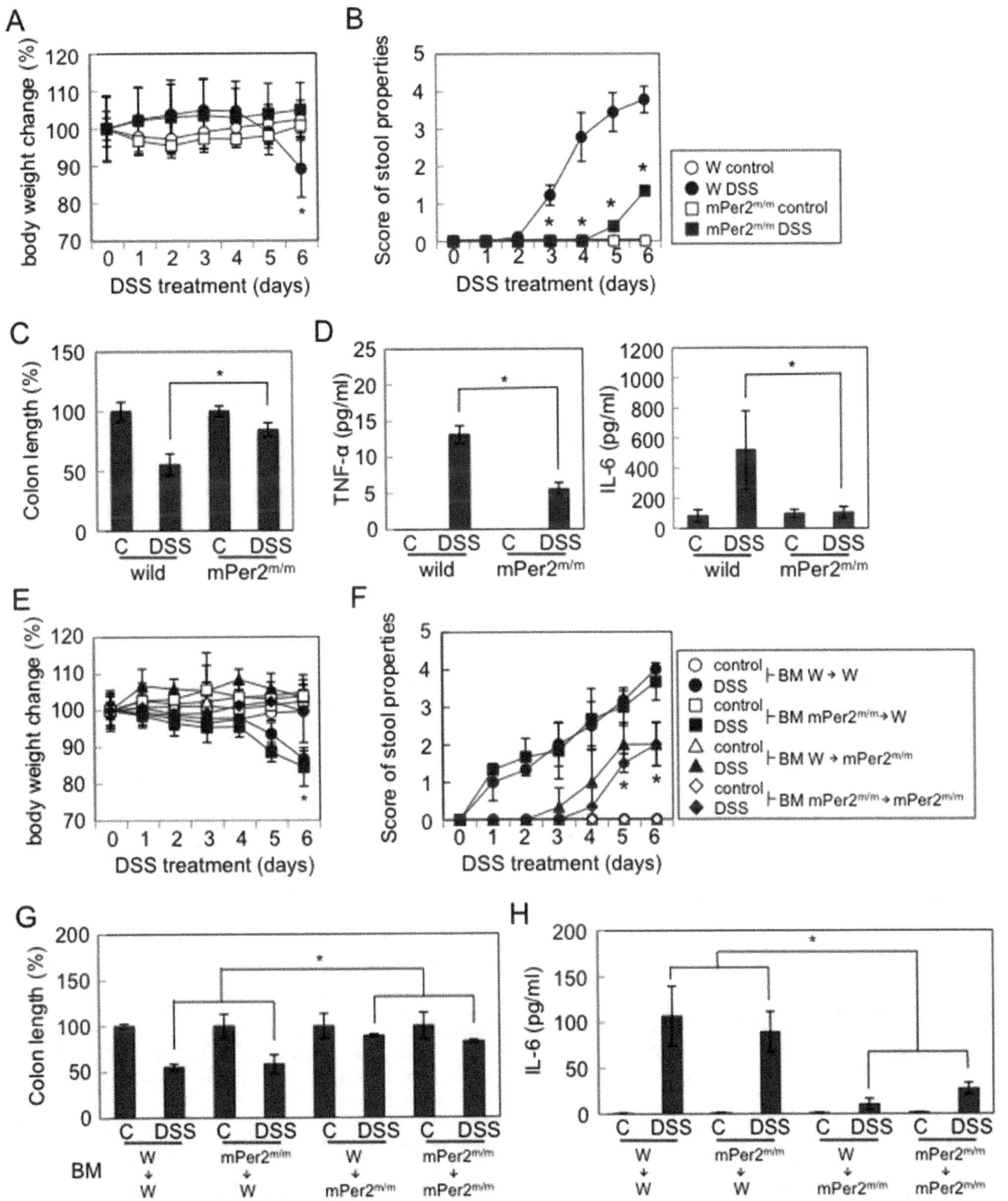

Figure 4. mPer2$^{m/m}$ mice show reduced susceptibility to DSS-induced colitis. (**A**) Body weight changes in mice for 6 days after administration of 5% DSS. (**B**) Stool scores in mice for 6 days after administration of 5% DSS. (**C**) Colon length in mice on day 7 after administration of 5% DSS. (**D**) TNF-α and IL-6 levels in the colon tissue samples measured by ELISA. The samples were obtained from the mice on day 7 after administration of 5% DSS. The susceptibility to DSS-colitis in wild/mPer2$^{m/m}$ bone marrow chimeras mice was shown (**E–H**). (**E**) Body weight changes in mice 6 days after administration of 5% DSS. (**F**) Stool scores in mice 6 days after administration of 5% DSS. (**G**) Colon length in mice on day 7 after administration of 5% DSS. (**H**) IL-6 levels measured by ELISA in the colon tissue samples obtained from the mice on day 7 after the administration of 5% DSS. n = 8 per group, *$p<0.05$. The mice were sacrificed at ZT4 (10:00 AM) in Fig. **5C, D, G** and **H**.

wild-type mice and they were comparable between wild-type and $mPer2^{m/m}$ mice (**Fig. S7**).

Discussion

The circadian clock plays an important role in the regulation of several physiological functions of the intestine as well as other organs [7–9]. Most recently, Summa *et al.* also suggested that the circadian clock regulated intestinal permeability although the precise mechanisms remain largely unknown [10]. The current study demonstrated that the expressions of TJ proteins Occludin and Claudin-1 in the large intestinal epithelium showed daily oscillations, which required normal Per2 activity and the temporal changes of the expression levels were inversely associated with colonic permeability and different susceptibility to DSS-induced colitis between wild-type and $mPer2^{m/m}$ mice. These results suggest that the circadian clock regulates a time of day-dependent variation in colonic TJ protein expression levels, thereby affecting intestinal permeability on a daily basis and also susceptibility to colitis.

One of the primary findings of this study was that 1) Occludin and Claudin-1 mRNAs showed daily oscillations, 2) Clock and Bmal1 bond directly to the E-box elements of Occludin and Claudin-1 promoters, and 3) Overexpression of Clock and Bmal1 activated Occludin and Claudin-1 promoters containing E-box elements (**Fig. 1 and 2**). These results suggest that Occludin and Claudin-1 are CCGs with E-box elements in the promoter region directly regulated by Clock/Bmal1 heterodimers. However, a recent study suggests that only 22% of mRNA cycling genes are driven by de novo transcription in mouse liver [24]. Thus, we can not exclude the possibility that posttranscriptional mechanisms may also underlie the circadian regulation of Occludin and Claudin-1 expression.

We showed that colonic permeability was under the circadian control, which was inversely associated with Occludin and Claudin-1 expression levels (**Fig. 3**). Claudins are defined as most important key factors for tight junction permeability and the tightness of TJ is determined by the number, composition, and the mixing ratio of Claudins [25–27]. Recent studies also suggest that Occludin is important for the maintenance and assembly of TJ proteins [28–30].

We also found that IL-1β and TNF-α mRNA levels did not show circadian oscillations in wild-type mice and they were comparable between wild-type and $mPer2^{m/m}$ mice (**Fig. S7**). Therefore, it is likely that Clock-Bmal1 heterodimers regulate colonic permeability in a circadian manner by timing the expression level of Claudin-1 and Occludin and affect TJ function. However, it remains to be determined whether Occludin and Claudin-1 expression change are indeed primarily responsible for daily changes of tight junction permeability and susceptibility to DSS-induced colitis.

It appears that the current findings are incompatible with the previous findings by Summa et al. [10]. They reported that there were no significant differences in Occludin mRNA expression in the colon between wild-type mice and mice with a mutation of Clock ($Clock^{\Delta19/\Delta19}$ mice) and there were increased cytoplasmic (i.e. decreased membrane-bound) Occludin protein levels in $Clock^{\Delta19/\Delta19}$ mice compared with those in wild-type mice [10]. However, they examined Occludin mRNA and cytoplasmic Occludin protein levels in the mouse colon at only one time point in wild-type and $Clock^{\Delta19/\Delta19}$ mice. They did not examine total Occludin protein levels, either. These experimental differences might explain the discrepancy between the current and previous findings. Actually, we found that the mRNA levels of Occludin and Claudin-1 in the colon showed a time of day-dependent variation in wild-type mice whereas the variation was absent in $Clock^{\Delta19/\Delta19}$ mice (**S-Fig. 6A**).

In addition, Summa et al. reported that $Clock^{\Delta19/\Delta19}$ mice had increased colonic permeability compared with wild-type mice [10]. Since Clock (a positive limb of the circadian clock machinery) and Per2 (a negative limb of the circadian clock machinery) functions as an opposite direction as "clock genes", it may be that $Clock^{\Delta19/\Delta19}$ mice have opposite circadian phenotypes to $mPer2^{m/m}$ mice. The current findings that $Clock^{\Delta19/\Delta19}$ mice were sensitive to DSS-induced colonic injury compared to wild-type mice in contrast to $mPer2^{m/m}$ mice (**Fig. S6**) may support this idea.

A dysfunction of TJ proteins weakens intercellular adhesion, promotes intestinal permeability, and inflammation [1,3]. Therefore, constitutively high Occludin and Claudin-1 protein expression levels in the large intestine are likely to be attributed the reduced susceptibility to DSS-induced colitis in $mPer2^{m/m}$ mice (**Fig. 4**). Although, it is possible that the reduced susceptibility to DSS-induced colitis in $mPer2^{m/m}$ mice may be due to some type of immune cell dysfunction, such as NK cells and macrophages, the chimeric mouse experiments strongly suggest that the Per2 mutation in non-hematopoietic cells is responsible for the protection against DSS-induced colitis (**Fig. 4**).

It is not clear about the half-life of Occludin and Claudin-1 proteins *in vivo*. *In vitro* studies showed that basal half-life of Occludin was about ~6 hours in primary human brain microvascular cells [31] and basal half-life of Claudin-1 was also about ~6 hours in human lung carcinoma cell line A549 cells [32]. Hence, we speculate that Occludin and Claudin-1 proteins might have relatively short half-life in the mouse colon and circadian regulation of these molecules at the transcriptional levels could indeed contribute to the changes of the protein levels *in vivo*.

In summary, we suggest that expressions of TJ proteins Occludin and Claudin-1 in the large intestinal epithelium are under control of the circadian clock, which is associated with temporal changes of colonic permeability and also susceptibility to colitis. To our knowledge, this is the first study showing a novel regulation of TJs by the circadian clock. The findings would provide new insights into the regulation of intestinal barrier function and pathophysiology of colitis.

Supporting Information

Figure S1 Occludin and Claudin-1 expressions exhibit a time of day-dependent variation in colonic epithelium (detailed kinetic analysis). (A) Real-time PCR analysis for Occludin and Claudin-1 mRNAs expression in the colonic epithelial cells samples obtained at the indicated time points from wild-type mice (n = 4 per group). **(B)** The quantitative analysis of Western blot pictures for Occludin and Claudin-1 expression in the colonic epithelial cell samples from wild-type mice obtained at the indicated time points (n = 4 per group).
(TIF)

Figure S2 Kinetics of major "clock genes" mRNAs expression in the mouse colon. Real-time PCR analysis for Per1, Per2, Per3, Clock, Bmal1 and Cry1 mRNAs expression in the colon tissue samples from wild-type mice and $mPer2^{m/m}$ mice obtained at the indicated time points (n = 8 per group).
(TIF)

Figure S3 Clock and Bmal1 bind to the E-box element in the promoter regions of Occludin and Claudin-1 genes and affect their transcriptional responses in Caco-2. (A)

CHiP assays for recruitments of Clock and Bmal1 to E-box elements in Occludin and Claudin-1 promoter region using Caco-2 cells (n = 3 per group). **(B)** Relative luciferase activity in Caco-2 cells transfected with Occludin and Claudin-1 promoter reporter plasmids together with Clock and Bmal1 expression vectors or a control empty vector (n = 3 per group). $^*p<0.05$.
(TIF)

Figure S4 mPer2$^{m/m}$ mice show reduced susceptibility to DSS-induced colitis. **(A)** Real-time PCR analysis for Mpo, Ho-1, Cox-2 and Pges1 mRNAs expression in the colon tissue obtained from the mice on day 7 after the administration of 5% DSS. **(B)** The amounts of drinking water in mice for 6 days after administration of 5% DSS. n = 8 per group, $^*p<0.05$. The mice were sacrificed at ZT4 (10:00 AM).
(TIF)

Figure S5 Per2 mutation in non-hematopoietic cells is critical for protection against DSS-induced colitis. Real-time PCR analysis for Ho-1, Cox-2 and Pges-1 mRNAs expression in the colon tissue obtained from the mice on day 7 after administration of 5% DSS. n = 8 per group, $^*p<0.05$. The mice were sacrificed at ZT4 (10:00 AM).
(TIF)

Figure S6 Clock$^{\Delta19/\Delta19}$ mice show enhanced susceptibility to DSS-induced colitis. **(A)** Real-time PCR analysis for Occludin and Claudin-1 mRNAs expression in the colon tissue samples from wild-type mice and Clock$^{\Delta19/\Delta19}$ mice obtained at the indicated time points (n = 4 per group). **(B–D)** The severity of DSS-colitis in the wild-type and Clock$^{\Delta19/\Delta19}$ mice; Body weight changes in mice for 5 days after administration of 5% DSS (**B**). Stool scores in mice for 5 days after administration of 5% DSS (**C**). Real-time PCR analysis for Ho-1 and Pges1 mRNAs expression in the colon tissue obtained from the mice on day 6 after the administration of 5% DSS (**D**). n = 4 per group, $^*p<0.05$. The mice were sacrificed at ZT4 (10:00 AM).
(TIF)

Figure S7 Kinetics of IL-1β and TNF-α mRNAs expression in the mouse colon. Real-time PCR analysis for IL-1β and TNF-α mRNAs expression in the colon tissue samples from wild-type mice and mPer2$^{m/m}$ mice obtained at the indicated time points (n = 4 per group).
(TIF)

Acknowledgments

We thank Ms. Natsumi Aoki, Tomoko Tohno, Yuko Ohnuma, and Mutsuko Hara for their assistance, and Dr. Fuyuki Sato (Hirosaki University, Aomori, Japan) for providing us with human Clock and Bmal1 expression plasmids.

Author Contributions

Conceived and designed the experiments: K. Oh-oka AN. Performed the experiments: K. Oh-oka HK KI. Analyzed the data: K. Oh-oka HK KI. Contributed reagents/materials/analysis tools: HO K. Okumura SS AN. Wrote the paper: K. Oh-oka AN.

References

1. Groschwitz KR, Hogan SP (2009) Intestinal barrier function: molecular regulation and disease pathogenesis. J Allergy Clin Immunol 124: 3–20.
2. Suzuki T (2013) Regulation of intestinal epithelial permeability by tight junctions. Cell Mol Life Sci 70(4): 631–659.
3. Turner JR (2009) Intestinal mucosal barrier function in health and disease. Nat Rev Immunol 9: 799–809.
4. Dibner C, Schibler U, Albrecht U (2010) The mammalian circadian timing system: organization and coordination of central and peripheral clocks. Annu Rev Physiol 72: 517–549.
5. Takahashi JS, Hong HK, Ko CH, McDearmon EL (2008) The genetics of mammalian circadian order and disorder: implications for physiology and disease. Nat Rev Genet 9: 764–775.
6. Hogenesch JB, Ueda HR (2011) Understanding systems-level properties: timely stories from the study of clocks. Nat Rev Genet 12: 407–416.
7. Mukherji A, Kobiita A, Ye T, Chambon P (2013) Homeostasis in intestinal epithelium is orchestrated by the circadian clock and microbiota cues transduced by TLRs. Cell 153(4): 812–827.
8. Hoogerwerf WA (2006) Biologic clocks and the gut. Curr Gastroenterol Rep 8(5): 353–359.
9. Pan X, Munshi MK, Iqbal J, Queiroz J, Sirwi AA, et al. (2013) Circadian regulation of intestinal lipid absorption by apolipoprotein AIV involves forkhead transcription factors A2 and O1 and microsomal triglyceride transfer protein. J Biol Chem 288(28): 20464–20476.
10. Summa KC, Voigt RM, Forsyth CB, Shaikh M, Cavanaugh K, et al. (2013) Disruption of the Circadian Clock in Mice Increases Intestinal Permeability and Promotes Alcohol-Induced Hepatic Pathology and Inflammation. PLoS One 8(6): e67102.
11. Takamura T, Harama D, Matsuoka S, Shimokawa N, Nakamura Y, et al. (2010) Activation of the aryl hydrocarbon receptor pathway may ameliorate dextran sodium sulfate-induced colitis in mice. Immunol Cell Biol 88: 685–689.
12. Komano H, Fujiura Y, Kawaguchi M, Matsumoto S, Hashimoto Y, et al. (1995) Homeostatic regulation of intestinal epithelia by intraepithelial gamma delta T cells. Proc Natl Acad Sci U S A 92(13): 6147–6151.
13. Mennigen R, Nolte K, Rijcken E, Utech M, Loeffler B, et al. (2009) Probiotic mixture VSL#3 protects the epithelial barrier by maintaining tight junction protein expression and preventing apoptosis in a murine model of colitis. Am J Physiol Gastrointest Liver Physiol 296(5): G1140–1149.
14. Kono H, Fujii H, Asakawa M, Yamamoto M, Matsuda M, et al. (2003) Protective effects of medium-chain triglycerides on the liver and gut in rats administered endotoxin. Ann Surg 237: 246–255.
15. Bishop BL, Lodolce JP, Kolodziej LE, Boone DL, Tang WJ (2010) The role of anthrolysin O in gut epithelial barrier disruption during Bacillus anthracis infection. Biochem Biophys Res Commun 394(2): 254–259.
16. Okayasu I, Hatakeyama S, Yamada M, Ohkusa T, Inagaki Y, et al. (1990) A novel method in the induction of reliable experimental acute and chronic ulcerative colitis in mice. Gastroenterology 98: 694–702.
17. Cooper HS, Murthy SN, Shah RS, Sedergran DJ (1993) Clinicopathologic study of dextran sulfate sodium experimental murine colitis. Lab Invest 69: 238–249.
18. Zheng B, Larkin DW, Albrecht U, Sun ZS, Sage M, et al. (1999) The mPer2 gene encodes a functional component of the mammalian circadian clock. Nature 400: 169–173.
19. Oishi K, Miyazaki K, Kadota K, Kikuno R, Nagase T, et al. (2003) Genome-wide expression analysis of mouse liver reveals CLOCK-regulated circadian output genes. J Biol Chem 278(42): 41519–41527.
20. Storch KF, Lipan O, Leykin I, Viswanathan N, Davis FC, et al. (2002) Extensive and divergent circadian gene expression in liver and heart. Nature 417(6884): 78–83.
21. Ikenouchi J, Matsuda M, Furuse M, Tsukita S (2003) Regulation of tight junctions during the epithelium-mesenchyme transition: direct repression of the gene expression of claudins/occludin by Snail. J Cell Sci 116(Pt 10): 1959–1967.
22. Martínez-Estrada OM, Cullerés A, Soriano FX, Peinado H, Bolós V, et al. (2006) The transcription factors Slug and Snail act as repressors of Claudin-1 expression in epithelial cells. Biochem J 394(Pt 2): 449–457.
23. Henderson P, van Limbergen JE, Schwarze J, Wilson DC (2011) Function of the intestinal epithelium and its dysregulation in inflammatory bowel disease. Inflamm Bowel Dis 17: 382–395.
24. Koike N, Yoo SH, Huang HC, Kumar V, Lee C, et al. (2012) Transcriptional architecture and chromatin landscape of the core circadian clock in mammals. Science 338(6105): 349–354.
25. Furuse M, Fujita K, Hiiragi T, Fujimoto K, Tsukita S (1998) Claudin-1 and -2: novel integral membrane proteins localizing at tight junctions with no sequence similarity to occludin. J Cell Biol 141(7): 1539–1550.
26. Furuse M, Sasaki H, Tsukita S (1999) Manner of interaction of heterogeneous claudin species within and between tight junction strands. J Cell Biol 147(4): 891–903.
27. Nitta T, Hata M, Gotoh S, Seo Y, Sasaki H, et al. (2003) Size-selective loosening of the blood-brain barrier in claudin-5-deficient mice. J Cell Biol 161(3): 653–660.
28. Saitou M, Fujimoto K, Doi Y, Itoh M, Fujimoto T, et al. (1998) Occludin-deficient embryonic stem cells can differentiate into polarized epithelial cells bearing tight junctions. J Cell Biol 141(2): 397–408.
29. Furuse M, Itoh M, Hirase T, Nagafuchi A, Yonemura S, et al. (1994) Direct association of occludin with ZO-1 and its possible involvement in the localization of occludin at tight junctions. J Cell Biol 127(6 Pt 1): 1617–1626.

30. Saitou M, Furuse M, Sasaki H, Schulzke JD, Fromm M, et al. (2000) Complex phenotype of mice lacking occludin, a component of tight junction strands. Mol Biol Cell 11(12): 4131–4142.
31. Ramirez SH, Fan S, Dykstra H, Rom S, Mercer A, et al. (2013) Inhibition of glycogen synthase kinase 3β promotes tight junction in brain endothelial cells by half-life extension of Occudin and Clausin-5. PLoS ONE 8: e55972.
32. Kovalenko OV, Yang XH, Hemler ME. (2007) A novel cysteine cross-linking method reveals a direct association between Claudinn-1 and tetaraspanin CD9. Mol Cell Proteomics 6: 1855–1867.

2

Curcuma longa Extract Exerts a Myorelaxant Effect on the Ileum and Colon in a Mouse Experimental Colitis Model, Independent of the Anti-Inflammatory Effect

Rita Aldini[1*❡], Roberta Budriesi[2*❡], Giulia Roda[3¤], Matteo Micucci[2], Pierfranco Ioan[2], Antonia D'Errico-Grigioni[4], Alessandro Sartini[3], Elena Guidetti[3], Margherita Marocchi[3], Monica Cevenini[3], Francesca Rosini[4], Marco Montagnani[3], Alberto Chiarini[2], Giuseppe Mazzella[3]

1 Ospedale Policlinico S.Orsola and Dipartimento di Scienza dei Metalli, Elettrochimica e Tecniche Chimiche, Università degli Studi di Bologna, Bologna, Italy, **2** Dipartimento di Scienze Farmaceutiche, Università degli Studi di Bologna, Bologna, Italy, **3** Dipartimento di Medicina Clinica, Università degli Studi di Bologna, Ospedale Policlinico S. Orsola, Bologna, Italy, **4** Dipartimento di Medicina Interna, dell'Invecchiamento e Malattie Nefrologiche, Università degli Studi di Bologna; Ospedale Policlinico S. Orsola, Bologna, Italy

Abstract

Background: Curcuma has long been used as an anti-inflammatory agent in inflammatory bowel disease. Since gastrointestinal motility is impaired in inflammatory states, the aim of this work was to evaluate if *Curcuma Longa* had any effect on intestinal motility.

Methods: The biological activity of Curcuma extract was evaluated against Carbachol induced contraction in isolated mice intestine. Acute and chronic colitis were induced in Balb/c mice by Dextran Sulphate Sodium administration (5% and 2.5% respectively) and either Curcuma extract (200 mg/kg/day) or placebo was thereafter administered for 7 and 21 days respectively. Spontaneous contractions and the response to Carbachol and Atropine of ileum and colon were studied after colitis induction and Curcuma administration.

Results: Curcuma extract reduced the spontaneous contractions in the ileum and colon; the maximal response to Carbachol was inhibited in a non-competitive and reversible manner. Similar results were obtained in ileum and colon from Curcuma fed mice. DSS administration decreased the motility, mainly in the colon and Curcuma almost restored both the spontaneous contractions and the response to Carbachol after 14 days assumption, compared to standard diet, but a prolonged assumption of Curcuma decreased the spontaneous and Carbachol-induced contractions.

Conclusions: Curcuma extract has a direct and indirect myorelaxant effect on mouse ileum and colon, independent of the anti-inflammatory effect. The indirect effect is reversible and non-competitive with the cholinergic agent. These results suggest the use of curcuma extract as a spasmolytic agent.

Editor: Daniel S. Sem, Concordia University Wisconsin, United States of America

Funding: This work was supported by grants from Fondazione del Monte di Bologna e Ravenna and from Alisal (Mazz100136- 2010). ALISAL is a project supported by the MINISTERO DELLE POLITICHE AGRICOLE, ALIMENTARI E FORESTALI, with D.M. 11008/7303/10, dated 17/05/2010. The title of the project is: Miglioramento delle proprietà igienico-sanitarie, salutistiche e funzionali di commodity per l'alimentazione dell'uomo e/o degli animali (Improvement of sanitary properties, healthy and functional food commodities for human and/or animals). Prof. Mazzella was supported with materials, reagents, animals. The funders had no role in study design, data collection and analysis, decision to publish, or preparation of the manuscript.

Competing Interests: The authors have declared that no competing interests exist.

* E-mail: rita.aldini@unibo.it (RA); roberta.budriesi@unibo.it (RB)

❡ These authors contributed equally to this work.

¤ Current address: Mount Sinai Hospital, New York, New York, United States of America

Introduction

Ulcerative colitis (UC) and Crohn's disease (CD) are chronic inflammatory conditions of the intestinal tract: they are the consequence of environmental influences, genetic disorders, intestinal microbiota alterations, leading to an abnormal immune response with inflammation [1,2]. A combination of all these factors is probably necessary for clinical expression of the disease [3]. Although the inflammation may remain limited to certain gastrointestinal segments, the function of the whole tract is altered [4,5,6]. Intestinal motility has been reported to be impaired in patients with Inflammatory Bowel Disease (IBD) [7,8]. Inflammation is associated with decreased colonic mixing and haustra formation, but increased propulsive motility, leading to diarrhea [9]. The physiopathology of dysmotility in IBD has not been completely elucidated: a selective hyperactivity 10] of the non-adrenergic, non-cholinergic inhibition has been documented in human colon. Disruption in intracellular Ca2+ mobilization and signaling [11], defective norepinephrine release [12], impairment of the protease-activated receptor 2 [13], defective inhibitory neuron dependent relaxation in the colon [14] have been reported in the experimental animal. Conventional therapy for IBD is hampered by toxicity, intolerance or slow onset of action [15]. Recently, anti-tumour necrosis factor alpha and other biologic agents have been introduced [3,16–18], but their safety in long term treatment has not been proved jet. Therefore, the use of natural substances with no side effects, though not so powerful effective as drugs so far employed, is encouraged, at least in the prevention and in the maintenance of remissions of IBD. Unfractionated or low-molecular-weight heparin, omega-3 polyunsaturated fatty acids, microbes and microbial products are currently under investigation [3].

Curcuma longa (turmeric) is a perennial herb, cultivated in the Southeast Asia [19]. In traditional medicine it has been used for centuries due to its antitumor, antimicrobial, anti-inflammatory, antioxidant properties and it presents acethylcholinesterase inhibitory activity [20–25].

Turmeric chemicals include curcumin (the primary constituent responsible for its yellow color), demethoxycurcumin, and bisdemethoxycurcumin, as well as volatile oils, sugars, proteins, and resins, curcumin (1,7-bis[4-hydroxy-3-methoxyphenyl]-1,6-heptadiene-3,5-dione) being the most studied compound [26]. The anti-inflammatory activity of curcumin has been investigated in various in vitro and in vivo studies [27–30]. In the experimental animal a turmeric extract has been shown to prevent the development of Trinitrobenzene Sulfonic Acid (TNBS)-induced colitis [28,31–33] through the inhibition of signal transduction pathways critical to inflammatory responses, such as AP-1, protein kinase C, and NF-κB [34,35–37]. Moreover, it has been shown to prevent inflammation through blockage of NF-κB in the mucosa in Dextran Sodium Sulphate (DSS) induced chronic colitis [38] and to inhibit immunostimulatory functions of dendritic cells by blocking MAPKs and NF-κB activation [39]. In addition, Curcuma, in a randomized, double-blind, placebo-controlled trial, has been shown to be effective and safe in maintaining ulcerative colitis remission, and to decrease active oxygen species production [30]. So far, many data are available about *Curcuma longa* anti-inflammatory properties, but little and conflicting information is available about the effect of *Curcuma longa* on intestinal motility [40–42]. The wide clinical use of *Curcuma longa* as an anti-inflammatory agent in IBD and its empiric use in diarrhea in eastern countries prompted the present investigation in order to evaluate whether Curcuma exerts some myorelaxant effect on intestinal ileal and colonic motility in healthy intestinal segments, whether this effect, if any, is also observed in DSS induced acute and chronic experimental colitis, and, finally, whether this effect is independent of the anti-inflammatory effect.

Methods

Animals

One hundred thirty male Balb/c mice (8 weeks old, 25–30 g b.w.) (Charles Rivers Laboratories, Calco, LC, Italy) were enrolled: a higher number of animals than required were recruited in order to compensate for the drops out in the course of the experiments, due to the severity of colitis compelling to stop the experiments, according to the Recommendations of the Ethical Committee of the University of Bologna for Animal Experiments. The animals were kept at constant light/dark cycling and constant room temperature of 22°C. They were fed the usual commercial diet and were allowed water *ad libitum*.

Mice were divided into 5 groups: a first group of healthy animals (n 15) was used as donors of intestinal segments in order to evaluate the in vitro effect of Curcuma extracton intestinal motility parameters by antagonism of Carbachol-induced contraction in isolated ileum and distal colon. In a second and a third group of animals Dextran Sodium Sulphate (DSS) (MP Biomedicals, Solon; OH, USA; m.w. 36.000–50.000) chronic (n 50) and acute(n 25) colitis (see below) respectively were induced and the effect of DSS on the Disease Activity parameters and intestinal motility were evaluated. After colitis induction, Curcuma extract was orally administered (200 mg/kg b.w./day) and, at fixed time intervals, (see below), the Disease Activity parameters and intestinal motility were evaluated. A fourth group of animals (n 14) was used as controls and a fifth group of mice (n 6) were used as Curcuma fed control, after oral administration of Curcuma over seven days. For all groups of animals, intestinal histology, spontaneously and Carbachol-induced motility were assessed. The effect of Atropine in Carbachol-induced contraction was also studied in order to get more insights into the mechanism of action of Curcuma extract on the ileal and colonic contraction.

Study protocol. *In vitro studies.* The in vitro effect of curcuma was evaluated on isolated mice ileum and distal colon segments.

In vivo studies. Chronic colitis: chronic colitis was induced in mice by oral administration of DSS (2.5%, w/v) in drinking water (see Text S1). Throughout the period, the animals were fed the usual commercial diet. After 52 days colitis induction, mice were divided into two groups: one group was switched to a Curcuma (200 mg/Kg b.w.) (Indena, Milan, Italy) added diet, the other continued the usual diet. Throughout the experiment, the Disease Activity Index (DAI) was evaluated. After colitis induction and after 7, 14, 21 days of either Curcuma extract added diet (200 mg/kg/b.w.) or standard diet administration, 6 mice of each group were sacrificed and the following parameters were evaluated: colon length, intestinal histology and motility. Acute colitis: acute colitis was induced in mice, by addition of DSS (5% w/v) in the drinking water for 7 days. After this period, the mice were randomly allotted to two groups, one group continued the standard usual diet, the other was switched to a diet similar to the previous but added with Curcuma (200 mg/kg b.w.); after 7 days, the animals were sacrificed. The same parameters as in the previous group were recorded. **Control animals.** 14 mice were studied as controls and the same parameters as above reported were evaluated.

Curcuma fed controls. 6 mice were fed Curcuma added diet over 7 days and thereafter sacrified and similarly studied. A schematic representation of the study is reported in Figure 1.

DSS Colitis Induction

Acute and chronic colitis were induced by DSS administration according to Wirtz [43] (see Text S1). The chronic colitis model has been shown to induce a long lasting colonic inflammation in mice [43].

Assessment of Colitis

Evaluation of disease activity index (DAI)and colon length. Disease Activity Index (DAI) was calculated for each animal as described by Fitzpatrick et al. [44]. The colon was individuated as the segment between the ileo-cecal valve and the rectum and the length was measured (see Text S1 and Table S1).

Curcuma Extract Administration

Mice were on a 4RF21diet (Mucedola S.r.l., Milan, Italy).The 4RF21 complete food was added with Curcuma (Indena Spa, Milan, Italy) extract at a final concentration of 1 g/kg. The

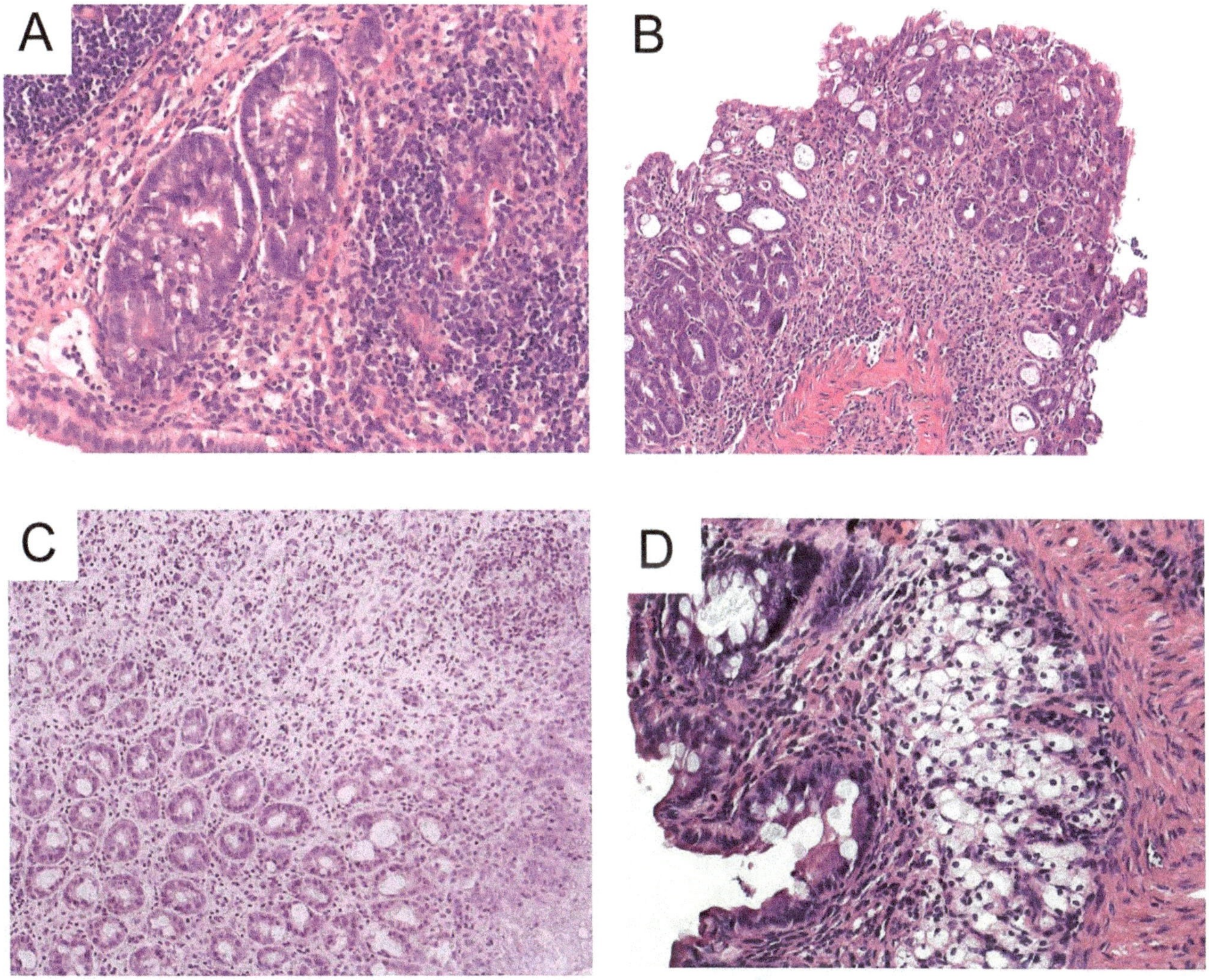

Figure 1. Photomicrographs of hematoxylin and eosin staining of Colon sections from DSS (5%w/v over 7 days) treated mice, before(a) and after 7 days Curcuma extract administration (b) and from DSS (2.5%,w/v, three cycles over 52 days) (c) and after 21 days Curcuma extract administration (d). (**a**) Intestinal mucosal with edema and marked/moderate acute inflammation composed by neutrophils, lymphocites and plasmacells. The intestinal glands show moderate regenerative hyperplasia.(H&E 10×). (**b**) Moderate mucosal inflammation composed by lymphocytes and some neutrophils; the intestinal glands show mild regenerative hyperplasia. (H&E 5×). (**c**) Chronic colitis. The mucosa shows a chronic infiltrate composed by lymphocytes and plasmacells. The glands show mild regenerative hyperplasia. (H&E 5×). (**d**) Intestinal mucosal with mild inflammation composed by lymphocytes, plasmacells and rare neutrophils. The submucosa shows many foam macrophages (H&E 20×).

delivery form of Curcuma used in the present study is a patented formulation of Curcumin (Free Curcumin; Curcuminglucuronide; Curcuminsulphate), a dietary phenolic, with soylecithin. The two compounds form a non-covalent adduct in a 1:2 weight ratio, and two parts of microcrystalline cellulose are then added to improve formulation (www.phytosomes.info).

The chemical preparation was proved to be 18–22% pure by HPLC total curcuminoids content. Each mouse received 200 mg/

Table 1. Histological score.

Grade	Morphological features
0	No inflammatory infiltration of neutrophyls and eosinophils in the lamina propria.
1	Mild and focal infiltrate of neutrophils and eosinophils in the lamina propria with mild crypt aggression.
2	Moderate infiltrate of neutrophils and eosinophils in the lamina propria with moderate crypt aggression.
3	Marked and diffuse infiltrate of neutrophils and eosinophils in the lamina propria with marked crypt aggression.

Table 2. Histological score of inflammatory damage of the colon in mice after acute and chronic DSS induced colitis and after curcuma extract (200 mg/kg/day) or standard diet administration: range of 6 animals.

		Histological Grading			
		After colitis induction	**After 7 days**	**After 14 days**	**After 21 days**
Controls		0	0	0	0
Acute colitis	**followed by standard diet**	3–3	2–3		
	followed by curcuma extract	3–3	1–2		
Chronic colitis	**followed by standard diet**	3–3	2–3	2–3	2–2
	followed by curcuma extract	2–3	2–2	1–2	0–1

The histological score was performed by blind pathology to the study design.

kg per day, i.e. the human equivalent dose for mice [45] (see Text S1).

Ethics statement. The work has been conducted according to relevant National and International Guidelines. All experiments were conducted in conformity with the Public Health Service Policy on Humane Care and use of Laboratory Animals and approved by the Ethical Committee of the University of Bologna(PR 22.03.10). The animals were kept at constant temperature, light/dark cycle. Whenever a mouse gave signs of discomfort, the experiment was interrupted and the animal was switched to plain water and the usual commercial diet and excluded from the study.

Experimental Procedure

Twenty four hours before the experiments, food was withdrawn and water was maintained *ad libitum.* The animals were sacrificed by cervical dislocation. The abdomen was opened by median laparotomy and exposed. A portion of jejunum, immediately after the Treitz was removed (1.5 cm) and retained for histological examination. A 1.5 cm length segment of the terminal ileum, immediately proximal to the ileo-cecal valve and a 2.5 cm region of the distal colon were identified, slightly cleaned with Krebs solution to remove fecal residues and dissected into two parts: one part was placed in 10% formalin for subsequent histological analysis, a second was retained for immediate in vitro motility

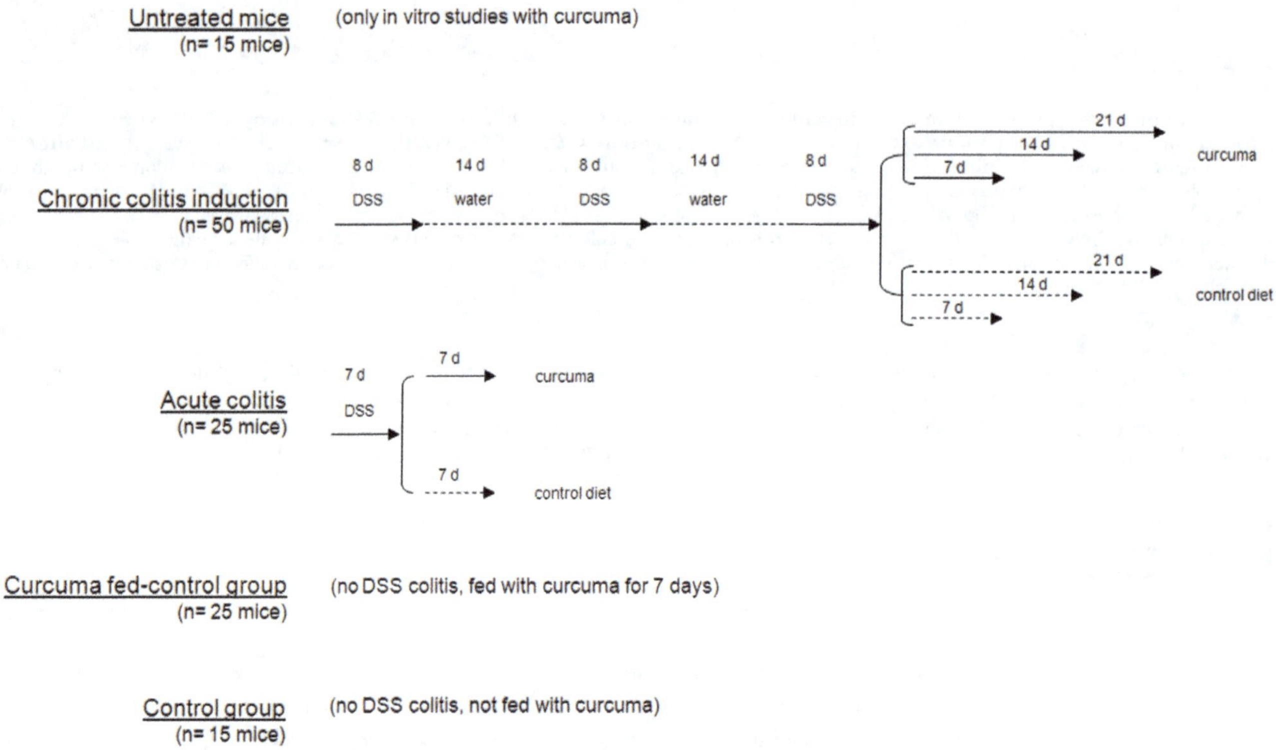

Figure 2. A schematic representation of the experimental design.

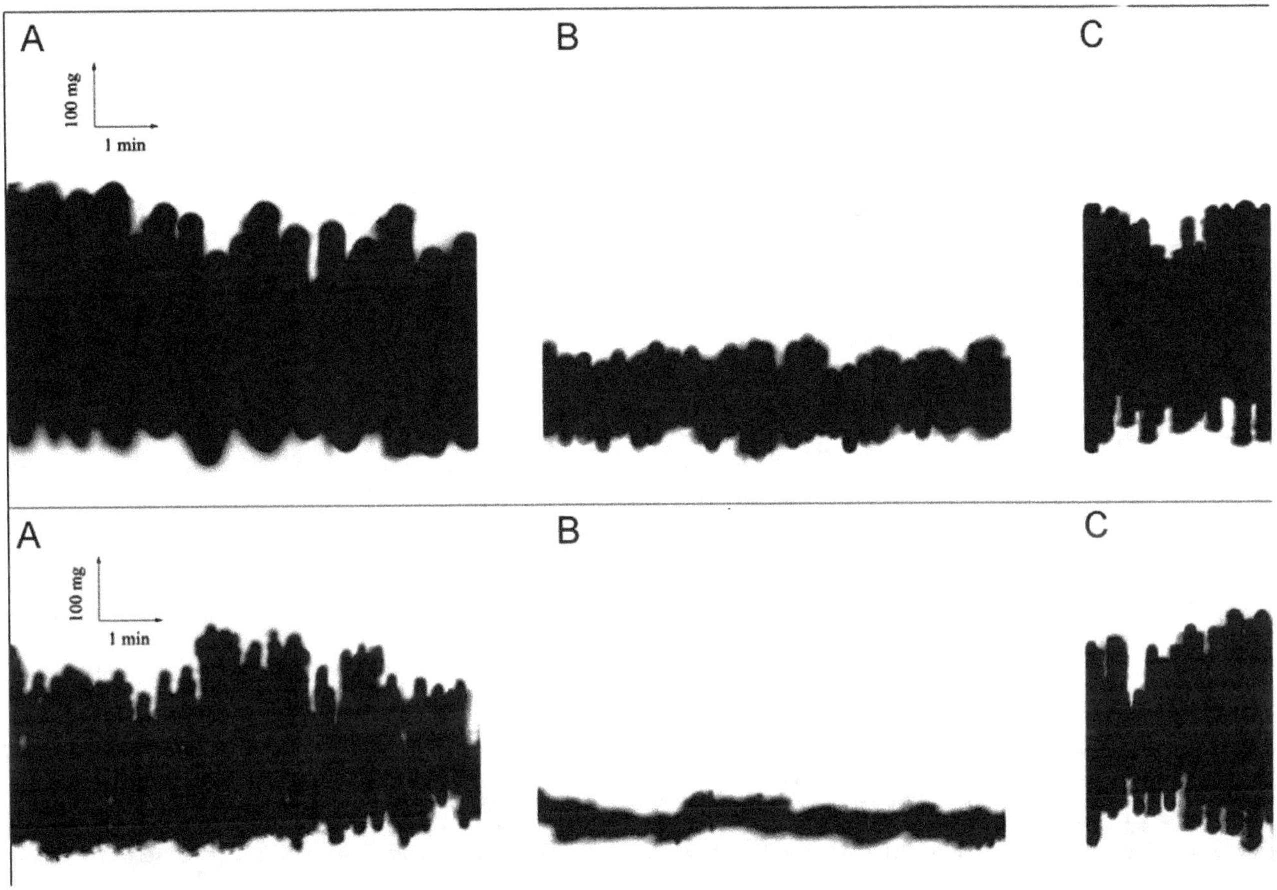

Figure 3. Inhibition of spontaneous motility of ileum (upper panel) and colon (lower panel) by curcuma extract. The segments were suspended in organ baths containing gassed warm Krebs solution under a load of 1 g maintained at 37°C. Tension changes in longitudinal muscle length were recorded. In control conditions (a), after curcuma extract additioned medium (b) and after washing (c).For details see Methods section.

studies (see below). Stools were analyzed for consistency and blood traces.

Histology

The sections of ileum and colon specimens were preserved in 10% neutral buffered formalin for about 48 hours and routinely processed. Five micron sections were cut and stained with Haematoxylin and Eosin (H&E).The histological preparations were examined histologically on a blinded basis.

Histological grading. Acute colitis is characterised by intense inflammatory cell infiltrate, crypt abscesses, mucin depletion, and surface ulceration, that are the main histological features of acute activity. The hallmark is the presence of neutrophils and eosinophils infiltrating lamina propria and crypt epithelium.

Chronic colitis is characterized chronic inflammatory cells, plasma cells and lymphocytes in the lamina propria, distortion of the normal architecture of colonic mucosa, including crypts branching and regeneration. These morphological features induce a variety of altered shapes and sizes of crypts and changes in surface contours. Basal accumulation of lymphocytes and plasma cells with hyperplasia of lymphoid tissue probably represents an early immunologic manifestation of the underlying disease.

Therefore, according to the amount of acute and chronic inflammatory cell infiltrate in colon and in small bowel slides colitis was classified in four grades as reported in Table 1.

Functional Studies

The animals were sacrificed by cervical dislocation, and the organ (ileum and distal colon) required was set up rapidly under a suitable resting tension in 15 mL organ bath containing appropriate physiological salt solution (PSS) consistent warmed (see below) and buffered to pH 7.4 by saturation with 95% O_2–5% CO_2 gas.

Mouse ileum. The terminal portion of ileum (immediately proximal to the ileo-caecal junction) was cleaned, and segments 1 cm long of ileum were set up under 1 g tension at 37°C in organ baths containing Tyrode solution of the following composition (mM): NaCl, 145; KCl, 2.6; $CaCl_2{\cdot}2H_2O$, 1.5; $MgCl_2{\cdot}6H_2O$, 0.73; $NaH_2PO_4{\cdot}2H_2O$, 0.33; $NaHCO_3$, 4.8; glucose, 11.1 [46]. Each segments was set up under 1 g tension in the longitudinal direction along the intestinal wall. Tissue were allowed to equilibrate for at list 30 min during which time the bathing solution was changed every 10 min. Concentration-response curves were constructed by cumulative addition of the agonist Carbachol (CCh). The concentration of agonist in the organ bath was added only after the response to the previous addition had attained a maximal level and remained steady. Contractions were recorded by means of displacement transducer (FT. 03, Grass Instruments, Quincy, MA) using Power Lab software (ADInstruments Pty Ltd, Castle Hill, Australia). In all cases, parallel experiments in which tissues did not receive any antagonist were run in order to check any variation in

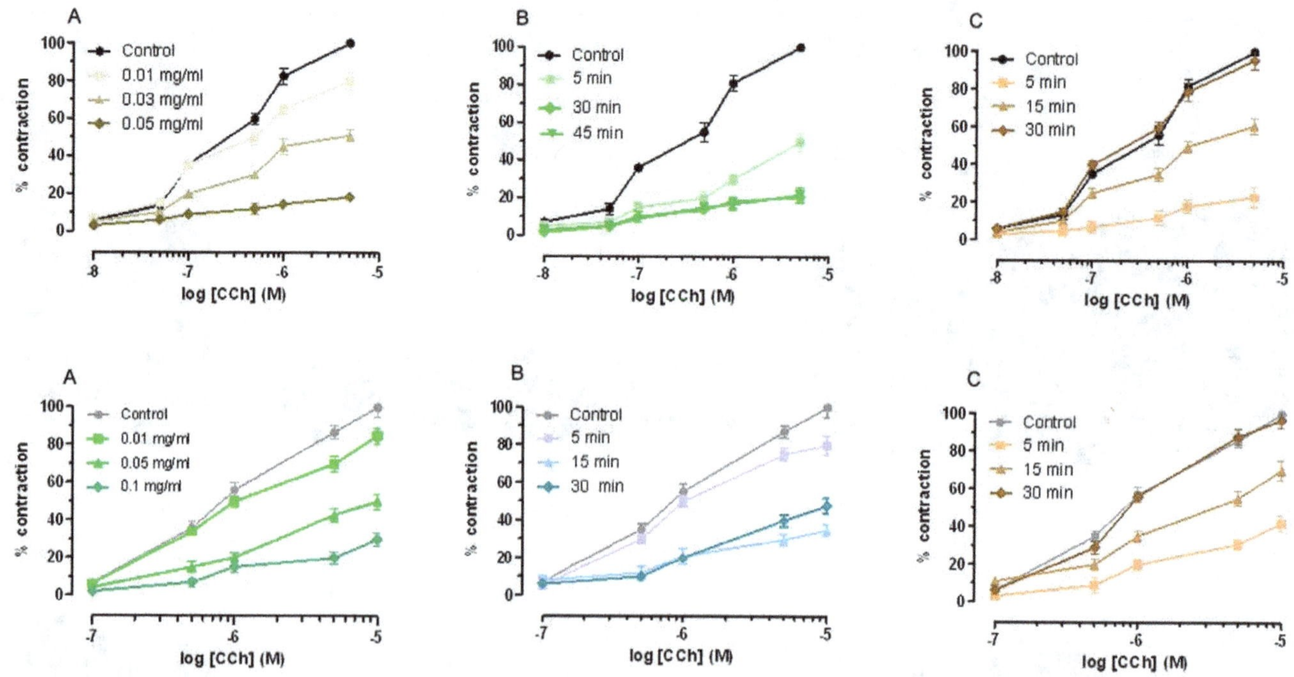

Figure 4. Effect of curcuma extract on carbachol-induced contraction in isolated mouse ileum (A) and distal colon (B). a) Cumulative concentration-response curves were obtained before and after exposure to curcuma extract for 30 min. Each point is the mean ± SEM (*n* =3–5). **b)** Time course of curcuma extract effect on Carbachol-induced contraction in isolated mouse ileum (**A**) or distal colon (**B**) (100%). Cumulative concentration-response curves were obtained before and after exposure to curcuma extract (0.05 mg/mL) for 5, 30 and 45 min. Each point is the mean ± SEM (*n* =3–5). **c)** Time course of curcuma extract (0.05 mg/mL) on carbachol-induced contraction in isolated mouse ileum (**A**) and distal colon (**B**). Cumulative concentration-response curves were obtained before and after exposure to curcuma extract (0.05 mg/mL) and following 5, 30 and 60 min washing. Data are the mean ± SEM (*n* =3–5). Where error bars are not shown, these are covered with the point itself.

sensitivity. Concentration–response curves to agonist were obtained at 30 min intervals, the first one being discarded and the second one used as control. A new concentration-response curve to agonist was obtained following incubation with the antagonist (Atropine or Curcuma extract). Tension changes were recorded isotonically.

Mouse distal colon. A segment of about 2 cm of the distal colon was transected, rinsed with Krebs solution of the following composition (mM): NaCl, 119; KCl, 4.5; $CaCl_2$, 2.5; $MgSO_4 \cdot 7H_2O$, 2.5; $KH_2PO_4 \cdot 2H_2O$, 1.2; $NaHCO_3$, 25; glucose, 11.1; the mesenteric tissue was removed. The segments were suspended in organ baths containing gassed warm Krebs solution under a load of 1 g maintained at 37°C. Tension changes in longitudinal muscle length were recorded. Tissues were allowed to equilibrate for at least 30 min during which time the bathing solution was changed every 10 min. Concentration–response curves to agonist Carbachol (CCh) were recorded isotonically and obtained at 30 min intervals, the first one being discarded and the second one taken as control. Following incubation with the antagonists (Atropine or Curcuma extract), a new concentration–response curve to agonist was obtained. Longitudinal muscle contractions were recorded isotonically by the mean of force displacement transducer (FT 03, Grass Instruments, Quincy, MA) using Power Lab software (ADInstruments Pty Ltd, Castle Hill, Australia). In all cases, parallel experiments in which tissues did not receive any antagonist were run in order to check any variation in sensitivity.

Statistical Analysis

Determination of Dissociation Constants. Functional activity of CCh and antagonism of Atropine and Curcuma extract *vs* CCh induced contraction, was determined in gut segments. The biological results of agonist CCh was expressed as pEC_{50} values. pEC_{50} values represent the $-logEC_{50}$. EC_{50} values are the means ± SE of at least four independent experiments and were calculated by a non-linear regression curve-fitting computer program [47].

In functional experiments, dose ratios at the EC_{50} values of the agonist were calculated at three to five antagonist concentrations, and each concentration was tested from two to four times. The results are expressed as pA_2 values [48,49]. Data are presented as means ± SE of *n* experiments. Differences between mean values were tested for significance by Student's *t*-test. *P* value less than 0.05 was considered significant.

The antagonism activity to CCh of curcuma extract was estimated by determining the concentration of the non-competitive antagonist that inhibited 50% of the maximum response to the agonist. Three different antagonist concentrations were used and each concentration was tested at least three times. A pharmacological computer program was used to analyze data [49]. It was always verified that EC_{50} values for the agonist in tissues receiving only the solvent were not significantly different ($P>0.05$) from control values. In other cases experiments were discarded. Figures were created using GraphPad software [50].

Materials

Carbachol, Atropine and all chemicals were obtained from Sigma (St. Louis, MO, USA). Curcuma was gently supplied by Indena (Indena Spa, Milan, Italy).

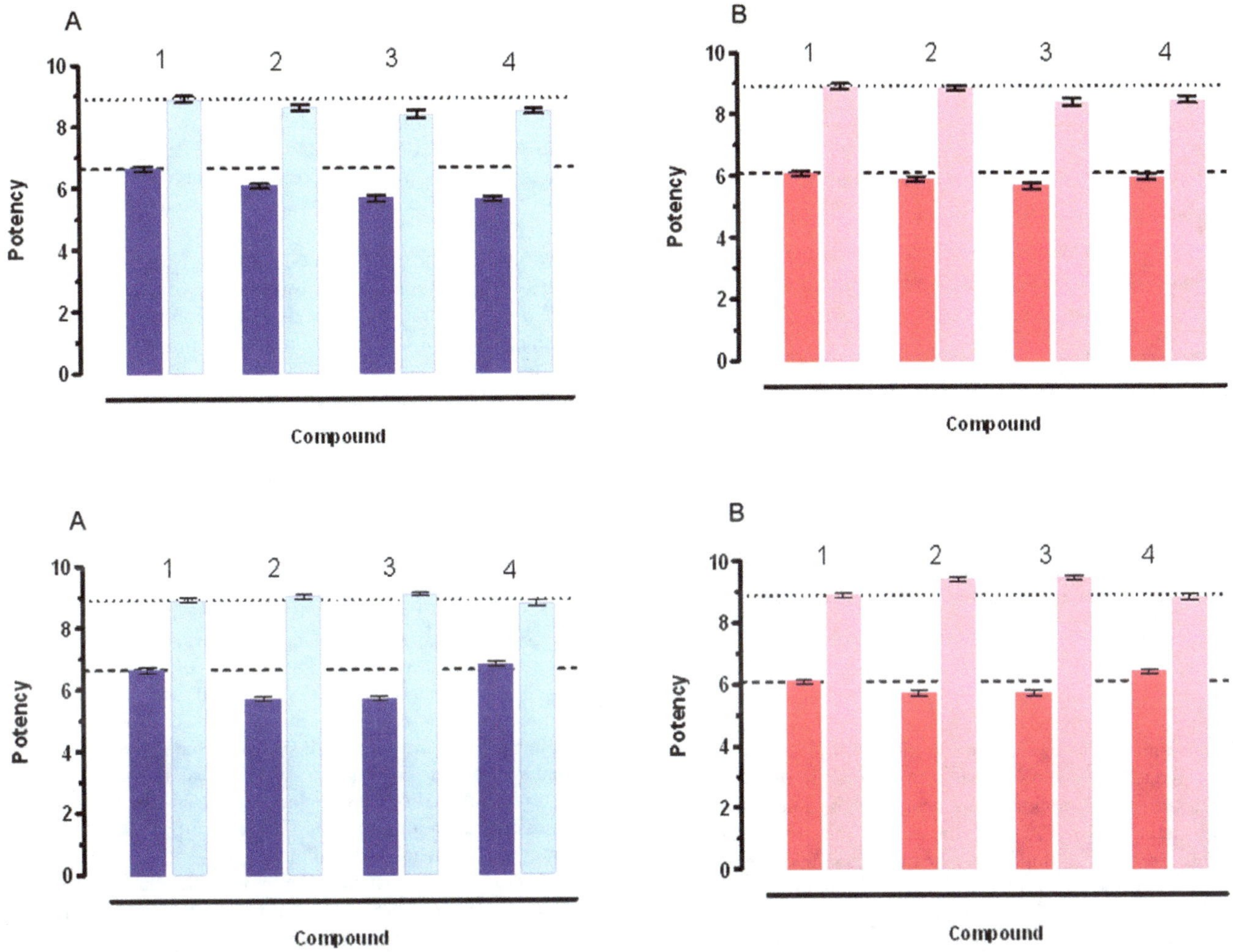

Figure 5. Potency of CCh (pEC_{50}) (dark blu) and atropine (pA_2) (light blu) on ileum (a) and on distal colon (red) and (pink) respectively. (1): control mice. (2): mice with acute DSS induced colitis; (3): acute colitis mice fed the usual diet over 7 days after stopping DSS; (4): acute colitis mice fed curcuma over 7 days after stopping DSS. The dashed line shows the control values for CCh pEC_{50}. The dotted line shows the control values for Atropine pA_2. When error bar are not shown these are covered by the point itself. The contraction induced by Carbachol and the antagonistic effects of Atropine were used as reference. In healthy animals Carbachol is by 3.55 times more potent on the ileum than on the colon. Atropine presents similar antagonistic activity on both tissues: these data have been used as a comparison with the effect of Carbachol and Atropine on tissues from acute colitis animals. Carbachol pEC_{50} decreased by 3.80 times in the ileum and 1.58 times in the colon and Atropine pA_2 was reduced by 1.86 and 1.12 times respectively in the ileum and the colon, compared with the corresponding intestinal segments of control mice. Curcuma administration improved the response to Carbachol in the colon, but not in the ileum, also if it did not completely restore the normal values.

Results

Induction of Acute and Chronic colitis Assessment of Acute and Chronic Colitis and Evaluation of the Response to Curcuma Extract (see Text S1)

Histological parameters. the histological score is reported in Table 2. Both the ileum and the distal colon of the control mice demonstrated a very mild lymphocytic infiltration, typical for the "physiological inflammation" observed in murine intestine under normal conditions [51].

Acute DSS-induced colitis is characterized by histological findings such as severe edema, infiltration of inflammatory cells with granulocytes into both the mucosa and the submucosa, with destruction of the epithelial cells: seven days after withdrawal of DSS, the histological analysis indicated that the severity of colitis was higher in DSS-treated mice assuming standard diet compared to Curcuma treated mice. In chronic DSS induced colitis, chronic inflammatory cells sometimes with mild neutrophil infiltrate were present in the mucosa and submucos; in some cases we observed a mild epithelial aggression. Twenty days after suspension of DSS, Curcuma extract administration improved the histological findings compared to the standard diet control group (Figure 2). Not any pathological alterations were found in the duodenum and jejunum.

Colon length and Disease Activity Index (DAI). the results are reported respectively in Figure S1, S2 and S3.

Functional Studies

Spontaneous motility in ileum and colon. In control mice, spontaneous contractions in the ileum and colon were constant in amplitude and frequency. The ileal and colonic contractions in basal conditions were considered as 100% and the contractions in pathological conditions were compared with the control motility. In vitro curcuma extract inhibited the spontaneous

Table 3. Agonist (carbachol) and antagonist (atropine) affinities expressed as pEC_{50} or pA_2 respectively on the isolated mice ileum and distal colon of control mice and mice fed Curcuma extract over seven days.

			Standard Diet[a]	CurcumaExt[b]
ileum	CCh	pEC_{50}[c]	6.63±0.04	6.40±0.03
	Atropine	pA_2[d]	8.89±0.03	9.16±0.02
colon	CCh	pEC_{50}[c]	6.08±0.01	6.00±0.01
	Atropine	pA_2[d]	8.89±0.01	9.47±0.02

[a]Tissues from healthy mice fed standard diet over seven days.
[b]tissues from healthy mice fed Curcuma extract over seven days.
[c]pEC_{50} = $-\log EC_{50}$. EC_{50} values are the means ± SE of at least four independent experiments and were calculated by a non linear regression curve-fitting computer program (47).
[d]pA_2 values ± SE were calculated from Schild plots [48] constrained to slope −1.0 [49]). pA_2 is the positive value of the intercept of the line derived by plotting log (DR −1) vs log [antagonist]. The log (DR −1) was calculated from three different antagonist concentrations, and each concentration was tested from four to six times. Dose-ratio (DR) values represent the ratio of the potency of the agonist carbachol (EC_{50}) in the presence of the antagonist and in its absence. Parallelism of concentration–response curves was checked by linear regression, and slopes were tested for significance ($p<0.05$).

intestinal contraction by 100% both in ileum and colon (Figure 3). In vivo, when orally administered over one week to healthy mice, the spontaneous motility in the ileum and colon was reduced by 30%; the contractions were constant in frequency and amplitude. In acute colitis, intestinal motility was increased by 230% in the ileum; the contractions were highly irregular in amplitude and frequency; they were reduced by 100% in the colon; Curcuma extract administration over one week to mice reduced the by 50% the spontaneous contraction in ileum without any significant effect on the colon, while standard diet administration did not modify significantly ileal and colonic contractions. In chronic DSS colitis, spontaneous contractions increased by 400%and 300% respectively in the ileum and colon. They were of irregular amplitude and frequency. Seven days after curcuma administration, a partial normalization was observed in both the ileum and the colon; 14 days after Curcuma administration the basal ileal and colonic motility were normalized and were of constant amplitude and frequency. A longer administration (21 days) inhibited the basal spontaneous activity of the ileum and colon. Standard diet administration did not substantially modify the intestinal basal motility since only a partial recovery was observed with time.

Response to Carbachol and Atropine. *Curcuma extract effect on isolated ileum and colon.* Initially we have evaluated the antispasmodic activity of *Curcuma longa Linn* Extract from rhizomes on ileum and distal colon. Experiments performed in mice ileum and colon showed that Curcuma extract inhibited the maximum response to Carbachol in a non-competitive manner. These results show that the extract produce a smooth muscle relaxation effect on mice ileum and colon, as previously described for Guinea Pig [42]. Furthermore, this blockade was reversed after 30 min tissue washing (Figure 3). The IC_{50} value for Curcuma extract was 0.03 mg/ml in ileum and 0.04 mg/min distal colon respectively (Table S2). In both cases, the agonist activity was comparable.

Effect of Carbachol and Atropine on ileum and colon from control mice. In order to evaluate the effects of Curcuma extract on the intestinal muscular layers of ileum and colon, we have used as reference the contraction induced by Carbachol and the antagonistic effects of Atropine. Figure 4 reports Carbachol pEC_{50} and Atropine pA_2 on ileum and colon respectively.

As it can be observed (for data see Table S3), Carbachol is by 3.55 times more potent on the ileum than on the colon. Atropine presents similar antagonistic activity on both tissues: these data have been used as a comparison with the effect of Carbachol and Atropine on tissues from DSS treated animals (acute and chronic colitis) and after Curcuma extract or placebo administration.

Functional Study in DSS Mice Smooth Muscle

Acute colitis. Acute colitis was induced with DSS (5%, w/v) over 7 days in the drinking water, after which one group went on assuming the usual commercial diet, the other was switched to curcuma (200 mg/kg/day) added diet for 7 days.

Carbachol induced contraction was reduced: in fact Charbacol pEC_{50} decreased by 3.80 times in the ileum and 1.58 times in the colon compared to the respective control intestinal segments (Figure 5; for data see Table S4). Similarly, the effect of Atropine was decreased: pA_2 was reduced by 1.86 and 1.12 times respectively in the ileum and the colon, compared with the corresponding intestinal segments of control mice. Both the effects were stronger in the ileum than in the colon: This finding is at variance with the histological damage, which is limited to the colon, resembling the histopathological features of UC. Seven days Curcuma extract administration improved the response to Carbachol in the colon, but not in the ileum, both in comparison with the response of colon from mice with acute disease and mice assuming control diet, also if it did not completely restore the normal values. The response to Atropine was decreased both in the Curcuma added diet group and in the controls. In the ileum, Curcuma extract administration did not even partially restore the response to Carbachol and Atropine.

In order to evaluate whether Curcuma extract had any effect on normal intestine and compare it, if any, with the effect of Curcuma on the intestine from mice with DSS induced acute colitis, we have administered Curcuma extract over 7 days to control mice. As shown in Table 3, Curcuma extract, when added to diet decreased the response to Carbachol in the ileum, by 1.69 and in the colon, by 1.20, while it increased in both the response to Atropine. As it can be observed, the effect was greater in the ileum.

Chronic colitis. Chronic colitis was induced in mice with DSS (2.5%w/v), three "8 days" cycles, with plain water between, for a total of 52 days, after which one group continued the control diet for 7 days, the other was switched to curcuma (200 mg/kg/day) over 7 days. After colitis induction, animals were either switched to curcuma extract administration or continued the usual diet. They were then sacrificed after 7, 14, 21 days and the two groups of animals were compared (Figure 6; for data see Table S5).

Discussion

Scanty data are available in literature about the effect of Curcuma on intestinal motility. In healthy humans, an indirect evidence that Curcuma activates bowel motility has been produced by hydrogen breath [40]. On the contrary, Curcuma increases intestinal transit time in albino rats and ileal motility in Guinea Pig, consistently with the traditional use of curcumin in disorders of altered intestinal motility [41–42]. The use of turmeric as an anti-inflammatory agent in IBD and the traditional empiric use of Curcuma as an antidiarrheal symptomatic drug in functional disorders of the gastrointestinal tract suggested an effect on intestinal motility.

The GI tract function is under neural control, extrinsic autonomic nerves influencing the activity of enteric neurons

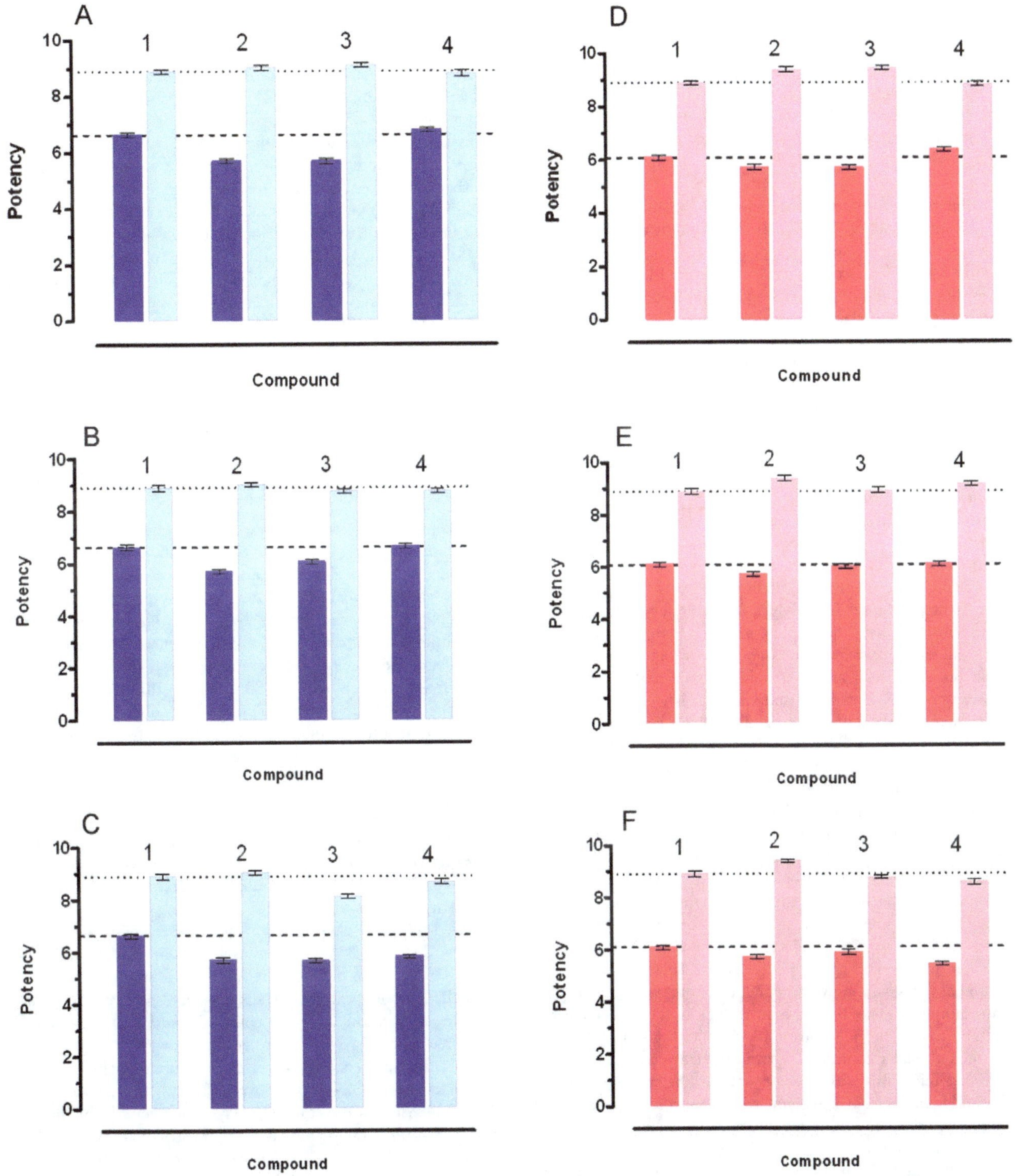

Figure 6. Potency of CCh (pD_2) and Atropine (pA_2) on the ileum (a, b, c) and on the colon (d, e, f) from mice with chronic colitis. 1: control mice, 2: chronic DSS induced colitis, 3: DSS chronic colitis mice assuming standard diet over 7 (a) 14 (b) and 21 (c) days after stopping DSS; 4: DSS chronic colitis mice assuming curcuma extract over 7 (a), 14 (b) and 21 (c) days after stopping DSS. The dashed line shows the control values for CCh pEC_{50}. The dotted line shows the control values for Atropine pA_2. When error bar are not shown these are covered with the point itself Carbachol. The contraction induced by Carbachol and the antagonistic effects of Atropine were used as reference. In healthy animals Carbachol is by 3.55 times more potent on the ileum than on the colon. Atropine presents similar antagonistic activity on both tissues: these data have been used as a comparison with the effect of Carbachol and Atropine on tissues from chronic colitis animals. After induction of chronic colitis, Charbacol pEC_{50} decreased by 8.71 times in the ileum and 2.34 times in the colon and Atropine pA_2 was increased by 1.35 and 3.09 times in the ileum and the colon respectively, compared with the corresponding intestinal segments of control mice. Curcuma administration improved the response to Carbachol in the ileum by 9.12 times and by 2.45 times in the colon after 14 days administration; Atropine pA_2 was decreased by 1.78 and 1.66 respectively in the two intestinal segments.

located within the wall of the gut [52,53]. Although the inflammation in IBD occurs in discrete regions of the gastrointestinal tract, the ensuing functional alterations, among which altered motility, are not limited to the inflamed segments [54,55] and a reduced sympathetic regulation in uninflamed intestinal tracts has been demonstrated [12]. The development of intestinal dysmotility may in turn result in abnormal growth of intestinal microflora, subsequently inducing a translocation of bacteria or bacterial products through the impaired mucosal barrier [56].

In humans, it is under debate whether IBD is associated with hyper or hypomotility [7,8,57]. Reduced haustra formation, but increased colonic propulsive motility and diarrhea seem to be present [58,59]. DSS colitis shares clinical and histopathological features of UC and reproduces a model of chemically driven colitis, where the damage of the epithelium is related to inflammation without an immune component. In our system, this model represents a good way to induce inflammation in the colon and to study its effect on motility. Conflicting data exist about the effect of DSS on intestinal motility in the experimental animal. Spontaneous phasic contractions and Carbachol-evoked contractions of distal colon smooth muscles have been found diminished by DSS [11,60–62]. Conversely, increased Carbachol-evoked contractions and colonic smooth muscle hypercontractility were reported [63]. These findings may correlate with differences in experimental conditions, strain and gender differences in the susceptibility of DSS-colitis. In view of the possible gene differences, we have used male Balb/c mice: Balb/c mice are a strain commonly used for all-purpose laboratory investigations. Moreover males have been preferred over females due to the phasic influences of sexual hormones on gastrointestinal motility. In the present investigation, DSS induces deep disturbances in basal motor activity of ileum and colon: it is worthwhile noting that in acute colitis a hyperexcitability of the ileum is observed associated with a depressed motor activity in the colon, while a severe hyperexcitability is present both in ileum and in colon in the chronic colitis model. The abolition of any motor activity of the colon in acute experimental colitis is in agreement with the clinical condition of the toxic megacolon. We have chosen as reference of disturbed motility the ileal and colonic response to Carbachol and the inhibitory effect of Atropine on the Carbachol induced contraction. Carbachol and Atropine are respective agonist and antagonist at cholinergic muscarinic receptors. Both agonist and antagonist bind to the cholinergic receptors M(2) and M(3), present in mice small intestine and colon cellular membrane. In the present investigation, we have induced both chronic and acute colitis in mice, since the chronic model is more suitable for Curcuma treatment. The muscarinic receptor agonist Carbachol generated a smaller contractile force in the DSS-treated mice than in normal mice: this was the case both in the inflamed colonic strips and in the normal ileal segments. The altered response to the antagonist is a further confirmation that the cellular membrane, where not anatomically altered, as is the case with the ileum, is functionally altered. In this study we show that, in control conditions, Carbachol effect is more potent in the ileum than in the colon, while the antagonistic effect of Atropine is similar. In vitro, Curcuma exerts an inhibition of intestinal basal and Carbachol induced contraction both in the ileum and the colon: this effect is non-competitive and reversible. The inhibition of basal intestinal motility demonstrates a direct effect on the intestinal muscular cells. The inhibition of Carbachol response is stronger in the ileum while the antagonistic effect of Atropine is increased in both. When orally administered to healthy animals, Curcuma has similarly shown a direct myorelaxant activity and an inhibition of Carbachol response on the ileum and colon, stronger on the former than on the latter. The effect of Atropine is conversely increased on both the intestinal tracts. To our knowledge, this is the first report of a myorelaxant effect of *Curcuma longa* both in the normal ileum and colon and in an experimental colitis model. The present experiments, in agreement with most of the authors, confirm that Carbachol-induced contractions are reduced in the colon in the DSS-mouse colitis model: in addition, in the present investigation, defective Carbachol evoked contractions have been documented also in the ileum. In acute and chronic colitis, Curcuma extract added diet improves the ileal and colonic motility: in the chronic colitis model, 14 days Curcuma administration restores the motility pattern in the colon and in the ileum, but after a longer Curcuma extract oral administration, once the mucosal repair is achieved, the myorelaxant effect of Curcuma is prevalent in both the intestinal segments and the inhibitory effect of Curcuma on the colonic muscular layers is predominant, showing that the inhibition on the muscular layers is independent of the anti-inflammatory effect. The potency of the inhibitory effect of Curcuma Longa on the intestinal motility is not powerful: this is not surprising since Curcuma is a natural substance and this should be considered in the translation from the animal model to human pathology.

In conclusion, Curcuma extract exerts a myorelaxant effect on the ileum and colon independent of the anti-inflammatory effect. The mechanism of action is due both to a direct myorelaxant effect on the intestinal muscle layers and to a non-competitive and reversible inhibition of the cholinergic agent. It was beyond the aim of the present paper to investigate the mechanism underlying this effect. The present study provides the rationale for the use of Curcuma Longa in motility disorders of IBD and suggests a possible application to functional motor disturbances of the gastrointestinal tract, due to the myorelaxant effect on the normal intestine, independent of the anti-inflammatory activity.

Supporting Information

Figure S1 Effect of acute (a) and chronic (b) DSS administration on colon length, followed by curcuma extract (200 mg/kg) or standard diet. In the acute colitis model mice received DSS (5%) in drinking water over 7 days followed by seven days water; in the chronic colitis model, they received DSS (2.5%) over 7 days followed by 14 days water per cycle, for a total of three cycles. After colitis induction they were fed either curcuma extract or standard diet respectively over 7 and 21 days. a1) control. a2) acute colitis.a3) acute colitis followed.by curcuma over 7 days. a4) acute colitis followed by standard diet over 7 days. b1) control. b2) chronic colitis. b3) chronic colitis followed by curcuma extract over 21 days. b4) chronic colitis followed by standard diet over 21 days. Each point is the mean ± SD (6 determinations). Significance: (**a**) 1*vs* 2: $p<0.005$; 1*vs* 3: $p<0.005$; 1*vs* 4: $p<0.001$; 2 *vs* 3: $p<0.05$; 2 *vs* 4: $p<0.05$; 3*vs* 4: p ns. (**b**) 1*vs* 2: $p<0.0001$; 1*vs* 3: $p<0.005$; 1*vs* 4: $p<0.0005$; 2 *vs* 3: $p<0.01$; 2 *vs* 4: $p<0.05$; 3 *vs* 4: p ns.

Figure S2 The Disease Activity Index in the acute (a) and chronic colitis (b) model. The DAIs were calculated as described in the Materials and Method section. Each point is the mean ± SD (6 determinations). Where error bars are not shown, these are covered by the point itself. Significance: (**a**) From day 4 on: DSS *vs* control tap water: $p<0.0001$. (**b**) From day 6 on: DSS *vs* control tap water: $p<0.0001$.

Figure S3 The DAI in mice fed curcuma (red) or standard diet (black) after acute (a) and chronic (b) colitis induction. The DAIs were calculated as described in the Materials and Method section. Each point is the mean ± SD (6 determinations). Significance: (**a**) 7 days after stopping DSS, Curcuma extract *vs* control diet, $p<0.0001$. (**b**) 14 days after stopping DSS, Curcuma extract *vs* standard diet: $p<0.05$; 21 days: $p<0.005$.

Table S1 Parameters investigated for the evaluation of the Disease Activity Index.

Table S2 Antagonist affinities, expressed as IC_{50} Values, in the different mouse gut smooth muscle segments.

Table S3 Potency of Chrabacol and Atropine on isolated mice tissues.

Table S4 Agonist (Carbachol) and antagonist (Atropine) affinities expressed as pEC_{50} or pA_2 respectively in the isolated mice ileum and distal colon.

Table S5 Agonist (Carbachol) and antagonist (Atropine) affinities expressed as pEC_{50} or pA_2 respectively in the isolated mice ileum and distal colon.

Text S1 Supporting information.

Acknowledgments

The authors thank Prof. Aldo Roda and Prof. Roberto De Giorgio for critical revision of the manuscript.

Author Contributions

Conceived and designed the experiments: RA RB GR GM AC. Performed the experiments: RA RB M. Montagnani PI AD AS EG MC FR M. Marocchi. Analyzed the data: M. Montagnani M. Marocchi RB. Contributed reagents/materials/analysis tools: GM AC M. Montagnani. Wrote the paper: RA RB GR. Critically revised the manuscript: RA RB.

References

1. Strober W, Fuss I, Mannon P (2007) The fundamental basis of inflammatory bowel disease. J Clin Invest 117: 514–521.
2. Xavier RJ, Podolsky DK (2007) Unravelling the pathogenesis of inflammatory bowel disease. Nature 448: 427–34.
3. Triantafillidis JK, Merikas E, Georgopoulos F (2011) Current and emerging drugs for the treatment of inflammatory bowel disease. Drug Des Devel Ther 5: 185–210.
4. Jacobson K, McHugh K, Collins SM (1995) Experimental colitis alters myenteric nerve function at inflamed and non-inflamed sites in the rat. Gastroenterology 109: 718–22.
5. Aube AC, Cherbut C, Barbier M, Xing JH, Roze C, et al. (1999) Altered myoelectrical activity in non-inflamed ileum of rats with colitis induced by trinitrobenzenesulphonic acid. Neurogastroenterol Motil 11: 55–62.
6. Blandizzi C, Fornai M, Colucci R, Antonioli L, Bernardini N, et al. (2003) Altered prejunctional modulation of intestinal cholinergic and noradrenergic pathways by alpha2-adrenoceptors in the presence of experimental colitis. Br J Pharmacol 139: 309–20.
7. Kohno N, Nomura M, Okamoto H, Kaji M, Ito S (2006) The use of electrogastrography and external ultrasonography to evaluate gastric motility in Crohn's disease. J Med Invest 53(3–4): 277–84.
8. Vrees MD, Pricolo VE, Potenti FM, Cao W (2002) Abnormal motility in patients with ulcerative colitis: the role of inflammatory cytokines. Arch Surg 137: 439–445; discussion 445–436.
9. Tomita R, Munakata K, Tanjoh K (1998) Role of non-adrenergic non-cholinergic inhibitory nerves in the colon of patients with ulcerative colitis. J Gastroenterol 33: 48–52.
10. Vasina V, Barbara G, Talamonti L, Stanghellini V, Tonini M, et al. (2006) Enteric neuroplasticity evoked by inflammation. Auton Neurosci 126–127: 264–72.
11. Qureshi S, Song J, Lee HT, Koh SD, Hennig GW, Perrino BA (2010) CaM kinase II in colonic smooth muscle contributes to dysmotility in murine DSS-colitis. Neurogastroenterol Motil 22: 186–186–95, e64.
12. Motagally MA, Neshat S, Lomax AE (2009) Inhibition of sympathetic N-type voltage-gated Ca2+ current underlies the reduction in norepinephrine release during colitis. Am J Physiol Gastrointest Liver Physiol 296: G1077–84.
13. Sato K, Ninomiya H, Ohkura S, Ozaki H, Nasu T (2006) Impairment of PAR-2-mediated relaxation system in colonic smooth muscle after intestinal inflammation. Br J Pharmacol1 48: 200–7.
14. Mizuta Y, Isomoto H, Takahashi T (2000) Impaired nitrergic innervation in rat colitis induced by dextran sulfate sodium. Gastroenterology 118: 714–23.
15. Mattar MC, Lough D, Pishvaian MJ, Charabaty A (2011) Current management of inflammatory bowel disease and colorectal cancer. Gastrointest Cancer Res 4: 53–61.
16. Lim AW, Panaccione R, Seow CH (2011) Exploring the role of monitoring anti-TNFα drug and antibody levels in the management of inflammatory bowel disease. Therap Adv Gastroenterol 4: 145–51.
17. Papadakis KA, Targan SR (2000) The role of chemokines and chemokine receptors in mucosal inflammation. Inflamm Bowel Dis 6: 303–13.
18. Rutgeerts P, Sandborn WJ, Feagan BG, Reinisch W, Olson A, et al. (2005)Infliximab for induction and maintenance therapy for ulcerative colitis. N Engl J Med 335: 2462–76.
19. Ammon HP, Wahl MA (1991) Pharmacology of Curcuma longa. Planta Med 57: 1–7.
20. Singh AK, Sidhu GS, Deepa T, Maheshwari RK (1996) Curcumin inhibits the proliferation and cell cycle progression of human umbilical vein endothelial cell. Cancer Lett 107: 109–15.
21. Negi PS, Jayaprakasha GK, Jagan Mohan Rao L, Sakariah KK (1999) Antibacterial activity of turmeric oil: a byproduct from curcumin manufacture. J Agric Food Chem 47: 4297–4300.
22. Jain SK (1994) Ethnobotany and research on medicinal plants in India. Ciba Found Symp 185: 153–64.
23. Huang TS, Lee SC, Lin JK (1991) Suppression of c-Jun/AP-1 activation by an inhibitor of tumor promotion in mouse fibroblast cells. Proc Natl Acad Sci USA 88: 5292–5296.
24. Xu YX, Pindolia KR, Janakiraman N (1997) Curcumin, a compound with anti-inflammatory and anti-oxidant properties, down-regulates chemokine expression in bone marrow stromal cells. Exp Hematol 25: 413–422.
25. Ahmed T, Gilani AH (2008) Inhibitory effect of curcuminoids on acetylcholinesterase activity and attenuation of scopolamine-induced amnesia may explain medicinal use of turmeric in Alzheimer's disease. Pharmacol Biochem Behav 91: 554–9.
26. Singh G, Kapoor IP, Singh P, de Heluani CS, de Lampasona MP, et al. (2010) Comparative study of chemical composition and antioxidant activity of fresh and dry rhizomes of turmeric (Curcuma longa Linn.).Food Chem Toxicol 48: 1026–31.
27. Camacho-Barquero L, Villegas I, Sánchez-Calvo JM, Talero E, Sanches-Fidalgo S, et al. (2007) Curcumin, a Curcuma longa constituent, acts on MAPK p38 pathway modulating COX-2 and iNOS expression in chronic experimental colitis. Int Immunopharmacol 3: 333–42.
28. Sugimoto K, Hanai H, Tozawa K, Aoshi T, Uchijima M, et al. (2002) Curcumin prevents and ameliorates trinitrobenzenesulfonic acid-induced colitis in mice. Gastroenterology 123: 1912–22.
29. Claramunt RM, Bouissane L, Cabildo MP, Cornago MP, Elguero J, et al. (2009) Synthesis and biological evaluation of curcuminoid pyrazoles as new therapeutic agents in inflammatory bowel disease: effect on matrix metalloproteinases. Bioorg Med Chem 171: 290–6.
30. Hanai H, Iida T, Takeuchi K, Watanabe F, Maruyama Y, et al. (2006) Curcumin maintenance therapy for ulcerative colitis: randomized, multicenter, double-blind, placebo-controlled trial,. Clin Gastroenterol Hepatol 12: 1502–6.
31. Jian YT, Mai GF, Wang JD, Zhang YL, Luo RC, Fang YX (2005) Preventive and therapeutic effects of NF-kappaB inhibitor curcumin in rats colitis induced by trinitrobenzene sulfonic acid. World J Gastroenterol 11: 1747–52.
32. Salh B, Assi K, Templeman V, Parhar K, Owen D, et al. (2003) Curcumin attenuates DNB-induced murine colitis. Am J Physiol, Gastrointest Liver Physiol 285: G235–43.
33. Ukil A, Maity S, Karmakar S, Datta N, Vedasiromoni JR, et al. (2003) Curcumin, the major component of food flavorturmeric, reduces mucosal injury in trinitrobenzenesulphonic acid induced colitis. Br J Pharmacol 139: 209–18.
34. Bharti AC, Donato N, Singh S, Aggarwal BB (2003) Curcumin (diferuloyl-methane) down-regulates the constitutive activation of nuclear factor-kappa B and IkappaBalpha kinase in human multiple myeloma cells, leading to suppression of proliferation and induction of apoptosis. Blood 101: 1053–62.

35. Han SS, Keum YS, Seo HJ, Surh YJ (2002) Curcumin suppresses activation of NF-kappaB and AP-1 induced by phorbol ester in cultured human promyelocytic leukemia cells. J Biochem Mol Biol 35: 337–42.
36. Singh S, Aggarwal BB (1995) Activation of transcription factor NF-kappa B is suppressed by curcumin (diferuloylmethane)[corrected]. J Biol Chem 270: 24995–25000.
37. Xu YX, Pindolia KR, Janakiraman N, Chapman RA, Gautam SC (1977) Curcumin inhibits IL1 alpha and TNF-alpha induction ofAP-1 and NF-kB DNA-binding activity in bone marrow stromal cells. Hematopathol Mol Hematol 11: 49–62.
38. Deguchi Y, Andoh A, Inatomi O, Yagi I, Bamaba S, et al. (2007) Curcumin prevents the development of Dextran Sulfate Sodium (DSS)-induced experimental colitis. Dig Dis Sci 52: 2993–8.
39. Kim GY, Kim KH, Lee SH,Yoon MS, Lee HJ, et al. (2005) Curcumin inhibits immunostimulatory function of dendritic cells: MAPKs and translocation of NF-kappa B as potential targets. J Immunol 174: 8116–24.
40. Shimouchi A, Nose K, Takaoka M, Hayashi H, Kondo T (2009) Effect of dietary turmericon breath hydrogen. Dig Dis Sci 54: 1725–9.
41. Kumar A, Purwar B, Shrivastava A, Pandey S (2010) Effects of curcumin on the intestinal motility of albino rats. Indian J Physiol Pharmacol 54: 284–8.
42. Itthipanichpong C, Ruangrungsi N, Kemsri W, Sawasdipanich A (2006) Antispasmodic effects of curcuminoids on isolated guinea-pig ileum and rat uterus. J Med Assoc Thai 86,Suppl 2: S2999–309.
43. Wirtz S, Neufert C, Weigmann B, Neurath MF (2007) Chemically induced mouse models of intestinal inflammation. Nat Protoc 2: 541–6.
44. Fitzpatrick LR, Wang J, Le M (2000) In vitro and in vivo effects of gliotoxin, a fungal metabolite: Efficacy against dextran sodium sulfate-induced colitis in rats. Dig Dis Sci 45: 2327–36.
45. Reagan-Shaw S, Nihal M, Ahmad N (2008) Dose translation from animal to human studies revisited. FASEB J 22: 659–61.
46. Takemasa K (1957) On the inorganic salts in the artificial nourishing fluid for isolated intestine. J Physiol Soc Japan 19: 1217–27.
47. Motulsky H, Christopoulos A (2003) Fitting Models to Biological Data Using Linear and Non Linear Regression, GrafhPad, La Jolla, CA, 2003. Available: www. graphpad.com/manual/Prism4/RegressionBook.pdf. Accessed 2010 May 10.
48. Arunlakshana D, Schild HO (1959) Some Quantitative Uses of Drug Antagonists. Br J Pharmacol 14: 48–58.
49. Tallarida RJ, Murray RB (1987) Manual of Pharmacologic Calculations with Computer Programs, 2nd ed.; Springer-Verlag: New York.
50. Version 3.0; GraphPad Software, Inc., San Diego, CA, USA.
51. Larmonier CB, Midura-Kiela MT, Ramalingam R, Laubitz D, Janikashvili N, et al. (2011) Modulation of neutrophil motility by curcumin: implications for inflammatory bowel disease. Inflamm Bowel Dis 17 (2): 503–15.
52. Furness JB (2008) The enteric nervous system: normal functions and enteric neuropathies. Neurogastroenterol Motil 20 (Suppl 1): 32–8.
53. Grundy D, Schemann M (2005) Enteric nervous system. Curr Opin Gastroenterol 21: 176–8.
54. Linden DR (2003) Colitis: it is not just for the colon anymore. Br J Pharmacol 139: 185–6.
55. Linden DR, Sharkey KA, Ho W, Mawe GM (2004) Cyclooxygenase-2 contributes to dysmotility and enhanced excitability of myenteric AH neurones in the inflamed guinea pig distal colon. J Physiol 557: 191–205.
56. Lomax AE, Fernandez E, Sharkey KA (2005) Plasticity o f the entericnervous system during intestinal inflammation. Neurogastroenterol Motil 17: 4–15.
57. Akiho H, Ihara E, Motomura Y, Nakamura K (2011) Cytokine-induced alterations of gastrointestinal motility in gastrointestinal disorders. World J Gastrointest Pathophysiol 15; 2(5): 72–81.
58. Reddy SN, Bazzocchi G, Chan S, Akashi K, Villanueva-Meyer J, et al. (1991)Colonic motility and transit in health and ulcerative colitis. Gastroenterology 101: 1289–97.
59. Kinoshita K, Sato K, Hori M, Ozaki H, Karaki H (2003) Decrease in activity of smooth muscle L-type Ca2+ channels and its reversal by NF-kappaB inhibitors in Crohn's colitis model. Am J Physiol - Gastrointestinal and Liver Physiology 285: G483–G493.
60. Myers BS, Martin JS, Dempsey DT, Parkman HP, Thomas RM, et al. (1997) Acute experimental colitis decreases colonic circular smooth muscle contractility in rats. Am J Physiol - Gastrointestinal and Liver Physiology 273: G928–G936.
61. Pazdrak K, Shi XZ, Sarna SK (2004) TNFα suppresses human colonic circular smooth muscle cell contractility by SP1- and NF-κB-mediated induction of ICAM1.Gastroenterology 127: 1096–109.
62. Ihara E, Beck PL, Chappellaz M, Wong J, Medlicott SA, et al. (2009) Mitogen-activated protein kinase pathways contribute to hypercontractility and increased Ca2+ sensitization in murine experimental colitis. Mol Pharmacol 75(5): 1031–41.
63. Kondo T, Nakajima M, Teraoka H, Unno T, Komori S, et al. (2011) Muscarinic receptor subtypes involved in regulation of colonic motility in mice: functional studies using muscarinic receptor-deficient mice. Eur J Pharmacol 670: 236–43.

3

HVEM Signalling Promotes Colitis

Corinne Schaer[1], Stefanie Hiltbrunner[1], Bettina Ernst[1], Christoph Mueller[2], Michael Kurrer[3], Manfred Kopf[1], Nicola L. Harris[4]*

1 Molecular Biomedicine, Institute of Integrative Biology, Swiss Federal Institute of Technology, Zurich, Switzerland, **2** Institute of Pathology, University of Bern, Bern, Switzerland, **3** Institute of Pathology, Cantonal Hospital Aarau, Aarau, Switzerland, **4** Swiss Vaccine Research Institute and Global Health Institute, Ecole Polytechnique Fédérale, Lausanne, Switzerland

Abstract

Background: Tumor necrosis factor super family (TNFSF) members regulate important processes involved in cell proliferation, survival and differentiation and are therefore crucial for the balance between homeostasis and inflammatory responses. Several members of the TNFSF are closely associated with inflammatory bowel disease (IBD). Thus, they represent interesting new targets for therapeutic treatment of IBD.

Methodology/Principal Findings: We have used mice deficient in TNFSF member HVEM in experimental models of IBD to investigate its role in the disease process. Two models of IBD were employed: i) chemical-induced colitis primarily mediated by innate immune cells; and ii) colitis initiated by $CD4^{+}CD45RB^{high}$ T cells following their transfer into immuno-deficient $RAG1^{-/-}$ hosts. In both models of disease the absence of HVEM resulted in a significant reduction in colitis and inflammatory cytokine production.

Conclusions: These data show that HVEM stimulatory signals promote experimental colitis driven by innate or adaptive immune cells.

Editor: Lena Alexopoulou, Centre d'Immunologie de Marseille-Luminy, CNRS-Inserm, France

Funding: N. Harris is supported by the Swiss Vaccine Research Institute (http://www.swissvaccineresearchinstitute.ch/). The project was funded by a research grant (no. TH-1407-3) from the Swiss Federal Institute of Technology (http://www.ethz.ch/index_EN). The funders had no role in study design, data collection and analysis, decision to publish, or preparation of the manuscript.

Competing Interests: The authors have declared that no competing interests exist.

* E-mail: nicola.harris@epfl.ch

Introduction

Members of the TNFSF play a central role in the regulation of immune responses by providing signals involved in differentiation, activation, survival and homeostasis of immune cells [1]. HVEM can promote T cell proliferation and IFNγ production [2,3], and has been linked to IFNγ production by human mucosal T cells [4]. HVEM has a widespread expression, being present on most hematopoietic cells in addition to some stromal and epithelial cells [5,6]. HVEM has multiple ligands, however LIGHT is thought to be the predominant ligand delivering stimulatory signals in vivo [7]. LIGHT is expressed by activated T cells, immature DCs and monocytes [3], and binds to both HVEM and lymphotoxin β receptor (LTβR) which is present on stromal cells and some hematopoietic cells including DCs and monocytes [7]. LIGHT has been shown to induce the maturation of DCs as well as NK cell proliferation [8,9]. LIGHT-deficient mice exhibit defective T cell proliferation and activation in vitro [3], and fail to reject MHC-mismatched cardiac allografts coinciding with decreased intragraft expression of IFNγ [10]. However, LIGHT-deficient mice display normal immune responses following infection with Mycobacterium tuberculosis [11] or influenza A [12], suggesting that LIGHT may regulate some cellular responses whilst being superfluous for others.

LIGHT is contained within a region of the human chromosome 19p13.3 identified as a susceptibility locus for IBD [13], and LIGHT mRNA transcripts are over-expressed in inflamed biopsies from IBD patients [14]. In an experimental model of IBD, transgenic over-expression of LIGHT on T cells resulted in a lymphoid proliferative disorder, widespread autoimmune disease and development of severe intestinal inflammation [15]. Intestinal inflammation driven by transgenic over-expression of LIGHT was found to involve signalling to both HVEM expressed by T cells and LTβR expressed by stromal cells [15]. Collectively, these data implicate, but do not prove, a role for HVEM stimulatory interactions in promoting intestinal inflammation.

In the current study we subjected mice deficient for LIGHT or HVEM to Dextran sulfate sodium (DSS)-induced colitis and investigated the impact of gene deficiency on diarrhea, ulcerations and cellular infiltration of the colon. Additionally, we compared the ability of wildtype C57BL/6 or $HVEM^{-/-}$ and $LIGHT^{-/-}$ $CD4^{+}CD45RB^{high}$ T cells to mediate experimental colitis following their transfer into immuno-compromised $RAG1^{-/-}$ hosts. Our data demonstrates that HVEM-mediated stimulatory signals are essential for promoting innate and adaptive immune cell activation, pro-inflammatory cytokine production and intestinal pathology.

Materials and Methods

Mice

C57BL/6 mice, $HVEM^{-/-}$ [16] mice and $LIGHT^{-/-}$ [10] mice were bred and maintained under specific pathogen-free (SPF) conditions at Bio-Support (Zürich, Switzerland). $HVEM^{-/-}$ and $LIGHT^{-/-}$ mice were backcrossed for 9 generations to C57BL/6 background. $RAG1^{-/-}$ (C57BL/6) mice were purchased from the Institute for Laboratory Animal Science, University of Zürich. Congenic CD45.1-allelic C57BL/6 mice were purchased from Jackson Laboratory. All mice used in this study were 5–8 weeks old. Mice from different genotypes were housed within the same cage or bedding from the cages of male mice was mixed for at least 2–3 weeks prior to all the experiments.

Ethics Statement

All animal procedures were approved by the local animal committee Kantonales Veterinäramt Zürich, protocol no. 3282, and performed in accordance with our institutional guidelines.

DSS- induced experimental colitis

Acute colitis was induced in age-matched C57BL/6, $HVEM^{-/-}$, $LIGHT^{-/-}$ and $RAG1^{-/-}$ mice, by oral administration of Dextran sulfate sodium (DSS) (MP Biomedicals) at a concentration of 5% (w/v) in drinking water for 4 days. Age-matched C57BL/6, $HVEM^{-/-}$ and $LIGHT^{-/-}$ mice receiving normal drinking water served as controls. Mice were evaluated daily for changes in body weight or the development of clinical symptoms. Six days after the induction of colitis mice were sacrificed by CO_2 inhalation, the abdominal cavity was exposed and the entire colon was removed from the cecum to the anus. As the distal colon is the main site of inflammation in the DSS model [17], the distal colon was analyzed for inflammation by mRNA expression for inflammatory cytokines and by histology.

Experimental colitis induced by $CD4^+$ T cells

T cell-mediated colitis was induced by transferring 4×10^5 $CD4^+CD25^-CD45RB^{high}$ T cells into $RAG1^{-/-}$ mice. Cells isolated from spleen cell preparations were labeled with anti-CD4 microbeads and separated by positive selection on a magnetic column, according to the manufacturer's instructions (Miltenyi Biotech). Purified $CD4^+$ T cells were then labeled with CD4, CD25 and CD45RB antibodies and sorted for $CD4^+CD25^-CD45RB^{high}$ population on a FACS Vantage (BD Biosciences). The purity of FACS sorted $CD4^+CD25^-CD45RB^{high}$ cells was routinely ≥98%. Mice were sacrificed at 14 days, 28 days, or 6–8 weeks post transfer. In preliminary experiments the colon was divided into 3 parts and each part analyzed for inflammation by mRNA expression for inflammatory cytokines and by histology. As the middle section was repeatedly the most inflamed section in all mice we only analyzed this portion in later experiments and data is shown only for this section.

Assessment of the clinical activity score during DSS-induced colitis

Assessment of body weight, stool consistency and the presence of occult/gross blood by a guaiac test (Hemoccult Sensa; Beckman Coulter) were determined at the day of sacrifice for all mice. Colitis was quantified with a clinical score, as described by Cooper et al. [17], using the parameters of weight loss, stool consistency and fecal blood. Briefly, weight loss was considered as negligible (0 points), 1–5% (1 point), 5–10% (2 points), 10–15% (3 points) or ≥15% (necessitating sacrifice and given 4 points). Stool character was characterized as normal (0 points), soft with well-formed pellets (2 points), or diarrhea (4 points). For occult blood, scores were given as an absence of blood (0 points), a positive hemoccult score (2 points) or gross bleeding (4 points). The scores for each individual parameter were then added together to give a total score between 0 and 12.

Histological assessment of colitis

Colonic specimens obtained as described were fixed in formalin for at least 24 hours, embedded into paraffin, and cut into 4–5 μm sections. Sections were then stained with hematoxylin and eosin (H&E) for blind microscopic assessment of mucosal lesions. Histological scoring for DSS colon sections was performed, with slight modifications, as previously described by Schenk et al. [18]. Briefly, for inflammation scores were given as rare inflammatory cells in the lamina propria (0 points), increased numbers of lymphocytes and granulocytes in the lamina propria (1 point), confluence of inflammatory cells extending into the submucosa (2 points), or transmural extension of the infiltrate (3 points). For crypt damage scores reflected intact crypts (0 points), loss of every third crypt (1 point), loss of two out of three crypts (2 points), complete crypt loss (3 points), or change of epithelial surface with epithelial erosion (4 points). For evaluation of the confluence of epithelial erosion scores reflected an absence of epithelial erosion (0 points), 1–2 foci of epithelial erosion (1 point), 3–4 foci (2 points), or confluent epithelial erosion (3 points). The scores for each individual parameter were then added together to give a total score between 0 and 10.

Histological scoring of colonic sections from the T cell transfer-induced colitis model was determined according to the following parameters. An estimated score was made based on first impression (score from 0–3), loss of goblet cells (score from 0–4), crypt abscesses (score from 0–3), mucosal thickness (score from 0–3), cellular infiltration (score from 0–3) and epithelial erosions (score from 0–2). The scores for each individual parameter were then added together to give a total score between 0 and 18.

Cell isolation and Flow cytometry

MLN single cell suspensions were obtained by mechanical disruption through a 40 μM cell strainer (BD Biosciences). Colon LP lymphocytes were isolated as previously described [19]. Briefly, colon tissue was cut into 0.5 cm pieces and incubated at 37°C for 30 min. in PBS containing 0.5% BSA, 2% HEPES, 1% NaPyruvate and 10 mM EDTA to remove epithelial cells. The remaining tissue was further digested in complete IMDM medium containing 10% FCS and 1.5 mg Collagenase VIII (Sigma Aldrich) for 20 min. at 37°C and then smashed through a cell strainer. Cells were stained with surface antibodies diluted in PBS with 0.5% BSA (Sigma Aldrich). For intracellular staining cells were fixed in BD lysis buffer (BD Biosciences), permeabilized using 0.5% Saponin (Sigma Aldrich) in 0.5% BSA/PBS and stained with intracellular antibodies in 0.5% Saponin in 0.5% BSA/PBS. For the analysis of cytokine production by intracellular staining cells were first stimulated with PMA (Sigma-Aldrich) and ionomycin (Sigma-Aldrich) for 4 h at 37°C in IMDM medium plus 7% FCS. For the final two hours, Brefeldin A (10 μg/ml) was added to the cultures to retain cytokines in the cytoplasm. Stained cells were analyzed on FACS Calibur (BD Bioscience) or Cyan (Dako Cytomation) flow cytometers using FlowJo software (Tree Star). Fluorescently conjugated mAbs directed against CD4 (L3T4), CD25 (PC61), CD45RB (C363-16A), CD45.1 (A20), Ki-67 (MOPC-21), IL-17A (TC11), IFNγ (XMG1.2) and Foxp3 (FJK-16s) were purchased from eBiosciences.

Detection of cytokine mRNA expression by quantitative RT-PCR

Total RNA was isolated from all colonic specimens obtained as described using TRI Reagent (Molecular Research Center, Inc.) and reverse transcribed using Superscript III RT kit (Invitrogen). Transcribed cDNA was used as a template for the PCR reaction.

Real-time RT-PCR was performed using Brilliant SYBR Green (Stratagene) and an iCycler (Bio-Rad Laboratories). Expression was normalized according to expression of the housekeeping gene β-Actin. Sequences of primers used: β-Actin; 5′-CTT TTC ACG GTT GGC CTT AG-3′ and 5′-CCC TGA AGT ACC CCA TTG AAC-3′, CCL3; 5′-AGA TTC CAC GCC AAT TCA TC-3′ and 5′-CCC AGG TCT CTT TGG AGT CA-3′, CCL4; 5′-TTC TGT GCT CCA GGG TTC TC-3′ and 5′-AGC AAA GAC TGC TGG TCT CA-3′, CCL5; 5′- CAA TCT TGC AGT CGT GTT TG-3′ and 5′- AGA ATC AAG AAA CCC TCT ATC-3′, IL-6; 5′-TTC CAT CCA GTT GCC TTC TTG-3′ and 5′-TCA TTT CCA CGA TTT CCC AGA G-3′, IFNγ; 5′-GCT CTG AGA CAA TGA ACG CTA C-3′ and 5′-TTC TAG GCT TTC AAT GAC TGT GC-3′, TNFα; 5-GAA CTG GCA GAA GAG GCA CT-3′ and 5′-AGG GTC TGG GCC ATA GAA CT-3′, CXCL9, 5′-GCA AAA GTG AGC TCC AGA AGG-3′ and 5′-AGC TTC CCA GAT CAC AGA GG-3′.IL-6; 5′-TTC CAT CCA GTT GCC TTC TTG-3′ and 5′-TCA TTT CCA CGA TTT CCC AGA G-3′, IL-12p40; 5′-TAC AGT TCA GGC GCC GGA T-3′ and 5′-AGA GTT AAC CTG AGG TCC GCA-3′, TNFα; 5-GAA CTG GCA GAA GAG GCA CT-3′ and 5′-AGG GTC TGG GCC ATA GAA CT-3′, IL-21R; 5′-TCT GGA CCA TCA CCT GTG TC-3′and 5′-TTG TGG CCA GAC CTG TGT AG-3′, IL23R; 5′-GCC AAG AAG ACC ATT CCC GA-3′ and 5′-TCA GTG CTA CAA TCT TCT TCA GAG GAC A-3′ and IL-6R; 5′-AAG AGT GAC TTC CAG GTG CC-3′ and 5′-GGT ATC GAA GCT GGA ACT GC-3′ .

Statistical Analysis

A two-tailed unpaired Student's t test with a confidence interval of 95% was performed on all data and are shown as p-values $p<0.05$ (*), $p<0.005$ (**), or $p<0.0005$ (***).

Results

HVEM is required for DSS-induced colitis

To investigate the role of HVEM signaling during intestinal inflammation mediated by innate immune cells, we examined the response of HVEM$^{-/-}$ mice to DSS-induced intestinal damage. In this model, administration of DSS in the drinking water results in weight loss, intestinal epithelial cell damage and immune-mediated colonic inflammation. As expected wild type C57BL/6 mice exhibited severe weight loss and intestinal inflammation following acute DSS administration (Figure 1A). In contrast HVEM$^{-/-}$ mice exhibited significantly reduced weight loss and reduced rectal bleeding following DSS treatment (Figure 1A&B). In addition, HVEM$^{-/-}$ mice showed attenuated intestinal immuno-pathology as determined by histological analysis of leukocyte infiltration, crypt destruction and epithelial erosion within the colon (Figure 1C&D). Importantly, the absence of inflammation in HVEM$^{-/-}$ mice was

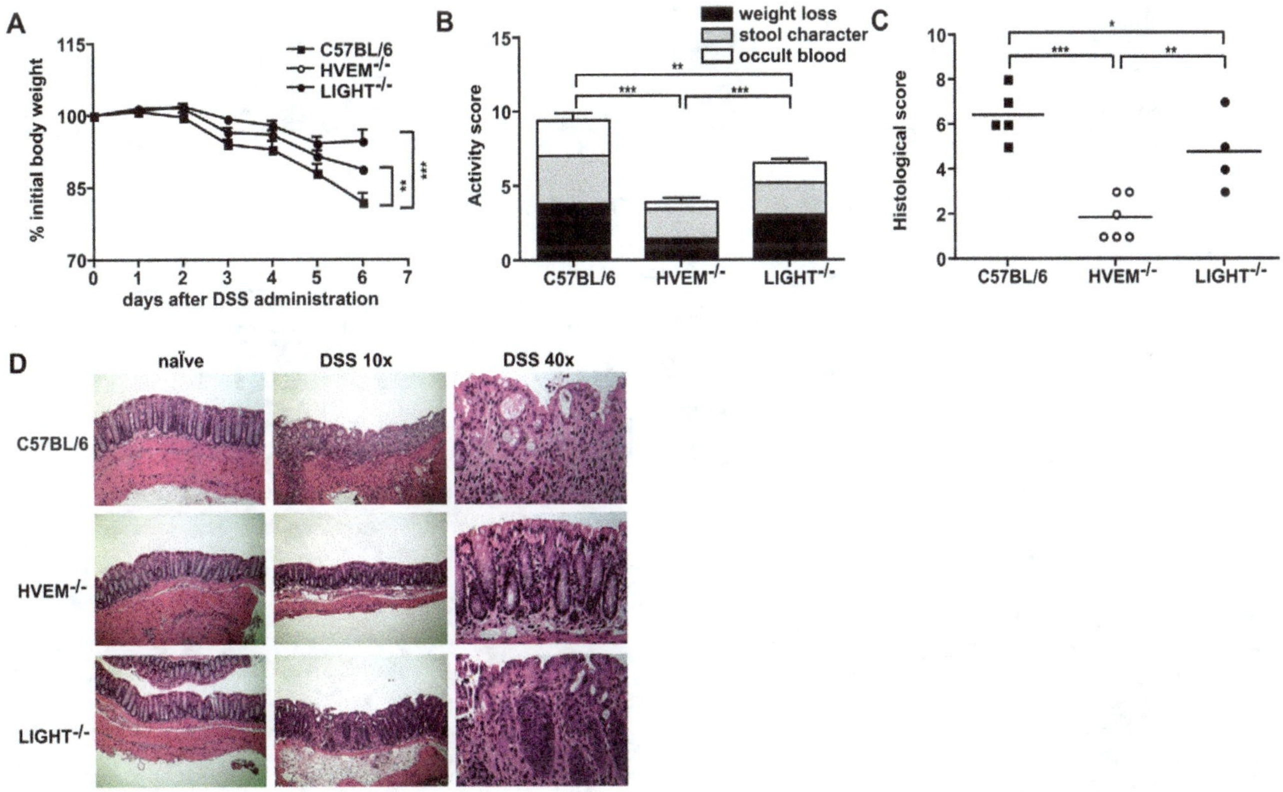

Figure 1. HVEM$^{-/-}$ mice are resistant to DSS-induced colitis. C57BL/6, HVEM$^{-/-}$ and LIGHT$^{-/-}$ mice were given 5% DSS in the drinking water for 4 days, then returned to normal drinking water and sacrificed at day 6. (A) Body weight loss was monitored daily and is expressed as percentage change from initial body weight at day 0 for C57BL/6 (closed squares), HVEM$^{-/-}$ (open circles) or LIGHT$^{-/-}$ (closed circles). (B) Clinical activity scores were assessed at the time of sacrifice by a combination of total weight loss, stool character and occult blood. (C) Histological scores indicating immuno-pathology were calculated as described in the Materials and Methods and are shown for the distal part of the colon of individual mice for C57BL/6 (closed squares), HVEM$^{-/-}$ (open circles) or LIGHT$^{-/-}$ (closed circles). (D) Representative H&E staining of distal colon tissue sections from control and DSS-treated mice. Scale bars are 10× magnification = 200 μm and 40× magnification = 0.05 μm. Data in (A), (B) and (C) represent the mean ± SD of one experiment (n = 4-6 mice per group) out of three independent experiments. Statistically significant differences between groups were assessed by a two tailed Student's t test: $^{*}p<0.05$, $^{**}p<0.005$, $^{***}p<0.0005$.

not due to a delayed response, as mice did not exhibit weight loss even at late time points following DSS administration. Although DSS-induced intestinal inflammation can lead to the activation and recruitment of T cells, the disease is mediated largely by the activation of innate immune cells [20,21]. Taken together, these data demonstrate that HVEM-mediated stimulatory signals are necessary to promote the activation of innate immune responses responsible for disease induction.

LIGHT is thought to represent a major HVEM stimulatory ligand. We therefore additionally investigated DSS-induced intestinal inflammation in LIGHT$^{-/-}$ mice. LIGHT$^{-/-}$ mice exhibited an intermediate phenotype showing less severe inflammation than C57BL/6 mice, but significantly more severe inflammation than that observed for HVEM$^{-/-}$ mice (Figure 1A–D).

To further assess the impact of HVEM on immunity during DSS-induced intestinal inflammation we analyzed the production of chemokines and pro-inflammatory cytokines within the intestine. DSS-induced production of CCL3 (MIP-1α), CCL4 (MIP-1β), CCL5 (RANTES), IFNγ, TNFα, IL-6 and CXCL9 was severely attenuated in the absence of HVEM (Figure 2A-G). These cytokines and chemokines are largely produced by local DC, monocytes and stromal cells, NK cells and/or T cells and their attenuation in the absence of HVEM indicates that HVEM is required for both innate and adaptive immune cell activation in this model. Chemokine and cytokine expression in LIGHT$^{-/-}$ mice was highly variable but overall there was a non-significant decrease compared to C57BL/6 mice, and a non-significant increase as compared to HVEM$^{-/-}$ mice (Figure 2A-G).

These data suggested that HVEM could signal directly to innate immune cells within the intestine to promote the production of pro-inflammatory cytokines and chemokines following DSS administration. The intermediate phenotype of LIGHT$^{-/-}$ mice - in terms of chemokine and cytokine expression, weight loss and intestinal immuno-pathology - indicated that LIGHT only partially accounts for HVEM-mediated stimulatory signals in our model and raises the possibility that additional HVEM-stimulatory ligands contribute to intestinal inflammation in vivo.

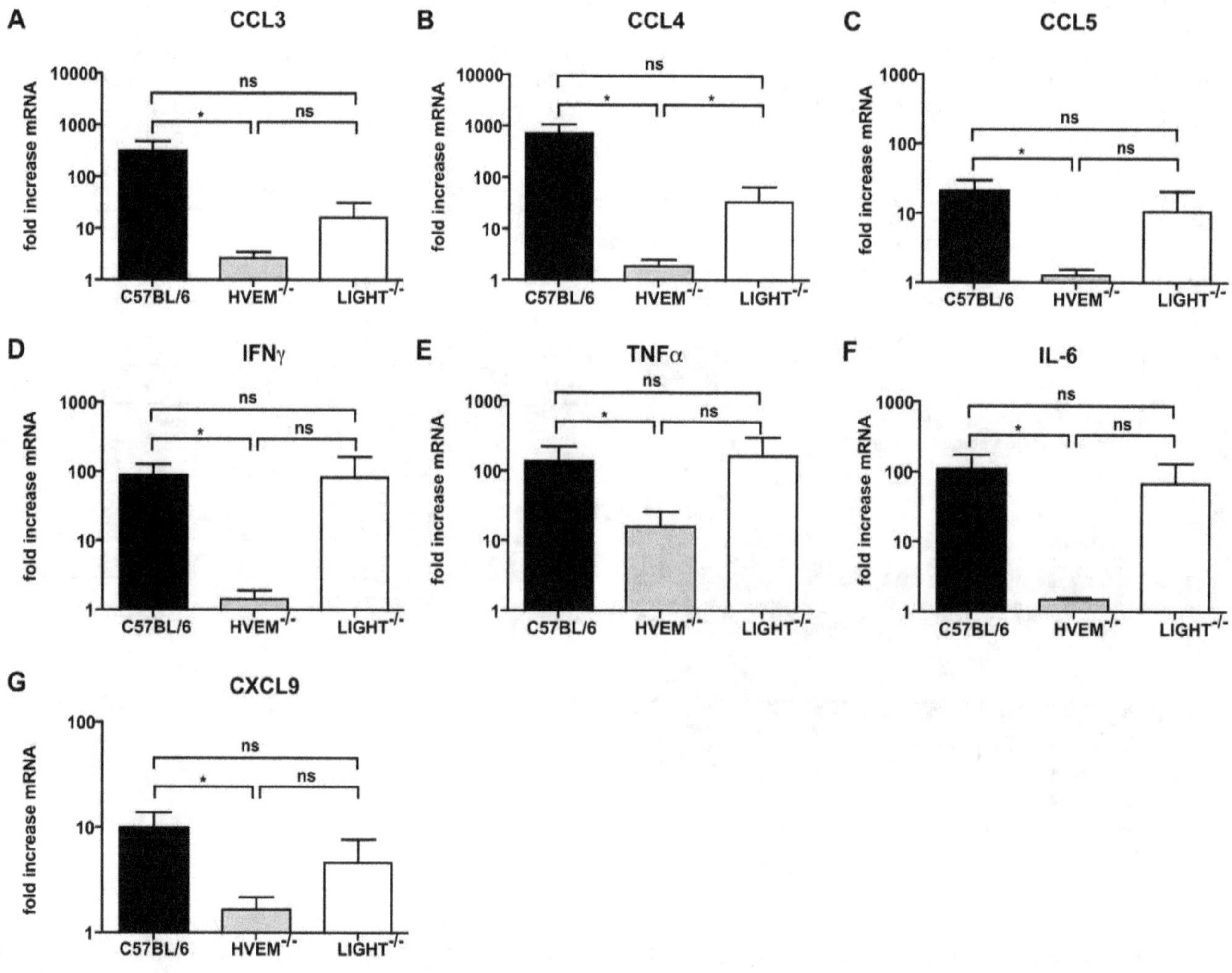

Figure 2. HVEM is required for DSS-induced pro-inflammatory cytokine and chemokine production. C57BL/6, HVEM$^{-/-}$ and LIGHT$^{-/-}$ mice were given 5% DSS in the drinking water for 4 days, then returned to normal drinking water. At day 6 mice were sacrificed and the colon removed for RNA isolation. (A) CCL3, (B) CCL4, (C) CCL5, (D) IFNγ, (E) TNFα, (F) IL-6 and (G) CXCL9 gene expression in the distal colon was analyzed by quantitative RT-PCR for C57BL/6 (black bar), HVEM$^{-/-}$ (grey bar) and LIGHT$^{-/-}$ (white bar) mice. For each individual sample, gene expression was normalized relative to β-Actin. Values represent fold increases in mRNA expression over the corresponding untreated controls. Means ± SD are shown for two independent experiments (n = 8–10 mice per group) out of three independent experiments. Statistically significant differences between groups were assessed by a two tailed Student's t test: $^{*}p<0.05$, $^{**}p<0.005$, $^{***}p<0.0005$.

HVEM stimulatory signals regulate T cell-mediated colitis

To directly investigate the role of HVEM-mediated signaling to $CD4^+$ T cells we used an experimental model whereby colitis is initiated by the transfer of $CD4^+CD45RB^{high}$ T cells into immuno-deficient hosts. $CD4^+CD45RB^{high}$ T cells were purified from the spleens of $HVEM^{-/-}$ or wildtype C57BL/6 mice and 4×10^5 cells injected intravenously into age and sex-matched $RAG1^{-/-}$ recipients. $RAG1^{-/-}$ recipients receiving $CD4^+CD45RB^{high}$ T cells from C57BL/6 mice exhibited weight loss and intestinal inflammation commencing between day 30 and 40 after transfer (Figure 3A–C). In contrast recipients of $HVEM^{-/-}$ $CD4^+CD45RB^{high}$ T cells

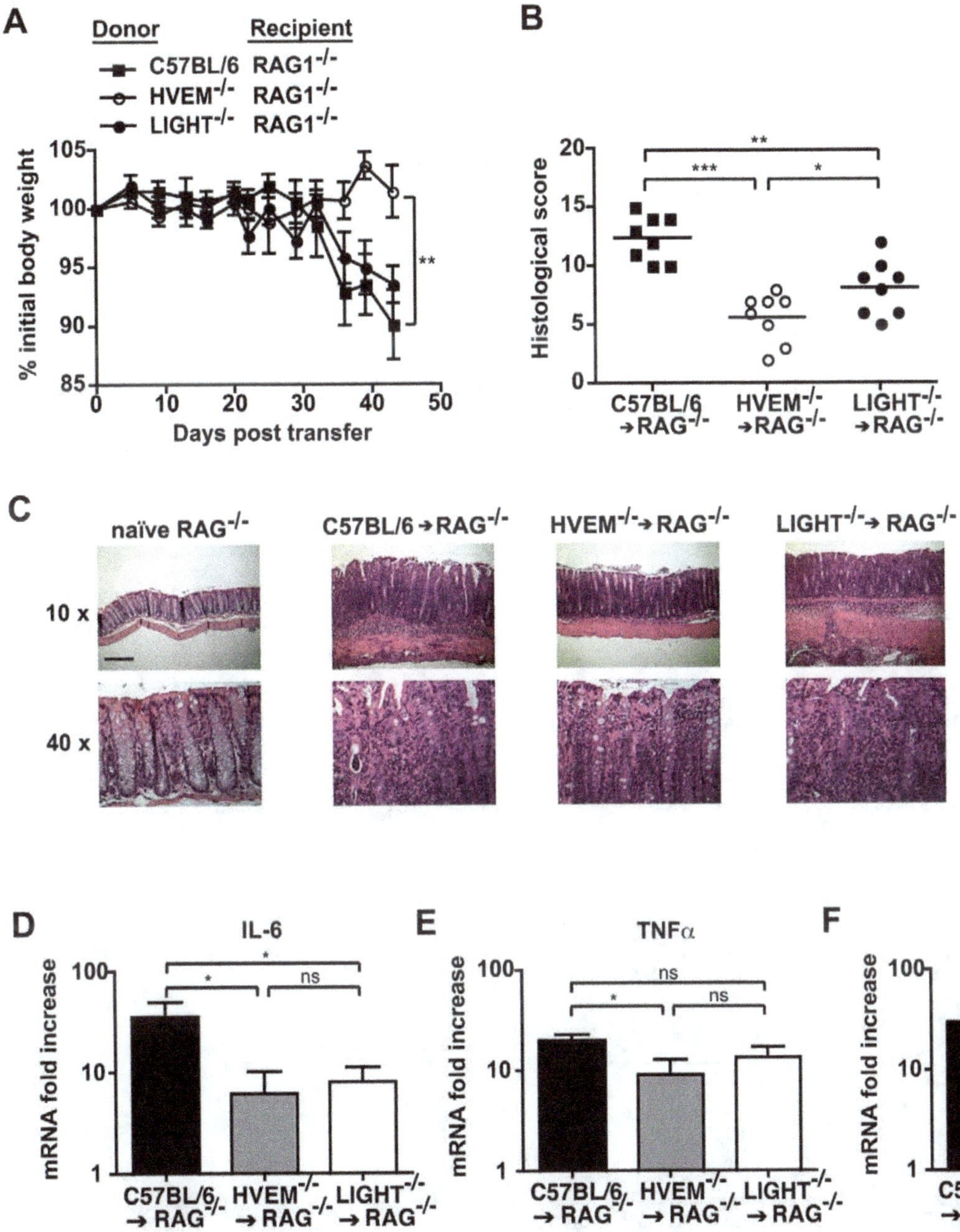

Figure 3. HVEM expression by $CD4^+$ T cells is required for T cell-mediated colitis. 4×10^5 $CD4^+CD25^-CD45RB^{high}$ T cells from C57BL/6, $HVEM^{-/-}$ or $LIGHT^{-/-}$ mice were injected intravenously into $RAG1^{-/-}$ hosts and recipients sacrificed 6-8 weeks later. (A) Body weight was monitored regularly and is expressed as percentage change from initial body weight at day 0 for C57BL/6 (closed squares), $HVEM^{-/-}$ (open circles) or $LIGHT^{-/-}$ (closed circles) T cells transferred into $RAG1^{-/-}$ mice (n = 8 mice per group). (B) Histological scores indicating immuno-pathology were calculated as described in the Materials and Methods section and are shown for the middle part of the colon. Symbols represent individual $RAG1^{-/-}$ animals receiving either C57BL/6 (closed squares), $HVEM^{-/-}$ (open circles) or $LIGHT^{-/-}$ (closed circles) $CD4^+CD25^-CD45RB^{high}$ T cells (n = 8 mice per group). (C) Representative H&E staining of middle colon tissue-sections from control $RAG1^{-/-}$ mice, and mice receiving either C57BL/6, $HVEM^{-/-}$ or $LIGHT^{-/-}$ $CD4^+CD25^-CD45RB^{high}$ T cells. Scale bars are 10× magnification = 200 μm and 40× magnification = 0.05 μm. Colon mRNA expression of (D) IL-6, (E) TNFα and (F) IL-12p40 was determined in the distal colon part in $RAG1^{-/-}$ hosts receiveing C57BL/6 (black bar), $HVEM^{-/-}$ (grey bar) and $LIGHT^{-/-}$ (white bar) $CD4^+CD25^-CD45RB^{high}$ T cells. Data from (A), (B), (D), (E) and (F) represents means ± SD of two pooled experiments (n = 8 mice per group) out of four independent experiments. Statistically significant differences between groups were assessed by a two tailed Student's t test: $^*p<0.05$, $^{**}p<0.005$, $^{***}p<0.0005$.

exhibited a clear resistance to weight loss (Figure 3A). Analysis of histopathology showed clear intestinal pathology in recipients of HVEM$^{-/-}$ CD4^{+}CD45RB^{high} T cells, however this was significantly reduced compared to RAG1$^{-/-}$ mice receiving C57BL/6 CD4^{+}CD45RB^{high} T cells (Figure 3B&C). The presence of some degree of intestinal inflammation in recipients of HVEM$^{-/-}$ CD4^{+}CD45RB^{high} T cells did not correlate with the absence of weight loss. However this was not unexpected as it is well described in this model that weight loss alone is not a reliable measure of intestinal inflammation [22].

Since T cells are known to be a major source of LIGHT [23], we additionally investigated the role of T cell-expressed LIGHT in promoting intestinal inflammation. Transfer of CD4^{+}CD45RB^{high} T cells from LIGHT$^{-/-}$ mice into RAG1$^{-/-}$ recipients did not impact on weight loss (Figure 3A) but did reduce intestinal inflammation (Figure 3B&C). Attenuated intestinal inflammation observed following transfer of LIGHT$^{-/-}$ T cells was significant when compared to mice receiving C57BL/6 T cells, but was not as dramatic as that observed for mice receiving HVEM$^{-/-}$ T cells, indicating that other sources of LIGHT, or additional HVEM stimulatory ligands must exist.

To validate the reduced intestinal inflammation observed in mice receiving HVEM$^{-/-}$ or LIGHT$^{-/-}$ CD4^{+}CD45RB^{high} T cells we additionally investigated the production of pro-inflammatory cytokines within the colon. All mice exhibited increased cytokine production as compared to naïve RAG1$^{-/-}$ controls (Figure 3D–F). However, mice receiving HVEM$^{-/-}$ T cells exhibited reduced levels of IL-6, TNFα and IL-12p40 as compared to recipients that received C57BL/6 naïve T cells, in the colon (Figure 3D, E&F). Mice receiving LIGHT$^{-/-}$ T cells exhibited an intermediate phenotype compared to both C57BL/6 and HVEM$^{-/-}$ CD4^{+}CD45RB^{high} T cell-transferred mice, with significantly reduced IL-6 plus IL-12p40 in the colon (Figure 3D&F) but normal levels of TNFα (Figure 3E). Overall these data correlate well with the relative degrees of intestinal immuno-pathology observed in the same animals (Figure 3A–C) and reinforce our observations that HVEM stimulatory signals to T cells promote development of intestinal inflammation.

We next investigated the impact of HVEM or LIGHT deficiency on the accumulation of T cells in the draining mesenteric lymph node (MLN) and their production of inflammatory cytokines. Mice receiving C57BL/6, HVEM$^{-/-}$ or LIGHT$^{-/-}$ CD4^{+}CD45RB^{high} T cells had similar percentages of CD4^{+} T cells in the MLN (Figure 4A), however those mice receiving HVEM$^{-/-}$ T cells had a decreased total number of CD4^{+} T cells present (Figure 4B). Both the percentage and total number of CD4^{+} T cells producing IFNγ or IL-17A was significantly decreased in mice receiving HVEM$^{-/-}$ T cells as compared to mice

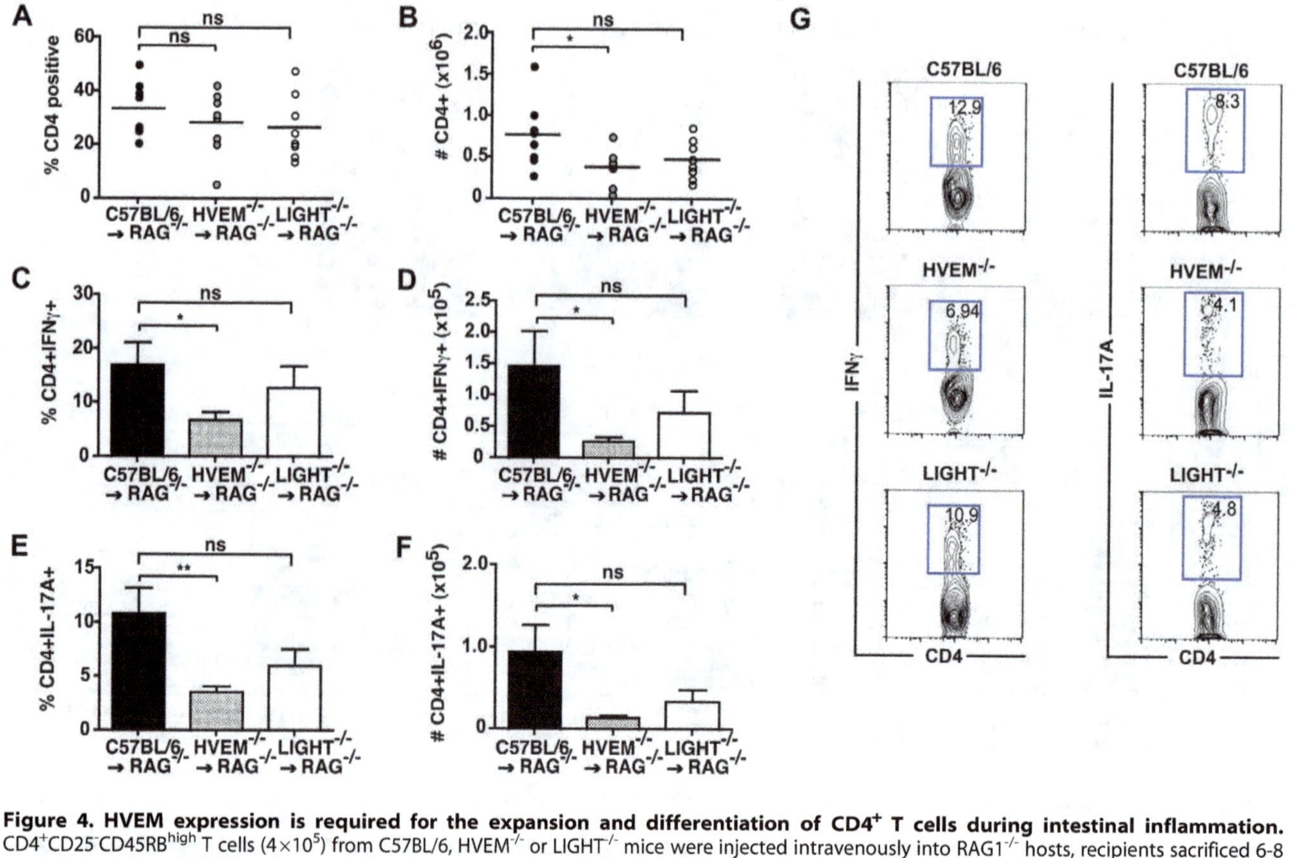

Figure 4. HVEM expression is required for the expansion and differentiation of CD4^{+} T cells during intestinal inflammation. CD4^{+}CD25^{-}CD45RB^{high} T cells (4×10^{5}) from C57BL/6, HVEM$^{-/-}$ or LIGHT$^{-/-}$ mice were injected intravenously into RAG1$^{-/-}$ hosts, recipients sacrificed 6-8 weeks later and total MLN lymphocytes isolated. Frequency of (A) CD4^{+}, (C) CD4^{+}IFNγ^{+} and (E) CD4^{+}IL-17A^{+} T cells in C57BL/6 (closed circles and black bar), HVEM$^{-/-}$ (grey circles and squattered bar) and LIGHT$^{-/-}$ (open circles and white bar) transferred RAG1$^{-/-}$ recipients were analyzed by flow cytometry using fluorescent marker-conjugated mAbs (n = 8 mice per group). Total numbers (indicated by # symbol) of (B) CD4^{+}, (D) CD4^{+}IFNγ^{+}, (F) CD4^{+}IL-17A^{+} T cells in the MLN of RAG1$^{-/-}$ mice receiving either C57BL/6 (black bar), HVEM$^{-/-}$ (striped bar) or LIGHT$^{-/-}$ (white bar) CD4^{+}CD25^{-}CD45RB^{high} T cells were calculated (n = 8 mice per group). (G) Representative FACS profiles for IFNγ and IL-17A production by C57BL/6, HVEM$^{-/-}$ or LIGHT$^{-/-}$ CD4^{+} T cells isolated from the MLN of RAG1$^{-/-}$ recipients. Symbols and bar graphs represent means (± SD) from two pooled experiments, and are representative of four independent experiments. Statistical analysis between groups was assessed by a two tailed Student's t test: $^{*}p<0.05$, $^{**}p<0.005$, $^{***}p<0.0005$.

receiving C57BL/6 T cells (Figure 4C–G). Selective deficiency of LIGHT on $CD4^+$ T cells did not impact significantly on the total number of $CD4^+$ T cells present in the MLN (Figure 4B), or on the percentage of $CD4^+$ T cells producing IFNγ (Figure 4C) or IL-17A (Figure 4E). Total numbers of $IFN\gamma^+$ or IL-$17A^+$ $LIGHT^{-/-}$ T cells were routinely observed to be decreased but this did not reach statistical significance (Figure 4D&F). By contrast, no differences in $CD4^+$ T cell number and cytokine production were seen in C57BL/6, $HVEM^{-/-}$ or $LIGHT^{-/-}$ $CD4^+$ T cells obtained from the spleen of transferred $RAG1^{-/-}$ recipient mice (data not shown). These findings indicated that HVEM expression by $CD4^+$ T cells is required for their expansion, activation or survival within the draining lymph nodes and for their effector function within the intestine during experimental colitis. Our data also demonstrated that the required HVEM-stimulatory signals were derived, at least in part, by T cell-expressed LIGHT.

Attenuated $CD4^+$ T cell expansion and cytokine production in the absence of HVEM stimulatory signals cannot be overcome by inflammatory conditions

We hypothesized that the decreased numbers of $HVEM^{-/-}$ $CD4^+$ T cells, and their inability to produce normal levels of inflammatory cytokines, may result from inadequate T cell-mediated DC activation and/or reduced production of pro-inflammatory cytokines in recipient mice. To address this we performed a co-transfer of equal numbers of $HVEM^{-/-}$ and congenic C57BL/6 $CD4^+CD45RB^{high}$ T cells into $RAG1^{-/-}$ recipients. Mice receiving both sets of T cells developed severe colitis similar to that observed in mice receiving C57BL/6 T cells alone (data not shown). However, both the percentage and total number of $HVEM^{-/-}$ $CD4^+$ T cells was markedly reduced in both the MLN (Figure 5A&B) and the spleen (Figure S1A&B) compared to their C57BL/6 counterparts. HVEM deficiency also resulted in reduced percentages and total numbers of $IFN\gamma^+$ or IL-$17A^+$ cells in the MLN (Figure 5C–G) and the spleen (Figure S1C–F). Thus, in contrast to our original hypothesis the co-transfer of C57BL/6 T cells allowed for the full development of inflammatory C57BL/6 T cells capable of initiating intestinal inflammation, but these cells acted in a competitive manner with $HVEM^{-/-}$ T cells to further reduce their expansion.

$HVEM^{-/-}$ $CD4^+$ T cells exhibit normal expansion at early time-points following their transfer into lymphopenic hosts

Our earlier findings indicated that HVEM deficiency on $CD4^+$ T cells results in an inherent defect in the ability of these cells to expand and produce effector cytokines. We next set out to determine whether this defect occurred due to a failure to undergo homeostatic and/or spontaneous expansion following their transfer into lymphopenic hosts, or whether it was related to a defect in T cell activation and differentiation into effector cells. For this purpose a time-course experiment was performed whereby $RAG1^{-/-}$ recipients receiving $HVEM^{-/-}$ $CD4^+$ T cells together with congenic wildtype C57BL/6 $CD4^+$ T cells were sacrificed at day 14, 28 and 50 following transfer. The percentage and total numbers of $CD4^+$ T cells was then determined and the fraction of $CD4^+$ T cells expressing the proliferation marker Ki-67 examined.

No differences in the percentage or total number of $HVEM^{-/-}$ versus wildtype $CD4^+$ T cells present in the draining MLN (Figure 6A&B) or colon (Figure S2A&B) were observed at day 14 following transfer. The fraction of $CD4^+$ T cells expressing Ki-67 was also similar for $HVEM^{-/-}$ and C57BL/6 cells (Figure 6C and Figure S2C). At day 28 following transfer the total numbers of $HVEM^{-/-}$ $CD4^+$ T cells, and the percentage of these cells expressing Ki-67 were not significantly different in the MLN (Figure 6D&F) or colon (Fig. S2D&F). However a significant reduction in the percentage of $CD4^+$ $HVEM^{-/-}$ T cells relative to C57BL/6 cells was noted for the MLN and colon at this time (Figure 6E and Figure S2E). In keeping with the data presented in Figure 5, both the percentage and total number of $HVEM^{-/-}$ T cells was reduced compared to wildtype cells by day 50 post-transfer (Figure 6G&H and Figure S2G&H). This correlated with a decreased fraction of $HVEM^{-/-}$ $CD4^+$ T cells expressing the proliferation marker Ki-67 (Figure 6I and Figure S2I), and attenuated production of IFNγ and IL-17A (Figure 5). No significant production of IFNγ or IL-17A was noted for either C57BL/6 or $HVEM^{-/-}$ T cells time-points earlier than day 50 (data not shown).

Taken together these data indicate that HVEM deficiency does not alter the ability of $CD4^+$ T cells to undergo expansion, or to survive, during the first few weeks following their transfer into lymphopenic hosts. Instead defective T cell responses in the absence of HVEM appear to occur at approximately the same time as inflammation begins, indicating that they result from a reduced capacity to maintain expansion and to differentiate into effector cells in the presence of ongoing intestinal inflammation.

Discussion

LIGHT-HVEM interactions have been previously implicated in IBD but the therapeutic potential of targeting this stimulatory pathway remains unclear. The aim of our study was to investigate how LIGHT- and HVEM-mediated stimulatory signals regulate intestinal immune responses during homeostasis or inflammation. For this purpose we used two mouse models of intestinal inflammation - where disease is driven primarily by innate cells or by $CD4^+$ T cells and thus replicate distinct components of human IBD. These studies have allowed us to reveal that HVEM-mediated co-stimulatory signals to both innate immune cells and $CD4^+$ T cells form an essential component of immune cell activation, proliferation, pro-inflammatory cytokine production and intestinal pathology.

Although we noted attenuated intestinal inflammation in the absence of HVEM, it is important to keep in mind that HVEM can also act as an inhibitory ligand. HVEM signaling to B and T lymphocyte attenuator (BTLA) [24] and CD160 [25] can result in an inhibition of T cell responses [24,25,26]. Indeed, inhibitory signals mediated by HVEM have been postulated to explain observations in $HVEM^{-/-}$ mice of increased mortality during ConA-mediated autoimmune hepatitis [27], and increased susceptibility to MOG peptide-induced experimental autoimmune encephalomyelitis (EAE) [27]. In addition Steinberg et al. reported a critical role for HVEM expression by stromal cells in preventing intestinal inflammation following T cell transfer to immunodeficient hosts [28]. In keeping with our own observations, these authors saw a clear reduction in the histopathological score in the colon of $RAG^{-/-}$ mice receiving HVEM or LIGHT deficient T cells [28]. However, they also reported an accelerated onset of intestinal inflammation following transfer of wildtype T cells into HVEM and RAG double deficient mice. This anti-inflammatory role of HVEM was determined to be mediated through T cell expressed BTLA [28]. Taken together with our own experiments these findings demonstrate that HVEM can mediate both pro- and anti-inflammatory signals during intestinal inflammation. We believe the most likely explanation of these collective data is that HVEM stimulatory signals are required to turn-on immune responses, whilst HVEM-mediated inhibitory signals function

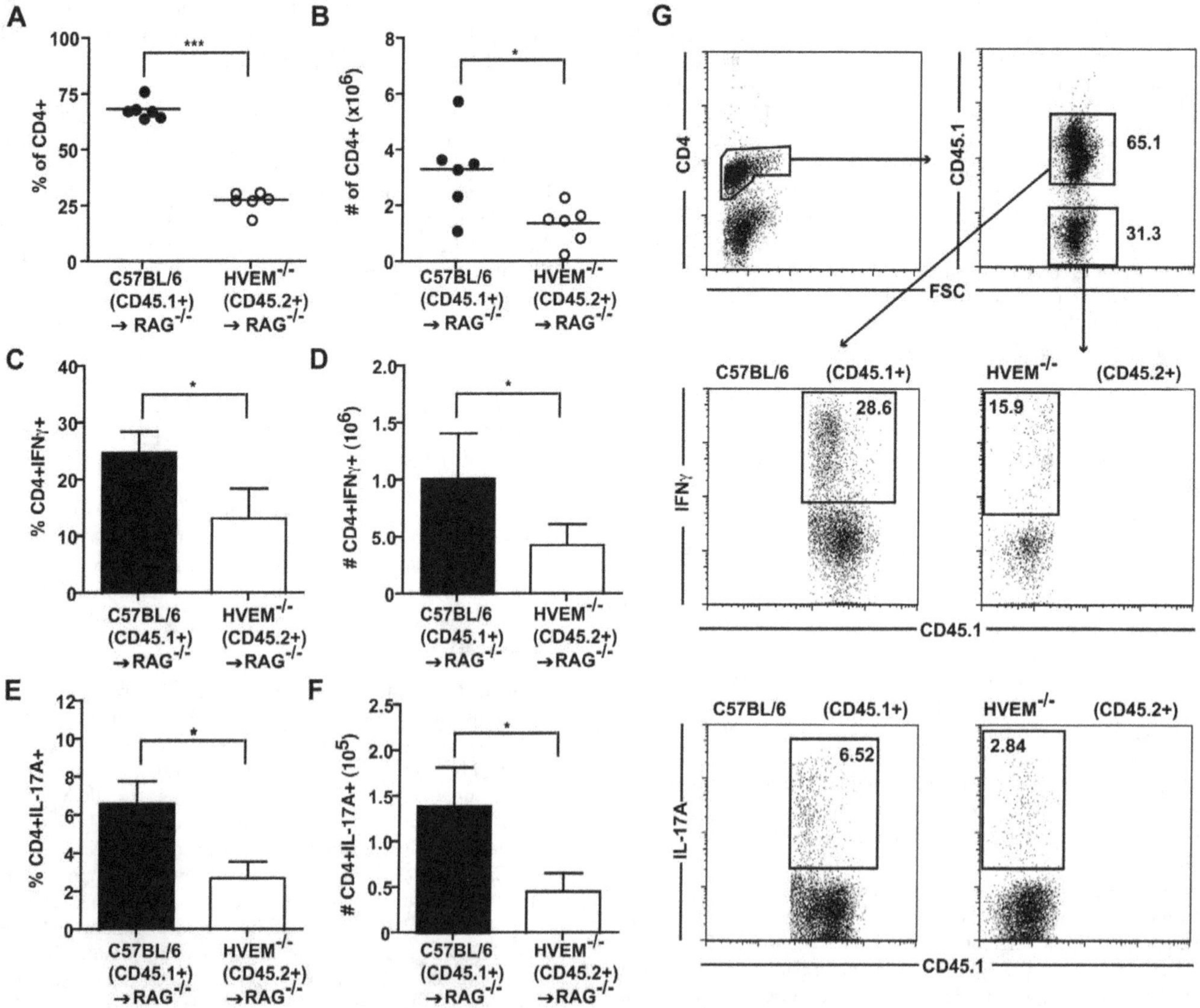

Figure 5. Attenuated HVEM$^{-/-}$ CD4$^+$ T cell expansion and cytokine production cannot be overcome by the presence of C57BL/6 CD4$^+$ T cells. Purified 4×10^5 CD4$^+$CD25$^-$CD45RB^{hight} T cells from congenic C57BL/6 (CD45.1$^+$) and HVEM$^{-/-}$ (CD45.1$^-$) mice were injected together at a 1:1 ratio (2×10^5 cells each genotype) into RAG1$^{-/-}$ recipients and mice were sacrificed 6-8 weeks later. Whole MLN cell suspensions from RAG1$^{-/-}$ recipients were analyzed by flow cytometry and percentages of C57BL/6 (closed circles and black bar) and HVEM$^{-/-}$ (open circles and white bar) (A) CD4$^+$, (C) CD4$^+$IFNγ^+ and (E) CD4$^+$IL-17A$^+$ T cell lymphocytes assessed (n = 6 mice per group). Total numbers (indicated by # symbol) of C57BL/6 (closed circles and black bar) or HVEM$^{-/-}$ (open circles and white bar) for (B) CD4$^+$, (D) CD4$^+$IFNγ^+ and (F) CD4$^+$IL-17A$^+$ T cells were calculated (n = 6 mice per group). (G) Flow cytometry plots showing gating strategy to distinguish C57BL/6 (CD45.1$^+$) from HVEM$^{-/-}$ (CD45.1$^-$) MLN CD4$^+$ T cells recovered from RAG1$^{-/-}$ recipients and representative plots of CD4$^+$ T cell IFNγ and IL-17A cytokine staining. Symbols and bar graphs represent means $\pm$ SD from two pooled experiments and are representative of three independent experiments. Statistical analysis between groups were calculated using the two tailed Student's t test: $^*p<0.05$, $^{**}p<0.005$, $^{***}p<0.0005$.

largely to switch-off immune responses. Support for this hypothesis comes from the finding that expression levels of the inhibitory ligands BTLA and CD160 are increased on T cells following their activation [24].

Although HVEM-mediated stimulatory signals were clearly required for the full activation of innate cells during DSS-induced colitis in our experiments, the exact identity of the stimulatory ligand(s) remains unclear. LIGHT is a known stimulatory ligand for HVEM, however LIGHT$^{-/-}$ mice only exhibited a partial defect in intestinal inflammation indicating that an alternative ligand must exist. LTα3 is produced by activated T-, B- and NK-cells and has been reported to bind to HVEM in vitro [29]. Although not formally proven, it was postulated that LTα3 delivers stimulatory signals to HVEM based on the finding that both LIGHT and LTα3 bind to the CRD2 and CRD3 regions of HVEM [30]. Thus LTα3 and LIGHT together may deliver the stimulatory signals necessary to promote inflammation. Paradoxically, LTα-deficient mice are reported to exhibit increased disease severity following DSS administration suggestive of a regulatory role for LTα in this model [31]. However, it should be kept in mind that delineating a clear role for LTα3-HVEM interactions in vivo is difficult as LTα forms a heterodimer with LTβ which acts to stimulate stromal cell-expressed LTβ receptor (LTβR), an interaction that is essential for lymphoid organogenesis and organization (reviewed in [32]).

It is also possible that ligands other than LIGHT are responsible for HVEM mediated stimulatory signals during T cell mediated intestinal inflammation. In our experiments an absence of LIGHT

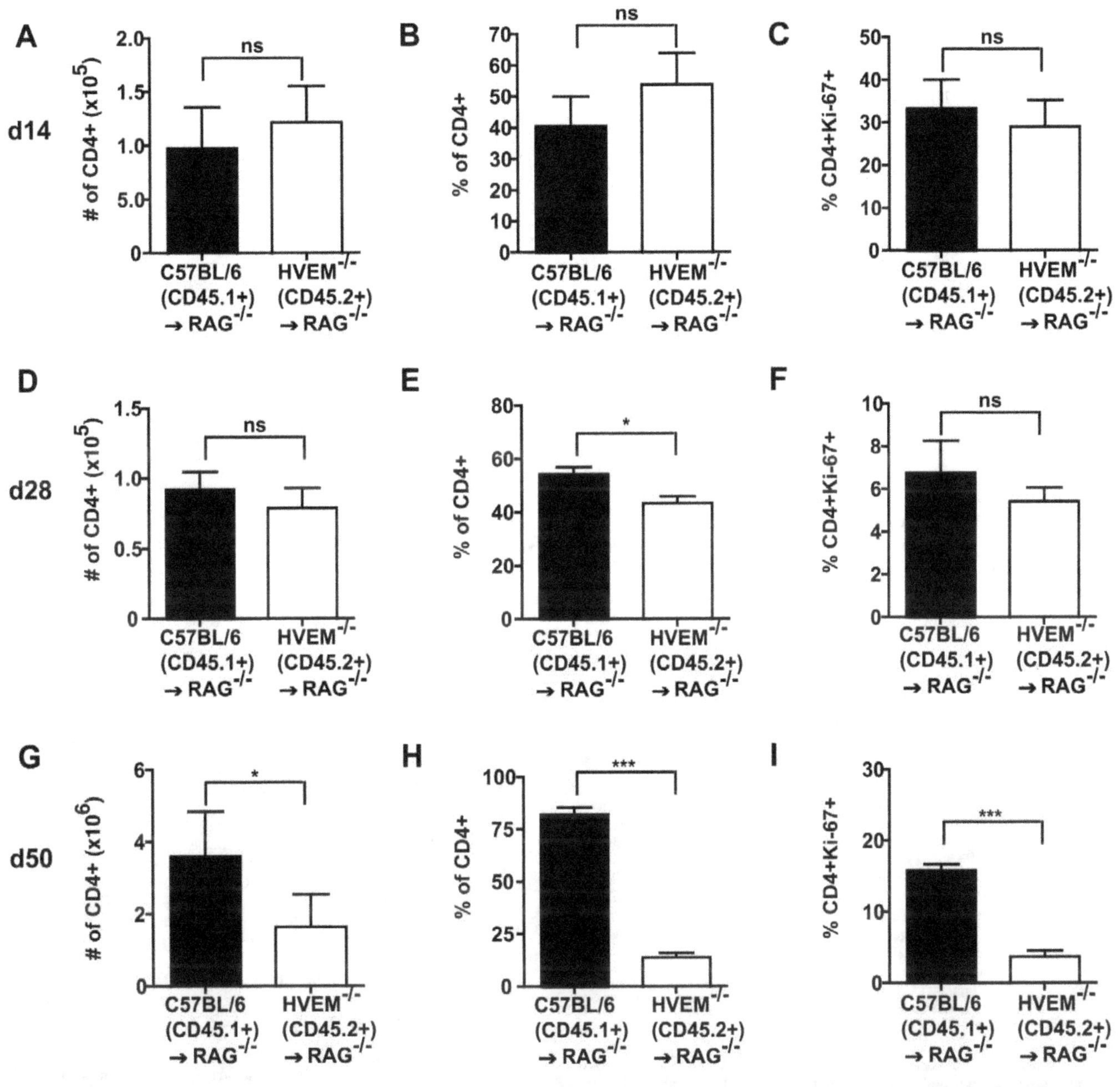

Figure 6. HVEM expression is required for the prolonged expansion of CD4$^+$ T cells and differentiation of effector cells. 4×10^5 CD4$^+$CD25$^-$CD45RB^{hight} T cells from congenic C57BL/6 (CD45.1$^+$) and HVEM$^{-/-}$ (CD45.1$^-$) mice were injected together at a 1:1 ratio (2×10^5 cells each genotype) into RAG1$^{-/-}$ recipients and mice were sacrificed at the indicated time points following transfer. MLN lymphocyte suspensions were counted and the total number (indicated by # symbol) of transferred C57BL/6 (CD45.1$^+$, black bar) or HVEM$^{-/-}$ (CD45.1$^-$, white bar) CD4$^+$ T cells determined. CD4$^+$ T cell numbers at (A) day 14, (D) day 28 and (G) day 50 post transfer into RAG1$^{-/-}$ recipient mice are shown. Frequencies of C57BL/6 (CD45.1$^+$, black bar) or HVEM$^{-/-}$ (CD45.1$^-$, white bar) CD4$^+$ T cells were assessed by flow cytometry at (B) day 14, (E) day 28 and (H) day 50 after injection into RAG1$^{-/-}$ mice. Expression of the proliferation marker Ki-67 by C57BL/6 (CD45.1$^+$, black bar) or HVEM$^{-/-}$ (CD45.1$^-$, white bar) CD4$^+$ T cells. Data represent means ± SD of two pooled experiments (n = 6 mice per group) and are representative of three independent experiments. Statistically significant differences between groups (n = 6 mice per group) were assessed by a two tailed Student's t test: $^*p<0.05$, $^{**}p<0.005$, $^{***}p<0.0005$.

on T cells did lead to a reduction in disease pathology but not to the same degree as T cell HVEM deficiency. Of course additional sources of LIGHT are likely to be present in the RAG1$^{-/-}$ recipients in the form of resident innate cells (DCs, NK cells, monocytes), and these sources may account for the remaining disease observed in RAG1$^{-/-}$ mice receiving LIGHT$^{-/-}$ CD4$^+$ T cells. Alternatively, CD4$^+$ T cells may be able to receive HVEM stimulatory signals from other ligands such as LTα3. Lastly, Although BTLA-HVEM signaling is recognized to deliver inhibitory signals via HVEM, BTLA was recently shown to play a role in the accumulation T cells following T cell transfer into immunodeficient hosts [33]. This finding was attributed to an ability of BTLA to provide intrinsic survival signals to T cells following ligation of HVEM in a cis-complex and indicates than an absence of BTLA-HVEM signals may also play a role in the inability of HVEM$^{-/-}$ T cells to promote intestinal inflammation [33].

Supporting Information

Figure S1 Reduced HVEM$^{-/-}$ CD4^{+} T cell expansion and cytokine production in spleen cannot be overcome by the presence of C57BL/6 CD4^{+} T cells. Purified 4×10^{5} CD4^{+}CD25^{-}CD45RB^{high} T cells from congenic C57BL/6 (CD45.1^{+}) and HVEM$^{-/-}$ (CD45.1^{-}) mice were injected together at a 1:1 ratio (2×10^{5} cells each genotype) into RAG1$^{-/-}$ recipients and mice were sacrificed 6-8 weeks later. Whole spleen cell suspensions from RAG1$^{-/-}$ recipients were analyzed by flow cytometry and percentages of C57BL/6 (closed circles and black bar) and HVEM$^{-/-}$ (open circles and white bar) (A) CD4^{+}, (C) CD4^{+}IFNγ^{+} and (E) CD4^{+}IL-17A^{+} T cell lymphocytes assessed (n = 6 mice per group). Total numbers (indicated by # symbol) of C57BL/6 (closed circles and black bar) or HVEM$^{-/-}$ (open circles and white bar) for (B) CD4^{+}, (D) CD4^{+}IFNγ^{+} and (F) CD4^{+}IL-17A^{+} T cells were calculated (n = 6 mice per group). Symbols and bar graphs represent means ± SD from one experiment. Statistical analysis between groups were calculated using the two tailed Student's t test: $^{*}p<0.05$, $^{**}p<0.005$, $^{***}p<0.0005$.

Figure S2 HVEM expression is required for the expansion of CD4^{+} T cells in the colon during intestinal inflammation. 4×10^{5} CD4^{+}CD25^{-}CD45RB^{hight} T cells from congenic C57BL/6 (CD45.1^{+}) and HVEM$^{-/-}$ (CD45.1^{-}) mice were injected together at a 1:1 ratio into RAG1$^{-/-}$ recipients and mice sacrificed at the indicated time points after transfer. Colon lamina propria suspensions were counted and the total number (indicated by # symbol) of transferred C57BL/6 (CD45.1^{+}, black bar) or HVEM$^{-/-}$ (CD45.1^{-}, white bar) CD4^{+} T cells calculated. CD4^{+} T cell number at (A) day 14, (D) day 28 and (G) day 50 post transfer into RAG1$^{-/-}$ recipient mice. Frequencies of C57BL/6 (CD45.1^{+}, black bar) or HVEM$^{-/-}$ (CD45.1^{-}, white bar) CD4^{+} T cells were assessed by flow cytometry at (B) day 14, (E) day 28 and (H) day 50 after injection into RAG1$^{-/-}$ mice. Expression of the proliferation marker Ki-67 by C57BL/6 (CD45.1^{+}, black bar) or HVEM$^{-/-}$ (CD45.1^{-}, white bar) CD4^{+} T cells was analyzed by flow cytometry at (C) day 14, (F) day 28 and (I) day 50 after injection. Data represent means ± SD of two pooled experiments (n = 6 mice per group) and are representative of three independent experiments. Statistically significant differences between groups (n = 6 mice per group) were assessed by a two tailed Student's t test: $^{*}p<0.05$, $^{**}p<0.005$, $^{***}p<0.0005$.

Acknowledgments

We thank Anthony J. Coyle for providing the HVEM$^{-/-}$ and LIGHT$^{-/-}$ mice.

Author Contributions

Conceived and designed the experiments: CS NLH. Performed the experiments: CS SH BE. Analyzed the data: CS NLH M. Kurrer CM. Contributed reagents/materials/analysis tools: M. Kopf. Wrote the paper: CS NLH.

References

1. Mackay F, Kalled SL (2002) TNF ligands and receptors in autoimmunity: an update. Curr Opin Immunol 14: 783–790.
2. Scheu S, Alferink J, Potzel T, Barchet W, Kalinke U, et al. (2002) Targeted disruption of LIGHT causes defects in costimulatory T cell activation and reveals cooperation with lymphotoxin beta in mesenteric lymph node genesis. J Exp Med 195: 1613–1624.
3. Tamada K, Shimozaki K, Chapoval AI, Zhai Y, Su J, et al. (2000) LIGHT, a TNF-like molecule, costimulates T cell proliferation and is required for dendritic cell-mediated allogeneic T cell response. J Immunol 164: 4105–4110.
4. Cohavy O, Zhou J, Granger SW, Ware CF, Targan SR (2004) LIGHT expression by mucosal T cells may regulate IFN-gamma expression in the intestine. J Immunol 173: 251–258.
5. Harrop JA, McDonnell PC, Brigham-Burke M, Lyn SD, Minton J, et al. (1998) Herpesvirus entry mediator ligand (HVEM-L), a novel ligand for HVEM/TR2, stimulates proliferation of T cells and inhibits HT29 cell growth. J Biol Chem 273: 27548–27556.
6. Pakala R, Liang CT, Benedict CR (2001) A peptide analogue of thrombin receptor-activating peptide inhibits thrombin and thrombin-receptor-activating peptide-induced vascular smooth muscle cell proliferation. J Cardiovasc Pharmacol 37: 619–629.
7. Ware CF (2008) Targeting lymphocyte activation through the lymphotoxin and LIGHT pathways. Immunol Rev 223: 186–201.
8. Morel Y, Truneh A, Sweet RW, Olive D, Costello RT (2001) The TNF superfamily members LIGHT and CD154 (CD40 ligand) costimulate induction of dendritic cell maturation and elicit specific CTL activity. J Immunol 167: 2479–2486.
9. Fan Z, Yu P, Wang Y, Wang Y, Fu ML, et al. (2006) NK-cell activation by LIGHT triggers tumor-specific CD8+ T-cell immunity to reject established tumors. Blood 107: 1342–1351.
10. Jiang HQ, Kushnir N, Thurnheer MC, Bos NA, Cebra JJ (2002) Monoassociation of SCID mice with Helicobacter muridarum, but not four other enterics, provokes IBD upon receipt of T cells. Gastroenterology 122: 1346–1354.
11. Ehlers S, Holscher C, Scheu S, Tertilt C, Hehlgans T, et al. (2003) The lymphotoxin beta receptor is critically involved in controlling infections with the intracellular pathogens Mycobacterium tuberculosis and Listeria monocytogenes. J Immunol 170: 5210–5218.
12. Sedgmen BJ, Dawicki W, Gommerman JL, Pfeffer K, Watts TH (2006) LIGHT is dispensable for CD4+ and CD8+ T cell and antibody responses to influenza A virus in mice. Int Immunol 18: 797–806.
13. Granger SW, Butrovich KD, Houshmand P, Edwards WR, Ware CF (2001) Genomic characterization of LIGHT reveals linkage to an immune response locus on chromosome 19p13.3 and distinct isoforms generated by alternate splicing or proteolysis. J Immunol 167: 5122–5128.
14. Cohavy O, Zhou J, Ware CF, Targan SR (2005) LIGHT is constitutively expressed on T and NK cells in the human gut and can be induced by CD2-mediated signaling. J Immunol 174: 646–653.
15. Castaneda FE, Walia B, Vijay-Kumar M, Patel NR, Roser S, et al. (2005) Targeted deletion of metalloproteinase 9 attenuates experimental colitis in mice: central role of epithelial-derived MMP. Gastroenterology 129: 1991–2008.
16. Tao R, Wang L, Murphy KM, Fraser CC, Hancock WW (2008) Regulatory T cell expression of herpesvirus entry mediator suppresses the function of B and T lymphocyte attenuator-positive effector T cells. J Immunol 180: 6649–6655.
17. Cooper HS, Murthy SN, Shah RS, Sedergran DJ (1993) Clinicopathologic study of dextran sulfate sodium experimental murine colitis. Lab Invest 69: 238–249.
18. Schenk M, Bouchon A, Seibold F, Mueller C (2007) TREM-1–expressing intestinal macrophages crucially amplify chronic inflammation in experimental colitis and inflammatory bowel diseases. J Clin Invest 117: 3097–3106.
19. Prestwood TR, Prigozhin DM, Sharar KL, Zellweger RM, Shresta S (2008) A mouse-passaged dengue virus strain with reduced affinity for heparan sulfate causes severe disease in mice by establishing increased systemic viral loads. J Virol 82: 8411–8421.
20. Axelsson LG, Landstrom E, Goldschmidt TJ, Gronberg A, Bylund-Fellenius AC (1996) Dextran sulfate sodium (DSS) induced experimental colitis in immunodeficient mice: effects in CD4(+) -cell depleted, athymic and NK-cell depleted SCID mice. Inflamm Res 45: 181–191.
21. Dieleman LA, Ridwan BU, Tennyson GS, Beagley KW, Bucy RP, et al. (1994) Dextran sulfate sodium-induced colitis occurs in severe combined immunodeficient mice. Gastroenterology 107: 1643–1652.
22. Ostanin DV, Bao J, Koboziev I, Gray L, Robinson-Jackson SA, et al. (2009) T cell transfer model of chronic colitis: concepts, considerations, and tricks of the trade. Am J Physiol Gastrointest Liver Physiol 296: G135–146.
23. Morel Y, Schiano de Colella JM, Harrop J, Deen KC, Holmes SD, et al. (2000) Reciprocal expression of the TNF family receptor herpes virus entry mediator and its ligand LIGHT on activated T cells: LIGHT down-regulates its own receptor. J Immunol 165: 4397–4404.
24. Hurchla MA, Sedy JR, Gavrieli M, Drake CG, Murphy TL, et al. (2005) B and T lymphocyte attenuator exhibits structural and expression polymorphisms and is highly Induced in anergic CD4+ T cells. J Immunol 174: 3377–3385.
25. Cai G, Anumanthan A, Brown JA, Greenfield EA, Zhu B, et al. (2008) CD160 inhibits activation of human CD4+ T cells through interaction with herpesvirus entry mediator. Nat Immunol 9: 176–185.
26. Gonzalez LC, Loyet KM, Calemine-Fenaux J, Chauhan V, Wranik B, et al. (2005) A coreceptor interaction between the CD28 and TNF receptor family members B and T lymphocyte attenuator and herpesvirus entry mediator. Proc Natl Acad Sci U S A 102: 1116–1121.

27. Wang Y, Subudhi SK, Anders RA, Lo J, Sun Y, et al. (2005) The role of herpesvirus entry mediator as a negative regulator of T cell-mediated responses. J Clin Invest 115: 711–717.
28. Steinberg MW, Turovskaya O, Shaikh RB, Kim G, McCole DF, et al. (2008) A crucial role for HVEM and BTLA in preventing intestinal inflammation. J Exp Med 205: 1463–1476.
29. Deppong C, Juehne TI, Hurchla M, Friend LD, Shah DD, et al. (2006) Cutting edge: B and T lymphocyte attenuator and programmed death receptor-1 inhibitory receptors are required for termination of acute allergic airway inflammation. J Immunol 176: 3909–3913.
30. Sarrias MR, Whitbeck JC, Rooney I, Ware CF, Eisenberg RJ, et al. (2000) The three HveA receptor ligands, gD, LT-alpha and LIGHT bind to distinct sites on HveA. Mol Immunol 37: 665–673.
31. Spahn TW, Herbst H, Rennert PD, Lugering N, Maaser C, et al. (2002) Induction of colitis in mice deficient of Peyer's patches and mesenteric lymph nodes is associated with increased disease severity and formation of colonic lymphoid patches. Am J Pathol 161: 2273–2282.
32. Drayton DL, Liao S, Mounzer RH, Ruddle NH (2006) Lymphoid organ development: from ontogeny to neogenesis. Nat Immunol 7: 344–353.
33. Cheung TC, Oborne LM, Steinberg MW, Macauley MG, Fukuyama S, et al. (2009) T cell intrinsic heterodimeric complexes between HVEM and BTLA determine receptivity to the surrounding microenvironment. J Immunol 183: 7286–7296.

4

Lysate of Probiotic *Lactobacillus casei* DN-114 001 Ameliorates Colitis by Strengthening the Gut Barrier Function and Changing the Gut Microenvironment

Zuzana Zakostelska[1], Miloslav Kverka[1*], Klara Klimesova[1], Pavel Rossmann[1], Jakub Mrazek[3], Jan Kopecny[3], Michaela Hornova[1], Dagmar Srutkova[2], Tomas Hudcovic[2], Jakub Ridl[4], Helena Tlaskalova-Hogenova[1]

1 Institute of Microbiology, Academy of Sciences of the Czech Republic, Prague, Czech Republic, **2** Institute of Microbiology, Academy of Sciences of the Czech Republic, Novy Hradek, Czech Republic, **3** Institute of Animal Physiology and Genetics, Academy of Sciences of the Czech Republic, Prague, Czech Republic, **4** Institute of Molecular Genetics, Academy of Sciences of the Czech Republic, Prague, Czech Republic

Abstract

Background: Probiotic bacteria can be used for the prevention and treatment of human inflammatory diseases including inflammatory bowel diseases (IBD). However, the nature of active components and exact mechanisms of this beneficial effects have not been fully elucidated. Our aim was to investigate if lysate of probiotic bacterium *L. casei* DN-114 001 (Lc) could decrease the severity of intestinal inflammation in a murine model of IBD.

Methodology/Principal Findings: The preventive effect of oral administration of Lc significantly reduces the severity of acute dextran sulfate sodium (DSS) colitis in BALB/c but not in SCID mice. In order to analyze how this beneficial effect interferes with well-known phases of intestinal inflammation pathogenesis *in vivo* and *in vitro*, we evaluated intestinal permeability using the FITC-labeled dextran method and analysed tight junction proteins expression by immunofluorescence and PCR. We also measured $CD4^+FoxP3^+$ regulatory T cells proportion by FACS analysis, microbiota composition by pyrosequencing, and local cytokine production by ELISA. Lc leads to a significant protection against increased intestinal permeability and barrier dysfunction shown by preserved ZO-1 expression. We found that the Lc treatment increases the numbers of $CD4^+FoxP3^+$ regulatory T cells in mesenteric lymph nodes (MLN), decreases production of pro-inflammatory cytokines TNF-α and IFN-γ, and anti-inflammatory IL-10 in Peyer's patches and large intestine, and changes the gut microbiota composition. Moreover, Lc treatment prevents lipopolysaccharide-induced TNF-α expression in RAW 264.7 cell line by down-regulating the NF-κB signaling pathway.

Conclusion/Significance: Our study provided evidence that even non-living probiotic bacteria can prevent the development of severe forms of intestinal inflammation by strengthening the integrity of intestinal barrier and modulation of gut microenvironment.

Editor: Bernhard Ryffel, French National Centre for Scientific Research, France

Funding: This work was supported by grants from Danone Institute of Czech Republic (2005–2006 and 2010–2011), the Czech Science Foundation (P304/11/1252, 310/08/H077, 305/08/0535 and 303/08/0367), http://www.gacr.cz/; the Academy of Sciences of Czech Republic (KJB500200904), http://www.gaav.cz/; the Ministry of Education, Youth and Sports of the Czech Republic (2B06155), http://www.msmt.cz; the Grant Agency of the Ministry of Health of the Czech Republic (IGA MZ NS10340), http://www.mzcr.cz/; and by Institutional Research Concept Grant AV0Z50200510, http://www.isvav.cz. The funders had no role in study design, data collection and analysis, decision to publish, or preparation of the manuscript.

Competing Interests: The authors have declared that no competing interests exist.

* E-mail: kverka@biomed.cas.cz

Introduction

Inflammatory bowel diseases (IBD), such as Crohn's disease and ulcerative colitis, are severe chronic inflammatory illnesses of the gastrointestinal tract. Although their etiology and pathogenesis are not fully understood, it is generally accepted, that the inflammation is a result of an aberrant immune response to antigens of resident gut microbiota in genetically susceptible individuals [1]. Moreover, dysbiosis, an imbalance in the intestinal bacterial ecosystem, has been found in IBD and linked to its pathogenesis [2]. It has been suggested that this microbial imbalances and an aberrant immune response could be restored by oral administration of certain beneficial bacterial species, probiotics [3].

When administered in adequate amounts, probiotics, defined as live microorganisms, confer a health benefit to the host [4], and have been successfully used in treatment of IBD [5]. Using animal models of IBD, three main mechanisms of how these beneficial microbes protect from intestinal inflammation have been described. A single probiotic bacterium could possess more than one mechanism depending on its unique specific metabolic activities and cellular structures [6]. First, probiotics may exclude or inhibit the growth of certain pathogens [7]; second, they may improve the gut barrier function [8]; and third, they can modulate mucosal and/or systemic immune response or metabolic functions [9]. The outcome of probiotic therapy also depends on the stage of the disease and the overall health status of the patient. Despite of the generally safe profile of the probiotic therapy, the use of live microorganisms may lead to severe infections, and therefore represents considerable risk especially in severely ill patients [10]. There is increasing evidence, that similar beneficial effects could be achieved with sterile lysates or components isolated from probiotic or even commensal microbes [11].

Colitis induced by dextran sulfate sodium (DSS) is a well established and reliable model of IBD because its clinical features resemble the ulcerative colitis [12]. Acute DSS colitis starts with epithelial cell barrier dysfunction which causes the antigens from the gut lumen to enter the lamina propria and stimulate the immune response. The dysfunction of the epithelial barrier starts as early as the first day after DSS treatment by gradual decrease in the tight junction protein ZO-1 production, which in turn leads to increased gut permeability [13,14]. In the acute phase, DSS-induced colitis is driven mainly by cells of innate immunity, because it also occurs in the absence of functional T, B and NK cells [15]. The functional adaptive immune system, however, plays an important role in the chronic phase of the inflammation and might be necessary for its preventive treatment with microbial antigens [11,16].

The most intensively studied and used probiotic bacteria are lactobacilli [17,18]. Oral treatment with probiotic bacterium *L. casei* DN-114 001 has been found to reduce the duration and severity of diarrhea and common infectious diseases in children [19]. Moreover, supernatant of this probiotic strain was described to exert immunological activities and strong inhibitory effect on epithelial cell adhesion of virulent *E. coli* strain [20] . These studies clearly show the beneficial potential of this bacterium, however, the clinical utility of such approach remains controversial, as neither the specific mechanisms of action nor the active component responsible for its beneficial properties has been established.

In our previous study, we have shown that the preventive treatment with live probiotic bacterium *L. casei* DN-114001 protects mice from subsequent acute DSS-induced colitis in BALB/c mice [21]. Here, we show that oral treatment with lysate of this bacterium (Lc) has a similar effect, and that this effect is associated with change in the intestinal microbiota composition, modulation of mucosal immune system, and induction of regulatory T cells in mesenteric lymph nodes (MLN). Our results show that even killed probiotic bacteria can decrease the severity of the intestinal inflammation, which represents safer and more practical therapeutic intervention than the use of live bacteria in the treatment of intestinal inflammation.

Materials and Methods

Preparation of bacteria

Lactobacillus casei DN-114 001 (Danone Institute, Palaiseau Cedex, France), *Lactobacillus plantarum* CCDM 185 (Culture Collection of Dairy Microorganisms, Milcom a.s., Prague), were grown in an anaerobic chamber in De Man, Rogosa, and Sharpe broth (Oxoid, Basingstoke, UK) at 37°C until the cultures were in the late log phase of growth. Both lactobacilli were harvested by centrifugation (4000× g, 30 min) and washed twice with sterile phosphate-buffered saline (PBS). After the treatment with the French press, lactobacilli were freeze-dried and diluted to a working concentration of 30 g/l. In order to kill all remaining viable bacteria, the lysate was heated to 60°C for 30 min and the sterility of all components was verified by both aerobic and anaerobic 48 hours cultivation before administration.

Animals

Ethics statement: All animal experiments were approved by the Animal Care and Use Committee of the Institute of Microbiology, Academy of Sciences of the Czech Republic, approval ID: 10/2005, 94/2008 and 211/2009. Female BALB/c mice (8–12 weeks old) or severe combined immunodeficient mice BALB/cJHanHsd-SCID (SCID) were obtained from a breeding colony at the Institute of Physiology (Academy of Sciences of the Czech Republic, Prague, Czech Republic) or at the Institute of Microbiology (Academy of Sciences of the Czech Republic, Novy Hradek, Czech Republic), respectively, and reared under conventional conditions.

Study design and DSS induced colitis

We administered 1.5 mg of Lc in 50 µl of sterile PBS, i.e. 6×10^8 CFU of heat killed bacteria, by gavage. To reduce proteolytic activity in the gut, the Lc components were co-administered with 1 mg of soybean trypsin inhibitor (Sigma-Aldrich, St. Louis, MO, USA) dissolved in 50 µl of 0.15 M sodium bicarbonate buffer (pH 8.0). Control mice were given only sterile PBS with soybean trypsin inhibitor in bicarbonate buffer. The administration of lysates was repeated every 7 days for a total number of 4 doses (on days 0, 7, 14 and 21). Acute colitis was induced 7 days later by 3% (wt/v) DSS (molecular weight 36–50 kDa; MP Biomedicals, Irvine, CA, USA) dissolved in tap water for 7 days, and on the last day of the experiment the colitis was evaluated by using a clinical activity score, colon length, and the histological scoring system as described previously [11]. Furthermore, to analyze if the protective effect of Lc could be achieved also by parenteral administration, four subcutaneus doses of Lc or PBS (25 µg per dose) were injected in incomplete Freund's adjuvant (Difco Laboratories, Detroit, MI, USA) before colitis induction. For chronic colitis, mice received four cycles of DSS as described previously [12].

Evaluation of intestinal barrier function

Intestinal permeability *in vivo*. The intestinal permeability was measured by determining the amount of FITC-dextran in blood after it was orally administered as described previously [22]. Briefly, each mouse received 440 mg/kg of body weight of FITC-dextran (molecular weight 4.4 kDa; Sigma-Aldrich) by gavage. A blood sample, obtained 5 h later, was first centrifuged (3,000 rpm at 4°C) for 30 min, and serum was collected and added to a 96-well microplate. The concentration of FITC-dextran was determined by spectrophotofluorometry (Safire^2, Tecan Group Ltd., Männedorf, Switzerland) with an excitation wavelength of 483 nm and an emission wavelength of 525 nm using serially diluted samples of the marker as standard.

Immunohistology. Segments of colon and terminal ileum were frozen in liquid nitrogen immediately after removal and stored at −80°C until used. Frozen sections (6 µm) were mounted on the poly-L-lysine-coated slides. Then the slides were dried and fixed in 4% buffered paraformaldehyde (pH 7.4) for 10 min at room temperature. Fixed sections were washed in PBS and blocked with 2% donkey serum (Sigma-Aldrich) in PBS for 20 min at room temperature. The slides were incubated with the rabbit polyclonal anti-mouse ZO-1 or occludin antibodies (both from Invitrogen, Camarillo, CA, USA) overnight at 4°C. The negative controls were performed similarly using 1% bovine serum albumin (BSA) in PBS instead of primary antibody. After washing, the sections were incubated with donkey anti-rabbit antibody conjugated either with

Texas Red or with DyLight 488 fluorochrome (both from Jackson ImmunoResearch Laboratories, West Grove, USA). Nuclei were counterstained using DAPI (4′,6-diamidino-2-phenylindole; Sigma-Aldrich) stain. Finally, the sections were mounted in Vectashield mounting medium for fluorescence (Vector Laboratories, Burlingame, CA, USA) and viewed with a fluorescence microscope Olympus AX-70 (Olympus, Tokyo, Japan).

Determination of ZO-1 mRNA expression in intestinal tissue. Intestinal mucosa from terminal ileum and colon was placed in RNAlater stabilization reagent (QIAGEN GmbH, Hilden, Germany). Total messenger RNA (mRNA) was extracted by using the RNeasy Mini isolation kit (QIAGEN GmbH) following the manufacturer's instructions. RNA integrity was determined by gel electrophoresis in 1.5% agarose gel stained with ethidium bromide. The purity of the RNA was assessed by the ratio of absorbance at 260 and 280 nm. RNA purity was within a range of 2.0–2.1. The total RNA concentration was estimated by spectrophotometric measurements at 260 nm assuming that 40 μg of RNA per mililitre equal one absorbance unit. Real time PCR was performed as described previously [23]. Briefly, RNA was converted to cDNA using Taq-Man reverse transcription reagents (Applied Biosystems, Foster City, CA, USA). Beta-actin was used as an endogenous control and its expression was similar in all tested samples. A reaction mix for real-time PCR was made with Taq-Man Universal PCR master mix, water, and assays on demand gene expression products for ZO-1 and β-actin (all Applied Biosystems, Foster City, CA, USA). The master mix (20 μl) was aliquoted to the wells on a real-time PCR plate; and each sample was analyzed in duplicate. A volume of 5 μl of cDNA was added to each well, and the PCR reaction was run on a 7300 real-time PCR System (Applied Biosystems, Foster City, CA, USA) using standard conditions. The data was analyzed with Genex software (version 4.3.8).

Production of cytokines

Intestinal tissue culture and measurement of cytokines. Sections of Peyer's patches (PP), ileum, cecum, and colon were taken from every mouse. The intestines were then opened longitudinally, washed in ice cold PBS containing antibiotics and cultivated for 48 hours at 37°C and 5% CO_2 in complete RPMI medium with 10% fetal bovine serum (Biochrom AG, Berlin, Germany) and 100,000 U/l penicillin, 100 mg/l streptomycin (Sigma-Aldrich), as described previously [11] . Commercially available ELISA sets were used to measure the levels of TNF-α, IFN-γ, TGF-β, IL-10 (Invitrogen Corp.) and IL-6 (R&D Systems Inc., Minneapolis, MN, USA) in these supernatants. All tests were performed according to the manufacturers' recommendations.

Determination of cytokine mRNA expression in intestinal tissue. The samples were processed as described above (see Determination of ZO-1 mRNA expression in intestinal tissue). Gene expression assays for IL-10, IL-6, TNF-α and β-actin were all purchased by Applied Biosystems, Foster City, CA, USA.

Determination of specific antibodies

Sera and small intestine washings were collected for specific antibody evaluation. Gut washings were obtained by flushing the content of isolated small intestine with 2 ml of sterile PBS containing a mixture of proteinase inhibitors (Sigma-Aldrich). The samples were then vortexed and centrifuged at 4°C, and the supernatant was collected and stored at −80°C until analysis. Indirect ELISA, optimized in our laboratory as previously described [11], was used to assess the specific antibody response against Lc in serum (IgG, IgM, and IgA) and gut washings (secretory IgA; SIgA). Briefly, Nunc MaxiSorp 96-well plates (Thermo Fisher Scientific Inc., Rochester, NY, USA) were coated overnight with Lc (100 μl/well at 10 mg/l in PBS) and blocked with 1% BSA (Sigma-Aldrich) in PBS. Serum and gut washing samples diluted 1:50 and 1:10 in 1% BSA, respectively, were added and incubated for 2 hours. As control sera normal reference serum purchased from Bethyl Laboratories (TX, USA) and hyperimmune serum prepared by four subcutaneous injections of Lc in incomplete Freund's adjuvant within 14 days intervals (50 μg of Lc in the each dose) were used. After washings (three times with PBS containing 0.05% Tween 20 (Sigma-Aldrich)), secondary antibodies (50 μl/well) were added and incubated for 1 hour at room temperature. Antibody combinations were used as follows: 1) rabbit anti-mouse SIgA (Uscn Life Science Inc., China) and horseradish peroxidase (HRP)-labeled anti-rabbit IgG (Cell Signaling Technology Inc., Danvers, MA, USA); 2) biotinylated anti-mouse IgA (Sigma-Aldrich) and streptavidin-HRP (R&D Systems Inc.); 3) HRP-labeled anti-mouse IgG; 4) HRP-labeled anti-mouse IgM (both The Binding Site Ltd, Birmingham, UK). All reagents were diluted in 1% BSA in PBS except anti-IgA antibody that was diluted in 1% BSA with 5% fetal bovine serum (BioClot GmbH, Aidenbach, Germany). The plates were developed with 3,3′,5,5′-tetramethylbenzidine (Sigma-Aldrich) and the optical density (OD) was measured at 450 nm. The OD of the background (1% BSA) was subtracted and resulting adjusted ODs of the treated groups were compared with those of PBS-treated groups.

Flow cytometry

Single-cell suspensions of spleens, MLNs and PPs were prepared and stained for T_{regs} using FoxP3 Staining Set (eBioscience, San Diego, CA, USA) with fluorochrome-labeled anti-mouse mAbs: CD4-Qdot® 605 (Invitrogen, Carlsbad, CA, USA), CD8-BD Horizon™ V500 (BD Biosciences, San Jose, CA, USA), CD3-FITC and FoxP3-Phycoerythrin (both from eBioscience) according to the manufacturer's recommendation.

RAW 264.7 cells were cultivated and stained for IL-7R-Alexa647 (a gift from Pavel Otahal, IMG AS CR, Prague, Czech Republic), CD206-PE (AbD Serotec, Oxford, UK), CD-11c-NC625 and F4/80-APC780 (both from eBioscience). Hoechst 33342 (Sigma-Aldrich) was used to determine cell viability. Flow cytometric analysis was performed on LSRII (BD Biosciences), and the data was analyzed using FlowJo software (Tree Star Inc., Ashland, OR, USA).

Evaluation of the anti-inflammatory properties of Lc *in vitro*

The LPS-activated macrophage cell line (RAW 264.7; ATCC TIB-71) was cultivated in the presence of different concentrations of bacterial lysate, as previously described [11]. Briefly, the cells were cultured for 24 hour at 37°C and 5% CO_2 in Dulbecco's modified Eagle's medium (Institute of Molecular Genetics AS CR, Prague, Czech Republic) containing 10% heat-inactivated fetal bovine serum (Biochrom AG), 4.5 g/l glucose, 1.5 g/l sodium bicarbonate, 4 mM glutamine (Institute of Molecular Genetics AS CR), 100,000 U/l penicillin and 100 mg/l streptomycin (both Sigma-Aldrich). The cells were cultured together with Lc, lysate of *L. plantarum* (Lp) or sterile PBS in the presence or absence of LPS (*Salmonella typhimurium*, 1 mg/l, Sigma-Aldrich). After cultivation, the concentration of TNF-α in the supernatant was measured with ELISA (Invitrogen). The nuclear proteins were extracted from stimulated RAW264.7 cells by a nuclear extract kit (Active Motif, Rixensart, Belgium) and used to quantify the DNA binding activity of p65 subunit using the TransAM NF-κB family transcription factor assay kit (Active Motif). In NF-κB assay, only the concentration with the strongest immunomodulatory properties of Lc was used, i.e. 10 pg/l. All assays were performed according to the manufacturer's recommendation.

Evaluation of microbiota changes by pyrosequencing

Stool samples from PBS or Lc-treated mice, on day 0, 28 (just before DSS administration) and 35 (the last day of experiment) were collected. Total DNA from these samples was then isolated with ZR Fecal DNA Kit™ (Zymo Research Corp., Orange, CA) according to the manufacturer's recommendation.

DNA was subsequently gel-purified and PCR was performed in triplicate for each primer pair, and pooled to minimize random PCR bias. The reaction mixture contained 1 µl of DNA (10 ng/µl), 1.5 mmol/l $MgCl_2$, 0.2 mmol/l of dNTPs, 1× PCR buffer and 1 U platinum TAQ DNA polymerase (Invitrogen) and 0.40 µmol/l of forward modified primer consisting of 454 adaptor A (5′-CCATCTCATCCCTGCGTGTCTCCGACTCAG-3′; Genome Sequencer FLX system), unique 10-base tag sequence (ATATCGCGAG, CGTGTCTCTA, CTCGCGTGTC, TAGTATCAGC, TCTCTATGCG) and universal broad-range bacterial primer 5′-AYTGGGYDTAAAGNG and 0.40 µmol/l of reverse primer consisting of adaptor B (5′-CCATCTCATCCCTGCGTGTCTCCGACTCAG-3′) and universal primer TACNVGGGTATCTAATCC. PCR conditions were as follows: 1×: 95°C, 3 min; 35×: 94°C, 50 sec; 40°C, 30 sec; 72°C, 60 sec; 1×: 72°C, 5 min and final hold at 4°C. The length of PCR product was checked on the agarose gel electrophoresis. PCR product was subsequently purified using magnetic beads (AMPure beads, Beckman Coulter Genomics, Danvers, USA). Concentration was measured on Qubit fluorometer (Invitrogen, Carlsbad, CA, USA). Equimolar amounts of PCR product from each sample were used for unidirectional 454 FLX amplicon pyrosequencing using LIB-L emPCR kits following the manufacturer's protocols (Roche Diagnostics, Basel, Switzerland).

Metagenomic data processing

Flowgrams were processed using amplicon analysis option in data processing software from Roche. The sequencing resulted in 161551 overall number of reads. Quality trimmed sequences obtained from the FLX sequencing run were processed using RDP pyrosequencing pipeline. Beforehand, data files were depleted of chimeras by Black Box chimera Checker [24] using default settings. Processing involved aligning of sequences with fast, secondary-structure aware Infernal aligner, subsequent clustering with max distance of 3% based on complete-linkage clustering method and classifying of incurred clusters by naïve Bayesian rDNA classifier [25]. Bootstrap cutoff was set to 50%, which was sufficient for accurate classification at the genus level. Generated designations of clustered sequences together with their relative abundances within the given samples were used for comparing bacterial diversity.

Statistical analysis

One-way analysis of variance (ANOVA) with Dennett's multiple comparison test was used to compare multiple experimental groups with the control group. Differences between two groups were evaluated using an unpaired two-tailed Student's t-test and deviation of values from hypothetical mean were calculated by one sample t-test. The data is presented as the mean ± standard deviation (SD) unless stated otherwise and differences were considered statistically significant at $P \leq 0.05$. GraphPad Prism statistical software (version 5.0, GraphPad Software, Inc., La Jolla, CA,USA) was used for analyses.

Results

Oral administration of lysate *L. casei* attenuate the acute colitis in BALB/c mice but not in SCID mice

In our previous study we showed that oral treatment with *L. casei* DN-114 001 attenuates the severity of acute experimental colitis [21]. To test if its lysate have similar activity, we pretreated mice with four weekly oral doses of Lc and induced colitis by DSS in BALB/c and SCID mice. Oral (Table 1A) but not parenteral (data not shown) administration of Lc is effective in preventing the acute DSS colitis in BALB/c mice, improving clinical and morphological markers of colitis. In contrast, when colitis was induced in SCID mice (Table 1A) pretreatment with Lc failed to improve acute colitis in all tested parameters. Also no significant effects of Lc were found when the model of chronic colitis was used (data not shown).

Lysate of *L. casei* prevents the increase in intestinal permeability and preserves ZO-1 expression in acute colitis

Increased intestinal permeability caused by impairment of the gut barrier function drives the pathogenesis of intestinal inflammation in both DSS-induced colitis and human IBD [26,27]. To investigate the effect of Lc on the gut barrier function in acute DSS-induced colitis, we administered a single dose of FITC–dextran by gavage and measured the intensity of fluorescence in mouse serum 5 h later. Oral pretreatment with Lc significantly decreased the intestinal permeability to macromolecules on the last day of DSS (day 35) to the same extent as found in healthy mice (Figure 1A). One possible mechanism by which this effect could be mediated is the reinforcement of tight junctions. Previous studies have demonstrated that DSS causes the extensive decrease in ZO-1 expression and occludin redistribution and that this effect could be prevented by live bacteria or their components in the murine colonic epithelium [28,29]. Therefore, we

Table 1. Lc improves the severity of DSS-induced colitis in BALB/c, but not in SCID mice.

Mouse strain	Experimental group	Disease activity index	Colon length (cm)	Histological grade
BALB/c	DSS/PBS	2.80±0.68	6.35±0.62	1.59±0.54
	DSS/Lc	1.67±1.09***	7.14±0.34***	1.20±0.51*
SCID	DSS/PBS	1.95±1.66	6.63±0.55	1.2±0,84
	DSS/Lc	1.99±1.54	7.17±1.21	1.26±0.85

Values are expressed as means ± SD (5 BALB/c mice per group) of one representative experiment out of three independent experiments. Unpaired Student's t-test in BALB/c mice was used to evaluate the significance of differences between experimental groups and the PBS-treated control group (*P<0.05, ***P<0.001).

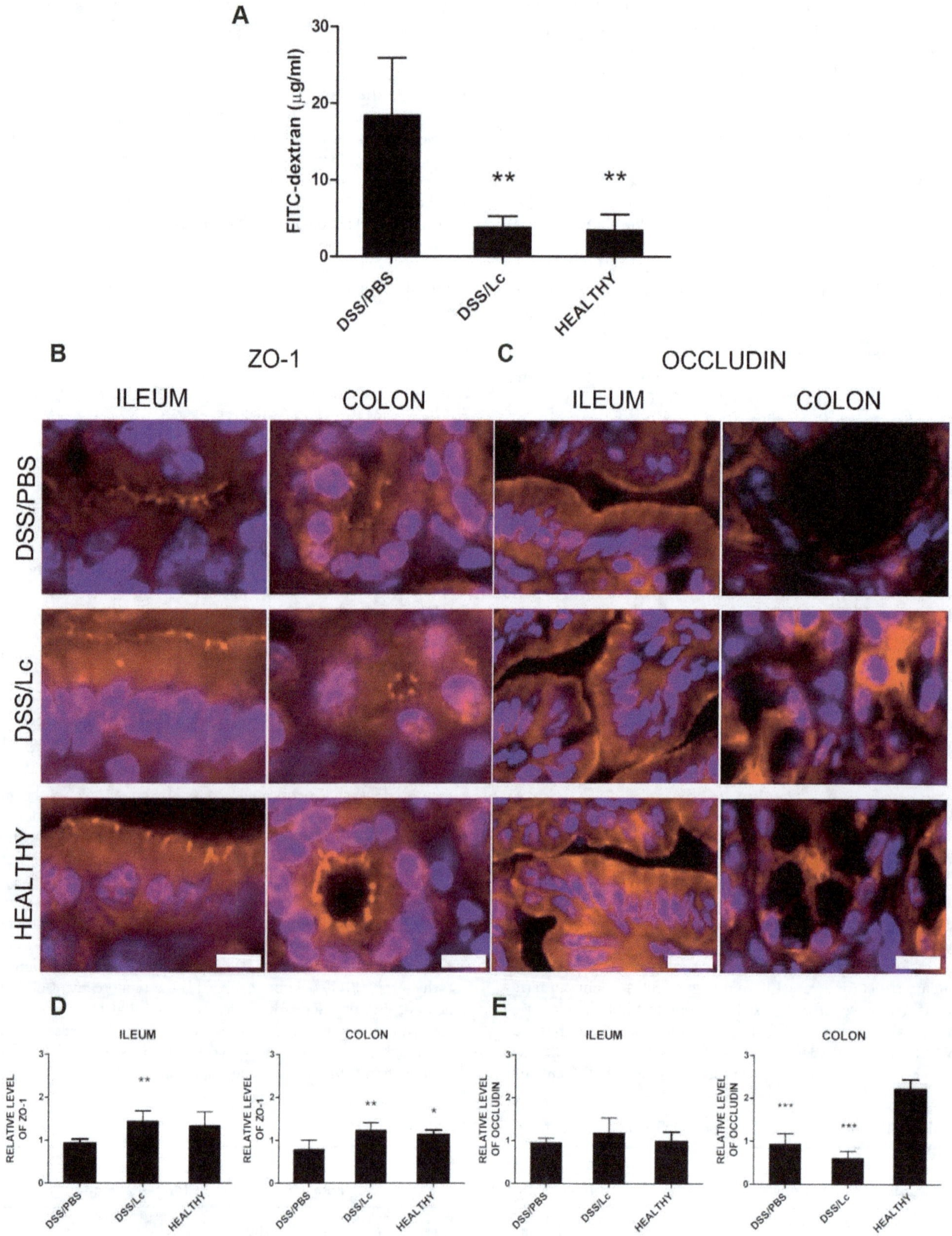

Figure 1. Oral treatment with Lc strengthens the gut barrier function as compared to PBS control mice. (A) Measurement of intestinal permeability by FITC-dextran. Serum levels of 4.4-kDa FITC-dextran 5 hour after administration by gavage in DSS/PBS, DSS/Lc-treated group and healthy controls. Immunohistological detection of tight junction proteins ZO-1 (B) and occludin (C) in representative sections of colon and terminal ileum from DSS/PBS-, DSS/Lc-treated group and healthy controls. Fluorescent signal of ZO-1 or occludin (red) is merged with DAPI counterstained nuclei (blue). mRNA expression of ZO-1(D) and occludin (E) evaluated in DSS/PBS, DSS/Lc treated group and healthy controls in colon and terminal ileum. RT-PCR was performed using TaqMan® gene expression assay for ZO-1. β-actin was used as the internal control. One-way ANOVA with

Dunnett's multiple comparison test was used to evaluate the significance of differences between experimental groups and the DSS/PBS-treated control group (*$P<0.05$, **$P<0.01$, ***$P<0.001$). Data represent means (bar) ± SD (whisker) of five mice of one representative experiment out of three independent experiments. Scale bars are 10 μm in ZO-1 and 20 μm in occludin figures.

investigated whether treatment with Lc interferes with changes in the tight junction proteins production and distribution. As shown by immunohistochemistry and RT-PCR, treatment with Lc could completely prevent the loss of expression and changes in distribution of ZO-1 in both colon and terminal ileum (Figure 1B and D). Interestingly, in PBS-treated mice with subsequent induction of colitis (DSS/PBS) or in Lc-treated mice with subsequent induction of colitis (DSS/Lc) was a substantial loss of occludin in colon but not in terminal ileum (Figure 1C and E). Nevertheless, its distribution in colon seems to be slightly less affected in DSS/Lc- as compared with DSS/PBS-treated mice. Thus, we are able to demonstrate that the expression of ZO-1 in the colon and terminal ileum was significantly preserved following Lc treatment and probably contributes to reduced permeability of FITC-dextran. These findings suggest that treatment with Lc enhances the intestinal barrier function.

Oral treatment with lysate of *L. casei* results in important changes in the gut microbial ecology

Changes in the intestinal gut microbial ecology are expected to be associated with the state of disease and could be influenced by probiotic treatment [30]. To determine the impact of oral treatment with Lc on the intestinal microbiota, we used pyrosequencing of segments of genes for bacterial 16S rRNA. We collected feces before the treatment (day 0), before the colitis induction (day 28), and at the end of the experiment (day 35). We found that oral treatment with Lc resulted in significant changes in the intestinal microbial ecology (Figure 2). The frequently present genus in our fecal samples was a little-studied genus *Barnesiella*, from the Bacteroidetes phylum, one of the most abundant phylum in intestinal microbiota. The next most abundant genus with very well described capability to ameliorate intestinal inflammation *Lactobacillus* increased in abundance after exposure to DSS and the Lc treatment. This increase in abundance was not observed in the control PBS group. The *Bacteroides*, known to be increased during DSS-induced colitis, proliferated after intestinal inflammation, was induced in Lc and PBS treated groups. Moreover, there is an increase in the biggest group of genera from Clostridium cluster: butyrate producing *Butyricicoccus*, *Coprococcus* and *Anaerostipes*. Butyrate is crucial for energy homeostasis of mammalian colonocytes, capable to prevent their autophagy [31]. Dynamic changes in microbiota composition were observed before and during DSS administration in both Lc-treated and PBS-treated control group. Therefore, we can suggest that these microbial changes lead to improvement in gut barrier function and decrease susceptibility to intestinal inflammation by producing active substances such as lactate and butyrate.

Oral administration of Lc changes the immune response of gut mucosa

Changes in cytokine microenvironment in the gut mucosa can influence the mucosal immune response to luminal antigens leading to the decrease of intestinal inflammation. Therefore, we investigated if the protective effect of Lc is associated with modifications in inflammatory response in the key compartments of the gut. We cultivated tissues from four distinct parts of the gut of either DSS/PBS or DSS/Lc-treated mice for 48 h and then measured the cytokines in supernatants by ELISA. We found that pretreatment with DSS/Lc decreased the production of pro-inflammatory cytokines (IL-6, IFN-γ) and anti-inflammatory cytokine IL-10 in PPs, cecum and colon as compared to DSS/PBS-treated mice (Figure 3). These results were confirmed at mRNA level by RT-PCR (data not shown).

Lc treatment increased the number of regulatory T cells

Since the intestinal inflammation in acute DSS-induced colitis is triggered by microbial antigens [32], the induction of oral tolerance to microbiota could be the one of the potential mechanisms of Lc protective effects. As the oral tolerance is maintained mainly at the periphery by T_{regs} , we analyzed the changes in $CD4^{+}FoxP3^{+}$ T_{regs} in the spleen, MLNs and PPs of DSS/PBS-, DSS/Lc-treated mice. We found a statistically significant increase in T_{regs} in MLN of DSS/Lc-treated mice as compared to DSS/PBS-treated mice. There were no statistically significant differences in the numbers of T_{regs} in spleen and PPs between these groups (Figure 4).

Lysate of *L. casei*, but not *L. plantarum*, decreases the production of TNF-α and down-regulates NF-κB activity in LPS-activated macrophages

Because probiotics have an immunomodulatory effect on cells involved in innate immunity [33] and because the macrophages play a role in the pathogenesis of DSS-induced colitis [12], we analyzed the anti-inflammatory effect of Lc in LPS-activated macrophages *in vitro*. We found that doses below 100 pg/l significantly decrease the production of TNF-α by LPS-stimulated RAW 264.7 cells *in vitro*, while similarly prepared Lp did not (Figure 5A). Using the FACS analysis of cultured cells, we found that neither Lc nor Lp changes the viability of RAW 264.7 cells (data not shown). The treatment with either lysate of bacteria in the absence of LPS did not change the TNF-α production (data not shown), this data is in agreement with a study using *L. casei* 3260 [34]. As published by others [34,35], this result suggests that Lc could interfere with the intracellular proinflammatory signaling cascade leading to activation of NF-κB transcription factor. To test this hypothesis, we isolated the nuclear extract from the untreated RAW 264.7 cells or from cells treated with either LPS (1 mg/l), or LPS with Lc and measured the activity of the NF-κB signaling pathway. Lc significantly decreased the NF-κB/DNA binding activity of p65 subunit as compared to the LPS-only or Lp+LPS treated cells (Figure 5B).

Since Lc treatment decreased production of TNF-α by LPS-activated macrophages, we decided to characterize macrophages further by investigating their stage of polarization by FACS. We found that M2 phenotype marker, the mannose receptor CD206 was significantly upregulated and M1 phenotype marker IL-7R downregulated in LPS+Lc treated macrophages as compared to either LPS or LPS+Lp treated macrophages. Therefore, Lc seems to counteract the LPS mediated M1 polarization. Neither Lc nor Lp without the addition of LPS changes the macrophage polarization.

Discussion

Oral treatment with probiotic bacteria has emerged recently as a potentially useful therapeutic strategy for human IBD [5,36]. However, the clinical utility of such approach remains controver-

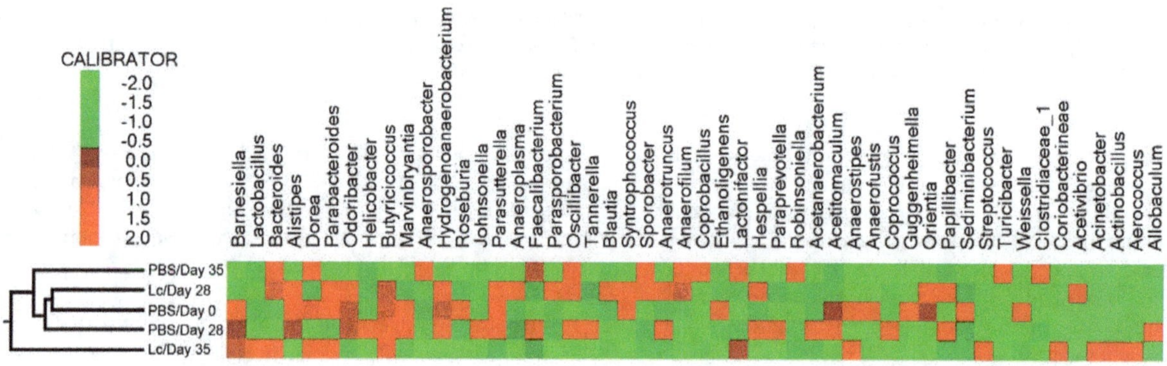

Figure 2. Oral treatment with Lc changes the intestinal microbiota composition. Normalized and z scored heat map and clustering dendrogram comparing relative abundance of the top 50 most abundant bacterial species in fecal microbiota of PBS (pool of 5 mice) and Lc-treated mice (pool of 5 mice) before the treatment (Day 0), before colitis induction (Day 28) and at the end of the experiment (Day 35). Horizontal columns represent the day of the experiment and or the treatment; vertical rows depict genus sorted from the most abundant species from left to right. The color scale for the heat maps is shown in upper left corner. The samples were clustered on the basis of their similarity by unsupervised clustering in the package CLUTO 2.1.1 (http://glaros.dtc.umn.edu/gkhome/cluto/cluto/download), as described previously [56].

sial, as the link between specific mechanisms of action and therapeutic effects of specific bacterium has been difficult to establish. We have shown previously that repeated oral administration of probiotic bacteria *L. casei* DN-114 001 protects BALB/c mice from severe forms of acute intestinal inflammation [21]. In this study we demonstrated that not only live probiotic bacteria, but also its lysate protects BALB/c, but not SCID, mice from severe forms of DSS-induced inflammation.

The lack of protective effect in SCID mice suggests that mechanisms of adaptive immunity are essential for the beneficial effect of Lc. We did not find any changes neither in Lc-specific serum IgA, IgG and IgM, nor in gut SIgA during our experiments (data not shown), so we analyzed another mechanism executed by adaptive immune response, oral tolerance. Major role in this mechanism is played by T_{regs}, whose protective role in inflammation control has been clearly established [37]. In this study, we found that Lc treatment leads to significant increase in T_{regs} in MLNs, but not PPs. This might be because MLNs are crossroads between mucosal and systemic immunity, because even naïve T cells (L-selectin expressing cells) can enter and after the

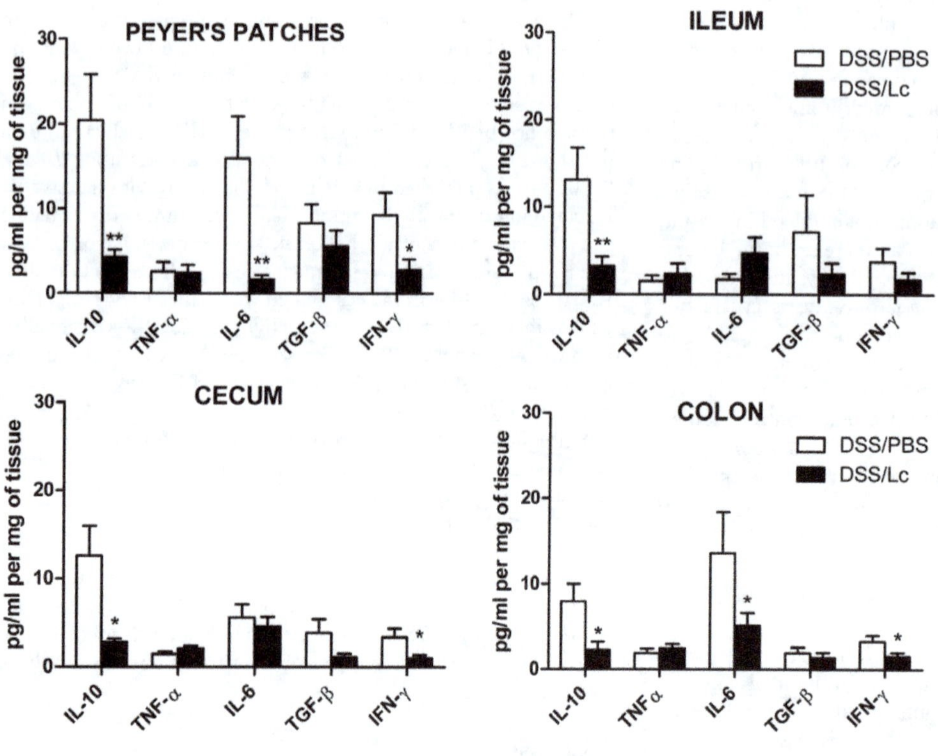

Figure 3. Pretreatment with Lc changes cytokine production in different parts of the gut. After DSS treatment and 24 hours cultivation, the production of cytokines TNF-α, TGF-β, IL-6, IL-10, IFN-γ differs in various parts of the gut as measured by ELISA. *P<0.05, **P<0.01 between DSS/PBS and DSS/Lc-treated mice in the same part of the gut was compared by unpaired Student's t-test (n = 10 per group).

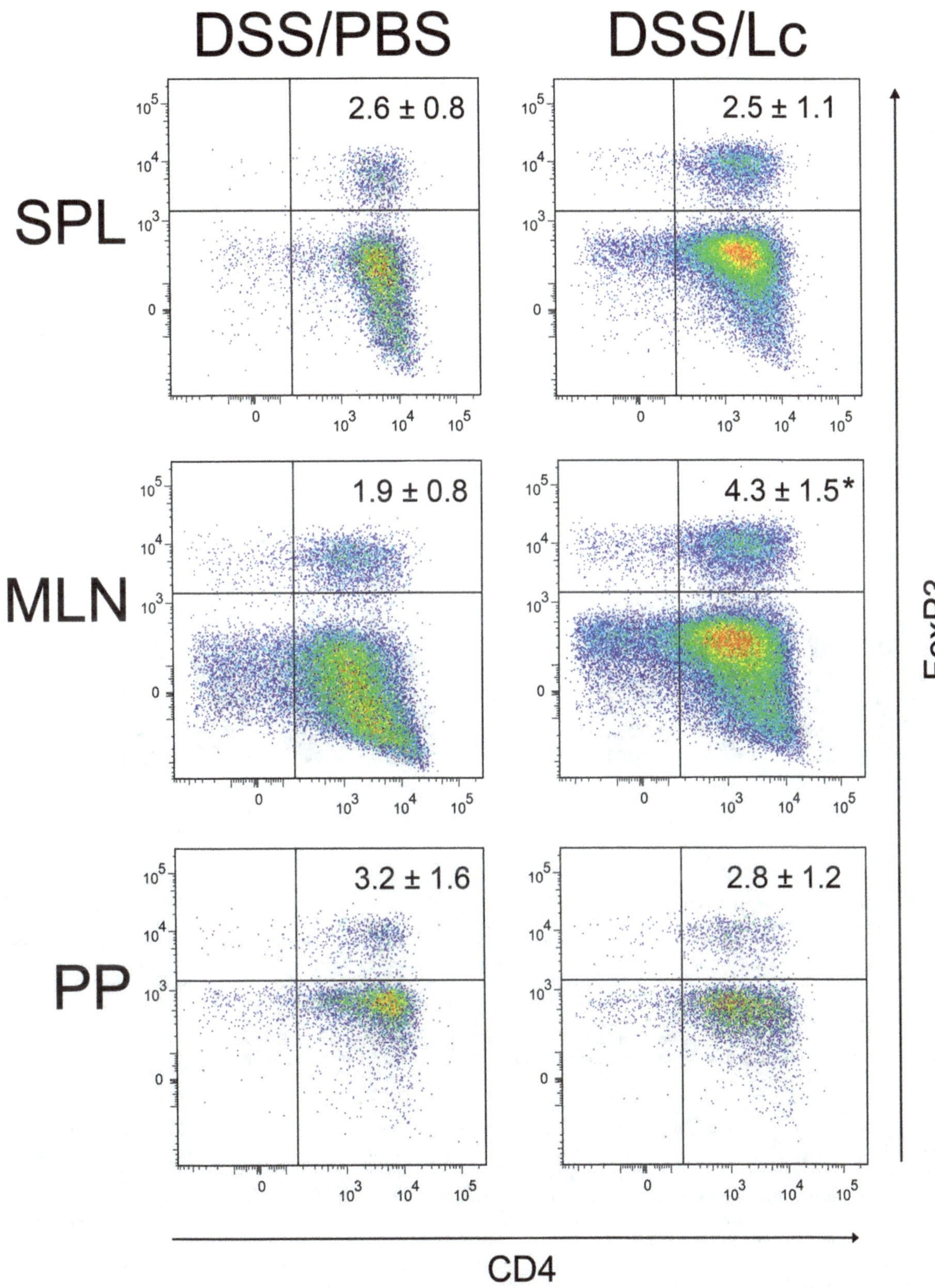

Figure 4. Oral treatment with Lc increases the number of CD4^{+}FoxP3^{+} T$_{regs}$ in MLNs. No significant changes were found in spleen or Peyer's patches. The plots shows the expression of CD4 *versus* FoxP3 on gated Th cells (CD3^{+}CD8^{-}), and the values within the plots represent the mean ± standard deviation of the total numbers of CD4^{+}FoxP3^{+} T cells from one representative experiment out of three independent experiments (3–5 mice per group). One-way ANOVA with Dunnett's multiple comparison test was used to evaluate the significance of differences in numbers of CD3^{+}CD8^{-}CD4^{+}FoxP3^{+} cells between DSS/Lc-treated groups and the DSS/PBS-treated (control) group (*$P<0.05$).

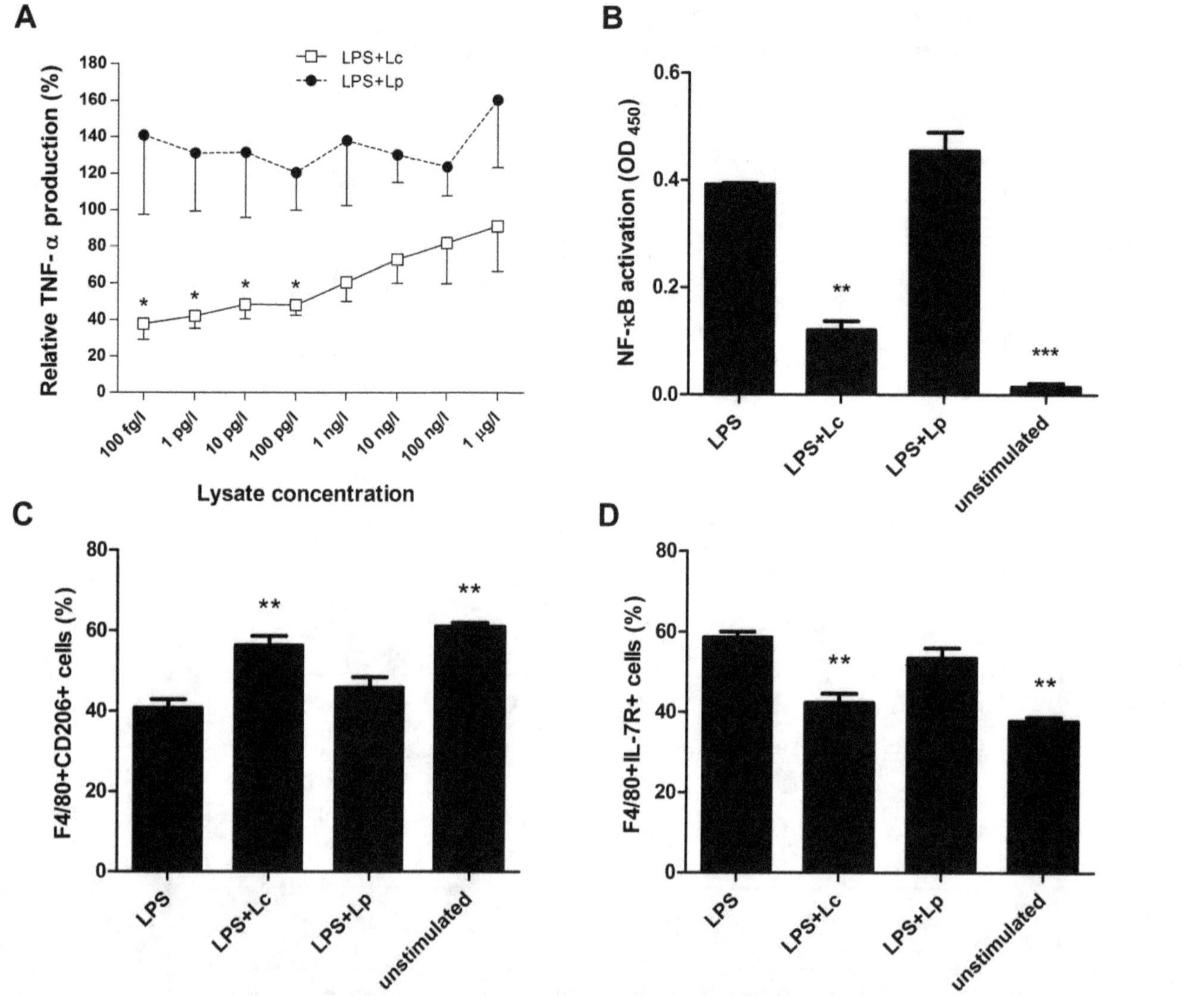

Figure 5. Lc exerts anti-inflammatory effect on LPS-activated macrophage cell line RAW 264.7. (A) Lc decreases the production of TNF-α in LPS-activated macrophages while Lp does not. TNF-α production by cells stimulated with 1 mg/l of LPS is set as 100% and data are expressed as means ± standard error of the mean of three independent experiments. *$P<0.05$: the means were compared against a hypothetical mean of 100% by one sample t-test (B) The effect of Lc on NF-κB binding activity in LPS-stimulated RAW 264.7 cells. Lc and Lp was co-cultured with LPS-activated cells for 24 h, and then the binding activity of NF-κB subunit p65 was analyzed by colorimetric assay. Data are expressed as mean ± standard deviation of three independent experiments. One-way ANOVA with Dunnett's multiple comparison test was used to evaluate the significance of differences between experimental groups and the LPS-treated cells group (**$P<0.01$, ***$P<0.001$). (C, D) Lc counteracts the LPS mediated M1 polarization. Expression of F4/80, CD206, IL-7R was determined by flow cytometry. One-way ANOVA with Dunnett's multiple comparison test was used to evaluate the significance of differences between experimental groups and the LPS-treated cells group (**$P<0.01$).

interaction with gut-committed cells (α4β7-integrin expressing cells) from intestine became T_{regs} [38].

The intestinal barrier prevents viable enteric bacteria and the microbiota derived components from excessive interaction with the immune system. Here, we demonstrated that increase in intestinal permeability and the decrease in local ZO-1 expression, typical for DSS-treated mice, are both significantly improved by oral application of Lc. These results are in agreement with several studies showing that *L. casei* and other probiotics can strengthen the gut barrier function [28,39]. Probiotic *E. coli* Nissle 1917 provided protection against DSS-mediated leakiness and was capable to produce specific up-regulation of ZO-1 expression in the intestinal epithelial barrier [29]. In addition, treatment with probiotic mixture VSL#3, where one of included bacterial strain is *L. casei*, prevents changes in expression and distribution of tight junction proteins ZO-1 and occludin [40]. It is well known that inadequate function of intestinal barrier could lead to inflammatory and neoplastic diseases [41,42]. The disruption of the gut barrier has been identified as one of the crucial steps in IBD pathogenesis, causing excessive host-microbiota interaction during the initial phases of the IBD [26]. Protection of the gut barrier from disruption by induction of changes in expression and distribution of tight junction proteins and mucus was proposed as a key mechanism of probiotic function [29,43].

Several studies showed that there is a marked difference in the gut microbiota composition in IBD patients ("dysbiosis") as compared to healthy individuals. These changes in microbiota composition, or presence of certain microbial species with increased virulence, cause or perpetuate the intestinal inflammation in IBD [44]. Here, we report that oral treatment with Lc significantly changes the composition of gut microbiota. Similar effects have been already described as mechanisms involved in the probiotics-mediated protection from intestinal inflammation [29,45]. Some of them are attributed to the fact, that probiotics can grow and colonize the gut, which could not be achieved with the non-living bacteria. The clear protective effect of bacterial lysate administration in intestinal inflammation is, therefore, rather indirect by shaping the gut microbial community or influencing the immune response. Nevertheless, similar mechanisms as in live bacteria could be involved to explain this effectiveness. Probiotics (or certain bacteria in general) can produce substances with antibiotic properties, such as bacteriocins, and molecules capable to signal to other members of the ecosystem to adjust their growth (quorum sensing modifiers), as recently reviewed [46]. These molecules could be present in the lysates of bacteria and, selectively modify the bacterial populations [47]. Moreover, certain probiotics can induce long-term production of anti-microbial peptides *in vivo*, which can shape the gut microbiota composition long time after the probiotic therapy has ended [48]. These mechanisms cause more favorable microbiota composition thus renders the Lc-treated mice less susceptible to intestinal inflammation.

By using the pyrosequencing technique we observed an increase in *Bacteroides* genus after induction of intestinal inflammation as shown previously [11]. DSS/Lc compared to DSS/PBS-treated group has shown a substantial increase in *Lactobacillus* genus which suggests that treatment with Lc promotes this genus among others. This effect could be caused by formation of niche ideal to lactobacilli. These and other differences in microbiota could be also explained by decreased inflammation in Lc-treated mice mediated by differing immunological mechanisms.

The cytokines produced in the gut mucosa greatly influence the resulting immunological outcome. The production of anti-inflammatory cytokines induces the mucosal unresponsiveness and tolerance and high levels of pro-inflammatory cytokines induce protective immune response and inflammation [49]. Here, we report that Lc treatment decrease the production of pro-inflammatory cytokines IL-6 and IFN-γ as well as anti-inflammatory cytokine IL-10 in both PP and the large intestine. This suggests that Lc can influence both the induction and effectors' functions of the mucosal immune system. We did not find significant decrease in local production of TNF-α, despite the clear differences in the colitis severity between Lc/DSS and PBS/DSS treated mice. This is consistent with our previous experiments, [11] and suggests that, despite being crucial pro-inflammatory cytokine produced by macrophages, TNF-α could be either exhausted or downregulated by IL-10, cytokine inhibiting TNF-α production, at this stage of colitis. Interestingly, since IFN-γ increases the gut permeability [50], a decrease in its local production can be responsible for strengthening of the gut barrier function as we found in Lc-treated mice. This is in agreement with findings that live *L. casei* can downregulate the pro-inflammatory mediators in the lamina propria of inflamed mucosa from Crohn's disease patients during *ex vivo* cultivation [51]. However, various strains of lactobacilli could differ in their immunological activities [52], and some lactobacilli are capable to induce T cells toward Th1 [53] or Th2 [54] immune responses.

Acute DSS colitis is believed to be driven initially by innate immunity mechanisms and, in particular, the role of macrophages has been proposed [12,15,32]. Therefore we tested the ability of bacterial lysates to decrease the inflammatory response of LPS-activated macrophages *in vitro*. We found that Lc, but not Lp, decreases the production of TNF-α, and the activation of NF-κB cascade and polarizes macrophages to M2 phenotype, suggesting a possible direct effect of Lc on the cells of the innate immunity. It is not excluded that negative regulators are involved in beneficial anti-inflammatory effects of probiotics [55].

In conclusion, our data provide evidence that even lysate of *L. casei* DN-114 001 can protect from induction of intestinal inflammation, thus confer a health benefit for the host. This is achieved by mechanisms that comprise: a) improvement in the gut barrier function, b) correction of the dysbiosis, and c) modulation of the mucosal immune response. These complex immunomodulatory properties of bacterial lysates may lead to the development of new therapeutic approaches for treatment of chronic intestinal inflammation. Moreover, oral administration of sterile bacteria, in contrast to live bacteria, may be safer in severely ill or immunocompromised patients.

Acknowledgments

We thank Prof. Jiri Mestecky for critical reading of this manuscript and his valuable advice. We also thank Jan Svoboda and Martin Kostovcik for excellent technical assistance.

Author Contributions

Conceived and designed the experiments: ZZ MK JR HT-H. Performed the experiments: ZZ MK KK PR JM JK MH DS TH JR. Analyzed the data: ZZ MK KK PR JM JK JR HT-H. Contributed reagents/materials/analysis tools: ZZ MK JK JR HT-H. Wrote the paper: ZZ MK KK PR JM JK MH DS TH JR HT-H.

References

1. Sartor RB (2006) Mechanisms of disease: pathogenesis of Crohn's disease and ulcerative colitis. Nat Clin Pract Gastroenterol Hepatol 3: 390–407.
2. Packey CD, Sartor RB (2009) Commensal bacteria, traditional and opportunistic pathogens, dysbiosis and bacterial killing in inflammatory bowel diseases. Curr Opin Infect Dis 22: 292–301.
3. Sheil B, Shanahan F, O'Mahony L (2007) Probiotic effects on inflammatory bowel disease. J Nutr 137: 819S–824S.
4. FAO/WHO (2001) Health and Nutritional Properties of Probiotics in Food including Powder Milk with Live Lactic Acid Bacteria. Cordoba (Argentina): Food and Agriculture Organization of the United Nations and World Health Organization. 34 p.
5. Bibiloni R, Fedorak RN, Tannock GW, Madsen KL, Gionchetti P, et al. (2005) VSL#3 probiotic-mixture induces remission in patients with active ulcerative colitis. Am J Gastroenterol 100: 1539–1546.
6. Lebeer S, Vanderleyden J, De Keersmaecker SC (2010) Host interactions of probiotic bacterial surface molecules: comparison with commensals and pathogens. Nat Rev Microbiol 8: 171–184.
7. Servin AL (2004) Antagonistic activities of lactobacilli and bifidobacteria against microbial pathogens. FEMS Microbiol Rev 28: 405–440.
8. Gupta P, Andrew H, Kirschner BS, Guandalini S (2000) Is lactobacillus GG helpful in children with Crohn's disease? Results of a preliminary, open-label study. J Pediatr Gastroenterol Nutr 31: 453–457.
9. Reiff C, Delday M, Rucklidge G, Reid M, Duncan G, et al. (2009) Balancing inflammatory, lipid, and xenobiotic signaling pathways by VSL#3, a biotherapeutic agent, in the treatment of inflammatory bowel disease. Inflamm Bowel Dis 15: 1721–1736.
10. Besselink MG, van Santvoort HC, Buskens E, Boermeester MA, van Goor H, et al. (2008) Probiotic prophylaxis in predicted severe acute pancreatitis: a randomised, double-blind, placebo-controlled trial. Lancet 371: 651–659.
11. Kverka M, Zakostelska Z, Klimesova K, Sokol D, Hudcovic T, et al. (2011) Oral administration of Parabacteroides distasonis antigens attenuates experimental murine colitis through modulation of immunity and microbiota composition. Clin Exp Immunol 163: 250–259.
12. Okayasu I, Hatakeyama S, Yamada M, Ohkusa T, Inagaki Y, et al. (1990) A novel method in the induction of reliable experimental acute and chronic ulcerative colitis in mice. Gastroenterology 98: 694–702.
13. Poritz LS, Garver KI, Green C, Fitzpatrick L, Ruggiero F, et al. (2007) Loss of the tight junction protein ZO-1 in dextran sulfate sodium induced colitis. J Surg Res 140: 12–19.
14. Yan Y, Kolachala V, Dalmasso G, Nguyen H, Laroui H, et al. (2009) Temporal and spatial analysis of clinical and molecular parameters in dextran sodium sulfate induced colitis. PLoS One 4: e6073.
15. Dieleman LA, Ridwan BU, Tennyson GS, Beagley KW, Bucy RP, et al. (1994) Dextran sulfate sodium-induced colitis occurs in severe combined immunodeficient mice. Gastroenterology 107: 1643–1652.

16. Dieleman LA, Palmen MJ, Akol H, Bloemena E, Pena AS, et al. (1998) Chronic experimental colitis induced by dextran sulphate sodium (DSS) is characterized by Th1 and Th2 cytokines. Clin Exp Immunol 114: 385–391.
17. Kleerebezem M, Vaughan EE (2009) Probiotic and gut lactobacilli and bifidobacteria: molecular approaches to study diversity and activity. Annu Rev Microbiol 63: 269–290.
18. Hanniffy S, Wiedermann U, Repa A, Mercenier A, Daniel C, et al. (2004) Potential and opportunities for use of recombinant lactic acid bacteria in human health. Adv Appl Microbiol 56: 1–64.
19. Merenstein D, Murphy M, Fokar A, Hernandez RK, Park H, et al. (2010) Use of a fermented dairy probiotic drink containing Lactobacillus casei (DN-114 001) to decrease the rate of illness in kids: the DRINK study. A patient-oriented, double-blind, cluster-randomized, placebo-controlled, clinical trial. Eur J Clin Nutr 64: 669–677.
20. Ingrassia I, Leplingard A, Darfeuille-Michaud A (2005) Lactobacillus casei DN-114 001 inhibits the ability of adherent-invasive Escherichia coli isolated from Crohn's disease patients to adhere to and to invade intestinal epithelial cells. Appl Environ Microbiol 71: 2880–2887.
21. Kokesova A, Frolova L, Kverka M, Sokol D, Rossmann P, et al. (2006) Oral administration of probiotic bacteria (E. coli Nissle, E. coli O83, Lactobacillus casei) influences the severity of dextran sodium sulfate-induced colitis in BALB/c mice. Folia Microbiol (Praha) 51: 478–484.
22. Wang Q, Fang CH, Hasselgren PO (2001) Intestinal permeability is reduced and IL-10 levels are increased in septic IL-6 knockout mice. Am J Physiol Regul Integr Comp Physiol 281: R1013–1023.
23. Zanvit P, Tichopad A, Havlickova M, Novotna O, Jirkovska M, et al. (2010) Adjuvant effect of *Bacillus firmus* on the expression of cytokines and toll-like receptors in mouse nasopharynx-associated lymphoid tissue (NALT) after intranasal immunization with inactivated influenza virus type A. Immunol Lett 134: 26–34.
24. Gontcharova V, Youn E, Wolcott RD, Hollister EB, Gentry TJ, et al. (2010) Black Box Chimera Check (B2C2): a Windows-Based Software for Batch Depletion of Chimeras from Bacterial 16S rRNA Gene Datasets. Open Microbiol J 4: 47–52.
25. Wang Q, Garrity GM, Tiedje JM, Cole JR (2007) Naive Bayesian classifier for rapid assignment of rRNA sequences into the new bacterial taxonomy. Appl Environ Microbiol 73: 5261–5267.
26. Munkholm P, Langholz E, Hollander D, Thornberg K, Orholm M, et al. (1994) Intestinal permeability in patients with Crohn's disease and ulcerative colitis and their first degree relatives. Gut 35: 68–72.
27. Kitajima S, Takuma S, Morimoto M (1999) Changes in colonic mucosal permeability in mouse colitis induced with dextran sulfate sodium. Exp Anim 48: 137–143.
28. Ewaschuk JB, Diaz H, Meddings L, Diederichs B, Dmytrash A, et al. (2008) Secreted bioactive factors from Bifidobacterium infantis enhance epithelial cell barrier function. Am J Physiol Gastrointest Liver Physiol 295: G1025–1034.
29. Ukena SN, Singh A, Dringenberg U, Engelhardt R, Seidler U, et al. (2007) Probiotic Escherichia coli Nissle 1917 inhibits leaky gut by enhancing mucosal integrity. PLoS One 2: e1308.
30. Fava F, Danese S (2011) Intestinal microbiota in inflammatory bowel disease: friend of foe? World J Gastroenterol 17: 557–566.
31. Donohoe DR, Garge N, Zhang X, Sun W, O'Connell TM, et al. (2011) The microbiome and butyrate regulate energy metabolism and autophagy in the mammalian colon. Cell Metab 13: 517–526.
32. Hudcovic T, Stepankova R, Cebra J, Tlaskalova-Hogenova H (2001) The role of microflora in the development of intestinal inflammation: acute and chronic colitis induced by dextran sulfate in germ-free and conventionally reared immunocompetent and immunodeficient mice. Folia Microbiol (Praha) 46: 565–572.
33. Mileti E, Matteoli G, Iliev ID, Rescigno M (2009) Comparison of the immunomodulatory properties of three probiotic strains of Lactobacilli using complex culture systems: prediction for in vivo efficacy. PLoS One 4: e7056.
34. Lee JM, Hwang KT, Jun WJ, Park CS, Lee MY (2008) Antiinflammatory effect of lactic acid bacteria: inhibition of cyclooxygenase-2 by suppressing nuclear factor-kappaB in Raw264.7 macrophage cells. J Microbiol Biotechnol 18: 1683–1688.
35. Matsumoto S, Hara T, Hori T, Mitsuyama K, Nagaoka M, et al. (2005) Probiotic Lactobacillus-induced improvement in murine chronic inflammatory bowel disease is associated with the down-regulation of pro-inflammatory cytokines in lamina propria mononuclear cells. Clin Exp Immunol 140: 417–426.
36. Kruis W, Fric P, Pokrotnieks J, Lukas M, Fixa B, et al. (2004) Maintaining remission of ulcerative colitis with the probiotic Escherichia coli Nissle 1917 is as effective as with standard mesalazine. Gut 53: 1617–1623.
37. Singh B, Read S, Asseman C, Malmstrom V, Mottet C, et al. (2001) Control of intestinal inflammation by regulatory T cells. Immunol Rev 182: 190–200.
38. Mowat AM, Donachie AM, Parker LA, Robson NC, Beacock-Sharp H, et al. (2003) The role of dendritic cells in regulating mucosal immunity and tolerance. Novartis Found Symp 252: 291–302; discussion 302–295.
39. Liu Z, Zhang P, Ma Y, Chen H, Zhou Y, et al. (2011) Lactobacillus plantarum prevents the development of colitis in IL-10-deficient mouse by reducing the intestinal permeability. Mol Biol Rep 38: 1353–1361.
40. Mennigen R, Nolte K, Rijcken E, Utech M, Loeffler B, et al. (2009) Probiotic mixture VSL#3 protects the epithelial barrier by maintaining tight junction protein expression and preventing apoptosis in a murine model of colitis. Am J Physiol Gastrointest Liver Physiol 296: G1140–1149.
41. Fasano A (2011) Zonulin and its regulation of intestinal barrier function: the biological door to inflammation, autoimmunity, and cancer. Physiol Rev 91: 151–175.
42. Tlaskalova-Hogenova H, Stepankova R, Kozakova H, Hudcovic T, Vannucci L, et al. (2011) The role of gut microbiota (commensal bacteria) and the mucosal barrier in the pathogenesis of inflammatory and autoimmune diseases and cancer: contribution of germ-free and gnotobiotic animal models of human diseases. Cell Mol Immunol 8: 110–120.
43. Chen HQ, Yang J, Zhang M, Zhou YK, Shen TY, et al. (2010) Lactobacillus plantarum ameliorates colonic epithelial barrier dysfunction by modulating the apical junctional complex and PepT1 in IL-10 knockout mice. Am J Physiol Gastrointest Liver Physiol.
44. Sokol H, Seksik P, Rigottier-Gois L, Lay C, Lepage P, et al. (2006) Specificities of the fecal microbiota in inflammatory bowel disease. Inflamm Bowel Dis 12: 106–111.
45. Tannock GW, Munro K, Harmsen HJ, Welling GW, Smart J, et al. (2000) Analysis of the fecal microflora of human subjects consuming a probiotic product containing Lactobacillus rhamnosus DR20. Appl Environ Microbiol 66: 2578–2588.
46. Boyer M, Wisniewski-Dye F (2009) Cell-cell signalling in bacteria: not simply a matter of quorum. FEMS Microbiol Ecol 70: 1–19.
47. Jamuna M, Jeevaratnam K (2004) Isolation and characterization of lactobacilli from some traditional fermented foods and evaluation of the bacteriocins. J Gen Appl Microbiol 50: 79–90.
48. Mondel M, Schroeder BO, Zimmermann K, Huber H, Nuding S, et al. (2009) Probiotic E. coli treatment mediates antimicrobial human beta-defensin synthesis and fecal excretion in humans. Mucosal Immunol 2: 166–172.
49. MacDonald TT, Monteleone G, Pender SL (2000) Recent developments in the immunology of inflammatory bowel disease. Scand J Immunol 51: 2–9.
50. Madara JL, Stafford J (1989) Interferon-gamma directly affects barrier function of cultured intestinal epithelial monolayers. J Clin Invest 83: 724–727.
51. Llopis M, Antolin M, Carol M, Borruel N, Casellas F, et al. (2009) Lactobacillus casei downregulates commensals' inflammatory signals in Crohn's disease mucosa. Inflamm Bowel Dis 15: 275–283.
52. Thomas CM, Versalovic J (2010) Probiotics-host communication: Modulation of signaling pathways in the intestine. Gut Microbes 1: 148–163.
53. Chuang L, Wu KG, Pai C, Hsieh PS, Tsai JJ, et al. (2007) Heat-killed cells of lactobacilli skew the immune response toward T helper 1 polarization in mouse splenocytes and dendritic cell-treated T cells. J Agric Food Chem 55: 11080–11086.
54. Delcenserie V, Martel D, Lamoureux M, Amiot J, Boutin Y, et al. (2008) Immunomodulatory effects of probiotics in the intestinal tract. Curr Issues Mol Biol 10: 37–54.
55. Biswas A, Wilmanski J, Forsman H, Hrncir T, Hao L, et al. (2011) Negative regulation of Toll-like receptor signaling plays an essential role in homeostasis of the intestine. Eur J Immunol 41: 182–194.
56. Zhao Y, Karypis G (2003) Clustering in life sciences. Methods Mol Biol 224: 183–218.

5

Dextran Sodium Sulfate (DSS) Induces Colitis in Mice by Forming Nano-Lipocomplexes with Medium-Chain-Length Fatty Acids in the Colon

Hamed Laroui[1]*, Sarah A. Ingersoll[1,2], Hong Chun Liu[3,4], Mark T. Baker[1], Saravanan Ayyadurai[1], Moiz A. Charania[1], Famina Laroui[2], Yutao Yan[1,2], Shanthi V. Sitaraman[3], Didier Merlin[1,2]

1 Department of Biology, Center Diagnostics and Therapeutics, Georgia State University, Atlanta, Georgia, United States of America, **2** Veterans Affairs Medical Center, Decatur, Georgia, United States of America, **3** Department of Medicine, Division of Digestive Diseases, Emory University, Atlanta, Georgia, United States of America, **4** Department of Gastroenterology, Zhongshan Hospital, Fudan University, Shanghai, China

Abstract

Inflammatory bowel diseases (IBDs), primarily ulcerative colitis and Crohn's disease, are inflammatory disorders caused by multiple factors. Research on IBD has often used the dextran sodium sulfate (DSS)-induced colitis mouse model. DSS induces *in vivo* but not *in vitro* intestinal inflammation. In addition, no DSS-associated molecule (free glucose, sodium sulfate solution, free dextran) induces *in vitro* or *in vivo* intestinal inflammation. We find that DSS but not dextran associated molecules established linkages with medium-chain-length fatty acids (MCFAs), such as dodecanoate, that are present in the colonic lumen. DSS complexed to MCFAs forms nanometer-sized vesicles ~200 nm in diameter that can fuse with colonocyte membranes. The arrival of nanometer-sized DSS/MCFA vesicles in the cytoplasm may activate intestinal inflammatory signaling pathways. We also show that the inflammatory activity of DSS is mediated by the dextran moieties. The deleterious effect of DSS is localized principally in the distal colon, therefore it will be important to chemically modify DSS to develop materials beneficial to the colon without affecting colon-targeting specificity.

Editor: Jan-Hendrik Niess, Ulm University, Germany

Funding: This work was supported by grants from the Department of Veterans Affairs and the National Institutes of Health of Diabetes and Digestive and Kidney by RO1-DK-071594. The funders had no role in study design, data collection and analysis, decision to publish, or preparation of the manuscript.

Competing Interests: The authors have declared that no competing interests exist.

* E-mail: hlaroui@gsu.edu

Introduction

Inflammatory bowel diseases (IBDs), principally ulcerative colitis (UC) and Crohn's disease (CD), are inflammatory disorders of the gastrointestinal tract caused by multiple genetic and environmental factors [1,2,3]. Various models of experimental IBD have been developed to investigate pathogenesis and to improve treatment options such as gene knockout (KO) models:interleukin (IL)-2/IL-2 receptor-alpha [4], IL-10 [5], T cell receptor [6], Tumor necrosis factor (TNF)-3′ untranslated region (UTR) [7] or transgenic models: IL-17 [8], HLA B27 [9]. Most commonly, experimental colitis is induced by the heparin-like polysaccharide DSS; this model is simple and affords a high degree of uniformity and reproducibility of most lesions in the distal colon [10,11]. By first interfering with intestinal barrier function, and next stimulating local inflammation, DSS is often used to induce a form of mouse colitis that mimics the clinical and histological features of IBDs that have characteristics of UC [12,13,14]. The typical features of colitis appear on day 3 and are maximally expressed by day 7 [15]. Notably, expression of pro-inflammatory cytokines and chemokines (IL-1, IL-6, KC, TNF-α, and Interferon-γ) are upregulated [15,16] whereas synthesis of anti-inflammatory cytokines, such as IL-10, is downregulated [16,17,18,19]. Other parameters such as decreases in body weight and colon length, elevation in myeloperoxidase level (suggestive of neutrophil infiltration into the epithelium), and higher histological and endoscopic scores characterize murine colitis [20,21,22]. DSS induces colitis, but the mechanism of action remains unknown. Miyazawa et al. [23] showed that DSS caused disruption of biological mechanisms (such as inhibitory effects on reverse transcriptase activities that affect major cellular functions), competing with poly(U) to this end [23]. Previously, it was shown that dextran sulfate inhibited ribonuclease action [24,25]. Other natural and synthetic polyanionic polymers play important roles in establishing the association of mRNA with ribosomes and can disturb mRNA translation [23]. But the mechanism of how DSS penetrates the cell is unknown as it could be through passive or active uptake by the cell via a specific receptor, or DSS could penetrate the cell after complexation with another molecular form (such as polycationic forms). Other studies have shown that DSS induced significant macrophage infiltration into the epithelium of the colon [26]. Our study attempted to correlate this last hypothesis by increasing medium-chain-length fatty acids (MCFAs) in the mouse colon. MCFAs are increased by a high fat diet. The role of MCFAs in inflammation is not clear as the size of the carbon chain is intermediate between small and long chains. The sodium salts of several MCFAs, particularly capric (C10) and lauric (C12) acids, have been shown to increase rectal drug absorption, presumably by causing alterations in intestinal tight junctions (TJ) barrier function. C10 has also been shown to lead to profound alterations in the barrier function of the TJ and has been investigated as an agent to enhance viral-mediated a gene transfer [27]. These agents are attractive as potential therapies to enhance absorption of gene transfer vectors due to the rapid onset of action (within minutes) and their relatively rapid recovery (within hours) after treatment [28,29,30,31] [27].

Although MCFAs have been widely investigated as agents to increase the delivery of therapeutic agents, relatively little is known regarding their primary mechanism of action. The ability of intercellular TJs to function as a barrier to the diffusion of macromolecules is dynamically regulated by numerous intracellular signals and the permeability properties of the TJ vary in response to changes in physiological state. Therefore, agents that regulate the TJ likely do so by direct or indirect actions on intracellular signals and/or the protein components of the TJ.

It has been extensively shown that short chain fatty acids, like butyrate, attenuate inflammation in DSS-induced colitis [32,33,34,35]. Conversely, long chain fatty acids, like palmitic acid (C16) or palmitic acid (monosaturated or polysaturated forms) have been shown to promote inflammation [26]. Kim et al. have shown that corn oil, mainly constituted with the long chain fatty acid cited above, have a significant effect on the aggravation of inflammation related colorectal cancer [26].

In the present study we investigated the mechanism of DSS action in the distal colon using *in vitro* and *in vivo* approaches.

Materials and Methods

Animal studies

All studies were performed in accordance with the Institutional Animal Care and Use Committee at Emory University (Atlanta, GA). All procedures were approved and are registered in the protocol IACUC ID: 156–2008, approval date 7/8/2010 to 7/8/2011. Strains, ages, and the number of animalsfollow the established protocol.

Female C57BL/6 mice (aged 8 weeks, weight 18–22 g, Jackson Laboratories, Bar Harbor, ME) used for this study were group-housed under controlled temperature (25°C) and photoperiod (12:12-hour light–dark cycle) conditions, and given unrestricted access to standard diet and tap water (or specified drinking solution). Mice were allowed to acclimate to these conditions for at least 7 days before inclusion in experiments.

High fat diet (60% kCal of fat, 20% kCal of protein, and 20% kCal of carbohydrate) and control diet (10% kCal of fat, 20% kCal of protein, and 70% kCal of carbohydrate) were purchased from Research Diets (New Brunswick, NJ). Supplementation of fat is provided by soybean oil (10%) and lard (90%).

Histology

Distal colonic sections were fixed in 10% formalin and embedded in paraffin. 5-μm sections were stained with H&E. Images were acquired using a Zeiss Axioskop 2 plus microscope (Carl Zeiss MicroImaging) equipped with an AxioCam MRc5 CCD camera (Carl Zeiss).

Histological score assessment of colitis

H&E-stained colonic sections were coded for blind microscopic assessment of inflammation (i.e., DSS-induced colitis). Histological scoring was based on 3 parameters. Severity of inflammation was scored as follows: 0, rare inflammatory cells in the lamina propria; 1, increased numbers of granulocytes in the lamina propria; 2, confluence of inflammatory cells extending into the submucosa; 3, transmural extension of the inflammatory infiltrate. Crypt damage was scored as follows: 0, intact crypts; 1, loss of the basal one-third; 2, loss of the basal two-thirds; 3, entire crypt loss; 4, change of epithelial surface with erosion; 5, confluent erosion. Ulceration was scored as follows: 0, absence of ulcer; 1, 1 or 2 foci of ulcerations; 2, 3 or 4 foci of ulcerations; 3, confluent or extensive ulceration. Values were added to give a maximal histological score of 11.

Endoscopic assessment of colitis

Direct visualization of DSS-induced colonic mucosal damage in vivo was performed using the Coloview (Karl Storz Veterinary Endoscopy, Tuttlingen, Germany). Mice were supplied with food and water until the endoscopy was performed. Mice were anesthetized with 1.5 to 2% isoflurane and 3 cm of the colon proximal to the anus was visualized after inflation of the colon with air. The endoscopic damage score was determined using a previously described scoring method with one modification: assessment of colon translucency (0–3 points), presence of fibrin attached to the bowel wall (0–3 points), granular aspect of the mucosa (0–3 points), morphology of the vascular pattern (0–3 points), and stool characteristic (normal to diarrhea; 0–3 points) [21]. Since this scoring method did not include assessment for the presence of blood in the lumen, we added this parameter (0 points: no blood; 1 point: slight bleeding; 2 points: frank bleeding) to generate a range in total score from 0–17 points.

Pro-inflammatory chemokine and cytokine analysis

Total RNA was extracted using TRIzol reagent (Invitrogen, Carlsbad, CA) and reverse-transcribed using the cDNA Synthesis kit (Fermentas, Glen Burnie, MD). RT-PCR was performed using the GeneJET Fast PCR kit (Fermentas, Glen Burnie, MD). Real-time RT-PCR was performed using an iCycler (Bio-Rad, Hercules, CA). Briefly, cDNA was amplified by 40 cycles of 95°C for 15 s and 60°C for 1 min, using the iQ SYBR Green Supermix system (Biorad, Hercules, CA) and the following specific primers:

KC sense 5′-TTGTGCGAAAAGAAGTGCAG-3′, KC antisense 5′-TACAAACACAGCCTCCCACA-3′,

IL-1β sense 5′-TCGCTCAGGGTCACAAGAAA-3′, IL-1β antisense 5′-CATCAGAGGCAAGGAGGAAAA C-3′;

TNF-α sense 5′-AGGCTGCCCCGACTACGT-3′, TNF-α antisense 5′-GACTTTCTCCTGGTATGAGATAGCAAA-3′;

IL-6 sense 5′-ACAAGTCGGAGGCTTAATTACACAT-3′, IL-6 antisense 5′-TTGCCATTGCACAACTCTTTT C-3′;

IFN-γ sense 5′-CAGCAACAGCAAGGCGAAA-3′, IFN-γ antisense 5′-CTGGACCTGTGGGTTGTTGAC-3′;

IL-10 sense 5′-ACCTGGTAGAAGTGATGCCCCAGGCA-3′ and 5′-CTATGCAGTTGATGAAGATGTCAAA-3′

18S sense 5′-CCCCTCGATGACTTTAGCTGAGTGT-3′, 18S antisense 5′-CGCCGGTCC AAGAATTTCACCTCT-3′;

mouse 36B4 sense 5′-TCCAGGCTTTGGGCATCA-3′, mouse 36B4 antisense 5′-CTTTATCAGCTGCACATCACT-CAGA-3′.

18S and 36B4 were used as housekeeping genes. Fold-induction was calculated using the Ct method, $\Delta\Delta CT = (Ct_{Target}\text{-}Ct_{housekeeping})_{infected} - (Ct_{Target}\text{-}Ct_{housekeeping})_{uninfected}$, and the final data were derived from $2^{-\Delta\Delta CT}$.

Myeloperoxidase (MPO) assay

Colonic tissue samples were homogenized in ice-cold potassium phosphate buffer (50 mM K2HPO4 and 50 mM KH2PO4, pH 6.0) containing 0.5% hexadecyltrimethylammonium bromide (Sigma). The homogenates were then sonicated, freeze-thawed three times, and centrifuged at 17,500 rcf for 15 min. Supernatants (20 μl) or MPO standard were added to 1 mg/mL *o*-

dianisidine hydrochloride (Sigma) and 0.0005% H_2O_2, and the change in absorbance at 450 nm was measured. One unit of MPO activity was defined as the amount that degraded 1 µmol peroxidase per minute. The results were expressed as relative MPO activity compared to water-treated mice (normalized to 1).

DSS-induced colitis

Colitis was induced by 3% (w/v) dextran sodium sulfate (DSS; molecular weight 42 kDa; ICN Biochemicals, Aurora, OH) added to the drinking water. Colonic inflammation was assessed 7 to 8 days after DSS treatment. Twelve mice were included in each group. To evaluate the effects of each drinking solution on induced colitis, the mice were given a bottle of each solution with equivalent number of moles of the studied molecules: DSS 30 g/L, dextran 14.9 g/L, glucose 17.33 g/L, and sulfate 25.99 g/L. The concentrations were obtained by calculating the concentration of dextran sodium sulfate: 6.98×10^{-4} mol.L^{-1}. The DSS supplier (MP Biomedicals) verified that the sulfate (SO3H) substitution rate was 1.9 groups per glycosyl residue of DSS. We approximated $\overline{M_n} = \overline{M_w} = 43000$ g/mol and calculated the degree of polymerization ($\overline{DP_n}$) of DSS:

$$\overline{DP_n} = \frac{\overline{M_n}}{\overline{M_0}}$$

$\overline{M_n}$ = numbered molecular mass of DSS

$\overline{M_0}$ = Molecular mass of a single glycosyl residue grafted with 1.9 sulfate group

$\overline{DP_n} = 43000/310.6 = 138$

In one polymer chain of DSS, there are 138 glycosyl residues. Equivalent concentrations for DSS associated molecules have to be calculated according to (DSS = 138 residues = 30 g/L; dextran = 138 residues = 14.9 g/L; sodium sulfate = 138*1.9 = 262.2 residues = 25.99 g/L; glucose = 138 residues = 17.33 g/L).

Osmolarity of mice feces

Feces was collected and dried in an incubator at 37°C (n = 6 per drinking solution treatment). 50 mg of feces was dissolved in 1 mL of NaCl (0.15 M). Osmolarity of water treated mice was set to 1 arbitrary unit (AU) as negative control. All osmolarities were then measured and calculated as relative osmolarity (Osmolarity of

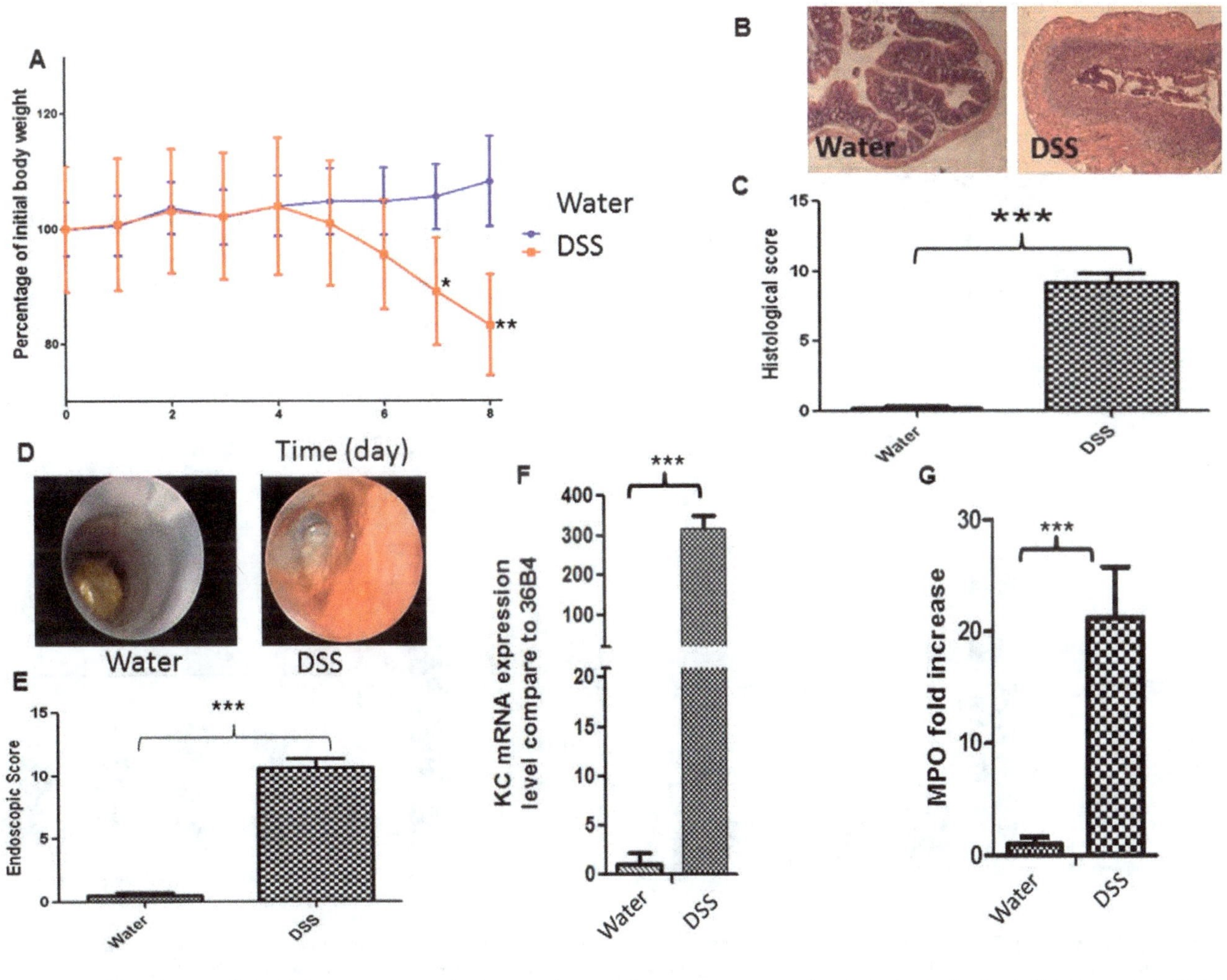

Figure 1. DSS induces colitis. (A) Mouse body weight changes during DSS treatment compared to that of control animals (drinking water). C57BL/6 mice were exposed to 3% (w/v) DSS in the drinking water for the indicated numbers of days. Body weight changes are shown as means±SEMs. * $P<0.05$, ** $P<0.01$. (B) Hematoxylin-stained colonic sections of mice treated with DSS; the mice were sacrificed on day 8. (C) Associated histological scores. *** $P<0.001$. (D) Macroscopic inflammation was assessed using a mouse colonoscope. Photographs were obtained on the day of sacrifice and (E) an endoscopic score was calculated. *** $P<0.001$. (F) KC mRNA expression was measured in test and control animals. *** $P<0.001$. (G) Determination of MPO enzymatic activity as an index of neutrophil infiltration into injured tissue. Results are expressed as MPO –fold increases compared to those of control mice and represent means±SEMs of three independent determinations. *** $P<0.01$.

sample feces/Osmolarity of water-treated mice feces). Osmolarity measurement was performed by an osmometer (Osmette III, Precision Systems, Natick, MA).

Epithelium resistance measurement by Electric Cell-substrate Impedance Sensing (ECIS)

For ECIS, cell-attachment assays were performed using ECIS technology (Applied BioPhysics, Troy, NY) [36]. The ECIS model 1600R (Applied BioPhysics) was used for these experiments. The measurement system consists of an 8-well culture dish (ECIS 8W1E plate), the surface of which is seeded with cell cultures. Each well contains a small, active electrode (area = 5.10^{-4} cm^2) and a large counter electrode (area = 0.15 cm^2) on the bottom of each well. A lock-in amplifier, with an internal oscillator, relays a signal to switch between the different wells, and a personal computer controls the measurement and stores the data. Attachment and spreading of cells on the electrode surface change the impedance in such a way that morphological information about the attached cells can be inferred. Caco2-BBE cells (1 million cells per mL) were seeded in ECIS 8W1E plates in DMEM (Invitrogen) supplemented with 10% (v/v) heat-inactivated fetal bovine serum (Invitrogen) and 1.5 µg/mL plasmocin (Invitrogen). Once cells reached confluence, the different solutions were added at a concentration given in the results section. Controls in DMEM medium cell cultures were used for each experiment. Basal resistance measurements were performed using the ideal frequency for Caco2-BBE cells, 500 Hz, and a voltage of 1 V.

Dextran-loaded nanoparticles synthesis

Poly (D,L-lactide) (PLA) was purchased from Sigma-Aldrich (St Louis, MO) ($\overline{M_w}$ of 75–120 kg/mol). The nanoparticles were produced by the double emulsion/solvent evaporation procedure previously described [37] for the elaboration of polyvinylic alcohol (PVA)-covered PLA nanoparticles. This method involves use of an

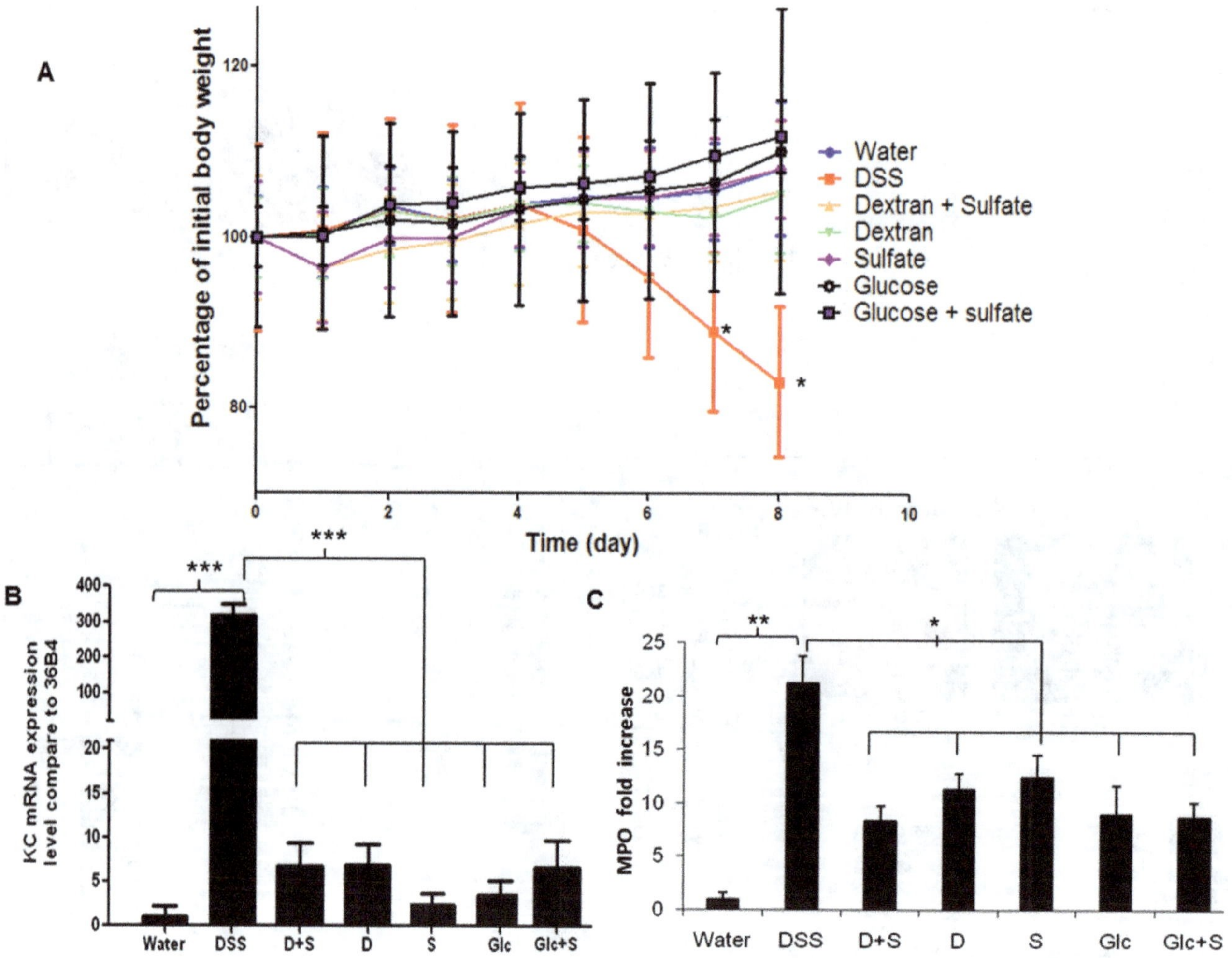

Figure 2. DSS but not DSS-associated molecules induce colitis. (A) Mouse body weight changes during consumption of water, DSS (3% w/v), dextran (1.49% w/v) in sulfate solution (2.6% w/v), dextran (1.49% w/v), sulfate solution (2.6% w/v), glucose (1.73% w/v), and glucose (1.73% w/v) in sulfate solution (2.6% w/v). C57BL/6 mice were given the various solutions as drinking water for the indicated numbers of days. Body weight changes are depicted as means±SEMs for each group. * P<0.05. (B) DSS significantly increased production of chemokine KC mRNA compared to the rises seen when DSS-associated molecules were given. KC mRNA expression was measured via qRT-PCR of extracts of colonic cells. *** P<0.001. (C) Determination of MPO enzymatic activity as an index of neutrophil infiltration into injured tissue. (D) Macroscopic observations of colons of mice treated with DSS-associated molecules [DSS = dextran sodium sulfate, D+S = dextran (1.49% w/v) in sulfate solution (2.6% w/v), D = dextran (1.49% w/v), S = sulfate solution (2.6% w/v), and Glc+S = glucose (1.73% w/v) in sulfate solution (2.6% w/v)] were made using a mouse colonoscope. Photographs were obtained from all treatment groups on the day of sacrifice. * P<0.05, ** P<0.01.

amphiphilic molecule as the surfactant of the secondary emulsion; however, in the present study, PVA was used, which was purchased from Aldrich (Milwaukee, WI) ($\overline{M_w}$ = 13,000–23,000 g/mol, hydroxylated at 87–89%). Typically, a primary water in oil emulsion (w/o) was prepared by mixing an organic phase (4 mL dichloromethane) containing PLA (25 g/L) with an internal aqueous phase (400 µL). The emulsion is stabilized by the bovine serum albumin (BSA; 50 g/L) of the internal aqueous phase. The internal phase also contains, or does not contain, dextran (2.5 g/L, $\overline{M_w}$ = 40 kDa). The mixture was stirred for 2 min with a Vortex mixer (Maxi Mix II, Thermolyne, USA), then sonicated (2 min, power 6, 50% active cycle, in an ice bath) using a Sonifier 450 (Branson, USA). This primary emulsion was poured into a second aqueous phase (8 mL) (external aqueous phase) containing an amphiphilic molecule (PVA 20 g/L). The water in oil in water emulsion (w/o/w) was then obtained by sonication (same conditions as those used for the primary emulsion). This double emulsion was then transferred to an aqueous 10^{-2} M $NaNO_3$ dispersing phase (40 mL) and stirred for 5 min. The organic solvent was evaporated under stirring and ambient air conditions and the collected solid nanospheres were resuspended in water then centrifuged again to remove the excess PVA. This purification procedure was repeated twice. The final suspension was then freeze-dried.

Particle size measurement

Diameters (nm) of NPs were measured by light scattering using 90 Plus/BI-MAS (Multi angle particle sizing, Brookhaven Instruments Corporation, Holtsville, NY, USA). The average and standard deviations of the diameters (nm) were calculated using 3 runs. Each run is an average of 10 measurements.

The effect of encapsulated dextran-loaded NPs on in vivo inflammation

To deliver the dextran-loaded NPs to C57BL/6 mice colonic lumen, we encapsulated them into a biomaterial comprised of alginate and chitosan at a ratio of 7/3 (wt/wt). We and others have previously shown that the biomaterial collapses in intestinal solution at pH 5 or 6, which is the colonic pH under inflamed and non-inflamed states [38,39,40]. C57BL/6 mice (8 per group) were gavaged daily for 4 days with encapsulated dextran-loaded or empty NPs as a negative control.

Cell Culture

Caco2-BBE cells were cultured to confluency in 75-cm^2 flasks at 37°C in a humidified atmosphere containing 5% CO_2. The culture medium used was DMEM/Ham's F-12 medium (Invitrogen, USA) supplemented with L-glutamine (2 mM), penicillin (100 units/mL), streptomycin (100 µg/mL), and heat-inactivated fetal calf serum (10%) (Invitrogen, USA).

Statistical analysis

Data are presented as average values and standard deviations from experiments performed in triplicate (n = 3), except *in vivo* experiments (n = 8). ANOVA tests were performed to obtain statistical comparisons between samples.

Results

Characterization of DSS-induced colitis in mice

The DSS-induced colitis murine model is commonly used to address the pathogenesis of IBD [15,20,41] and to test the efficacy of therapies such as nanotechnology-based drug release systems

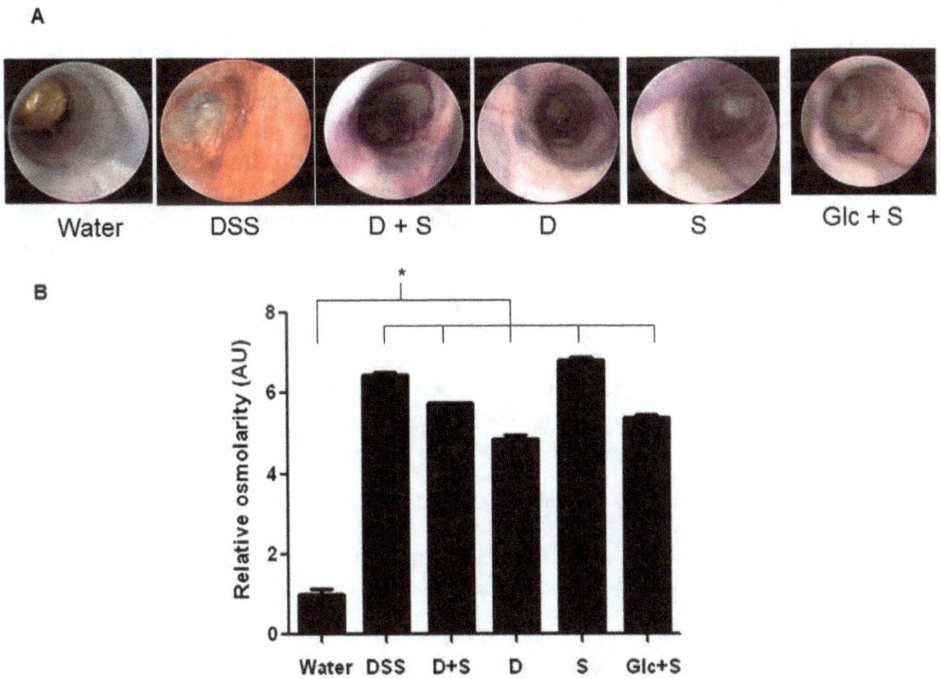

Figure 3. DSS and DSS-associated molecules affect luminal intestinal osmolarity. (A) Macroscopic observations of the effects of DSS-associated molecules [DSS = dextran sodium sulfate, D+S = dextran (1.49% w/v) in sulfate solution (2.6% w/v), D = dextran (1.49% w/v), S = sulfate solution (2.6% w/v), and Glc+S = glucose (1.73% w/v) in sulfate solution (2.6% w/v)] on colonic epithelium were assessed using a mouse colonoscope. Photographs were obtained from all treatment groups on the day of sacrifice. (B) Fecal relative osmolarity values (means±SEM, ANOVA statistical test, * $P<0.05$).

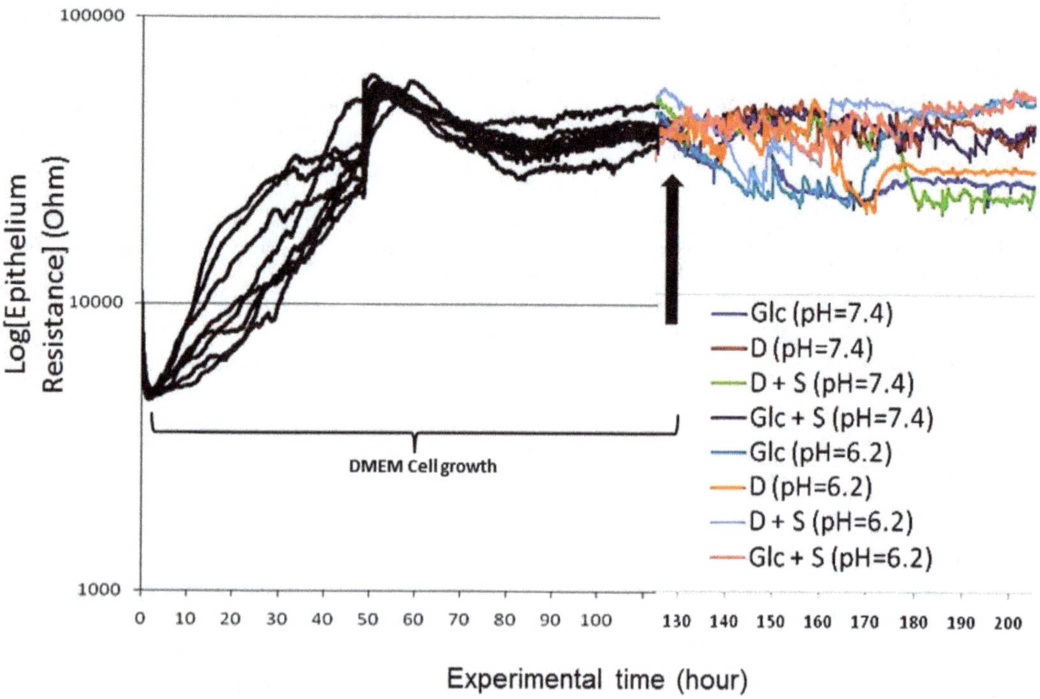

Figure 4. DSS-associated molecules do not affect the resistance of Caco2-BBE monolayers. Confluent cultures of Caco2-BBE cells were obtained after 48 h (dark lines) and epithelial resistance was assessed by conduct of continuous resistance measurements at pH 7.4 (cellular pH) and pH 6.2 (colonic pH). Resistance (Ohm) of Caco2-BBE cells was measured at $\Omega = 500$ Hz and $V = 1$ V by electrical impedance sensing method (ECIS) on ECIS 8W1E electrodes. After confluence (colored lines), DMEM-based solutions containing glucose 17.33 g/L (Glc), dextran 14.9 g/L (D), dextran 14.9 g/L and sodium sulfate 25.99 g/L (D+S) and glucose 17.33 g/L and sulfate 25.99 g/L (Glc+S) were added at both pH. Data represent means of n = 3/condition.

[39,40,42]. C57BL/6 mice were given 3% (w/v) DSS in drinking water for 8 days. Significant weight loss was evident in the DSS-treated group compared to the negative control (Figure 1A). About 20% of initial weight was lost after 8 days of DSS treatment (Figure 1A). During this treatment, inflammation was enhanced, as shown by rises in the extent of diarrhea and rectal bleeding. Colonic inflammation was also examined by histology (Figure 1B); hematoxylin-stained day 8 colon sections of DSS-treated mice showed severe lesions throughout the mucosa, alteration of epithelial structure, high-level neutrophil and lymphocyte infiltration into the mucosal and submucosal areas, and loss of crypts (Figure 1B). All alterations observed were combined to obtain histological scores (Figure 1C). The score calculated after DSS treatment was significantly higher than that of control mice; 9.2±1.5 versus 0.2±0.4, respectively. Histological observations were confirmed by macroscopic inflammation assessment using a mouse colonoscope. Photographs were obtained on the day of sacrifice (thus after 8 days of DSS treatment; Figure 1D); the colon was inflamed. Colon photographs after DSS treatment revealed bloody stools, diarrhea, ulcers, and mucosal inflammation; control animals had healthy mucosa. Figure 1E shows the endoscopic scores obtained upon analysis of the photographs; DSS-treated mice scored significantly higher than did control animals (10.6±1.3 versus 0.7±0.8). These macroscopic observations were confirmed by estimation of biological parameters relevant to inflammation. We measured expression of KC, a chemokine. DSS significantly increases KC production [43,44,45]. Expression of mRNA encoding KC was measured in DSS-treated and control mice. The extent of KC mRNA expression was 300-fold higher in DSS-treated animals compared to control animals (Figure 1F). MPO enzymatic activity (an index of neutrophil infiltration into the colonic mucosa) increased 20-fold in DSS-treated mice compared to controls (Figure 1G). The mouse DSS-induced colitis model can thus be used to address the pathogenesis of IBD.

Specificity of DSS for induction of colitis

We explored how DSS, a negatively charged polymer of glucose with engrafted sulfate groups, induced colitis in mice. As DSS is composed of successive glucose units substituted with sulfur groups ($-SO_3H$), we decided to test each DSS component separately. Thus, we explored the effects of dextran dissolved in water, dextran dissolved in a sulfate salt solution, sulfate salt dissolved in water, glucose dissolved in water, and glucose dissolved in a sulfate salt solution. To be consistent, the ratios of glucose, dextran, or sulfate molecules were identical to those in DSS. All concentrations were based on a 3% (w/v) DSS solution (mol. wt. 42 kDa; 17% by weight of engrafted sulfate groups). As shown in Figure 2A, DSS given in drinking water for 8 days increased colonic inflammation, as measured by body weight loss, however there was no observable inflammation in the other treated groups. Also, we did not observe diarrhea or rectal bleeding in mice treated with DSS-associated molecules (data not shown). DSS induction of KC-encoding mRNA was 300-fold higher than the control value whereas the maximum increase afforded by ingestion of DSS-associated molecules did not exceed 7-fold (Figure 2B). Determination of MPO enzymatic activity as an index of neutrophil infiltration into intestinal mucosa revealed a 20-fold increase in MPO activity in DSS-treated mice compared to controls (Figure 2C). A 10-fold increase in MPO level after treatment with DSS-associated molecules was observed compared to the control

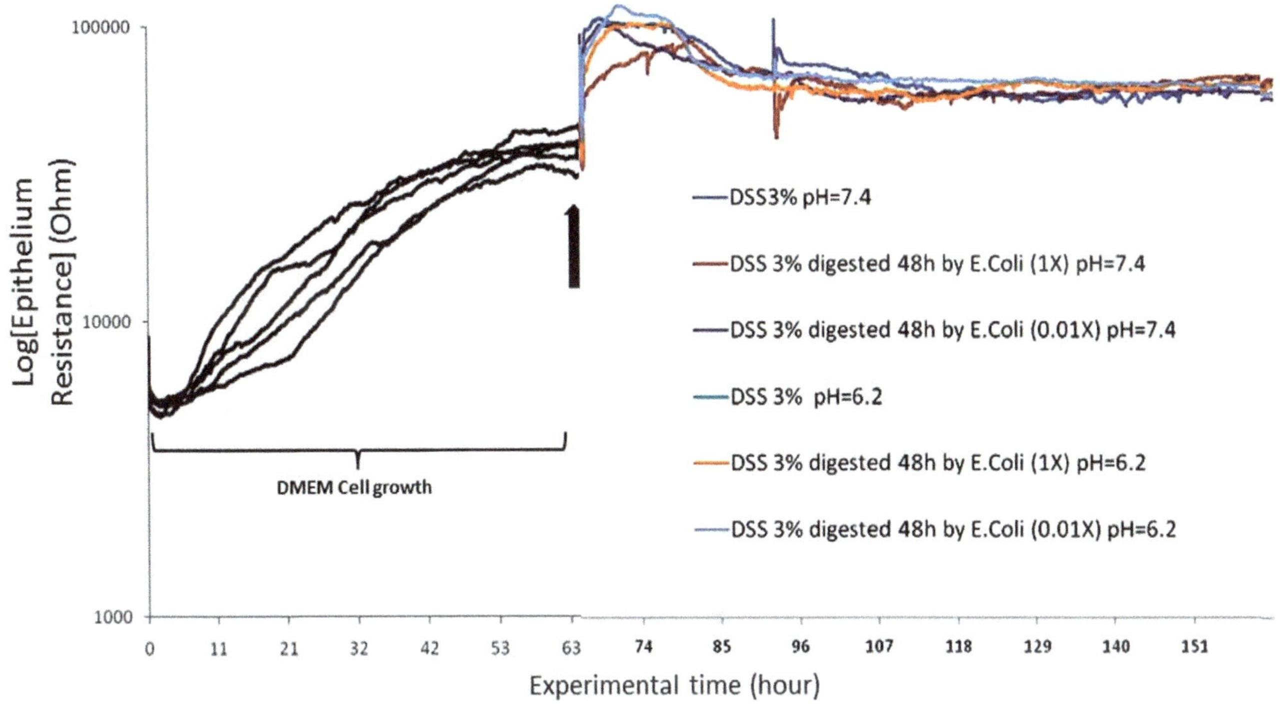

Figure 5. DSS and DSS sub-products obtained when DSS is digested by *E. coli* do not affect the resistance of Caco2-BBE monolayers. Confluent cultures of Caco2-BBE cells were obtained after 48 h (dark lines) and epithelial resistance was assessed by conduct of continuous resistance measurements at pH 7.4 (cellular pH) and pH 6.2 (colonic pH). Resistance (Ohm) of Caco2-BBE cells was measured at $\Omega = 500$ Hz and $V = 1$ V by electrical impedance sensing method (ECIS) on ECIS 8W1E electrodes. After confluence (colored lines), DMEM-based solutions containing potential sub-products of the digestion of DSS (3%) by Escherichia coli at high concentration (4.10^{11} CFU/mL, 1×) or diluted (4.10^{9} CFU/mL, 0.01×) were added at both pH. Data represent means of n = 3/condition.

value (Figure 2C). Macroscopic features of inflammation were assessed using a mouse colonoscope. In contrast to DSS, DSS-associated molecules did not induce the common characteristics of an inflamed colon (Figure 3A). However, whereas intestinal mucosa treated with DSS-associated molecules was intact, hemorrhagic vessels were observed in the submucosal layer after ingestion of all DSS-associated molecules (Figure 3A). We hypothesize that a local increase in osmolarity may affect the integrity of blood vessels (Figure 3A). To verify this hypothesis, we measured the osmolarity of feces. We found that mice treated with DSS and DSS-associated molecules had higher fecal osmolarity than did control animals (Figure 3B). This is consistent with the observed vessel degradation and submucosal bleeding in such animals, and the subsequent increase in neutrophil infiltration into the mucosa, as shown by MPO measurement (Figure 2C). Together, the data show that DSS is specific in terms of colitis induction in mice. No DSS-associated molecule tested induced colitis after 1 week of treatment. However, we suggest that DSS-associated molecules can cause development of hemorrhagic vessels mainly because of the change of colonic osmolarity in these groups.

DSS and DSS-associated molecules do not affect the electrical resistance of Caco2-BBE cell monolayers

As shown in Figure 4, using ECIS, we obtained confluent Caco2-BBE monolayer cells as assessed by attainment of a plateau with a high resistance value (R = 36,000 Ω; dark lines of Figure 4).

After adding the DMEM-based solution containing glucose 17.33 g/L (Glc), dextran 14.9 g/L (D), dextran 14.9 g/L and sodium sulfate 25.99 g/L (D+S) and glucose 17.33 g/L and sulfate 25.99 g/L (Glc+S) to the confluent Caco2-BBE monolayer of cells, the resistance plateau values (R = 36 kΩ) did not decrease (colored lines of Figure 4). Interestingly, no DSS-associated molecules affected monolayer resistance when the extracellular medium was at pH 7.4 or pH 6.2 (Figure 4). This shows that the *in vivo* ability of DSS, compared to DSS-associated molecules, to induce colitis, is lost *in vitro*. This suggests that some permissive *in vivo* "factor" must be present to allow DSS to induce colitis. The lack of a DSS effect on resistance *in vitro* suggests that DSS does not interact with an intestinal epithelial receptor (Figure 5).

DSS sub-products produced by Escherichia coli action do not affect Caco2-BBE cell monolayer resistance

When DSS is given to mice, DSS may interact with colonic bacteria. We considered that DSS might be chemically modified by such bacteria, producing a sub-product affecting intestinal barrier function. To test this hypothesis, we supplemented bacterial medium with 3% (w/v) DSS and grew *Escherichia coli* in the medium for 48 h at 37°C at a high concentration (saturated growth medium, 4.10^{11} CFU/mL, 1×) and at diluted concentration (4.10^{9} CFU/mL, 0.01×). The culture supernatant was collected and the pH adjusted to pH 7.4 or pH 6.2.

As shown in Figure 5, using ECIS, we obtained confluent Caco2-BBE monolayer cells as assessed by attainment of a plateau with a high resistance value (R = 42,000 Ω; dark lines of Figure 5).

Next, supernatant samples were added to confluent Caco2-BBE monolayers and online measurement of epithelial resistance was performed using ECIS (colored lines of Figure 5). As shown in Figure 5, supernatant at pH 7.4 or 6.2, containing DSS and presumably DSS sub-products, did not affect Caco2-BBE monolayer resistance as the value of the resistance did not change.

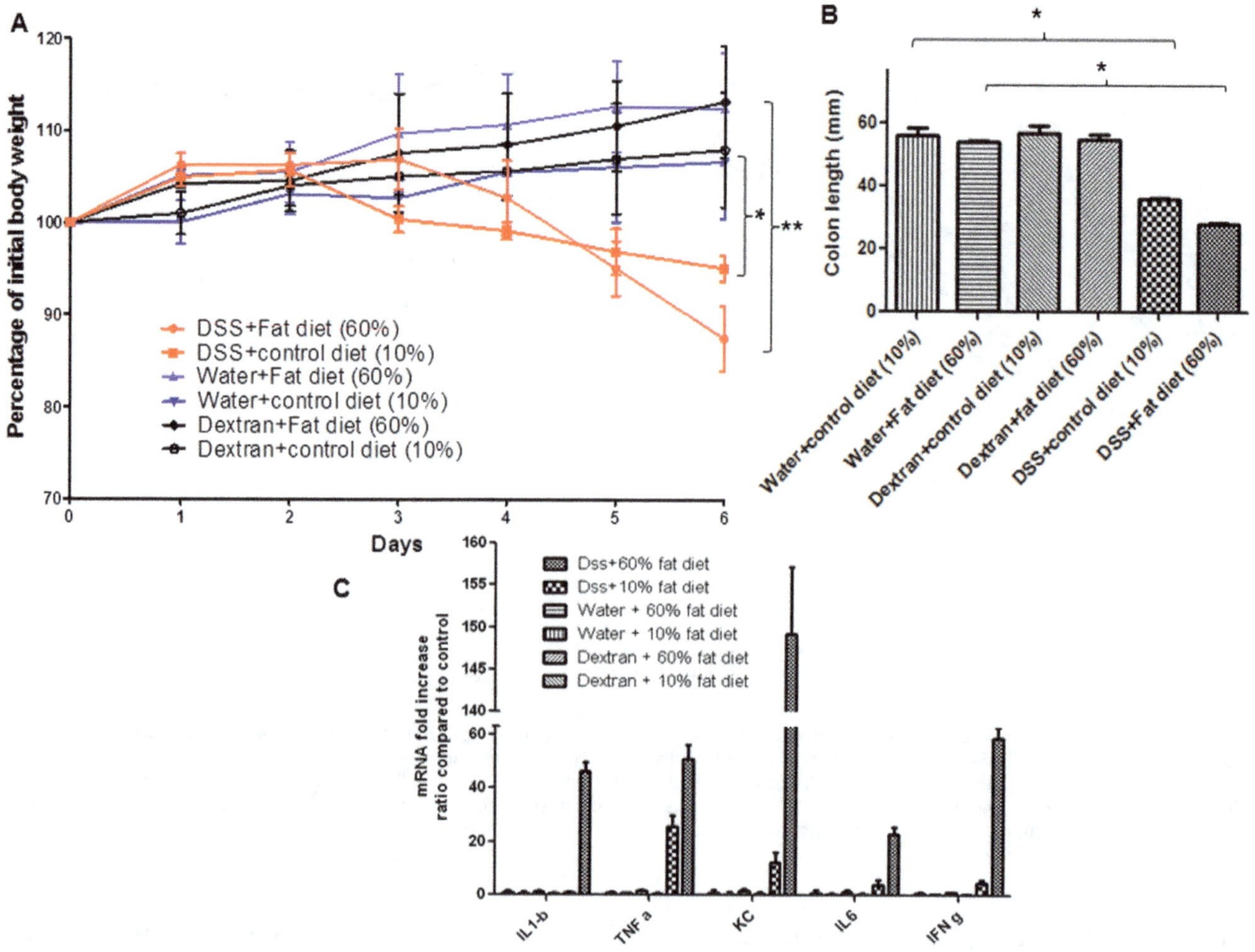

Figure 6. A high-fat diet increases the efficacy by which DSS induces colitis in mice. (A) Body weight changes in C57BL/6 mice on regular chow or a high-fat diet, drinking either a 3% (w/v) dextran or a 3% (w/v) DSS solution, for 6 days. Body weight changes are shown as means±SEMs. * $P<0.05$, ** $P<0.01$. (B) Determination of colon length (an index of colonic inflammation). Results are expressed in mm and represent means±SEMs of three independent determinations. * $P<0.05$. (C) Consumption of DSS and a high-fat diet significantly increases production of pro-inflammatory cytokines and chemokine mRNAs compared to what is seen in animals consuming DSS but (otherwise) regular chow. * $P<0.05$, ** $P<0.01$, *** $P<0.001$.

This showed that bacteria are not the permissive "factor" mediating the *in vivo* specificity of DSS in induction of colitis.

A high-fat diet increases the efficacy by which DSS induces colitis in mice

The above experiments showed that DSS did not interact directly with epithelial cells via a specific receptor, nor was inflammation induced by sub-products generated from DSS by bacterial degradation/modification. We next explored whether a high fat diet affected the efficacy of DSS in terms of inducing colitis in mice. As shown in Figure 6, ingestion of 3% (w/v) DSS and a high-fat diet (60% [w/w] fat) worsened colitis, as assessed by weight loss (Figure 6A), compared to use of DSS and the normal mouse chow (<10% fat). The observed effect was caused by the DSS/fatty diet combination because mice drinking regular drinking water and eating the high-fat diet showed no significant weight loss compared to mice with access to regular drinking water and regular chow after 6 days of treatment (Figure 6A). Also, ingestion of the high-fat diet increased the inflammation seen after DSS treatment compared to that noted when DSS was given together with regular diet. Thus, comparing the mice given a high-fat diet and DSS versus a regular diet coupled with DSS, the colon length was further reduced (28 mm versus 36 mm in Figure 6B) and pro-inflammatory cytokine expression levels were increased (46-fold increase in IL-1β mRNA level; 50-fold versus 25-fold in TNFα mRNA level; 23-fold versus 3.7-fold in IL6 mRNA level; 58.6-fold versus 4.7-fold in INFγ mRNA level; and 150-fold in KC mRNA level versus 10-fold in mice given regular chow) (Figure 6C). Interestingly, the high-fat diet acted in a manner similar to a cofactor, exacerbating the effect of DSS. These results were not observed when mice had access to regular water and a high-fat diet (Figure 6; A, B, and C). The results suggest that fatty acids specifically exacerbated DSS-induced colitis in mice. We propose that a potential electrostatic association between fatty acids and DSS, mediated via dicationic ions (Ca^{++}, Mg^{+}) or positively charged molecules, could result in formation of DSS-loaded vesicles which, via the hydrophobic domains, might fuse with the membranes of colonic cells and subsequently deliver DSS into such cells. Once in the cytosol, DSS would activate pro-inflammatory cascades. Several examples of inflammation caused by DSS have been reported. Interestingly, Miyazawa et al. [23] showed that DSS caused disruption of biological mechanisms

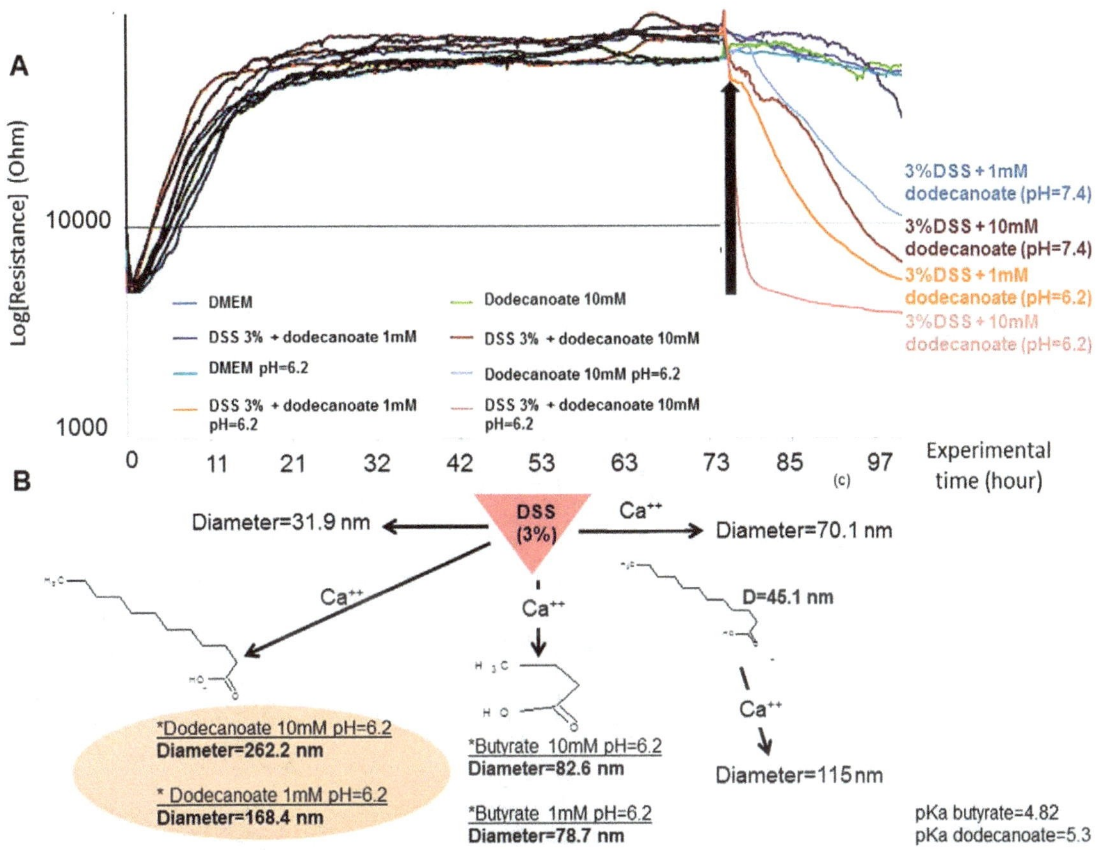

Figure 7. DSS and fatty acids form nano-lipocomplexes that disrupt Caco2-BBE monolayer resistance. (A) Confluent cultures were obtained after 48 h of growth and epithelial resistance was assessed by continuous resistance measurement at pH 7.4 (cellular pH) or pH 6.2 (colonic pH). The epithelial resistances of cultures treated with dodecanoate alone (10 mM) or with 3% (w/v) DSS (1 or 10 mM dodecanoate), at pH 6.2 or pH 7.4, were assessed by ECIS. (B) Light scattering measurement of the diameters (nm) of particles formed by DSS (3% w/v) alone; DSS (3% w/v) with Ca^{++} (1 mM); and DSS (3% w/v) with Ca^{++} (1 mM) and butyrate (1 or 10 mM) or dodecanoate (1 or 10 mM).

(such as inhibitory effects on reverse transcriptase activities that affect major cellular functions), competing with poly(U) to this end [23]. Previously, it was shown that dextran sulfate inhibited ribonuclease action [24,25]. Other natural and synthetic polyanionic polymers play important roles in establishing the association of mRNA with ribosomes and can disturb mRNA translation [23].

DSS associated with fatty acids disrupts Caco2-BBE monolayer resistance

Using ECIS, we showed that 3% (w/v) DSS did not affect *in vitro* intestinal barrier function (Figure 4). We also checked that the supplementation of the medium with 5% fetal bovine serum (FBS) had no effect on the epithelial barrier disruption (data not shown). Next, we investigated the effects of fatty acids (dodecanoate and butyrate salts) on the ability of DSS to disrupt *in vitro* intestinal barrier function. Caco2-BBE monolayer resistance in DMEM at pH 7.4 (cellular pH) and pH 6.2 (colonic pH) was assessed by ECIS. Butyrate did not significantly affect resistance (data not shown). As shown in Figure 7A, dodecanoate alone (10 mM) had no effect on epithelial resistance. However, addition of 3% (w/v) DSS supplemented with dodecanoate (10 mM, pH 6.2) to Caco2-BBE monolayers caused a rapid decrease (89%) in monolayer resistance, from 47,790 Ω to 5,420 Ω after 3 h (Figure 7A). Interestingly, under the same conditions but at pH 7.4, a slower and smaller decrease in resistance was observed (a 77% decrease after 23 h). This may be explained by variation in the hydrophobicity of vesicles at pH 7.4 and pH 6.2. Vesicles at pH 6.2 carry fewer negative charges than at pH 7.4 and can therefore engage in a higher level of interaction with the plasma membrane, which is generally negatively charged.

Next, we explored whether a mixture of DSS and fatty acids could form vesicles. DSS mixed with dodecanoate but not butyrate, in the presence of calcium, formed nanometer-sized vesicles (Figure 7B) 262 nm and 168 nm in diameter, respectively, when dodecanoate was used at 10 mM and 1 mM. No other DSS/fatty acid combination tested formed vesicles. Smaller vesicles were formed when DSS was complexed with calcium only (diameter 70 nm) or butyrate only (115 nm). Our data suggest that DSS (likely via the sulfate groups) engages in electrostatic interactions with carboxylate groups of medium or long fatty acids, involving bridging by Ca^{++} ions. Once vesicles are formed, they fuse with cell membranes and deliver DSS into the cytoplasm.

Dextran-loaded nanoparticles induce colitis

We thus showed that DSS/dodecanoate formed nanometer-sized vesicles taken up by Caco2-BBE monolayers. We speculated that the limiting step in *in vivo* colitis development induced by DSS was formation of nanometric vesicles via association of DSS and fatty acids. As dextran-loaded lipid vesicles are difficult to deliver to the colon, we decided to investigate the effects of dextran-loaded

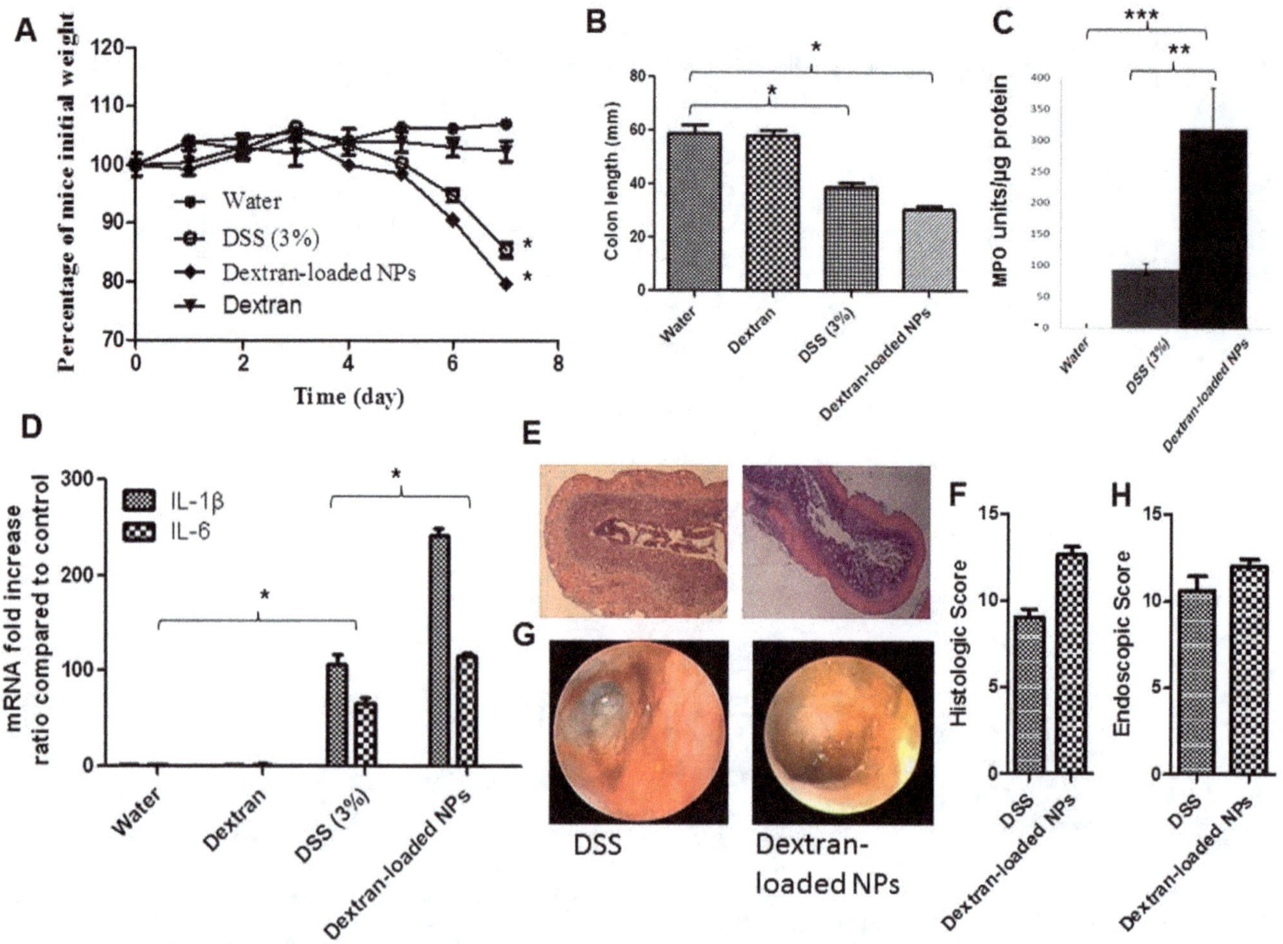

Figure 8. Dextran-loaded nanoparticles but not free dextran induce colitis. Mouse body weight changes during treatment with DSS supplemented with dextran-loaded NPs ("dextran-loaded NPs") or empty NPs ("DSS 3%") compared to those of control mice gavaged with empty NPs suspended in water. C57BL/6 mice drank a 3% (w/v) DSS solution, or water, for the indicated numbers of days. (A) Body weight changes are shown as means±SEMs. * $P<0.05$. (B) Colon length (mm) of DSS-treated mice given dextran-loaded or empty NPs, compared to that of control animals (drinking water only). * $P<0.05$. (C) Determination of MPO enzymatic activity as an index of neutrophil infiltration into injured tissue. Results are expressed as units of MPO per µg of protein, are compared to the values in control mice, and are means±SEMs of three independent determinations. ** $P<0.01$, *** $P<0.001$. (D) Dextran-loaded NPs can significantly increase production of IL-1β and IL-6, compared to use of empty NPs, in animals drinking DSS (3% w/v). mRNA expression was measured in test and control animals. * $P<0.05$. (E) Hematoxylin-stained colon sections of mice receiving daily gavage with dextran-loaded or empty NPs ("DSS") in the interval during which the drinking water contained DSS (3% w/v); thus on day 7. (F) Histological scores. (G) Macroscopic inflammation was assessed using a mouse colonoscope. Photographs were obtained on the day of sacrifice and, (H), endoscopic scores were calculated.

nanoparticles (NPs) *in vivo*. In previous studies, we have shown that we can deliver such NPs into the colon [39,40,42,46]. We chose to deliver dextran to the colon because dextran does not form vesicles in the presence of dodecanoate and does not induce colitis *in vivo*. We found that dextran-loaded NPs, but not free dextran, given by gavage over 8 days, increased measures of inflammatory parameters, such as weight loss (at day 7, 23% for mice given dextran-loaded NPs versus 17% for those given 3% [w/v] DSS) (Figure 8A), decreased colon length (Figure 8B) (to 28 mm versus 38 mm for DSS-treated mice), increased MPO activity (Figure 8C) (312 MPO units/µg protein for dextran-loaded nanoparticle-treated mice versus 96 MPO units/µg protein for DSS-treated mice), and increased the levels of pro-inflammatory cytokines (Figure 8D) (2.6-fold increase in IL-1β level and a 1.5-fold increase in IL-6 level for mice treated with NPs versus DSS alone). Again, all of these observations were confirmed by histology and endoscopy (Figures 8E and 8F). Finally, induction of colitis was more severe using dextran-loaded NPs compared to DSS alone (Figure 8A to 8H). The results suggest that dextran may be the active motif of the DSS molecule in terms of induction of colitis.

Discussion

During DSS treatment, inflammation is enhanced, as shown by rises in the extent of diarrhea and rectal bleeding. Colonic inflammation is also characterized by severe lesions throughout the mucosa, alteration of epithelial structure, high-level neutrophil and lymphocyte infiltration into the mucosal and submucosal areas, and loss of crypts. We explored how DSS, a negatively charged polymer of glucose with engrafted sulfate groups, induces colitis in mice. We tested different components of the molecule of DSS such as glucose, sulfate sodium, dextran and association of each. DSS-associated molecules had no proinflammatory effects. We did not observe any signs of inflammation (loss of barrier functions, apoptosis, etc.) *in vitro* in Caco2-BBE monolayer cells nor during *in vivo* study. Conversely, we showed that a high-fat diet increases the efficacy by which DSS induces colitis in mice. From those observations, we tested the effect of DSS on Caco2-BBE monolayer cells but with cell medium containing MCFAs (C12). We showed the ability of DSS associated with MCFAs to disrupt *in vitro* intestinal barrier function whereas butyrate (small chain fatty acid) did not significantly affect resistance. Next, we showed that DSS mixed with dodecanoate but not butyrate, in the presence of calcium, formed nanometer-sized vesicles.

It has been shown in the literature that claudins have significant interaction with MCFAs, and so could be involved in the "transport" of DSS through the epithelium, explaining the loss of membrane integrity shown in our article. *In vivo*, several MCFAs, particularly capric (C10) and lauric (C12) acids, have been shown to increase rectal drug absorption, presumably by causing alterations in intestinal TJ barrier function. C10 has also been shown to lead to profound alterations in the barrier function of the TJ and has been investigated as an agent to enhance viral-mediated gene transfer [27].

Conclusion

In the present study we have made progress toward elucidating the mechanism of action of DSS in terms of induction of colitis. Our findings suggest that DSS associates with medium-chain-length fatty acids (MCFAs) such as dodecanoate in the colonic lumen prior to induction of colitis. Interestingly, it is known that MCFAs are present at high concentrations in the colonic lumen and that the colonic epithelium absorbs and partially metabolizes MCFAs [47]. DSS complexed to MCFAs form nanometer-sized vesicles ~200 nm in diameter that fuse with colonocyte membranes. The arrival of such vesicles in the cytoplasm affects major epithelial cell pathways and consequently reduces intestinal barrier functions that initiate intestinal inflammatory signaling cascades. We also suggest that the inflammatory activity of DSS is afforded by the dextran moiety. This idea is supported by the fact that, when dextran is delivered to the cytoplasm, intestinal inflammatory signaling pathways are activated. The deleterious activity of dextran may be explained by the molecule having an inhibitory effect on reverse transcriptase activities that affect major cellular functions. The deleterious effects of DSS are targeted principally to the distal colon. It will be useful to chemically modify DSS molecules, rendering the molecule beneficial to the colon, without affecting targeting specificity.

Acknowledgments

We dedicate this article to the memory of Dr. Shanthi V. Sitaraman, a brilliant scientist, dedicated physician, passionate humanitarian and dearest friend.

Author Contributions

Conceived and designed the experiments: HL DM SVS. Performed the experiments: HL SAI SVS FL HL YY MAC. Analyzed the data: HL DM SVS. Contributed reagents/materials/analysis tools: HL DM SVS. Wrote the paper: HL DM. Proof read the manuscript: MB SA.

References

1. Orholm M, Munkholm P, Langholz E, Nielsen OH, Sorensen TI, et al. (1991) Familial occurrence of inflammatory bowel disease. N Engl J Med 324: 84–88.
2. Lowe AM, Roy PO, M BP, Michel P, Bitton A, et al. (2009) Epidemiology of Crohn's disease in Quebec, Canada. Inflamm Bowel Dis 15: 429–435.
3. Brant SR (2011) Update on the heritability of inflammatory bowel disease: the importance of twin studies. Inflamm Bowel Dis 17: 1–5.
4. Skewis LR, Reinhard BM (2010) Control of colloid surface chemistry through matrix confinement: facile preparation of stable antibody functionalized silver nanoparticles. ACS applied materials & interfaces 2: 35–40.
5. Riva G, Wiederhold BK, Mantovani F, Gaggioli A (2011) Interreality: the experiential use of technology in the treatment of obesity. Clinical practice and epidemiology in mental health : CP & EMH 7: 51–61.
6. Schlitt HJ, Mornex F, Shaked A, Trotter JF (2011) Immunosuppression and hepatocellular carcinoma. Liver transplantation: official publication of the American Association for the Study of Liver Diseases and the International Liver Transplantation Society.
7. Magitta NF, Pura M, Wolff ASB, Vanuga P, Meager A, et al. (2008) Autoimmune polyendocrine syndrome type I in Slovakia: relevance of screening patients with autoimmune Addison's disease. European journal of endocrinology/European Federation of Endocrine Societies 158: 705–709.
8. Hu Y, Mak JF, Lu WW, Cheung KM, Luk KD (2004) Visualization of lumbar muscle contraction synergy using surface electromyography (sEMG) streaming topography. Conference proceedings : Annual International Conference of the IEEE Engineering in Medicine and Biology Society IEEE Engineering in Medicine and Biology Society Conference 3: 2337–2340.
9. Walsh DA, McWilliams DF (2006) Tachykinins and the cardiovascular system. Current drug targets 7: 1031–1042.
10. Pinho RA, Silveira PC, Silva LA, Luiz Streck E, Dal-Pizzol F, et al. (2005) N-acetylcysteine and deferoxamine reduce pulmonary oxidative stress and inflammation in rats after coal dust exposure. Environmental research 99: 355–360.
11. Toth G, R FM, Lovas S (2001) Stabilization of local structures by pi-CH and aromatic-backbone amide interactions involving prolyl and aromatic residues. Protein engineering 14: 543–547.
12. Miyazawa F, Olijnyk OR, Tilley CJ, Tamaoki T (1967) Interactions between dextran sulfate and Escherichia coli ribosomes. Biochimica et biophysica acta 145: 96–104.
13. Nakamura T, Katori R, Watanabe T, Miyazawa K, Murai M, et al. (1967) Quantitation of left-to-right shunt from a single earpiece dye-dilution curve. Journal of applied physiology 22: 1156–1160.
14. Nakamura T, Katori R, Miyazawa K, Oda J, Ishikawa K (1967) Measurement of bronchial blood flow in tetralogy of Fallot. Circulation 35: 904–912.
15. Yan Y, Kolachala V, Dalmasso G, Nguyen H, Laroui H, et al. (2009) Temporal and spatial analysis of clinical and molecular parameters in dextran sodium sulfate induced colitis. PLoS One 4: e6073.
16. Rogler G, Andus T (1998) Cytokines in inflammatory bowel disease. World J Surg 22: 382–389.
17. Kennedy RJ, Hoper M, Deodhar K, Erwin PJ, Kirk SJ, et al. (2000) Interleukin 10-deficient colitis: new similarities to human inflammatory bowel disease. Br J Surg 87: 1346–1351.
18. Steidler L, Hans W, Schotte L, Neirynck S, Obermeier F, et al. (2000) Treatment of murine colitis by Lactococcus lactis secreting interleukin-10. Science 289: 1352–1355.
19. Hofstetter C, Kleen M, Habler O, Allmeling AM, Krombach F, et al. (1998) Recombinant human interleukin-10 attenuates TNFalpha production by porcine monocytes. Eur J Med Res 3: 299–303.
20. Cooper HS, Murthy SN, Shah RS, Sedergran DJ (1993) Clinicopathologic study of dextran sulfate sodium experimental murine colitis. Lab Invest 69: 238–249.
21. Cooper HS, Murthy SN, Shah RS, Sedergran DJ (1993) Clinicopathologic study of dextran sulfate sodium experimental murine colitis. Laboratory investigation; a journal of technical methods and pathology 69: 238–249.
22. Dignass A, Preiss JC, Aust DE, Autschbach F, Ballauff A, et al. (2011) [Updated German Guideline on Diagnosis and Treatment of Ulcerative Colitis, 2011.]. Zeitschrift fur Gastroenterologie 49: 1276–1341.
23. Miyazawa F, Olijnyk OR, Tilley CJ, Tamaoki T (1967) Interactions between dextran sulfate and Escherichia coli ribosomes. Biochim Biophys Acta 145: 96–104.
24. Fellig J, Wiley CE (1959) The inhibition of pancreatic ribonuclease by anionic polymers. Arch Biochem Biophys 85: 313–316.
25. Philipson L, Zetterqvist O (1964) The Presence of DNA in Human Erythrocyte Membranes. Biochim Biophys Acta 91: 171–173.
26. Kim IW, Myung SJ, Do MY, Ryu YM, Kim MJ, et al. (2010) Western-style diets induce macrophage infiltration and contribute to colitis-associated carcinogenesis. Journal of gastroenterology and hepatology 25: 1785–1794.
27. Coyne CB, Kelly MM, Boucher RC, Johnson LG (2000) Enhanced epithelial gene transfer by modulation of tight junctions with sodium caprate. American journal of respiratory cell and molecular biology 23: 602–609.
28. Lindmark T, Nikkila T, Artursson P (1995) Mechanisms of absorption enhancement by medium chain fatty acids in intestinal epithelial Caco-2 cell monolayers. The Journal of pharmacology and experimental therapeutics 275: 958–964.
29. Lindmark T, Soderholm JD, Olaison G, Alvan G, Ocklind G, et al. (1997) Mechanism of absorption enhancement in humans after rectal administration of ampicillin in suppositories containing sodium caprate. Pharmaceutical research 14: 930–935.
30. Tomita M, Hayashi M, Awazu S (1995) Absorption-enhancing mechanism of sodium caprate and decanoylcarnitine in Caco-2 cells. The Journal of pharmacology and experimental therapeutics 272: 739–743.
31. Tomita M, Hayashi M, Awazu S (1996) Absorption-enhancing mechanism of EDTA, caprate, and decanoylcarnitine in Caco-2 cells. Journal of pharmaceutical sciences 85: 608–611.

32. Andoh A, Bamba T, Sasaki M (1999) Physiological and anti-inflammatory roles of dietary fiber and butyrate in intestinal functions. JPEN Journal of parenteral and enteral nutrition 23: S70–73.
33. Venkatraman A, Ramakrishna BS, Pulimood AB, Patra S, Murthy S (2000) Increased permeability in dextran sulphate colitis in rats: time course of development and effect of butyrate. Scandinavian journal of gastroenterology 35: 1053–1059.
34. Venkatraman A, Ramakrishna BS, Shaji RV, Kumar NS, Pulimood A, et al. (2003) Amelioration of dextran sulfate colitis by butyrate: role of heat shock protein 70 and NF-kappaB. American journal of physiology Gastrointestinal and liver physiology 285: G177–184.
35. Vieira EL, Leonel AJ, Sad AP, Beltrao NR, Costa TF, et al. (2011) Oral administration of sodium butyrate attenuates inflammation and mucosal lesion in experimental acute ulcerative colitis. The Journal of nutritional biochemistry.
36. Charrier L, Yan Y, Driss A, Laboisse CL, Sitaraman SV, et al. (2005) ADAM-15 inhibits wound healing in human intestinal epithelial cell monolayers. Am J Physiol Gastrointest Liver Physiol 288: G346–353.
37. Laroui H, Grossin L, Leonard M, Stoltz JF, Gillet P, et al. (2007) Hyaluronate-covered nanoparticles for the therapeutic targeting of cartilage. Biomacromolecules 8: 3879–3885.
38. Lamprecht A, Yamamoto H, Takeuchi H, Kawashima Y (2005) A pH-sensitive microsphere system for the colon delivery of tacrolimus containing nanoparticles. J Control Release 104: 337–346.
39. Laroui H, Dalmasso G, Nguyen HT, Yan Y, Sitaraman SV, et al. (2010) Drug-loaded nanoparticles targeted to the colon with polysaccharide hydrogel reduce colitis in a mouse model. Gastroenterology 138: 843–853 e841–842.
40. Laroui H, Theiss AL, Yan Y, Dalmasso G, Nguyen HT, et al. (2011) Functional TNFalpha gene silencing mediated by polyethyleneimine/TNFalpha siRNA nanocomplexes in inflamed colon. Biomaterials 32: 1218–1228.
41. Vowinkel T, Kalogeris TJ, Mori M, Krieglstein CF, Granger DN (2004) Impact of dextran sulfate sodium load on the severity of inflammation in experimental colitis. Dig Dis Sci 49: 556–564.
42. Theiss AL, Laroui H, Obertone TS, Chowdhury I, Thompson WE, et al. (2011) Nanoparticle-based therapeutic delivery of prohibitin to the colonic epithelial cells ameliorates acute murine colitis. Inflamm Bowel Dis 17: 1163–1176.
43. Shea-Donohue T, Thomas K, Cody MJ, Aiping Z, Detolla LJ, et al. (2008) Mice deficient in the CXCR2 ligand, CXCL1 (KC/GRO-alpha), exhibit increased susceptibility to dextran sodium sulfate (DSS)-induced colitis. Innate Immun 14: 117–124.
44. te Velde AA, de Kort F, Sterrenburg E, Pronk I, ten Kate FJ, et al. (2007) Comparative analysis of colonic gene expression of three experimental colitis models mimicking inflammatory bowel disease. Inflamm Bowel Dis 13: 325–330.
45. Mitsuyama K, Tsuruta O, Tomiyasu N, Takaki K, Suzuki A, et al. (2006) Increased circulating concentrations of growth-related oncogene (GRO)-alpha in patients with inflammatory bowel disease. Dig Dis Sci 51: 173–177.
46. Laroui H, Wilson DS, Dalmasso G, Salaita K, Murthy N, et al. (2011) Nanomedicine in GI. Am J Physiol Gastrointest Liver Physiol 300: G371–383.
47. Schmidt C, Dignass A, Hartmann F, Huppe D, Kruis W, et al. (2011) [IBD Ahead 2010 - Answering Important Questions in Crohn's Disease Treatment]. Zeitschrift fur Gastroenterologie 49: 1246–1254.

6

Increased Susceptibility to Dextran Sulfate Sodium Induced Colitis in the T Cell Protein Tyrosine Phosphatase Heterozygous Mouse

Syed-Wajahat Hassan[1,2], Karen M. Doody[1,3], Serge Hardy[1], Noriko Uetani[1], Denis Cournoyer[1,2,4], Michel L. Tremblay[1,2,3]*

1 Rosalind and Morris Goodman Cancer Centre, McGill University, Montreal, Canada, **2** Department of Medicine, Division of Experimental Medicine, McGill University, Montreal, Canada, **3** Department of Biochemistry, McGill University, Montreal, Canada, **4** Department of Oncology, McGill University, Montreal, Canada

Abstract

T cell protein tyrosine phosphatase (TC-PTP / PTPN2) is an enzyme that is essential for the proper functioning of the immune system and that participates in the control of cell proliferation, and inflammation. We previously observed that TC-PTP$^{-/-}$ mice display various immunodeficiencies, hypersensitivity to LPS and die within three weeks of birth due to anemia and widespread inflammation. A recent analysis of the Wellcome Trust Case Control Consortium (WTCC) genome wide scan data, reported in 2007, indicated a potential role for TC-PTP in inflammatory bowel disease (IBD). To further investigate the potential role of TC-PTP in IBD, we studied heterozygous TC-PTP mutant mice challenged with dextran sulfate sodium (DSS) in their drinking water. In comparison to control animals, we observed significant changes in the colon mucosa of DSS-treated TC-PTP$^{+/-}$ mice, in the ratio of colon to body weight, as well as an up-regulation of mRNA transcripts for IL-6, IL-23, 1L-12β, IFN-γ, TNF-α. Moreover, up-regulation of serum IL-6 levels in DSS-treated TC-PTP$^{+/-}$ mice confirms that mice with a single copy of the TC-PTP gene display increased susceptibility to systemic inflammation due to bowel epithelial erosion resulting from DSS challenge. Our findings support the lack of modulation of Janus kinases 1 and 3 (Jak1, Jak3), and the downstream signal transducer and activator of transcription 1,3 and 5 (Stat1, Stat3, Stat 5) by PTPN2 in the development of IBD like condition. Pathological and molecular analysis reveal that the deficiency of TC-PTP results in pro-inflammatory condition in the bowel of heterozygous TC-PTP$^{+/-}$ mice. These novel findings in TC-PTP hemi-deficiency support the hypothesis that TC-PTP is an important regulator of inflammatory cytokine signaling and that it may be implicated in the pathophysiology of IBD.

Editor: Derya Unutmaz, New York University, United States of America

Funding: This work has been supported by the Canadian Cancer Society (NCIC#015200) grant to MLT. The funders had no role in study design, data collection and analysis, decision to publish, or preparation of the manuscript.

Competing Interests: The authors have declared that no competing interests exist.

* E-mail: michel.tremblay@mcgill.ca

Introduction

Ulcerative colitis and Crohn's disease are the main two types of inflammatory bowel disease (IBD). Colitis is a well established risk factor for the development of colorectal cancer, the 3rd leading cause of cancer in North America in both men and women with respect to both the incidence rate and estimated death rates [1,2]. IBD is associated with both colitis and ileitis. [1,3–7]. The cause(s) of colitis in IBD remains unknown, although many theories have been proposed, and links with genetic loci have been postulated. Individuals with IBD tend to have abnormalities of the immune system. More than 1 million Americans and more than 2 millions Europeans suffer from IBD [1]. Crohn's Disease, the 3rd ranking disease in a genome-wide association study performed by the Wellcome Trust Case Control Consortium (WTCC) in 2007 [2], was found associated with a SNP in a region of chromosome 18p11 with the only gene lying in this region being *PTPN2*, the encoding locus for the T-cell protein tyrosine phosphatase (TC-PTP) [2]. Moreover, other recent genetic studies have also shown links between IBD and the TC-PTP (*PTPN2*) locus [1–7].

TC-PTP is a classical non-receptor protein tyrosine phosphatase that can regulate pro-inflammatory cytokine signaling [8]. *PTPN2*-knockout mice have altered hematopoiesis affecting several lineages [9] and develop severe inflammation within two weeks of birth [8–11]. TC-PTP was one of the first members of the PTP gene family identified. Although originally cloned from a T cell cDNA library, it is ubiquitously expressed at all stages of mammalian development and in most embryonic and adult tissues [12]. The mouse isoform of TC-PTP was later cloned in 1992 [13]. *PTPN2* is located on chromosomal region 18p11.2–11.3 in humans and in a syntenic region in mice [14]. The 45 kDa form of TC-PTP (45 kDa) contains a nuclear localization signal N-terminal to its catalytic domain, and is encoded by the main detectable splice form in mice [13].

The systemic inflammation in TC-PTP$^{-/-}$ mice and various genetic studies focusing on the association of the *PTPN2* locus with IBD led to the hypothesis that the absence of the enzymatic activity or decreased expression of TC-PTP may play a role in many chronic inflammatory conditions. We evaluated the role of TC-PTP as a modulator of inflammation in IBD relevant conditions *in vivo*, using a dextran sulfate sodium (DSS)-induced colitis mouse model. DSS causes direct damage to the epithelial barrier of the colon leading to cellular dysfunction, impaired epithelial repair and altered epithelial barrier [15,16]. We compared TC-PTP $^{+/-}$ and wild-type mice treated with dextran sulfate sodium verses non-treated controls [15,16]. We observed that TC-PTP $^{+/-}$ mice were more sensitive to DSS treatment than TC-PTP$^{+/+}$ mice as shown by histopathological alterations of large bowel, increased cytokine expression in serum and cytokine signaling in the large bowel. Heterozygosity of TC-PTP may thus prime the immune system to respond more readily to irritants such as DSS resulting in a more severe inflammatory condition. This may partially explain the association of TC-PTP with chronic inflammatory diseases such as IBD [1–7]. TC-PTP is a key modulator in inflammation, and by detecting or controlling its expression or downstream events we may open new avenues in the diagnosis and treatments of inflammatory bowel diseases like colitis.

Results

Increased Weight Loss and Decreased Colon Weight of TC-PTP $^{+/-}$ Mice during DSS-Induced Colitis

To evaluate the role of TC-PTP in bowel inflammation, we treated wild type (WT) and heterozygous TC-PTP $^{+/-}$ mice with DSS to induce colitis. We compared four groups of animals: DSS-treated TC-PTP $^{+/-}$ and TC-PTP$^{+/+}$ mice, and non-treated TC-PTP $^{+/-}$ and TC-PTP$^{+/+}$ mice. TC-PTP$^{-/-}$ mice were not subjected to DSS-treatment as they die shortly after weaning [8–11] and cannot live long enough to complete the course of DSS treatment. However, untreated TC-PTP$^{-/-}$ mice were used as controls in some experiments.

We observed a significant decrease in the body weight of DSS-treated TC-PTP$^{+/-}$ mice compared to DSS-treated TC-PTP$^{+/+}$ mice (*$p<0.001$). In addition there was a decrease in body weight in DSS-treated TC-PTP $^{+/-}$ mice, throughout the course of DSS treatment, in comparison to non-treated TC-PTP $^{+/-}$ (*$p<0.001$) and TC-PTP$^{+/+}$ (***$p<0.0002$) (Figure 1A). Furthermore the ratio of colon to body weight of DSS-treated TC-PTP$^{+/-}$ mice was significantly lower than those of DSS-treated TC-PTP$^{+/+}$ mice (* $p<0.05$) (Figure 1B). Similarly, a significant decrease in colon to body weight ratio was observed in DSS-treated TC-PTP$^{+/-}$ mice in comparison to non-treated TC-PTP$^{+/-}$ mice (*** $p<0.001$), as well as in DSS-treated TC-PTP$^{+/+}$ compared to non-treated TC-PTP$^{+/+}$ mice (*** $p<0.001$).

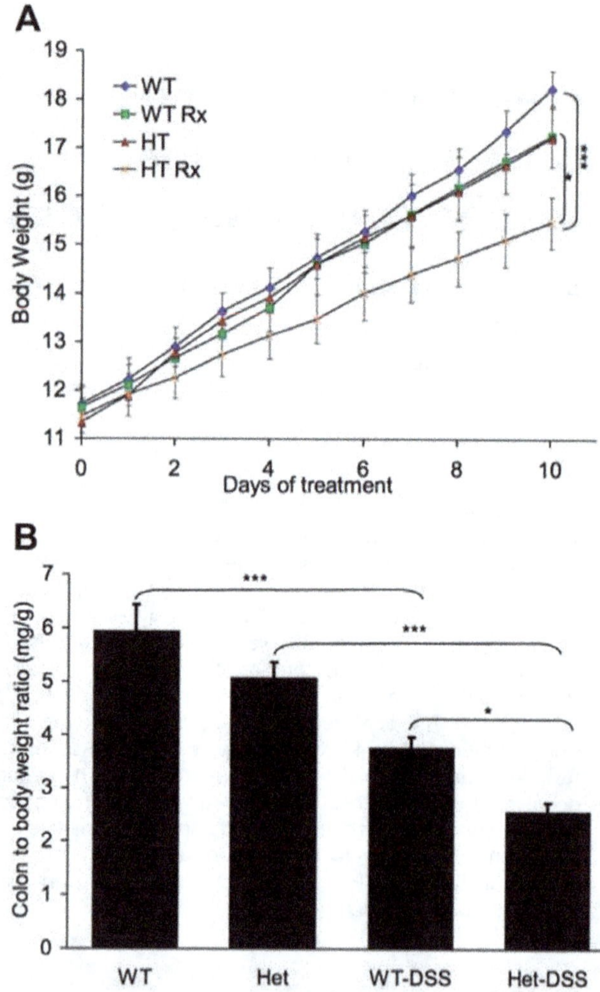

Figure 1. Increased response to DSS treatment in the presence of only one allele of TC-PTP. A. Increased weight loss of TC-PTP $^{+/-}$ mice during DSS-induced colitis. At 19 days of age mouse body weight was 11–12 g followed by DSS treatment. Body weight of DSS-treated TC-PTP $^{+/-}$ (Het-DSS) (2.58±0.4) mice were significantly lower than, TC-PTP$^{+/-}$ (Het) (5.0±0.8) and TC-PTP$^{+/+}$ (WT-DSS) (3.78±0.5) mice ***$p<0.0002$. DSS-treated TC-PTP$^{+/-}$ mice compared to DSS-treated TC-PTP$^{+/+}$ mice *$p<0.001$. Data represent the mean of three groups of three animals each (N = 9). **B.** Ratio of colon weight of DSS-treated TC-PTP $^{+/-}$ (Het-DSS) mice were significantly lower than DSS-treated TC-PTP$^{+/+}$ (WT-DSS) mice $p<0.05$. In the case of TC-PTP$^{+/-}$ (Het) vs. DSS-treated TC-PTP$^{+/-}$ (WT-DSS) mice $p<0.001$, and $p<0.001$ in comparison of TC-PTP$^{+/+}$ vs. DSS-treated TC-PTP$^{+/+}$ mice.

DSS-Treated TC-PTP$^{+/-}$ Colons Display Histological Alterations and Elevation of Peripheral Blood Lymphocytes and Neutrophils

To further investigate the phenotypes seen in DSS-treated TC-PTP heterozygous mice, we evaluated the degree of inflammatory activity by histo-pathological examination of the colons from animals with the different genotypes. Colon tissue sections on WT controls demonstrated normal crypt parallelism and intact surface epithelium (Figure 2A, B and C). Tissues collected from DSS-treated mice demonstrated crypt distortion and neutrophilic infiltration (Figure 2A, B and C). Alterations in morphology during colonic injury in DSS-treated TC-PTP$^{+/-}$ mice compared to DSS-treated TC-PTP$^{+/+}$, non-treated TC-PTP$^{+/-}$ and non-treated TC-PTP$^{+/+}$ mice showed significant increase in epithelial erosion and crypt damage, as shown in (Figure 2C). Colons from DSS-treated TC-PTP$^{+/-}$ mice also showed significantly more pronounced decrease in number of crypts ($p<0.001$), crypt width ($p<0.003$), crypt height ($p<0.005$) and epithelial height ($p<0.0002$) as compared to DSS-treated TC-PTP$^{+/+}$, as shown in Figure 2C. Histo-pathological scoring for assessment of inflammatory changes was 32 out of a maximum of 40 in DSS-treated TC-PTP $^{+/-}$ mice, compared to 12 in DSS-treated TC-PTP$^{+/+}$, ($p<0.0003$), as shown in Figure 3B. Likewise, differential peripheral white blood cell counts revealed a significant increase in lymphocyte ($p<0.0114$) and neutrophils ($p<0.0001$) counts in DSS-treated TC-PTP $^{+/-}$ mice compared to DSS-treated TC-PTP$^{+/+}$ (Figure 3A).

Hyperactivation of STAT and JAKs in TC-PTP$^{+/-}$ Colon upon DSS-Treatment

Key signaling molecules involved in the inflammatory process includes the janus kinases (Jaks) and the downstream effectors signal transducers and activators of transcription (STATs). Since

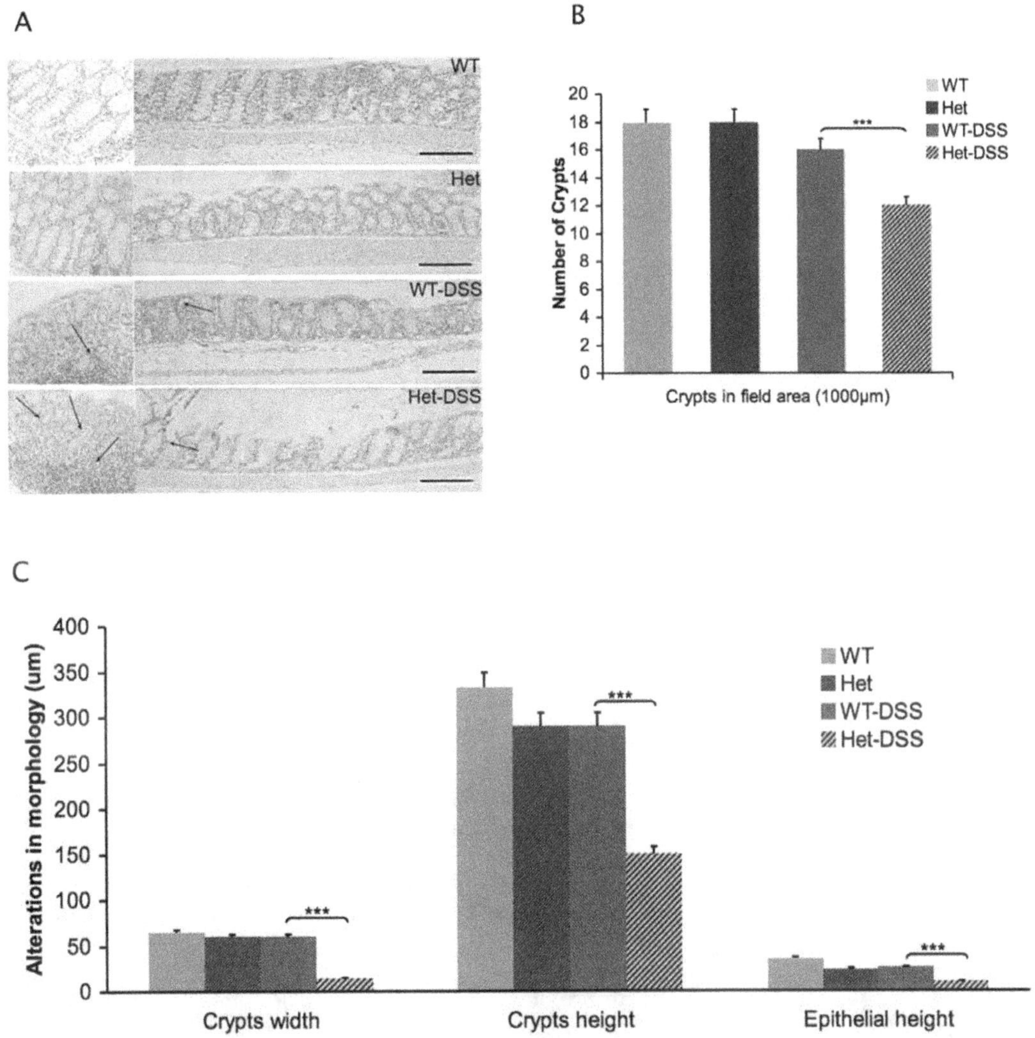

Figure 2. Loss of colorectal crypt-villi. A. Histopathological features of the mouse colon in association with colitis. Bar = 1000 μm. From top to bottom: TC-PTP$^{+/+}$(WT), TC-PTP$^{+/-}$ (Het), DSS-treated TC-PTP$^{+/+}$(WT-DSS) and DSS-treated TC-PTP$^{+/-}$ (Het-DSS). In TC-PTP$^{+/+}$(WT) crypts are straight and the base of the glands reach the muscularis mucosae. Crypt-villus axes are normal and epithelium layer is intact. In DSS-treated TC-PTP$^{+/-}$ (Het-DSS) mice ingestion of DSS caused crypt destruction, Numerous neutrophils were present in the section (arrows). Loss of the surface epithelial layer is obvious, while changes in crypt-villus axis and colon tissue architecture are observed. **B.** The number of crypts per field, field is 1000 μm in colorectal section of bowel. The number of crypts in DSS-treated TC-PTP$^{+/-}$ (Het-DSS) mice were significantly lower than DSS-treated TC-PTP$^{+/+}$ (WT-DSS) mice $p<0.002$. **C.** Crypts in field, crypts width, crypts height and epithelial height were quantified. Data represent mean and SD of three groups of three animal each (N = 9).

TC-PTP has been shown to be a major regulator of this pathway, and given that DSS-induced colitis is known to trigger inflammation in the bowel and activate these pathways [8–11], we examined the phosphorylation status of various Jaks and STATs in colonic cells from mice of various TC-PTP genotypes challenged with DSS treatment. Hence, bowel sections were isolated for immunoblotting. DSS treatment in TC-PTP$^{+/-}$ mice results in hyper-phosphorylation of JAK1, JAK3, STAT1, STAT3 and STAT5 while there was a decrease in JAK2 activity (Figure 4). Interestingly, both TC-PTP$^{+/+}$ and TC-PTP$^{+/-}$ mice showed a decrease in protein levels of TC-PTP in the bowel following DSS treatment with levels being at the limit of detection by Western blotting in treated TC-PTP$^{+/-}$ mice.

Up-Regulation of Pro-Inflammatory Cytokines in the Colon of DSS-Treated TC-PTP $^{+/-}$ Mice

Since there was hyper-activation of several STATs and JAKs mediators, we measured the expression of several corresponding downstream pro-inflammatory cytokines using RT-PCR. Colonic extracts from heterozygous TC-PTP mice treated with DSS showed up-regulation of TNFα, IFNγ, IL-12 β, IL-23R and IL-6 (Figure 5). Levels of these cytokines were significantly higher in DSS-treated TC-PTP$^{+/-}$ mice and untreated TC-PTP$^{-/-}$ (KO, used as a control) mice compared to WT mice, TC-PTP$^{+/-}$ (DSS non treated) and WT (DSS-treated).

Based on published evidence that Jaks and STAT pathways negatively regulate inflammatory bowel diseases like colitis in Crohn's disease and ulcerative coloitis [1–7], we pursued the possibility that DSS treatment was also initiating systemic inflammation in TC-PTP$^{+/-}$ mice. Therefore, we measured the levels of IL-6, IL-12p40, IFN-γ and TNF-α in the serum of DSS-treated TC-PTP $^{+/-}$ and TC-PTP$^{+/+}$ mice as well as non-treated control animals. Of the cytokines analyzed, we were able to detect a 4.2-fold increase in serum IL-6 concentration in the TC-PTP$^{+/-}$ mice treated with DSS compared to TC-PTP$^{+/+}$ mice treated with DSS ($p<0.05$) (Figure 6).

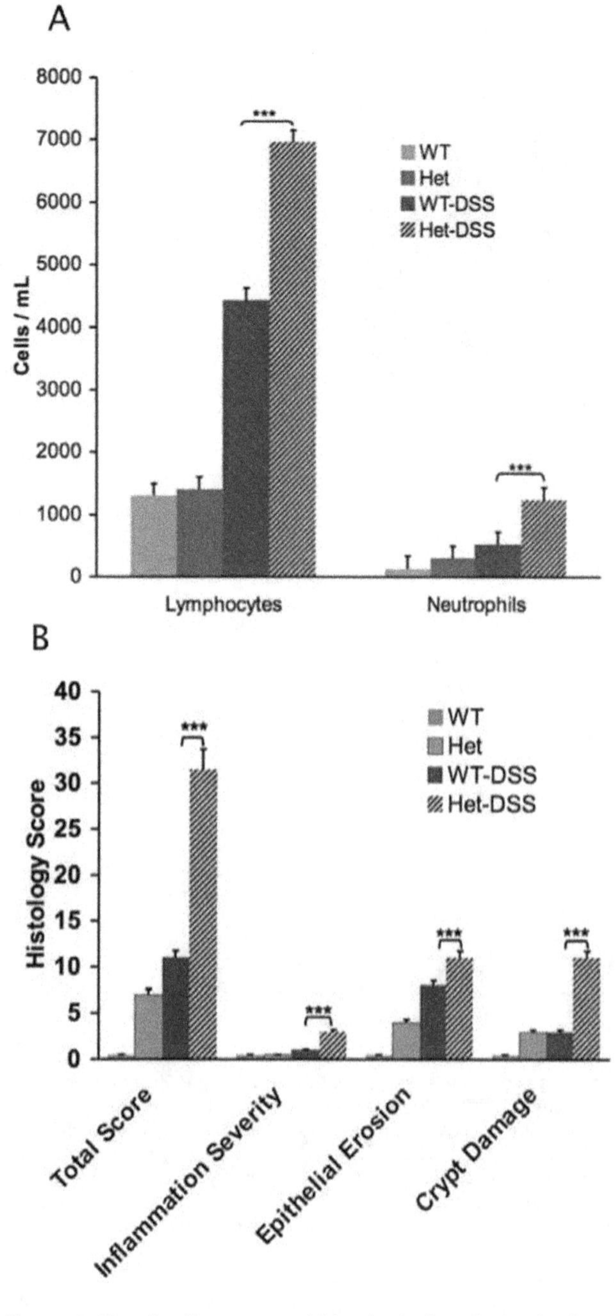

Figure 3. Blood cell counts and histological analysis of colons. **A.** Increase in numbers of lymphocytes $p<0.0114$ and neutrophils $p<0.0001$ in DSS-treated TC-PTP $^{+/-}$ mice compared to DSS-treated TC-PTP$^{+/+}$. **B.** The mean histology activity scores of colon tissue sections of TC-PTP$^{+/+}$(WT) (0.3 ± 0.34), TC-PTP$^{+/-}$ (Het) (7 ± 0.55), DSS-treated TC-PTP$^{+/+}$(WT-DSS) (12 ± 0.48) and DSS-treated TC-PTP$^{+/-}$(Het-DSS) (32 ± 0.67) mice. Analysis was performed blinded by pathologist on a scale from 0 to 40 (see Methods).

Discussion

Much effort has recently been invested in identifying new associations between gene expression and complex disease traits such as in IBD. Recently, the Wellcome Trust Case Control Consortium and other groups identified SNPs associated with IBD in close proximity to the TC-PTP locus [1–7]. Given these results, and the systemic inflammatory phenotype identified in

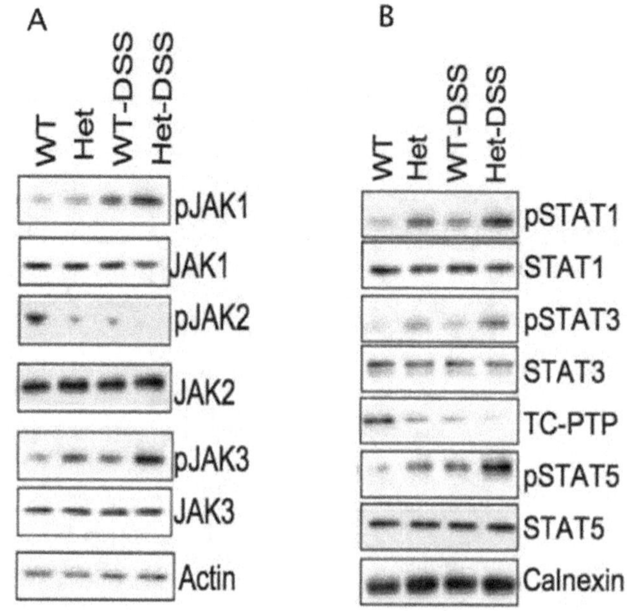

Figure 4. Jak/Stat signaling pathways. Immunoblotting was used to observe total protein levels and protein phosphorylation levels of JAK1, JAK3, STAT1, STAT3 and STAT5.

TC-PTP$^{-/-}$ mice [8], we used a well established model of experimental colitis to study the role of TC-PTP in bowel inflammation. Since the homozygous TC-PTP$^{-/-}$ phenotype is lethal at approximately 3 weeks of age, we focused our efforts on the hemizygous TC-PTP knock-out animals [8]. The gene dosage reduction of TC-PTP enzyme in heterozygous mice was associated with an increased susceptibility to DSS-induced colitis. DSS-treated TC-PTP$^{+/-}$ mice lost more body and bowel weight than control animals (Figure 1). They showed more pronounced decrease in number, height and width of colonic crypts (Figure 2), and higher histo-pathological scoring of colonic inflammatory changes (Figure 3). Also, DSS-treatment in TC-PTP$^{+/-}$ mice was found to result in colonic hyper-phosphorylation of the transduction pathway mediators JAK1, JAK3, STAT1, STAT3 and

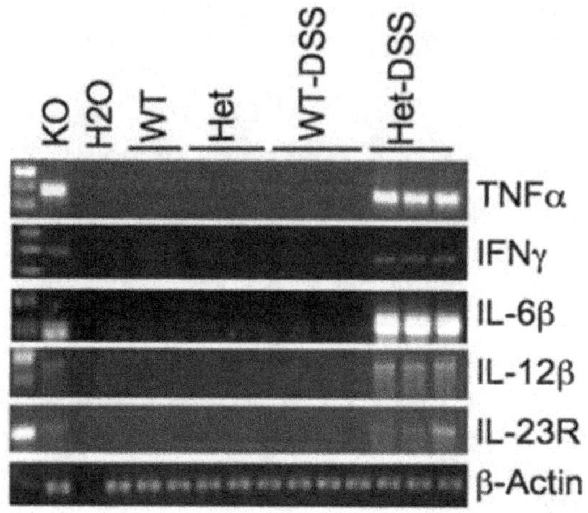

Figure 5. Colonic up-regulation of cytokines mRNA expression. DSS-treated TC-PTP$^{+/-}$(Het-DSS) mice showed up-regulation of TNFα, IFNγ, IL-12 β, IL-23R and IL-6. Untreated TC-PTP$^{-/-}$ (null) mouse colon mRNA was used as a control.

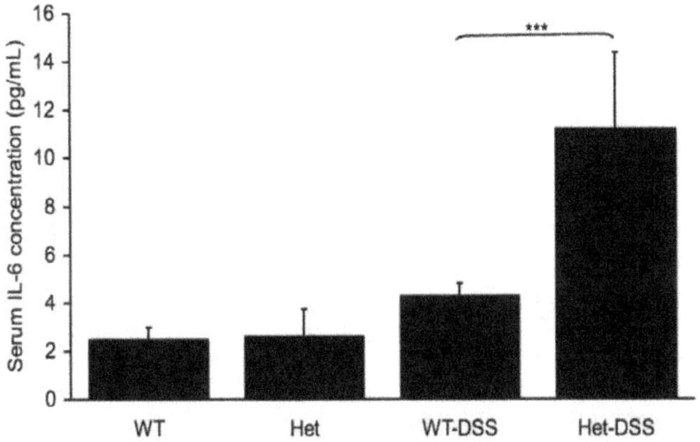

Figure 6. IL-6 serum level in DSS-treated and control mice. Serum was collected at the time of euthanasia and analyzed for cytokine levels using Mouse Cytokine Multiplex Assay. A 4.2-fold increase in serum IL-6 concentration in the TC-PTP$^{+/-}$(Het-DSS) (11.6±7.6 pg/ml) compared to TC-PTP$^{+/+}$ (WT-DSS) (2.6±2.4 pg/ml) mice ($p<0.05$).

STAT5, and further decrease in TC-PTP protein levels (Figure 4), as well as up-regulation of mRNA transcripts for TNFα, IFNγ, IL-12 β, IL-23R and IL-6 (Figure 5). Systemically, we detected a significant increase in peripheral blood lymphocyte and neutrophil counts (Figure 3) and a significant increase in serum IL-6 concentration in the DSS-treated TC-PTP$^{+/-}$ mice.

Taken together, these novel results indicate that DSS colitis inflammation is more severe in TC-PTP $^{+/-}$ mice than in control animals. This is accompanied by a marked increase in local expression of TC-PTP regulated inflammation mediators and a concomitant further decrease in TC-PTP expression. This local inflammation is associated with a systemic inflammatory response characterized by an elevation in serum IL-6 levels and increased peripheral blood. Thus, not only TC-PTP$^{+/-}$ mice are more sensitive to DSS-induced colitis, but they also respond more severely to DSS-treatment both at the local and systemic levels.

Noteworthy, the overexpression of mRNA transcripts of IFN-γ, TNF-α and IL-12, and the systemic increase in IL-6 serum levels observed in DSS-treated TC-PTP$^{+/-}$ mice are similar to those observed in control TC-PTP$^{-/-}$ mice. The over-expression of T_{H1} cytokines has previously been associated with Crohn's disease [8] [17]. Increased levels of those pro-inflammatory cytokines are a major factor in organ-specific autoimmune inflammation [3,7]. Looking at events downstream from cytokine production, analysis of the status of signal transducers revealed increased phosphorylation of Jak1 and Jak3 and of their substrates STAT1, STAT3 and STAT5 in DSS-treated TC-PTP$^{+/-}$ mice in a manner reminiscent to what is observed in TC-PTP$^{-/-}$ mice [8].

In the DSS-induced colitis mouse model, initial injury leads to its disruption and to the entry of bacteria into the intestinal wall and into the blood stream. Supporting evidence for this comes from rats treated with DSS which demonstrated higher level of endotoxin in the portal blood than control animals [18]. Bacterial invasion of the colonic wall and consequent production of endotoxins such as LPS in turn cause the recruitment and activation of inflammatory cells and result in the upregulation of multiple inflammatory cytokines (Figure 5) [18] [17,19]. One phenomenon occurring in DSS-treated TC-PTP$^{+/-}$ mice as well as in patients with Crohn's disease is the over-production of IL-6 [20] [21] [22]. Indeed, levels of IL-6 correlate with disease severity in humans [23]. Binding of IL-6 to its receptor initiates cellular events, including activation of Jak kinases. Jaks are a class of tyrosine kinases that associate with cytokine receptors and are able to phosphorylate and activate STAT proteins, which then dimerize and enter the nucleus to activate the transcription of target genes [24]. Jaks 1 and 3 have been identified as substrates of TC-PTP downstream of IL-2 signaling in substrate-trapping experiments using hematopoietic cell lines [25]. Downstream of Jak activation, STATs are phosphorylated and can thus be modified by PTPs to downregulate their action [26]. For instance, IL-6-induced activation of STAT3 was suppressed by over expression of the nuclear isoform of TC-PTP [27]. Thus, TC-PTP function has an important impact on the sensitivity of the innate immune system to bacterial antigens such as LPS [8], TC-PTP$^{-/-}$ macrophages are hypersensitive to LPS and respond by producing exaggerated amounts of interferon-alpha (IFN-α), tumor necrosis factor-gamma (TNF-γ), interleukin-12 (IL-12), and nitric oxide (NO) [28]. Likewise, cells lacking TC-PTP produced increased levels of IL-6 upon TNF-alpha (TNF-α) treatment [29]. TC-PTP$^{-/-}$ bone marrow-derived macrophages have elevated levels of phosphorylated Jak 1 upon IFN-gamma (IFN-γ) stimulation [25].

Here we show that a gene dosage reduction of TC-PTP enzyme in heterozygous TC-PTP$^{+/-}$ mice directly affects the intensity of the inflammatory response to colonic mucosal injury. This is mediated by an increased production of cytokines, including IL-6, which in all likelihood results directly from the hemi-deficiency in TC-PTP. Increased cytokine levels result in increased phosphorylation of Jaks tyrosine kinases, which in turn phosphorylate/activate signal transducers and activators of transcription (STATs). Owing to the hemi-deficiency of TC-PTP in TC-PTP$^{+/-}$ mice, normal targets for TC-PTP dephosphorylation, i.e. Jak-1, Jak3, and STAT1, STAT3 and STAT5 [9] , remain aberrantly activated, leading to an exaggerated inflammatory response. Our novel findings open the way for future studies examining the unexpected decrease in TC-PTP$^{+/-}$ protein levels following DSS treatment, as well as identifying specific mechanisms leading to the loss of epithelial cells in this animal model of IBD. Furthermore we will be able to investigate whether epithelial cell death is secondary to the decreased expression of TC-PTP in hemi-deficiency using isolated colonic epithelial cells and in particular, mucosal immune cells (lamina propria mononuclear cells/LPMC or lamin propria Tcells/LPT). By inference, human beings with a constitutively less active or less abundant TC-PTP enzyme might be more susceptible to exaggerated bowel inflammation in case of bowel mucosal injury. This hypothesis is consistent with WTCC's observation of Crohn's disease being associated with SNPs mapping near the TC-PTP gene locus.

Materials and Methods

Animal Model

Mice. Experiments were performed with Balb/c mice [10]. TC-PTP$^{+/+}$ and TC-PTP$^{+/-}$mice were obtained from heterozygous mating and genotyped by Southern blotting as previously described [10]. All mice were kept in specific pathogen-free housing in the animal care facility.

Ethics Statement

All procedures were reviewed and approved from the McGill University Animal Care Ethics committee.

Induction of Colitis

TC-PTP $^{+/+}$ and TC-PTP $^{+/-}$ mice, 19 days old and 11–12g in body weight, were administered 5% dextran sulfate sodium (DSS) dissolved in filter-purified and sterilized drinking *ad libitum* for 10 days, after which hydration with regular water was resumed for 1 day before they were weighted and humanely sacrificed (approx. age 30 days) [15,16]. Animals were weighed daily and monitored for rectal bleeding, diarrhea, and general signs of morbidity. Control animals were given normal drinking water.

Histology

Evaluation of inflammation activity. The large intestine was excised, and the colon weight was measured. The distal (2.2~2.4 cm) of the colon was transected, flushed with PBS and areas of redness for gross inflammation were recorded. The macroscopic appearance of the colon was scored in a blinded fashion as follows: 0, no evidence of inflammation; 1, erythema only; 2, erythema and small erosions; 3, 2 or more bleeding ulcers and/or inflammation and/or moderate adhesions [30]. Tissues were then fixed with 4% formaldehyde overnight. After overnight dehydration and paraffin impregnation, tissues were embedded in a paraffin block and serially sectioned. The 5-μm-thick sections were cut and stained with hematoxylin and eosin (H & E) .The sections were microscopically examined for histopathological changes, inflammation severity was scored by a blinded pathologist.

Blood Count

Blood samples were taken at the end of the experiments by cardiac puncture (heart blood) for blood count using an automatic cytometer following manufacturer protocol (Beckmann Coulter, Germany).

Histological Scoring

Analysis was performed blinded by pathologist and each specimen was scored on a scale from 0 to 40 as follows: severity of inflammation (0–3: none, slight, moderate, severe), epithelial erosion (0–3: none, none, slight, moderate, severe), and crypt damage (0–4: none, basal 1/3 damaged, basal 2/3 damaged, only surface epithelium intact, entire crypt and epithelium lost). Each score was then multiplied by a factor equivalent with the percentage of tissue involvement (×1: 0–25%, ×2: 26–50%, ×3: 51–75%, ×4: 76–100%) [31] [32].

Immunoblotting

Large bowel lysate was collected after crushing tissues in liquid nitrogen. Protein samples were resolved on 10% sodium dodecyl sulfate-polyacrylamide gel electrophoresis (SDS-PAGE) and subjected to immunoblotting. TC-PTP was detected using a monoclonal antibody 3E2 as described in [33]. Phosphorylated Jak1, Jak2, Jak3, Stat1, Stat3 and Stat5 proteins were detected using polyclonal antibodies (Cell Signaling Technology). Total Jak1, Jak2, Jak3, Stat1, Stat3 and Stat5 proteins were detected using polyclonal antibodies (Cell Signaling Technology). Calnexin and β-Actin monoclonal antibody were used as loading control for protein samples (Sigma, Oakville, ON, Canada). Primary antibodies were followed by horseradish peroxidase-conjugated goat anti–rabbit or mouse IgG (Perkin Elmer, Boston, MA) as appropriate. Proteins were detected by enhanced chemiluminescent substrate (Perkin Elmer, Boston, MA). Mean intensity values were calculated using ImageJ software (http://rsbweb.nih.gov/ij/).

RT-PCR of mRNA

Total RNA was extracted from tissues using TRIzol (Invitrogen) according to the manufacturer's specifications. mRNA was transcribed using the Super ScriptIII (Invitrogen) reverse transcriptase-polymerase chain reaction (RT-PCR) kit (Qiagen, Mississauga, ON, Canada) and the PCR machine (Roche Diagnostics, Laval, QC, Canada).

Primers

Oligo-nucleotides were synthesized by Sigma (Sigma, Oakville, ON, Canada) and sequences are as follows:

β-Actin was used as control of 187bp as forward, 5′-AGGTGACAGCATTGCTTCTG-3′ and reverse, 5′-GCTGC-CTCAACACCTCAAC-3′. Interleukin-6 (IL-6) forward, 5′- TC-CAGTTGCCTTCTTGGGAC -3′ and reverse, 5′- GTGTAAT-TAAGCCTCCGACTTG-3′ with size of fragment as 140 bp. Tumor necrosis factor-alpha (TNF-α) forward 5′- CCTGTAG-CCCACGTCGTAGC -3′ and reverse, 5′- TTGACCTCAG-CGCTGAGTTG -3′ with size of fragment as 373 bp. Interferon-gamma (IFN-γ) forward 5′-TGGAGGAACTGGCAAAAGG-ATG -3′, and reverse 5′-CGCTTCCTGAGGCTGGATTC -3′, with size of fragment as 289 bp. Interleukin-12β-p40 (IL-12β-p40) forward 5′-AGATGACATCACCTGGACCTCAG -3′, and reverse 5′- ACGTGAACCGTCCGGAGTAA -3′, with size of fragment as 230 bp.

Interleukin 23 receptor (IL-23R) forward, 5′-TCCACTGACT-CACTGCAAGG -3′ and reverse 5′-GTTCGTGGGAT-GATTTTGCT -3′, with size of fragment as 500 bp.

Serum Cytokine Analysis

Serum levels for IL-6, TNF-α, IFN-γ, and IL-12p40 were measured using Bio-Plex Pro Mouse Cytokine Multiplex Assay (Bio-Rad Laboratories, Hercules, CA, USA) as per manufacturer's protocol with some minor modifications. In brief, 25 μl of pre-mixed beads coated with capture antibodies were added to a 96-well plate. Beads were washed twice and 25 μl of standards and serum (diluted 4-fold) were added to the wells before incubating on a microtiter plate shaker at 300 rpm, protected from light, for one hour at room temperature. Beads were washed three times, followed by the addition of 12.5 μl of detection antibodies. The plate was incubated as before. After three washes, 25 μl of streptavidin-phycoerythrin were added to each well and incubated as before for only 10 minutes. Beads were resuspended in 62.5 μl Bio-Plex Assay buffer on the shaker at 300 rpm. Beads were read using the Bio-Plex Reader (Bio-Rad Laboratories, Hercules, CA) and data was analyzed with Bio-Plex Manager 2.0 software (Bio-Rad Laboratories, Hercules, CA).

Statistical Analysis

A linear-mixed model was employed and log likelihood was used to test significance between genotypes by treatment over time using R Statistical Package (R Development Core Team, http://www.r-project.org/).

Histograms represent mean ± standard error of the mean (SEM). *P* values were determined using a one-way ANOVA using Tukey-Kramer Multiple Comparisons.

Acknowledgments

The authors would like to thank Dr Claudio Fiocchi for constructive comments on this manuscript as well as Dr. Vicky Marcus for pathological analysis, Mr Joseph J. Bowden for statistical analysis, Dr Laurent Lessard and Ms. Marianne Filion for their help in providing the immunohistochemistry protocol, Mrs. Ailsa C. Lee Loy and members of the Tremblay laboratory for critical support and helpful discussions.

Author Contributions

Conceived and designed the experiments: SWH DC MLT. Performed the experiments: SWH KMD SH. Analyzed the data: SWH KMD SH NU DC MLT. Contributed reagents/materials/analysis tools: NU DC MLT. Wrote the paper: SWH DC MLT.

References

1. Franke A (2007) Systematic association mapping identifies NELL1 as a novel IBD disease gene. PLoS ONE 2(8): e691.
2. The Wellcome Trust Case Control Consortium (2007) Genome-wide association study of 14,000 cases of seven common diseases and 3,000 shared controls. Nature 447: 661–678.
3. Franke A (2008) Replication of signals from recent studies of Crohn's disease identifies previously unknown disease loci for ulcerative colitis. Nat Genet.
4. Glinsky G (2008) An SNP-guided microRNA map of fifteen common human disorders identifies a consensus disease phenocode aiming at principal components of the nuclear import pathway. Cell Cycle 7: 2570–2583.
5. Wu F (2008) MicroRNAs are differentially expressed in ulcerative colitis and alter expression of macrophage inflammatory peptide-2 alpha. Gastroenterology 135: 1624–1635.
6. Barrett JC (2008) Genome-wide association defines more than 30 distinct susceptibility loci for Crohn's disease. Nat Genet.
7. Fisher S (2008) Genetic determinants of ulcerative colitis include the ECM1 locus and five loci implicated in Crohn's disease. Nat Genet.
8. Heinonen KM, Nestel FP, Newell EW, Charette G, Seemayer TA, et al. (2004) T-cell protein tyrosine phosphatase deletion results in progressive systemic inflammatory disease. Blood 103: 3457–3464.
9. Doody KM, Bourdeau A, Tremblay ML (2009) T-cell protein tyrosine phosphatase is a key regulator in immune cell signaling: lessons from knockout mouse model and immplications in human disease. Immunological Reviews 228: 325–341.
10. You-Ten KE (1997) Impaired Bone Marrow Microenvironment and Immune Function in T Cell Protein Tyrosine Phosphatase–deficient Mice. J Exp Med 186: 683–693.
11. Heinonen KM, Dube N, Bourdeau A, Lapp WS, Tremblay ML (2006) Protein tyrosine phosphatase 1B negatively regulates macrophage development through CSF-1 signaling. Proc Natl Acad Sci U S A 103: 2776–2781.
12. Cool DE, Tonks NK, Charbonneau H, Walsh KA, Fischer EH, et al. (1989) cDNA isolated from a human T-cell library encodes a member of the protein-tyrosine-phosphatase family. Proc Natl Acad Sci USA 86: 5257–5261.
13. Mosinger B Jr, Tillmann U, Westphal H, Tremblay ML (1992) Cloning and characterization of a mouse cDNA encoding a cytoplasmic protein-tyrosine-phosphatase. Proc Natl Acad Sci USA 89: 499–503.
14. Sakaguchi AY, Sylvia VL, Martinez L, Smith EA, Han ES, et al. (1992) Assignment of tyrosine-specific T-cell phosphatase to conserved syntenic groups on human chromosome 18 and mouse chromosome 18. Genomics 12: 151–154.
15. Sasaki S, Yoneyama H, Suzuki K, Suriki H, Aiba T, et al. (2002) Blockade of CXCL10 protects mice from acute colitis and enhances crypt cell survival. Eur J Immunol 32: 3197–3205.
16. Malago JJ, Nondoli H (2008) Sodium arsenite reduces severity of dextran sulfate sodium-induced ulcerative colitis in rats. J Zhejiang Univ Sci B 9(4): 341–350.
17. Nielsen OH, Kirman I, Rudiger N, Hendel J, Vainer B (2003) Upregulation of interleukin-12 and -17 in active inflammatory bowel disease. Scand J Gastroenterol 38: 180–185.
18. Horie Y, Ma T (2004) Endotoxin-mediated disturbance of hepatic cytochrome P450 function and development of endotoxin tolerance in the rat model of dextran sulfate sodium-induced experimental colitis. Drug Metabolism and Disposition 32: 437–441.
19. Balding J, Livingstone WJ, Conroy J, Mynett-Johnson L, Weir DG, et al. (2004) Inflammatory bowel disease: the role of inflammatory cytokine gene polymorphisms. Mediators Inflamm 13: 181–187.
20. Podolsky DK (2002) Inflammatory bowel disease. N Engl J Med 347: 417–429.
21. Shanahan F (2002) Crohn's disease. Lancet 359: 62–69.
22. Atreya R, Mudter J, Finotto S, Mulberg J, Jostock T, et al. (2000) Blockade of IL-6 transsignalling abrogates established experimental colitis in mice by suppression of T cell resistance against apoptosis. Journal of Allergy and Clinical Immunology 105: S29–S29.
23. Mudter J, Neurath MF (2007) Il-6 signaling in inflammatory bowel disease: pathophysiological role and clinical relevance. Inflamm Bowel Dis 13: 1016–1023.
24. Kerr J (1995) Jaks and Stats in signaling by the cytokine receptor superfamily. Trends Genet 11: 69–74.
25. Simoncic PD, Loy A-L, Barber DL, Tremblay ML, McGlade CJ (2002) The T cell protein tyrosine phosphatase is a negative regulator of janus family kinases 1 and 3. Curr Biol 12: 446–453.
26. ten Hove J, de Jesus Ibarra-Sanchez M, Fu Y, Zhu W, Tremblay ML (2002) Identification of a nuclear Stat1 protein tyrosine phosphatase. Mol Cell Biol 22: 5662–5668.
27. Yamamoto T, Sekine Y, Kashima K, Kubota A, Sato N, et al. (2002) The nuclear isoform of protein-tyrosine phosphatase TC-PTP regulates interleukin-6-mediated signaling pathway through STAT3 dephosphorylation. Biochem Biophys Res Commun 297: 811–817.
28. Heinonen KM, Nestel FP, Newell EW, Charette G, Seemayer TA, et al. (2004) T-cell protein tyrosine phosphatase deletion results in progressive systemic inflammatory disease. Blood 103(109): 3457–3464.
29. van Vliet C, Bukczynska PE, Puryer MA, Sadek CM, Shields BJ, et al. (2005) Selective regulation of tumor necrosis factor-induced Erk signaling by Src family kinases and the T cell protein tyrosine phosphatase. Nat Immunol 6: 253–260.
30. Fitzpatrick LR Wang J, Le M (2000) In vitro and in vivo effects of gliotoxin, a fungal metabolite: Efficacy against dextran sodium sulfate-induced colitis in rats. Dig Dis Sci 45:45: 2327–2336.
31. McCafferty DM, Miampamba M, Sihota E, Sharkey KA, Kubes P (1999) Role of inducible nitric oxide synthase in trinitrobenzene sulphonic acid induced colitis in mice. Gut 45: 864–873.
32. Roviezzo F, Bucci M, Delisle C, Brancaleone V, Di Lorenzo A, et al. (2006) Essential requirement for sphingosine kinase activity in eNOS-dependent NO release and vasorelaxation. Faseb J 20: 340–342.
33. Gu F (2003) Protein tyrosine phosphatase 1B attenuates growth hormone-mediated JAK2-STAT signaling. Mol Cell Biol. pp 3753–3762.

7

Opposite Role of Tumor Necrosis Factor Receptors in Dextran Sulfate Sodium-Induced Colitis in Mice

Ke Wang[1,2], Gencheng Han[2], Yan Dou[3], Yi Wang[2], Guijun Liu[4], Renxi Wang[2], He Xiao[2], Xinying Li[2], Chunmei Hou[2], Beifen Shen[2], Renfeng Guo[5], Yan Li[2], Yanchun Shi[4]*, Guojiang Chen[2]*

1 Department of Immunology, School of Basic Medical Sciences, Central South University, Changsha, P. R. China, **2** Department of Immunology, Institute of Basic Medical Sciences, Beijing, P. R. China, **3** Department of Gastroenterology, General Hospital of PLA, Beijing, P. R. China, **4** Center of Molecular Biology, Inner Mongolia Medical College, Hohhot, P. R. China, **5** InflaRx GmbH, Jena, Germany

Abstract

Tumor necrosis factor-α (TNF-α) is a key factor for the pathogenesis of inflammatory bowel diseases (IBD), whose function is known to be mediated by TNF receptor 1 (TNFR1) or 2. However, the precise role of the two receptors in IBD remains poorly understood. Herein, acute colitis was induced by dextran sulfate sodium (DSS) instillation in TNFR1 or 2−/− mice. TNFR1 ablation led to exacerbation of signs of colitis, including more weight loss, increased mortality, colon shortening and oedema, severe intestinal damage, and higher levels of myeloperoxidase compared to wild-type counterparts. While, TNFR2 deficiency had opposite effects. This discrepancy was reflected by alteration of proinflammatory cytokine and chemokine production in the colons. Importantly, TNFR1 ablation rendered enhanced apoptosis of colonic epithelial cells and TNFR2 deficiency conferred pro-apoptotic effects of lamina propria (LP)-immune cells, as shown by the decreased ratio of Bcl-2/Bax and enhanced nuclear factor (NF)-κB activity.

Editor: Hiroyasu Nakano, Juntendo University School of Medicine, Japan

Funding: This work was supported by grants from the National Key Basic Research Program of China (2007CB512406; 2009CB522408) and the National Natural Science Foundation of China (30801029, 81072475 and 81172800). The funders had no role in study design, data collection and analysis, decision to publish, or preparation of the manuscript.

Competing Interests: The authors have the following interests. Renfeng Guo is an employee of InflaRx GmbH. There are no patents, products in development or marketed products to declare.

* E-mail: guogangch@yahoo.com (GC); ycshi5388@yahoo.com.cn (YS)

These authors contributed equally to this work.

Introduction

Tumor necrosis factor (TNF) plays a crucial role in immune response at physiological and pathological states, which is based on its pleiotropic function on differentiation, growth and apoptosis of both immune and non-immune cell populations [1,2]. Numerous studies have demonstrated that TNF is tightly implicated in the pathogenesis of inflammatory diseases and autoimmunity such as rheumatoid arthritis, multiple sclerosis and inflammatory bowel diseases (IBD) [3]. It is well established that the biological function of TNF is exerted through binding as a trimer to either TNF receptor (TNF-R) 1 or 2. TNF-R1, which is expressed on most cell types, contains a death domain that mediates apoptotic signaling through caspase activation and activates nuclear factor (NF)-κB, resulting in transcription of proinflammatory cytokines and chemokines as well as anti-apoptotic peptides [4]. TNF-R2, which is expressed predominantly by haematopoietic cells, lacks the death domains but delivers apoptotic signaling through the kinase receptor-interacting protein (RIP) [5].

Increasing data have been shown to support the intimate relationship of TNF-R expression with the pathogenesis of IBD. During active stages of the disease, TNF-R2 expression by colonic epithelial cells is increased in patients suffering from IBD and in mice with experimental colitis [6,7]. Furthermore, the polymorphisms in the TNF-R2 gene have been reported to be associated with a higher susceptibility to Crohn's disease (CD) [8]. These observations strongly support a disease-promoting role of TNF signaling via TNF-R2 during IBD development. However, a study demonstrates recently that the transfer of colitogenic $CD4^{+}CD45^{hi}TNF\text{-}R2^{-/-}$ T cells into RAG−/− recipients leads to acceleration of the onset of overt disease and to aggravated severity of intestinal inflammation [9], indicating an opposite effect of TNF-R2 expression by $CD4^{+}$ T cells on the course of colitis. The paradoxicality on the role of TNF signaling via TNF-R1 in IBD also exists. Ebath et al. [10] reported that TNF-R1-deficient C57Bl/6 mice had more weight loss and increased mortality after trinitrobenzene sulphonic acid (TNBS) instillation. In contrast, Nakai et al. [11] demonstrated that TNF-R1 ablation attenuated tissue damage after TNBS, which was related to reduced NF-κB activity. Our recent study has shown that TNF signaling via TNF-R1or TNF-R2 play a pathogenic role in TNBS-induced colitis [12]. Overall, these studies underline the complexity of TNF bioactivity via TNF-R1 or 2 during the onset and perpetuation of intestinal inflammation, which may be affected by different TNF-R expression patterns and distinct colitis models used.

The studies on the function of TNF signaling via TNF-R1 or 2 on the course of DSS-induced colitis, which is another widely used murine model of IBD and closely resembles UC, is relatively few. Recently, Stillie et al. reported that, although ablation of TNF-

R1or 2 had an effect on some parameters of DSS colitis in C57Bl/6 mice, TNF signaling via either of its receptors appeared to play a redundant role in the pathology of intestinal inflammation [13]. The exact role of TNF signaling via TNF-R1 or 2 in the course of DSS colitis in other strains and underlying mechanisms, however, remains poorly understood. In this study, we investigated the effect of TNF-R1 or 2 knockout on DSS-induced acute colitis in BALB/c strains. Ablation of TNF-R1 or 2 had opposite influence on the course of colitis. That is, TNF-R1 deficiency accelerated the onset of overt diseases, while TNF-R2 knockout attenuated the severity of colitis. This disagreement can be resolved by that TNF-R1 deficiency led to augmented production of proinflammatory cytokines in the lesions, while TNF-R2 knockout did not. Furthermore, enhanced apoptosis of colonic epithelial cells (CEC) was found in TNF-R1-deficient mice after DSS. In contrast, immune cells in the lamina propria (LP) had a trend to programmed death in TNF-R2-knockout rodents after DSS.

Materials and Methods

Animals

BALB/c wild type (WT) mice were purchased from Jackson Laboratory (Bar Harbor, Maine). TNFR1$^{-/-}$ and TNFR2$^{-/-}$ mice from Dr. Zhihai Qin [National Laboratory of Biomacromolecules, Institute of Biophysics, Chinese Academy of Sciences, Beijing, China] were backcrossed for 12 generations onto the BALB/c background [14]. Animals were housed in specific pathogen-free conditions with an alternating light/dark cycle. All experiments were performed using 6- to 8-week-old male mice. Care, use and treatment of mice in this study was in strict agreement with international guidelines for the care and use of laboratory animals and approved by Animal Ethics Committee of Institute of Basic Medical Sciences.

Colitis Induction

Acute colitis was induced in mice by adding 3% DSS (MW 36, 000–50, 000; MP Biochemicals, USA) to their drinking water and allowing them drink ad libitum, starting from day 0 for 8 days. Weights were measured before induction of colitis and daily thereafter. At the end of the experiments mice were sacrificed by cervical dislocation under anesthesia.

Histology

Colons removed from mice at indicated time of death were fixed in 10% neutral-buffered formalin solution and then embedded in paraffin, cun into tissue sections, and stained with hematoxylin and eosin. Stained sections were examined for evidence of colitis using as criteria: the presence of lymphocyte infiltration, elongation and/or distortion of crypts, frank ulceration, and thickening of the bowel wall. The degree of inflammation on microscopic cross-sections of the colon was graded semiquatitatively from 0 to 4 (0, no evidence of inflammation; 1, low level of lymphocyte infiltration with infiltration seen in <10% high-power field (hpf), no structural changes observed; 2, moderate lymphocyte infiltration with infiltration seen in 10–25% hpf, crypt elongation, bowel wall thickeningwhich does not extend beyond mucosal layer, no evidence of ulceration; 3, high level of lymphocyte infiltration with infiltration seen in 25–50% hpf, high vascular density, thickening of bowel wall which extends beyond mucosal layer; and 4, marked degree of lymphocyte infiltration with infiltration seen in >50% hpf, high vascular density, crypt elongation with distortion, transmural bowel wall thickening with ulceration).

Isolation of Colonic Epithelial Cells and Lamina Propria-immune Cells

The entire length of colon was opened longitudinally, washed with PBS, washed with PBS containing 100 μg/ml gentamycin, and cut into small pieces. The dissected mucosa was incubated with Ca^{2+}, Mg^{2+}-free HBSS supplemented with 10% fetal bovine serum, 5 mM EDTA, 15 mM HEPES, 100 μg/ml gentamycin under shaking at 37°C for 20 min then repeated for 4 times. The supernatants containing colonic epithelial cells were centrifuged at 800 g for 10 min at 4°C. the deposit was collected as colonic epithelial cells (purity>80%, identified by CK-18 staining). The remaining was washed with HBSS, followed by digestion in RPMI 1640 medium containing 100 U/ml collagenase D (Roche Diagnostics) under shaking at 37°C for 1 h then repeated for 2 times. The total of digested supernatants was centrifuged at 800 g for 10 min at 4°C and washed with PBS. The pellet was layered on a 40%/100% Percoll gradient (Pharmacia) and spun at 1,800 rpm for 5 min to collect the lymphocyte-enriched population at the 40%/100% Percoll interface as LP-immune cells.

Detection of Apoptotic Cells

For detection of apoptotic cells in tissues, labeling of degraded DNA specific to apoptotic cells was performed using a modification of the terminal deoxynucleotidyl transferase-mediated deoxyuridine triphosphate nick end-labeling (TUNEL) technique by application of the *in situ* cell death detection kits (Roche Diagnostics, Indianapolis, IN) according to the manufacturer's instructions. In this method, residues of digoxigenin-labeled nucleotides are added to the ends of DNA fragments by terminal deoxynucleotidyl transferase, then peroxidase-labeled antidigoxigenin antibodies and 3,3′-diaminobenzidine are added in turn; the latter are oxidized by the bound peroxidase to generate visible signals from the apoptotic cells.

Colon Homogenates

A 1 cm segment was divided from the distal 4 cm of the harvest colon. Wet weight was recorded separately for the whole distal 4 cm and the portion taken for homogenation. Colon tissue samples were homogenized in PBS containing a cocktail of protease inhibitors (1 μl to 20 mg of tissue according to the manufacturer's protocol, Roche) with a Polytron homogenizer and centrifuged at 12 000 *g* for 10 min. The supernatants were stored at −20°C until used for ELISA analysis.

Determination for Colon Edema

Colons were dissected at indicated timepoint after TNBS. A piece of the affected colon was then collected, weighed, placed in an 80°C oven for 24 h, then reweighed, and the wet-to-dry weight ratio was determined as a measure of colon edema [15].

Measurement of Myeloperoxidase Activity

Tissue MPO activity was determined by a standard enzymatic procedure as described previously [16], with minor modifications. Briefly, after the samples has been weighed, a tissue sample (approximately 300 mg) was homogenized in a buffer (0.5% hexadecyltrimethylammonium bromide in 50 Mm potassium phosphate buffer, pH 6.0) three times for 30 s each on ice. The sample was centrifuged at 20,000 g for 20 min at 4°C and the supernatant was collected. The supernatants (100 μl) was then added to 2.9 ml of 50 mM phosphate buffer (pH 6.0) containing 0.167 mg/ml O-dianisidine hydrochloride and 0.0005% hydrogen peroxide, and absorbances were measured using a spectrometer at

25°C. Results for colon MPO content were converted to absorbance units per gram of tissue.

Immunoblotting

Samples were homogenized and sonicated in RIPA lysis buffer (Santa Cruz Biotechnology Inc.), supplemented with protease inhibitors. After centrifugation at 20,000 *g* for 15 min, 30 μg of the supernatants were separated on 10% SDS-polyacrylamide gel and transferred onto an Immunobilon-P Transfer membrane (Millipore). After being blocked with 5% skim milk, the membrane was incubated with antibodies to Bcl-2 (1:1000), Bax (1:1000), or IκBα (1:1000). Rabbit anti-actin antibody (1:1000) was used as an internal control. ImmunoPure peroxidase-conjugated anti-rabbit IgG were used as secondary antibodies. The blotted membrane was then treated with the Super Signal West Dura Extended Duration Substrate (Pierce Biotechnology Inc.) and signals were detected by LAS-3000 mini CCD camera (Fuji Film). Primary antibodies used for immunoblotting were purchased from *e*Bioscience.

Cytokine Analysis

Colonic IL-6, IL-1β, MCP-1, IL-17A were measured by ELISA according to the manufacturers' instructions. ELISA kits were purchased from *e*Bioscience.

Flow Cytometry

Single cell suspension was prepared from spleen by passing them through nylon mesh or colonic tissues as described above and stained with appropriate antibodies in PBS with 2% heat-inactivated fetal calf serum and 0.1% sodium azide on ice for 25 minutes. The antibodies used are following: fluorescein isothiocyanate (FITC)-labeled anti-murine Gr-1 (RB6-8C5, Biolegend), F4/80 (CI:A3-1, Biolegend) antibody, phycoerythrin (PE)-labeled anti-murine TNF-R1 (55R-286, Biolegend), TNF-R2 (TR75-89, Biolegend) antibody. These cells were fixed using PBS with 1% paraformaldehyde. For detecting apoptosis, double staining with annexin V and propidium iodide (PI) (eBioscience) was performed according to manufacturer's instructions. Data collection and analysis were performed on a FACS Calibur flow cytometer using CellQuest software (Becton Dickinson).

Real-time Reverse Transcriptase-polymerase Chain Reaction (RT-PCR)

RNA extracted from colon tissues was reverse-transcribed into cDNA using the SuperScript III First Strand cDNA synthesis system (Invitrogen). cDNA was synthesized from 0.5 μg RNA using random hexamer primers and SuperScript III(Invitrogen). Real-time RT-PCR was performed on a Bio-Rad iCycler to quantify mRNA levels. The primers for real-time were as follows: CXCL-1 forward primer 5′-ACT GCA CCC AAA CCG AAG TC-3′ and reverse primer 5′-TGG GGA CAC CTT TTA GCA TCT T-3′; CXCL-2 forward primer 5′-GCG CCC AGA CAG AAG TCA TAG-3′ and reverse primer 5′-AGC CTT GCC TTT GTT CAG TAT C-3′; CCL-3 forward primer 5′-TGT ACC ATG ACA CTC TGC AAC-3′ and reverse primer 5′-CAA CGA TGA ATT GGC GTG GAA-3′; GAPDH forward primer 5′-TGA AGG TCG GAG TCA ACG GAT TTG GT-3′ and reverse primer 5′-CAT GTG GGC CAT GAG GTC CAC CAC-3′. All reactions were performed in triplicate. The data were analyzed using Q-Gene software and expressed as fold change mean normalized expression (MNE) from control value. MNE is directly proportional to the amount of RNA of the target gene relative to the amount of RNA of the reference gene, GAPDH.

Data Analysis

Student *t* test and 1-way analysis of variance (ANOVA) was used to determine significance, with $P<0.05$ considered significant. Kaplan-Meier was used for survival analysis with log rank $P<0.05$ to determine significance. Statistics were performed using SPSS 10.0 for Macintosh, and graphs were made on Deltagraph (SPSS, Chicago, I11.).

Results

TNF Signaling via TNF-R1 or 2 has Distinct Effects on Weight Loss and Mortality after DSS

Acute colitis was established in wild-type (WT) and TNF-R-knockout mice by continuous drinking of 3% DSS for eight days, respectively. WT mice lost an average of 11.8±4.3% of their baseline weight 8 days after DSS. TNF-R1−/− and TNF-R2−/− mice lost 28.8±2.6% and 4.4±2.3% at the same timepoint, respectively (Fig. 1A). Furthermore, in TNF-R1−/− group, acceleration of weight loss was initiated on day 5. In accord with this, at day 8, 57% (16/28) of TNF-R1−/−, 86% (31/36) of TNF-R2−/− mice had survived, whereas survival was 80% (16/20) in WT mice (Fig. 1B). Taken together, these results indicate that TNF-R1−/− mice exhibit more weight loss and mortality, while TNF-R2 deficiency attenuates the symptoms of colitis.

Deficiency of TNF-R1 or 2 Affects Colon Injury Differently after DSS

Next, the influence of TNF-R1 or 2 knockout on macroscopic and microscopic damage of colons after DSS was examined. WT mice displayed remarkable shortening and thickening of the colon 8 day after DSS (). TNF-R1 ablation led to more severe pathology of the target tissues. In contrast, the colon from TNF-R2−/− mice did not show considerable injury, resembling the colon of control mice (Fig. 2A). Moreover, wet-to-dry weight ratios of the colon from TNF-R1−/− group were significantly increased compared to WT mice after DSS (Fig. 2B). Whereas, the edema in TNFR2−/− colons was reduced obviously, which was comparable to the controls. Consistent with macroscopic changes, WT mice after DSS showed marked infiltration of inflammatory cells and ulceratic injury. TNF-R1 ablation rendered more severity of histopathological features of colitis (Fig. 2C). TNF-R2−/− colons, however, showed much less severity of intestinal damage. When quantified by histological system for evidence of inflammation and injury, these histological alterations were highly significant (Fig. 2D).

Mice Lacking TNF-R1 or 2 have Higher or Lower Levels of MPO in Colons after DSS

Neutrophil infiltrate is a key event for initiation and promotion of inflammatory responses in many inflammatory diseases including IBD [17–19]. To determine mild or severe signs of colitis in mice lacking TNF-R1 or 2 are partially attributed to decreased or increased infiltrate of neutrophil, we detected the levels of MPO, indices for neutrophil infiltration, in the colon 8 days after DSS. Levels of MPO in the colons of WT colitis mice were significantly higher than control mice (Fig. 3). In mice lacking TNF-R1, the levels of colonic MPO were increased remarkably compared to WT mice after DSS. The levels of MPO in the colon of TNF-R2−/− mice, in contrast, were reduced to similar levels to those of control animals (Fig. 3).

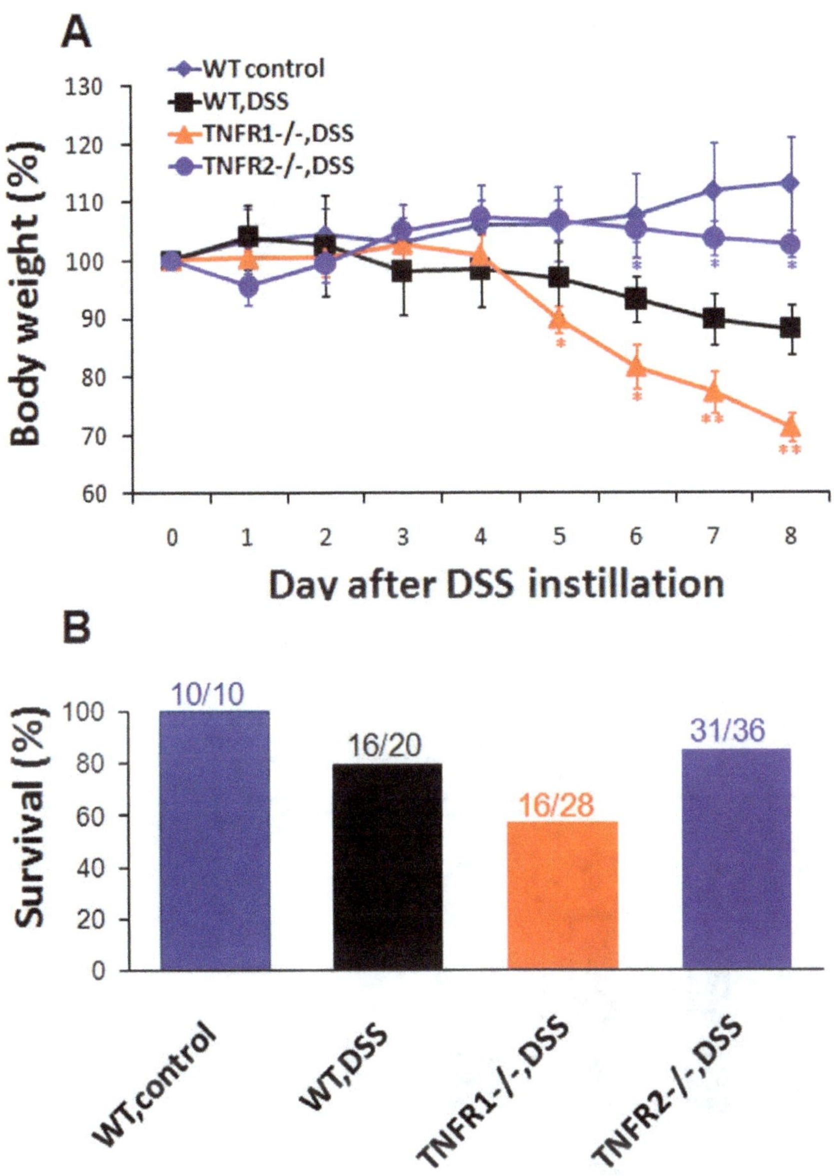

Figure 1. TNF-R1 or 2−/− mice have more or less weight loss and mortality after DSS. DSS colitis was established as described in Materials and methods. (A) Weight in each group was monitored daily at 8-day intervals. Weight was presented as percentage of the initial weight at day 0. (B) Survival rate was calculated at the end of experiments. Data are pooled from three independent experiments (n = 10–30 mice per group). *$P<0.05$, **$P<0.01$ vs WT mice after DSS.

TNF-R1 or 2 Ablation Up-regulates or Down-regulates the Colonic Production of Proinflammatory Cytokines after DSS

To determine whether opposite effects of TNF-R1 or 2 deficiency on pathological changes after DSS is associated with the alteration of expression of colitis-related proinflammatory cytokines and chemokines, the section of colons was dissected, homogenized and assayed at day 8 after DSS. Compared to WT colitis mice, lack of TNF-R1 resulted in significant up-regulation of IL-6, IL-1β, MCP-1, IL-17A levels in the colon tissues (Fig. 4A). In sharp contrast, the production of these cytokines in the lesions was decreased drastically (Fig. 4A). These results were in agreement with the data of colitis scores. Furthermore, the colonic expression of neutrophil-chemoattractant chemokines CXCL-1, CXCL-2, CCL-3 was increased in TNF-R1−/− mice, while was reduced in TNF-R2−/− counterparts (Fig. 4B). This result may explain the observation of the widespread infiltration of neutrophil in target tissues of TNF-R1-deficient mice instead of TNF-R2−/− mice.

Lack of TNF-R1 Augments Systemic Inflammatory Responses

It has been recognized that systemic inflammatory response is hallmark of DSS-induced colitis [20,21]. Thus, we examined the influence of TNF-R1 or 2 knockout on the disease parameters. 8 days after DSS, WT mice exhibited visible splenomeagly as indicated by the weight of spleen. This effect was more pronounced in mice lacking TNF-R1 (Fig. 5A), indicating that TNF-R1 ablation led to augmented systemic inflammatory reaction. However, the weight of spleen in mice lacking TNF-

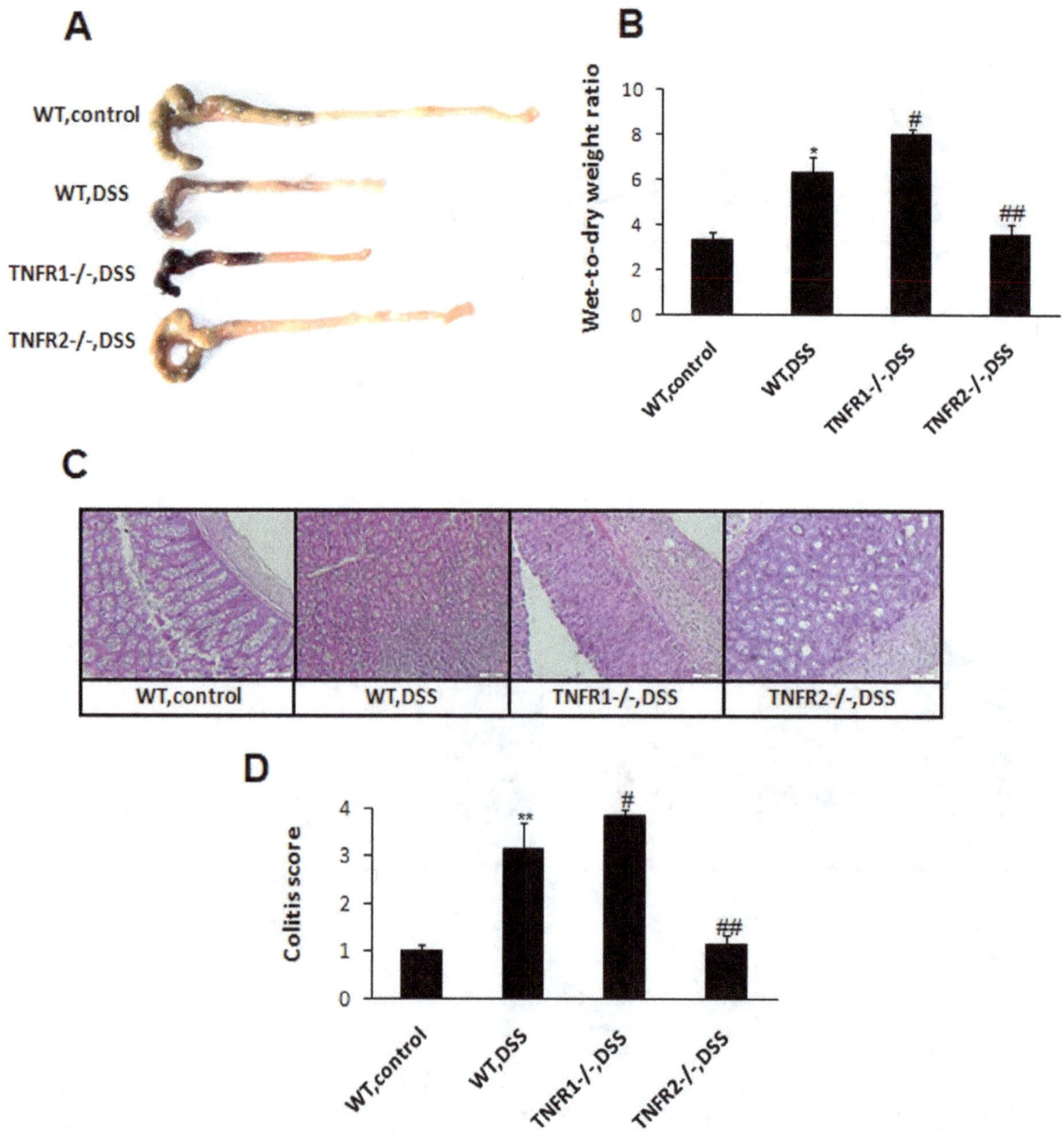

Figure 2. TNF-R1 or 2 deficiency exacerbates or ameliorates mucosal damage after DSS. Colons from each group were collected at day 8 after DSS instillation. (A) Macroscopic images of the colons are shown. (B) Colon edema was determined by wet-to-dry weight ratios. (C) Microscopic images of the colons are shown by haematoxylin and eosin staining. Magnification: ×200. (D) Colitis score was determined as described in Materials and methods. Data represent the mean±SD of eight to ten mice per group. *P<0.05, **P<0.01 vs WT control mice; #P<0.05, ##P<0.01 vs WT mice after DSS.

R2 was comparable to controls, suggesting that absence of TNF-R2 inhibits local and systemic inflammatory responses after DSS.

Next, we defined the characteristics of this systemic inflammatory response induced by DSS administration. FACS analysis for frequency of granulocytes and monocytes in spleen was performed. The percentage of granulocytes (Gr-1$^+$) was increased in WT, TNF-R1 or 2-knockout DSS-instilled mice compared to untreated controls (Fig. 5B), which was most pronounced in TNF-R1−/− group. Monocyte percentage, however, was sharply increased in WT and TNF-R1−/− groups, which was more significant in TNF-R1−/− mice. TNF-R2 deficiency did restrain the proliferation of monocytes in the spleen after DSS (Fig. 5C). These findings indicate that TNF signaling via TNF-R2 instead of TNF-R1 is required for systemic inflammatory responses.

TNF-R1 or 2 Deficiency Reduces Anti-apoptotic Bcl-2 Expression and Enhances NF-κB Activity in Different Cell Types in the Colons after DSS

To determine the mechanisms underlying aggravated or attenuated intestinal damage in absence of TNF-R1 or 2 when DSS colitis was established, we speculate that lacking TNF signaling via TNF-R1 or 2 leads to alteration of apoptosis of

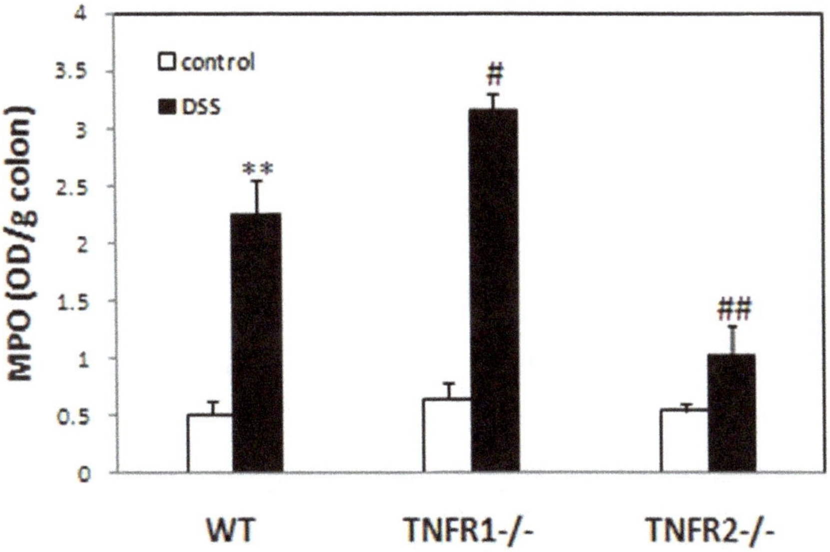

Figure 3. TNF-R1 or 2−/− mice have increased or reduced infiltrates of neutrophils into the colons after DSS. Levels of myeloperoxidase (MPO) in the colons of mice in each group were measured at day 8 after colitis induction. Data represent the mean±SD of four to six mice per group. **P<0.01 vs WT control mice; #P<0.05, ##P<0.01 vs WT mice after DSS.

colonic epithelial cells and/or lamina propria-residing immune cells. To address this issue, we first examined the expression of TNF-R1 and 2 on epithelial cells and LP-immune cells respectively. The result showed that TNFR1 was expressed only on CEC but not on LP-immune cells (Fig. 6A). Subsequently, colon samples from WT and TNF-R knockout groups were stained using the TUNEL methods. The apoptotic cells in colonic mucosa of WT control mice were almost invisible. Upon the establishment of DSS-induced colitis, numerous apoptotic cells in the epithelium were observed (Fig. 6B). In agreement with the grade of mucosal damage, TNF-R1−/− mice, which had higher colitis scores, showed significant increase of apoptotic epithelial cells (Fig. 6B). Interestingly, when TUNEL staining was done in the colon sample of DSS-instilled TNF-R2−/− mice, the enhanced apoptosis of LP-mononuclear immune cells rather than epithelial cells was seen (Fig. 6B). To further address this issue, we detected the apoptosis of colonic epithelial cells and LP-immune cells by annexin V/PI staining respectively. Significantly increased apoptosis of colonic epithelial cells was observed in TNF-R1−/− mice after colitis induction. While, TNFR2 deficiency led to increased number of apopototic LP-immune cells, instead of CEC, upon colitis establishment (Fig. 6C).

Next, we examine whether increase in apoptosis of colonic epithelial cells or LP-immune cells in TNF-R1or 2 knockout mice after DSS is associated with reduced anti-apoptotic signals. The results showed that DSS instillation drastically reduced the

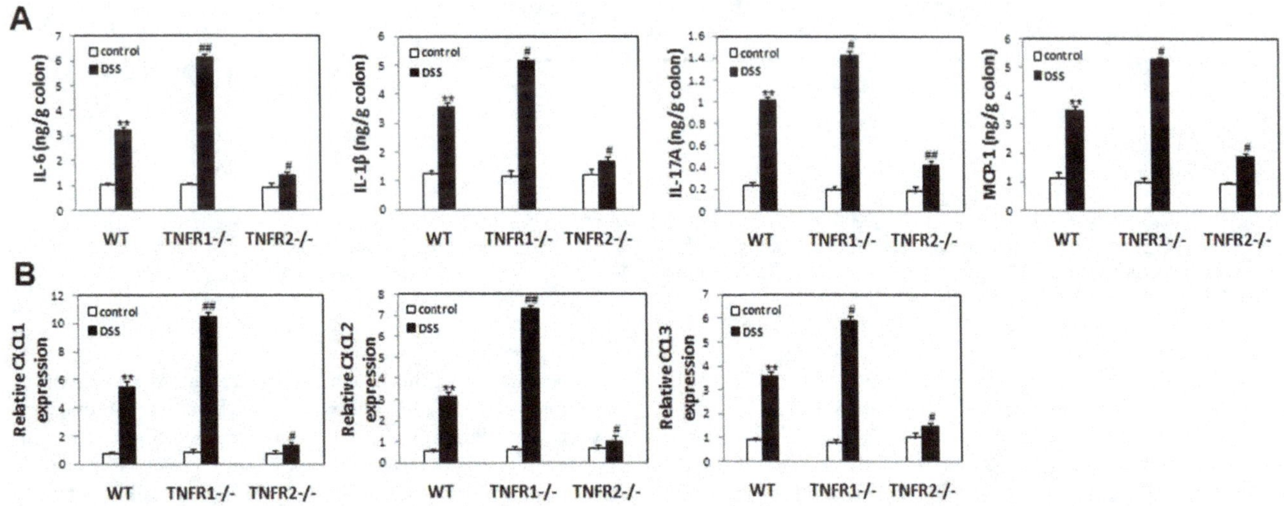

Figure 4. Lack of TNF-R1 or 2 increases or reduces proinflammatory mediator production in the colons after DSS. Colons were isolated and homogenized at day 8 after colitis induction. (A) IL-6, IL-1β, MCP-1, and IL-17A concentrations in the supernatants of homogenates were determined by ELISA. (B) mRNA were isolated from homogenates and CXCL1/2, CCL3 expression was examined by quantitative RT-PCR. Data represent the mean±SD of six to eight mice per group from two independent experiments. **P<0.05 vs WT control mice; #P<0.05, ##P<0.01 vs WT mice after DSS.

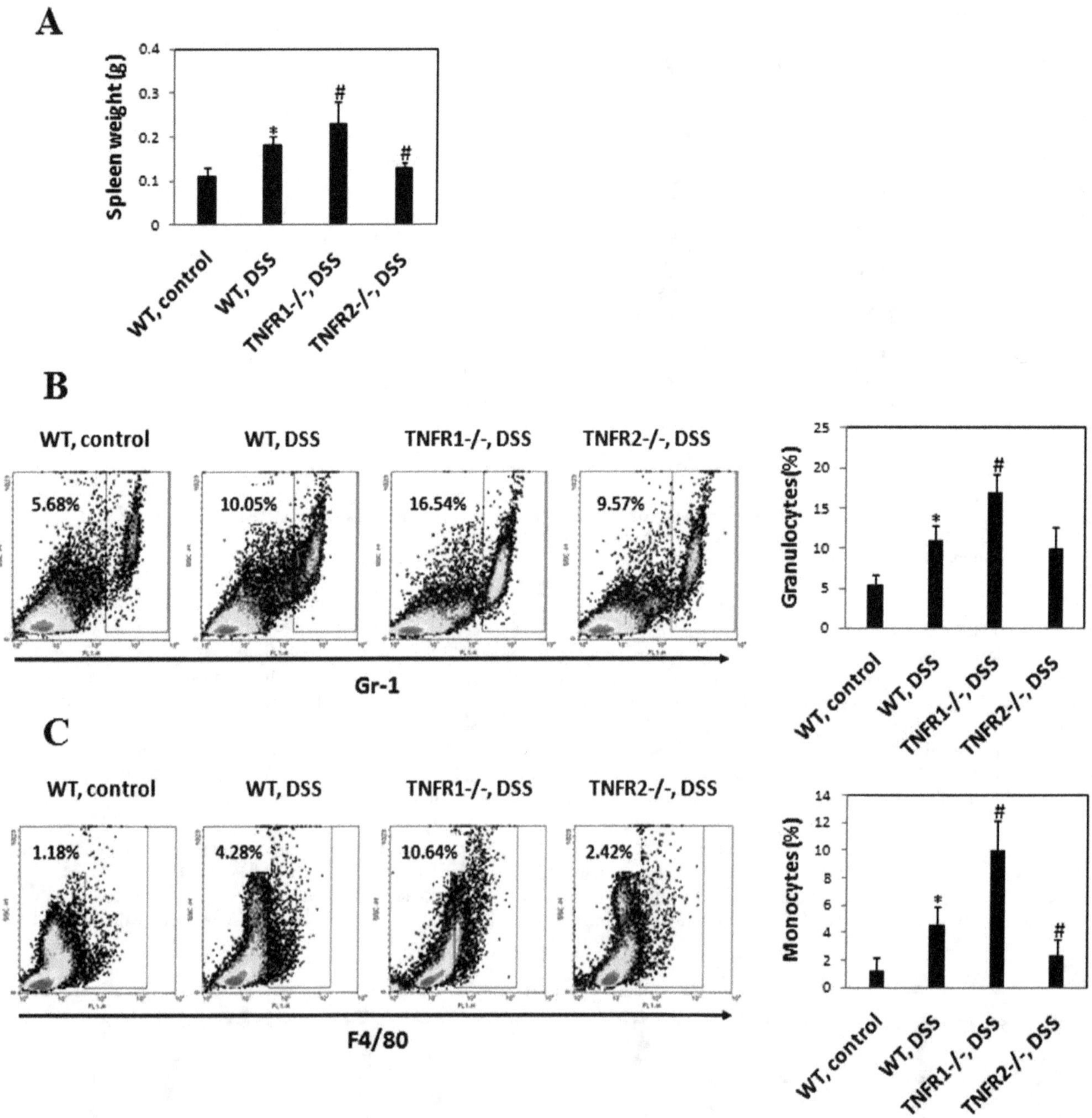

Figure 5. Systemic inflammatory response in TNF-R−/− and WT mice after DSS. (A) Spleen was isolated and weighed at day 8 after colitis induction. The percentage of granulocytes (Gr-1$^+$) (B) or monocytes (F4/80$^+$) (C) in the spleens were examined by flow cytometry. Representative plots were shown. Data represent the mean±SD of four to six mice per group from three independent experiments. *P<0.05 vs WT control mice; #P<0.05, ##P<0.01 vs WT mice after DSS.

expression of anti-apoptotic factor Bcl-2 in CEC of WT mice (Fig. 6D). This effect was more significant in TNF-R1−/− mice (Fig. 6D). Consistent with the data from TUNEL staining, reduction of Bcl-2 contents was found in LP-immune cells of TNFR2−/− mice (Fig. 6E). Furthermore, densitometry analysis showed that the ratio of Bcl-2/Bax in TNF-R1−/− or TNF-R2−/− mice was pronouncedly lower than in WT mice after DSS (Fig. 6E). Further, to elucidate the effects of TNF-R deficiency on NF-κB activity, we detected IκBα expression in the CEC or LP-immune cells after DSS. The amounts of IκBα in CEC for TNF-R1−/− mice or in LP-immune cells for TNF-R2−/− mice were much lower than those in WT DSS-treated mice (Fig. 6D and E), indicating that NF-κB activity was enhanced in CEC and LP-immune cells respectively. Thus, cell type-specific reduction in anti-apoptotic proteins and enhanced NF-κB activity may account for exacerbation or amelioration of colitis in TNFR1 or 2−/− mice after DSS.

Discussion

TNF plays a critical role in the immunopathogenesis of IBD. Blocking TNF using specific monoclonal antibody has been

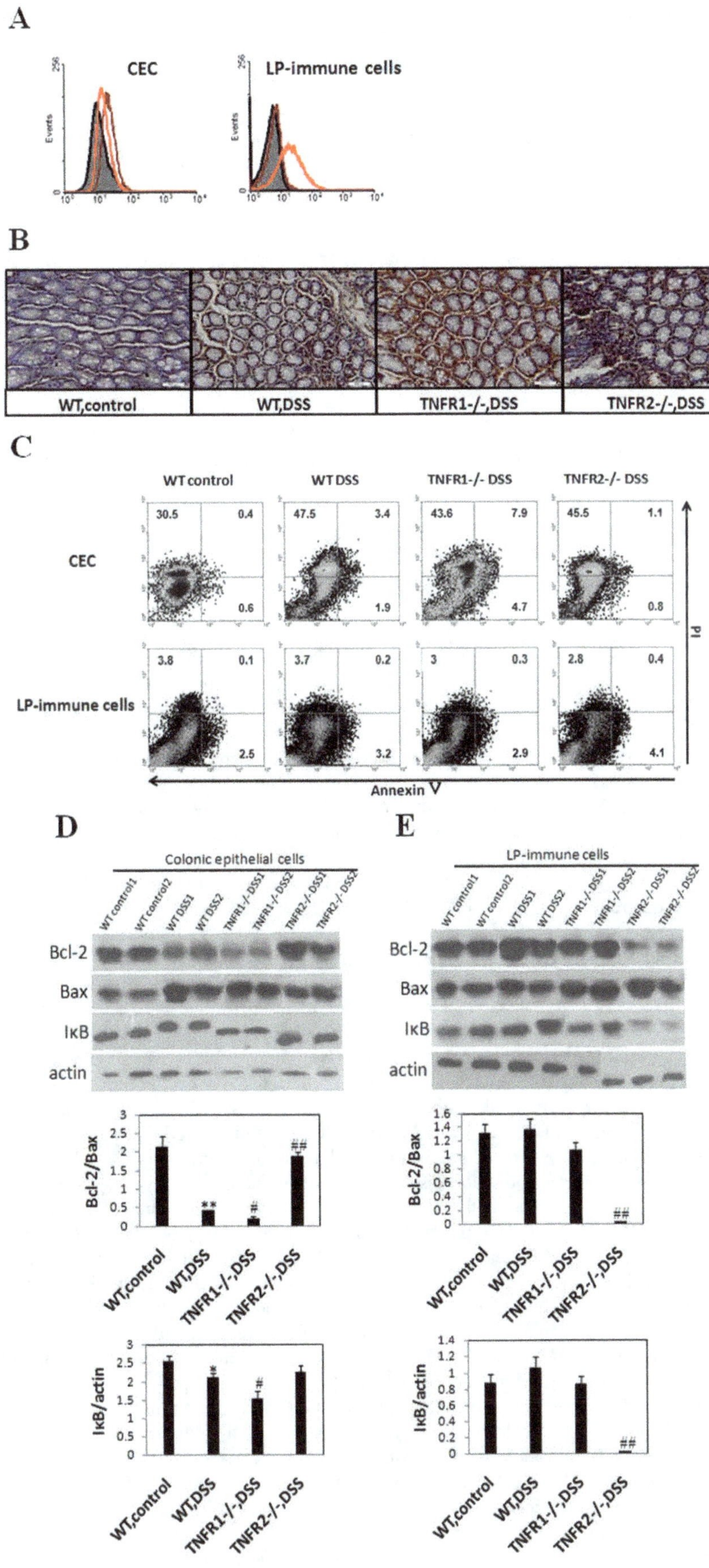
A
CEC
LP-immune cells
Events
B
WT,control
WT,DSS
TNFR1-/-,DSS
TNFR2-/-,DSS
C
WT control
WT DSS
TNFR1-/- DSS
TNFR2-/- DSS
CEC
30.5
0.4
0.6
47.5
3.4
1.9
43.6
7.9
4.7
45.5
1.1
0.8
LP-immune cells
3.8
0.1
2.5
3.7
0.2
3.2
3
0.3
2.9
2.8
0.4
4.1
Annexin V
PI
D
Colonic epithelial cells
WT control1
WT control2
WT DSS1
WT DSS2
TNFR1-/- DSS1
TNFR1-/- DSS2
TNFR2-/- DSS1
TNFR2-/- DSS2
Bcl-2
Bax
IκB
actin
Bcl-2/Bax
IκB/actin
WT,control
WT,DSS
TNFR1-/-,DSS
TNFR2-/-,DSS
E
LP-immune cells
Bcl-2
Bax
IκB
actin
Bcl-2/Bax
IκB/actin
WT,control
WT,DSS
TNFR1-/-,DSS
TNFR2-/-,DSS

Figure 6. TNF-R1 or 2 ablation affects apoptosis of colonic epithelial cells or infiltrating immune cells differently after DSS. Colons were dissected at day 8 after colitis induction. (A) Colonic epithelial cells and LP-immune cells were isolated as described in Materials and methods. TNF-R1 (brown line) and 2 (red line) expression in these cells was examined by flow cytometry. (B) Apoptosis was determined by terminal deoxynucleotidyl transferase-mediated deoxyuridine triphosphate nick end-labeling (TUNEL) staining (brown nuclei). Magnification: ×400. Histology is representative for more than 10 mice per group. (C) Colonic epithelial cells and LP-immune cells were stained with annexin V and PI. Their apoptosis was detected by flow cytometry. (D,E) Colonic epithelial cells (D) and lamina propria-immune cells (E) were isolated respectively and the proteins were extracted. Bcl-2, Bax, and IκBα expression was examined by western blotting. Glyceraldehyde 3-phosphate dehydrogenase (GAPDH) was used as internal control. Changes in quantity of expression of these factors were determined by densitometric assays. Data are representative of three independent experiments. $^*P<0.05$ vs WT control mice; $\#P<0.05$, $\#\#P<0.01$ vs WT mice after DSS.

identified to be beneficial for treatment of patients suffering from IBD [22]. Blockade of TNF, however, has been associated with the reactivation of tuberculosis and the possible development of other opportunistic infections such as histoplasmosis, listeriosis and pneumocystis [23]. Thus, it is very necessary to dissect the role of TNF signaling via TNF-R1 or 2 in experimental colitis, given that the beneficial outcome of complete blocking TNF may be achieved from blocking the signaling from only one of the two receptors. In this report, we provide evidence that TNF signaling via TNF-R1 or 2 has opposite effects on the pathogenesis of DSS-induced colitis. That is, TNF-R1-mediated signaling ameliorated the severity of colitis, while TNF-R2-mediated signaling was detrimental for the course of colitis. The data presented in this paper strongly support that blocking the interaction of TNF with its receptor 2 alone is sufficient to treat IBD.

It is worthy to note that the data presented in our study are incompletely consistent with a previous report that TNF signaling via TNF-R1 or 2 is redundant for the pathogenesis of DSS colitis in C57Bl/6 mice [13]. This discrepancy may be resolved by the fact that different mouse strains were used in these studies, as BALB/c strains used in our study are well known to be predisposed to a Th2 response, while C57Bl/6 strains do not. Interestingly, TNF signaling via TNF-R1 or 2 also appears to have distinct effects on different models of experimental colitis. Our previous study demonstrated that deficiency of TNF-R1 or 2 attenuated intestinal damage and improved the symptoms of TNBS-instilled colitis [12]. This may be explained by that different mechanisms are responsible for the initiation and progression of DSS and TNBS-induced experimental colitis respectively [24]. Interestingly, it is well accepted that intestinal inflammation induced by TNBS in BALB/c strains displays human CD-like features, while the pathogenesis of DSS colitis resembles ulcerative colitis in human [24]. Therefore, these data have implications for potential regimens targeting TNF-R1 or 2 to treat CD or UC in clinic.

The harmful or beneficial outcome of lack of TNF-R1 or 2 on DSS-induced colitis is tightly related to alteration of production of proinflammatory cytokines in the attacked tissues. This result indicates that interference with TNF signaling affects other putatively colitis-related cytokine expression, for example IL-6. Indeed, TNF can directly induce IL-6 production by NF-κB-, NF-IL-6-, and AP-1-dependent mechanisms [25], it also can facilitate the recruitment and survival of proinflammatory immune cells capable of IL-6 production [3]. The data in our paper extend these findings. IL-6 production induced by TNF is mediated mainly by TNF signaling via TNF-R2, as lacking TNF-R1 led to significant up-regulation of IL-6 expression in the colon, while TNF-R2 deficiency did not. Furthermore, the mutual regulation of TNF-R1 and 2-mediated signaling is orchestrated on proinflammatory cytokine production thereby signs of colitis, because TNF signaling via TNF-R1 dampens TNF-R2-mediated pathogenic responses, as shown by the fact that ablation of TNF-R1 dramatically aggravated TNF-R2-mediated colonic inflammation. The details, however, need further investigation.

One of the hallmarks of intestinal inflammation is the infiltration of neutrophils into colons and release of large amounts of oxgen radicals [18]. Our results showed significant increase of neutrophil infiltrates in sites of inflammation in TNF-R1−/− mice when DSS-induced colitis was established. Whereas, TNF-R2-deficient mice exhibited reduced infiltration of neutrophils, which may account for blunted intestinal inflammatory responses. Thus, we believe that the absence of TNF signaling via TNF-R1 or 2 affects neutrophil recruitment differently into colonic tissues upon the establishment of colitis. Intriguingly, these results are incompletely consistent with our previous study showing that TNF-R1 or 2−/− TNBS-instilled mice displayed restricted recruitment of neutrophils into inflamed colons, which may reflect the difference in the virtue of inflammation induced by DSS and TNBS. Increased infiltration of neutrophil in the colon of TNF-R1−/− colitic mice may be due to up-regulated expression of several putatively neutrophil-chemoattractant chemokines in local compartment, although the underlying mechanisms remain unclear [26]. Notably, it has been reported that TNF is able to induce integrin CD11b/CD18 up-regulation on human neutrophils, enhance cell adhesion and recruit as well as retain leukocytes in inflammatory sites [27]. Thus, TNF signaling may affect directly and indirectly the recruitment of neutrophils into inflamed tissues, thereby provoke or resolve inflammation in TNF-R1 or 2-deficient mice.

Mucosal damage is a key event for DSS-induced colonic inflammation. TNF is an important factor in this process, as in pathological settings TNF is released largely and has deleterious effects on epithelial cells [1]. Our results showed that DSS administration led to apoptosis of colonic epithelial cells by reducing expression of anti-apoptotic protein Bcl-2 and enhancing NF-κB activity. Lack of TNF signaling via TNF-R1 could accelerate this apoptosis-promoting process and rendered increased death of epithelial cells, finally resulted in more severity of mucosal injury. Interestingly, the absence of TNF signaling via TNF-R2 influenced mildly apoptosis of CEC, but drastically enhanced programmed cell death of LP-immune cells, which may account for resolution of inflammation in TNF-R2−/− mice. These data indicate that, in the setting of intestinal inflammation, colonic epithelial cells and inflammatory immune cells have different susceptibility to TNF-mediated apoptosis through TNF-R1 or 2. This concept is supported by the previous studies showing that TNF-R1 is dominantly functional to mediate TNF signaling in endothelial cells [28], myofibroblast [29], and infected host cells [30], while TNF function on immune cells is predominantly through TNF-R2 [31,32]. Although the pathways involved in TNF-mediated apoptosis of CEC and LP-immune cells need to be elucidated further, the present data indicate that enhanced apoptosis of CEC or LP-immune cells is one of the reasons for exacerbated or ameliorated inflammation in TNF-R1 or 2−/− mice after DSS.

In the current study, we demonstrated an opposite role of TNF-R1 or 2 in the course of DSS-induced colitis, which is associated with alteration in several parameters, including infiltration of granulocytes, release of proinflammatory mediators and apoptosis of epithelial cells as well as inflammatory immune cells. These data suggest that targeting TNF-R2 rather than TNF-R1 specifically might be an alternative approach to therapy for patients with UC, considering that TNF is a key factor in host defense against microbe infection [33]. Although TNF-R2 deficiency failed to expand monocyte population specifically after DSS, TNF signaling via TNF-R2 had minor role in anti-mycobacterial immunity [34]. So blockade of TNF-R2 specifically may be an alternative and promising approach to treat IBD. The studies in TNBS or DSS-induced experimental colitis suggest that the exact role of TNF signaling via TNF-R1 or 2 may depend on model of colitis and mouse strains used and need to be interpreted carefully. Further investigation in other models and in humans is warranted.

Acknowledgments

The authors would like to thank Prof. Zhihai Qin for supplying TNFR-knockout mice.

Author Contributions

Conceived and designed the experiments: GC YS. Performed the experiments: YW GH YD YW GL. Analyzed the data: RW HX BS RG YL. Contributed reagents/materials/analysis tools: XL CH. Wrote the paper: KW YC GC.

References

1. Hehlgans T, Pfeffer K (2005) The intriguing biology of the tumour necrosis factor/tumour necrosis factor receptor superfamily: players, rules and the games. Immunology 182: 1281–1290.
2. Papadakis KA, Targan SR (2000) Role of cytokines in the pathogenesis of inflammatory bowel disease. Annu Rev Med 51: 289–298.
3. Kallias G, Douni E, Kassiotis G, Kontoyiannis D (1999) On the role of tumor necrosis factor and receptors in models of multiorgan failure, rheumatoid arthritis, multiple sclerosis and inflammatory bowel disease. Immuol Rev 169: 175–194.
4. MacEwan DJ (2002) TNF receptor subtype signaling: differences and cellular consequences. Cell Signal 14: 477–492.
5. Pimental-Munios FX, Seed B (1999) Regulated commitment of TNF signaling: a molecular switch for death or activation. Immunity 11: 783–793.
6. Holtmann MH, Douni E, Schutz M, Zeller G, Mudter J, et al. (2002) Tumor necrosis factor receptor 2 is up-regulated on lamina propria T cells in Crohn's disease and promotes experimental colitis *in vivo*. Eur J Immunol 32: 142–151.
7. Mizoguchi E, Mizoguchi A, Takedatsu H, Cario E, de Jong YP, et al. (2002) Role of tumor necrosis factor receptor 2 (TNFR2) in colonic epithelial hyperplasia and chronic intestinal inflammation in mice. Gastroenterology 122: 134–144.
8. Sashio H, Tamura K, Ito R, Yamamoto Y, Bamba H, et al. (2002) Polymorphisms of the TNF gene and the TNF receptor superfamily member 1B gene are associated with susceptibility to ulcerative colitis and Crohn's disease, respectively. Immunogenetics 53: 1020–1027.
9. Schneider JD, Seibold I, Saxer-Sekulic N, Paredes BE, Saurer L, et al. (2009) Lack of TNFR2 expression by $CD4^{+}T$ cells exacerbates experimental colitis, Eur J Immunol 39: 1743–1753.
10. Ebach DR, Newberry R, Stenson W. (2005) Differential role of tumor necrosis factor receptors in TNBS colitis. Inflamm Bowel Dis 11: 533–540.
11. Nakai M, Sudo K, Yamada Y (2005) The role of the tumor necrosis factor receptor in 2,4,6-trinitrobenzene sulfonic acid (TNBS)-induced colitis in mice. Dig Dis Sci 50: 1669–1676.
12. Yang Y, Wang H, Dou Y, Wang Y, Han G, et al. (2011) Colitogenic role of tumour necrosis factor (TNF) receptors in trinitrobenzene sulphonic acid colitis: TNF-R1 ablation does not affect systemic inflammatory response. Clin Exp Immunol 165: 372–382.
13. Stillie R, Stadnyk AW (2009) Role of TNF receptors, TNFR1 and TNFR2, in dextran sodium sulfate-induced colitis. Inflamm Bowel Dis 15: 1515–1525.
14. Zhao X, Mohaupt M, Jiang J, Liu S, Li B, et al. (2007) Tumor necrosis factor receptor 2-mediated tumor suppression is nitric oxide dependent and involves angiostasis. Cancer Res 67: 4443–4450.
15. Rachmilewitz D, Simon PL, Schwartz LW, Griswold DE, Fondacaro JD, et al. (1989) Inflammatory mediators of experimental colitis in rats. Gastroenterology 97: 326–337.
16. Krawisz JE, Sharon P, Stenson WF (1984) Quantitative assay for acute intestinal inflammation based on myeloperoxidase activity. Assessment of inflammation in rat and hamster models. Gastroenterology 87: 1344–1350.
17. Mantovani A, Cassatella MA, Costantini C, Jaillon S (2011) Neutrophils in the activation and regulation of innate and adaptive immunity. Nat Rev Immunol 11: 519–531.
18. Grisham MB, Yamada T (1992) Neutrophils, nitrogen oxides, and inflammatory bowel disease. Ann N Y Acad Sci 664: 103–115.
19. Lochman I, Kral V, Lochmanova A, Lupac J, Cebecauer L (2011) ANCA in the diagnosis of neutrophil-mediated inflammation. Autoimmun Rev 10: 295–298.
20. Sydora BC, Albert EJ, Foshaug RR, Doyle JS, Churchill TA, et al. (2012) Intravenous injection of endogenous microbial components abrogates DSS-induced colitis. Dig Dis Sci 57: 345–354.
21. Westbrook AM, Schiestl RH (2010) Atm-deficient mice exhibit increased sensitivity to dextran sulfate sodium-induced colitis characterized by elevated DNA damage and persistent immune activation. Cancer Res 70: 1875–1884.
22. Blam ME, Stein RB, Lichtenstein GR (2001) Integrating anti-tumor necrosis factor therapy in inflammatory bowel disease: current and future perspectives. Am J Gastroenterol 96: 1977–1997.
23. Weisman MH (2002) What are the risks of biological therapy in rheumatoid arthritis? An update on safety. J Rheumatol Suppl 65: 33–38.
24. Strober W, Fuss IJ, Blumberg RS (2002) The immunology of mucosal models of inflammation. Annu Rev Immunol 20: 495–549.
25. Legrand-Poels S, Schoonbroodt S, Piette J (2000) Regulation of interleukin-6 gene expression by pro-inflammatory cytokines in a colon cancer cell line. Biochem J 349: 765–773.
26. Kobayashi Y (2008) The role of chemokines in neutrophil biology. Front Biosci 13: 2400–2407.
27. Montecucco F, Steffens S, Burger F, Da Costa A, Bianchi G, et al. (2008) Tumor necrosis factor-alpha (TNF-α) induces integrin CD11b/CD18 (Mac-1) up-regulation and migration to the CC chemokine CCL3 (MIP-1α) on human neutrophils through defined signaling pathways. Cell Signal 20: 557–568.
28. Zhou Z, Connell MC, MacEwan DJ (2007) TNFR1-induced NF-κB, but not ERK, P38MAPK or JNK activation, mediates TNF-induced ICAM-1 and VCAM-1 expression on endothelial cells. Cell Signal 19: 1238–1248.
29. Lai CF, Shao JS, Behrmann A, Krchma K, Cheng SL, et al. (2012) TNFR1-activated reactive oxidative species signals up-regulate osteogenic Msx2 programs in aortic myofibroblasts. Endocrinology 153: 3897–3910.
30. Paland N, Bohme L, Gurumurthy RK, Maurer A, Szczepek AJ, et al. (2008) Reduced display of tumor necrosis factor 1 at the host cell surface supports infection with Chlamydia trachomatis. J Biol Chem 283: 6438–6448.
31. Xu J, Chalrabarti AK, Tan JL, Ge L, Gambotto A, et al. (2007) Essential role of the TNF-TNFR2 cognate interaction in mouse dendritic cell-natural killer cell crosstalk. Blood 109: 3333–3341.
32. Aspalter RM, Eibl MM, Wolf HM (2003) Regulation of TCR-mediated T cell activation by TNF-RII. J Leukoc Biol 74: 572–582.
33. Ellerin T, Rubin RH, Weinblatt ME (2003) Infections and anti-tumor necrosis factor α therapy. Arthritis Rheum 48: 3013–3022.
34. Jacobs M, Brown N, Allie N, Chetty K, Ryffel B (2000) Tumor necrosis factor receptor 2 plays a minor role for mycobacterial immunity. Pathobiology 68: 68–75.

8

Modelling of Mouse Experimental Colitis by Global Property Screens: A Holistic Approach to Assess Drug Effects in Inflammatory Bowel Disease

Johan Gottfries[1], Silvia Melgar[2], Erik Michaëlsson[3]*

1 Department of Chemistry, University of Gothenburg, Gothenburg, Sweden, 2 Alimentary Pharmabiotic Centre, University College Cork, National University of Ireland, Cork, Ireland, 3 Department of Bioscience, Cardiovascular and Gastrointestinal IMED, AstraZeneca R&D Mölndal, Mölndal, Sweden

Abstract

Preclinical disease models play an important role in the establishment of new treatment paradigms, identification of biomarkers and assessment of drug efficacy and safety. However, the accuracy of these models in context of the human disease are sometimes questioned, e.g. due to trials failing to confirm efficacy in humans. We suggest that one reason behind this gap in predictability may relate to how the preclinical data is analyzed and interpreted. In the present paper, we introduce a holistic approach to analyze and illustrate data in context of one of the most commonly used colitis models, i.e. the mouse dextran sulphate sodium (DSS) colitis model. Diseased mice were followed over time along disease progression and by use of tool pharmacological compounds activating nuclear hormone receptors, respectively. A new multivariate statistics approach was applied including principal component analysis (PCA) with treatment prediction subsequent to establishing the principal component analysis model. Thus, several studies could be overlaid and compared to each other in a new, comprehensive and holistic way. This method, named mouse colitis global property screening, appears applicable not only to any animal modelling series of studies but also to human clinical studies. The prerequisites for the study set up and calculations are delineated and examples of new learnings from the global property screening will be presented.

Editor: Markus M. Heimesaat, Charité, Campus Benjamin Franklin, Germany

Funding: The study was funded by and performed at AstraZeneca R&D, Molndal, Sweden. The study design, generation of data, analysis of data, decision to publish as well as preparation of the manuscript were performed by the authors, of which E.M. is employed by AstraZeneca R&D.

Competing Interests: J.G. is an employee at the University of Gothenburg and is also founder and owner of the consulting company Gottfries Medicinal. S.M. is employed by GlaxoSmithKline. E.M. is employed by AstraZeneca R&D. None of the authors have competing interests as consultants, pending patents, or to products in development or at market related to the topic of the present paper.

* E-mail: erik.michaelsson@astrazeneca.com

Introduction

Inflammatory Bowel Disease (IBD), Crohn's disease (CD) and ulcerative colitis (UC), are multifactorial, complex, lifelong diseases with a broad spectrum of manifestations. The pathophysiology of IBD is still unclear but it is well acknowledged that multiple factors, including genetic, environmental and immunological, contribute to the occurrence and perpetuation of the disease. Furthermore, the patients on occasion also present with extraintestinal manifestations, such as cholangitis, uveitis, peri-anal and oral lesions. The disease severity is quantified by grading symptoms, which are then compiled in a univariate fashion to generate disease activity scores, such as the Crohn's disease activity index (CDAI).

Evaluating the outcome of new drugs in a clinical study is traditionally performed by statistical univariate methods created to discover statistically significant improvements for the treated patient group, in an unbiased way. However, univariate methods need high object inclusion numbers to meet their significance dependency and, in addition, some correlations are of truly multivariate nature [1]. In terms of complex diseases such as IBD, there is also a risk of overseeing clinically meaningful treatment effects. Such treatment effects may be diluted and masked by unrelated phenomena that are involved in the score, but not in the targeted pathophysiology. On one hand, these approaches are obviously required for drug development, both from ethical and business aspects and the regulatory authorities delineate stringent guidelines (see FDA guidelines), which the industry follows for good reasons. The above perspective relates mainly to the later development phase, i.e. clinical phase III studies, Research and early development studies, on the other hand, could benefit from parallel approaches, frontloading biological or physiological relevance versus statistical significance. Several studies [2,3,4] have indicated that multivariate analyses provide more in depth knowledge than significance test statistics on the physiology and at the systems biology level, and could therefore be applied to the study designs. Such holistic methods can for instance describe how individual animals alter their physiological pattern when they develop disease or when they are subjected to pharmacological treatment.

In terms of preclinical models for IBD, more than fifty models have been described including genetically modified, chemically induced, adoptive transfer of T cells and also few spontaneous models (reviewed in [5,6]). It should be noted that none of these models fully represent any form of human IBD. Rather, they can be viewed upon as mechanistic models illustrating different physiological and pathophysiological mechanisms occurring in the gastrointestinal tract. As such, the models have contributed greatly to our current understanding of the underlying mechanisms of gastrointestinal inflammation and disease pathogenesis. However, the complexity of gastrointestinal inflammation is seldom illustrated in these studies. Rather, there is a bias towards symptom scoring that are compiled into univariate composite indices. Similar to the human situation [7], these composite disease activity indices may not be informative for the severity of the local inflammation, and may therefore not be optimal endpoints for understanding the underlying mechanisms behind the disease.

For both ethical and scientific reasons it is always important to seek new ways to make the best use of any sacrificed animal, which will lead to higher accuracy in ensuing clinical studies [8]. In line with this thought we, by the current paper, want to present a new way towards a holistic and robust modelling of animal data, as exemplified on the murine dextran sodium sulphate (DSS) model of colitis. This has been achieved by a global property screening (GPS) approach, using a new way to set up data matrices for principal component analyses (PCA), applied to the characterization of the mouse model *per se*, but also to pharmacological treatments with small molecules.

Results

The present study includes two independent series of experiments using DSS-induced colitis in mice and thus two ways of using multivariate modelling in experimental IBD. The first series represents a description of the disease process over time in two mouse strains and the second series how one of the mouse strains respond to treatments with new chemical entities. The PCA models were calculated by inclusion of healthy control mice in combination with DSS-treated and DSS-treated plus placebo-treated animals. The animals undertaking any intervention, e.g. drug administration, were not used for building the model, but subsequently predicted into the scores space using the established PCA model.

Multivariate modelling of the disease dynamics in two genetic backgrounds

The first validation data set included DSS-treated C57BL/6 as well as BALB/c mice and the resulting PCA model provided models including 3 principal components. The mouse strain comparison between C57BL/6 versus BALB/c is depicted in Figure 1, previously shown to behave differently following exposure to DSS [9]. Indeed, the two strains behaved differently after the DSS challenge. This was observed by inspection of the individual animal positioning in the PCA scores plot. The PCA scores are generated by estimation of the object inter-related positioning in a scatter space comprising all collected biomarker data. The method implements each biomarker data as an individual and uniquely directed axis. In the example shown in Figure 1, 21 different biomarkers were assessed, thus generating 21 uniquely directed axes. Thereafter, the PCA least squares procedure was initiated, including the estimation of new vector dimensions adhering to minimized sum of squared distance from each data point to the generated vector, and thus the first PC is generated. In cases when the model needs more than a one-dimensional structure, a second and third and etc., component can be generated using the residual data (i.e. after removal of the data supporting the previously generated component). The validation for PCA model complexity was in the present study estimated by the cross-validation procedure as described in material and methods. Analysis of the present dataset yielded four significant PCs by the SIMCA P+ software. However, the fourth component explained less that 7% of the total data variance and comprised a negative contribution to Q^2 (i.e. the predictivity as assessed by cross validation) and was therefore removed. The remaining three PCs explained 73% (i.e. $R2 = 0.732$ for the X matrix) of the data with $Q^2 = 0.47$. The model scores, i.e. individual animal sample data scores, illustrating their time resolved reaction to the DSS treatment as assessed by biomarkers, are shown in Figure 1.

Evidently both strains were clustering together at day 0, i.e. all being healthy mice, after which the strain related property path diverted, which thus illustrated a tangible way towards mouse strain dependence to DSS response. Both strains revealed overlapping disease profiles throughout the initial week (d7). However, during the recovery phase the BALB/c mice moved, in the PCA projection scores system, in a close to inverse direction compared to the disease direction. After one week of recovery, these animals were apparently healthy and their individual position in the 3-dimensional score space were overlapping with that of healthy control BALB/c mice, illustrating complete recovery. C57BL/6 mice, on the other hand, did not recover towards a healthy phenotype, as seen in the PCA scores plot (Figure 1). Instead, they ended up in an orthogonal direction compared to the trajectory towards the healthy profile of the controls, but still different from the initial state induced by acute DSS-treatment, illustrating the chronic inflammation they suffered from.

In parallel, the influence from the primary biomarker variable correlation pattern on the property paths in the DSS experiment was inspected. This is achieved by use of the PCA inherent calculation of loadings, which are obtained by the assessment of the space angle between the direction of the original biomarker co-ordinate axis and the resulting PCs, respectively (PC1, PC2 and PC3 in the present example). A small space angle between a PC and a biomarker original axis indicates high correlation to the tested PC, and vice versa. Indeed the cosine of the obtained angle coincides with the correlation coefficient between the two axes. These estimates are called loadings (i.e. biomarker loadings in the present study), which are highly instrumental for entailing interpretation of observed individual animal trajectories and strain clustering seen in the PCA of data from the DSS induced colitis model (Figure 1).

Thus, we can conclude that the transition from health to acute disease (day 0 to 7) was characterised by the presence of blood in faeces and decreased biomarker loadings for colon levels of PGE_2 in both BALB/c and C57BL/6 mice. In C57BL/6 mice, the transition from day 7 to 12 was characterised by high diarrhoea scores, increased weight loss, increased macroscopical signs of colitis and peak colon levels of IL-1β, CCL2, CXCL2/3 and CCL4. From day 19 and further on, the colon biomarker loadings for cytokine levels and macroscopical signs of colitis remained high. In addition, there were increased levels of CXL10 and IFNγ. Also, these time points were characterised by increased spleen weights and recovered body weights. Thus, for short term studies (up to 7 days) the two strains behave similarly and appeared equally relevant for drug intervention studies, whereas for chronicity studies the C57BL/6 mice should be used.

Evaluation of new chemical compounds using PCA modeling

By pharmacological intervention we illustrate how the present approach can be used in drug discovery. In this example, a defined DSS-challenged mouse strain (BALB/c) was assessed for inflammatory biomarkers and other endpoints measured after treatment with three different nuclear hormone receptor agonists (i.e. LXR,

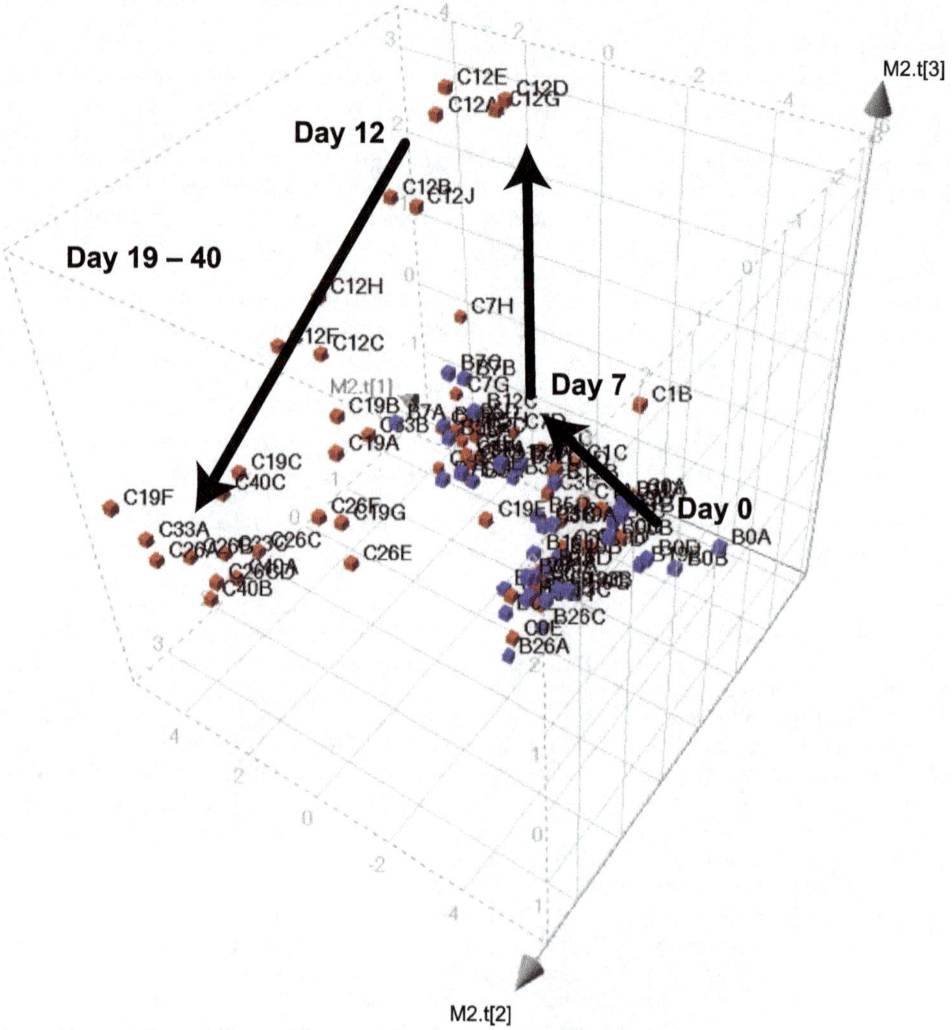

Figure 1. Multivariate projection of DSS-colitis development in BALB/c (Blue indicators, B) and C57BL/6 (Red indicators, C) mice. Each cube represents an individual animal. The number next to the cubes indicates the number of days since the initiation of DSS-treatment (from day 0 to day 40). Data were generated using a three-component principal component analysis (i.e. t1–t3 are plotted) based on the assessed variables according to Materials and Methods. Arrows indicate disease progression in C57BL/6 mice.

PPARα and PPARγ). Nuclear hormone receptor agonists have been shown to possess anti-inflammatory action, possibly via mechanisms involving sequestration of and/or competition for NF-κB cofactors [10,11].

First, a PCA-model was established using DSS- and placebo-treated and healthy control mice, respectively, with the aim to predict the data from animals receiving an additional compound treatment. This is possible for any PCA model given that the same variables, i.e. colitis biomarkers in the present study, are measured coherently. The data alignment aspect is depicted in Figure 2 and such prediction is straight-forward once a PCA model has been created. The expected advantages from this approach relates to standardization. Firstly, we provide a basic model that does not change in scale, biomarker loading correlation pattern towards the model PCs, or any other model property [12]. Secondly, when the PCA model is used for prediction of a pharmacological compound in treated animals (with or without DSS-pre-treatment) one can assess the cohort clustering and interpret their systems pharmacology positioning via the scores plot as compared to the healthy and DSS-treated cohort distributions (see Figure 3). However, in this step it is of outmost importance over time to include model animal objects to reveal any drift in the healthy and DSS treated animal clustering, be it for animal phenotype due to e.g. health status or response to DSS etc, or for drift in the analytical measures settings (data not shown). Thirdly, over time it is possible to combine any number of treatments and any comparison combination, including reference and tool compound treatments, for drug target and pharmacological mechanism investigation. By using the PCA prediction mode for new samples, i.e. predicting treated animal property positions into the initial model including the sample data from healthy and diseased animals, a robust model that facilitates interpretation between treatments over time is provided.

The resulting systems pharmacology model on the present study is illustrated in Figure 3A, comprising 2 significant principal components. The reason for the lower model complexity compared to the previous example, where two mouse strains with DSS colitis were validated, was the restricted time used for the pharmacological intervention, i.e. 7 days, and thus the modelling of the "chronic" phase observed in C57BL/6 mice was omitted.

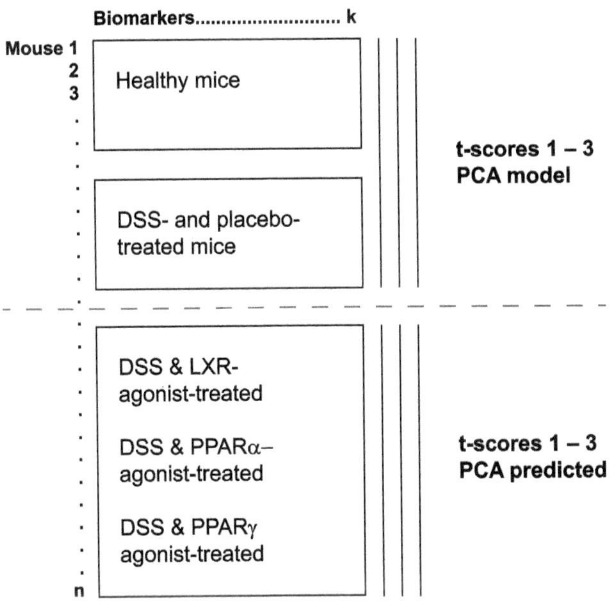

Figure 2. Schematic overview of matrix relation for the GPS calculations. The PCA model include healthy as well as placebo treated DSS-exposed mice. The distribution of these mice in the PCA model is shown in Figure 3A. The mice positioned into the PCA-model were treated with DSS- together with a LXR-agonist, PPARα-agonist or PPARγ-agonist. The positions of these mice are shown in Figure 3B.

Thereafter, the drug treated animals were positioned into the PCA model by prediction, illustrating the efficacies of three different nuclear hormone receptor agonists (see Figure 2 and Figure 3B). The biomarker and endpoint correlation pattern is depicted in Figure 3C. Figures 3A and B show the model based on healthy and vehicle-treated diseased mice. As shown in Figure 3A, mouse V3, V10, V17, V19 and V23 responded poorly to the DSS treatment ("low responders"), whereas the rest were classified as "diseased", but not "high responders". From the biomarker loadings (see Figure 3C), it was evident that all parameters except adiponectin and liver weight, were described by the first principal component, and this component was also what discriminated healthy from diseased mice. When the compound-treated animals were predicted into the model, it showed that treatment with the three NHR agonists generated three distinct patterns. Mice treated with the PPARγ agonist clustered towards the left-hand side along principal component 1 in the scores plot (i.e. negative scores, see Figure 3B), which represents higher plasma levels of haptoglobin (acute phase protein) and local markers of inflammation. Compared to PPARγ treated mice, LXR-treated mice comprised somewhat lower principal component 1 scores, demonstrating better anti-inflammatory efficacy. Finally, the PPARα-treated mice demonstrate the highest degree of disease amelioration of the three groups. However, the PPARα-treated mice also had low scores in the second component, due to high level biomarker loadings for liver weights in combination with low for plasma levels of adiponectin. From the loadings plot one can also conclude that the increased liver weight, which is a well-known effect by PPARα agonists [13], as well as the increased plasma levels of adiponectin, occurred independently from the anti-inflammatory action. Such interpretation can be drawn since adiponectin (and liver weight) loadings mapped orthogonally against the inflammatory biomarkers in the loadings plot (Figure 3C). Finding such uncoupled phenomena by orthogonal distributions of biomarker loadings illustrates an inherent property of multivariate analysis and unfolding the same pattern by univariate data analysis is less obvious. Rather, univariate analyses would, somewhat misleadingly, have suggested that liver weight increases occurs along with anti-inflammatory action (as illustrated in Figure 4).

Discussion

In the present paper, we have exemplified how multivariate analysis can be used to illustrate complex disease processes in a holistic manner and also document effects of pharmacological interventions on experimental colitis.

One hurdle for using PCA-analysis in inter-experimental comparisons is the mathematical rotation along principal components (i.e. mirror images of t-scores) that can occur. Although a mirror image of the t score is mathematically as valid as the original t score, it precludes comparison with data based on the original t score However, by using a holistic global property screening (GPS) approach with fixed principal components as presented herein, such rotations along principal components are avoided. Thus, pharmacological models (Figure 1) and compound treatment (Figure 3) can be compared to each other without scores and loadings scale alterations or rotations. These procedures standardize the interpretations over time of sequential analyses and contribute to holistic knowledge gain, which is the core property of GPS modelling concept [12]. Thus, it provides a background template system, in which instilled perturbations, e.g. pharmacological compounds, strain shifts including mutations, and housekeeping studies for robustness testing, etc, can be monitored. In other words, the GPS will help any user to simplify any comparisons of phenotypic perturbation, be it from disease model aspects or compound distribution for disease amelioration purposes, as long as the data structure complies with each other's format regarding measurements of biomarkers and other characterizing variables (see Figure 2).

Extrapolating the surplus findings provided by the GPS approach in the present study makes it tempting to conjecture that similar modelling of human clinical phase II data [14] could provide new important and ethically relevant insights by global comparability. This would add to Chalmers' [15] well formulated arguments regarding the importance of transparency of clinical data for ensuing translational information exchange. Regarding the possible translation by GPS-modelling to clinical data one must keep in mind the importance of maintained ethical considerations and that study design must be strictly regulated. However, we envision that parallel application of multivariate methodology could lead to synergistic learnings in clinical data analysis, for instance by contextualisation of biomarker data. First, PCA is an excellent tool to find the unforeseen. Unlike traditional data univariate analysis, PCA is not hypothesis-driven, but a tool to discover correlations in an unbiased manner. Second, the holistic principles of PCA will identify synergistic processes that often occur in biological systems, which would not necessarily be unveiled using traditional null-hypothesis based, univariate data-analysis. Along the same line, the PCA will also readily pinpoint parallel, independent processes that may occur in biological systems, such as the effect of PPARα-agonism on liver weight vs. intestinal inflammation as shown in the present paper. This means that PCA could provide useful knowledge and be a means to deal with the publication bias in which inconclusive or negative data are not published [8,15]. There are of course limitations with GPS. One considerable hurdle during implementation relates to the relatively abstract nature of the multivariate space. It can be

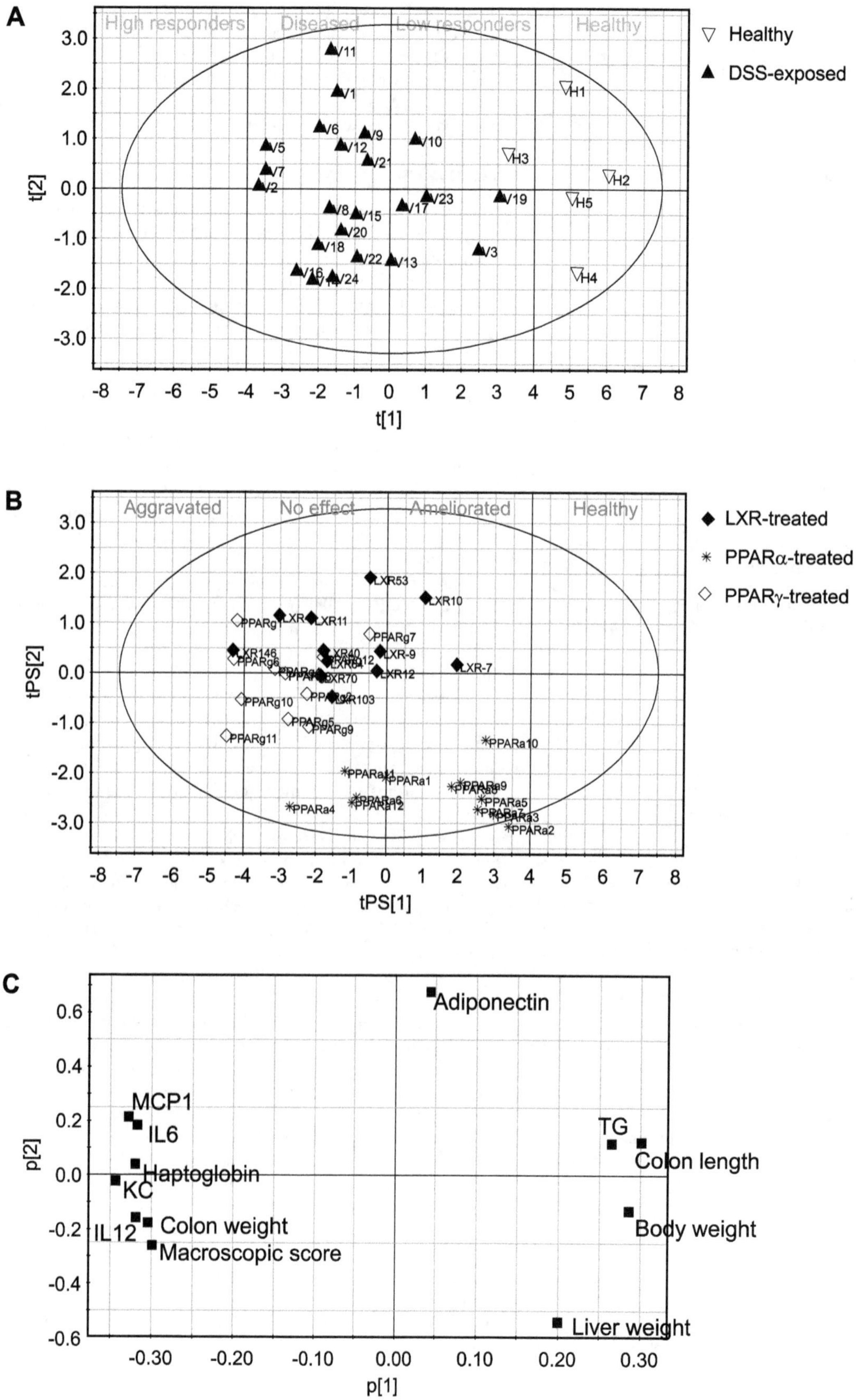
A
High responders
Diseased
Low responders
Healthy
Healthy
DSS-exposed
t[2]
t[1]
B
Aggravated
No effect
Ameliorated
Healthy
LXR-treated
PPARα-treated
PPARγ-treated
tPS[2]
tPS[1]
C
Adiponectin
MCP1
IL6
Haptoglobin
KC
IL12
Colon weight
Macroscopic score
TG
Colon length
Body weight
Liver weight
p[2]
p[1]

Figure 3. Evaluation of new chemical compounds using PCA modelling. A. Mouse colitis GPS model as generated from healthy control mice (open triangles) and placebo treated DSS-exposed mice (closed triangles) (see upper part of matrix in Figure 1). Based on the distance from the healthy control along the t(1) axis (i.e. the severity of the colitis) the mice are either classified as low responders, diseased or high responders. B. Mouse colitis GPS model including predictions for mice given nuclear hormone receptor agonists (dosing regimen as described in Materials and Methods), with receptor specificity as indicated (LXR (closed diamonds), PPARα (stars) and PPARγ (open diamonds)). Based on the position along the tPS(1) axis relative to the placebo-treated animals shown in Figure 3A, the effect of the treatment on the disease is either classified as ameliorated, no effect or aggravated. C. Individual variable correlation structure (i.e., loadings p1 versus p2 for PCA generated for objects in A) superimposable for interpretation of clustering in Figure 3A and B. The variables were plasma levels of haptoglobin, adiponectin and triglycerides (TG), colon levels of MCP1, KC, IL-6 and IL-12p40, colon weight, body weight, liver weight, colon length and macroscopic colon score. For example the PPARα-agonist treated animals in (B) are clustering in the lower end of principal component 2, due to high liver weight (and low adiponectin levels) and low principal component 1 due to reduced colitis.

challenging to understand why data, which at first glance appear to be un-structured, suddenly provide useful information and therefore should not be discarded. Secondly, the GPS-method is constrained to a pre-selected finite set of endpoints. As soon as one, or several variables are excluded or new variables are added into the data matrix (such as newly identified biomarkers), there is a risk of skewing and thereby limited predictive value of the model.

In conclusion, GPS modelling provides a good overview of data from complex measurements of biological systems, including holistic views on population distributions, definition of outlier individuals, and entailing model interpretation abilities to pinpoint serendipitous observanda, not the least by use of the additional GPS properties. This includes a potential for treatment stratification support [16,17] due to the straight forward pattern recognition properties via scores and biomarker loadings interpretation with opportunities for generation of multivariate stratification criteria. Finally, given that both animals and clinical patients undergo intervention with the same compound, a data structure with inherent properties for concatenation between animal models and human disease might come closer in sight [4].

Materials and Methods

Ethics statement

The procedures described herein were approved by the local animal ethics committee in Gothenburg, Sweden (approvals 220/2002 and 62/2004). The mice were housed in an environment enriched with chewing sticks, nest material and egg cartons. During the experiment, the general condition of the mice was monitored at least twice daily and individuals that displayed a significantly impaired state of health, i.e. were inactive, had ruffled fur or were unwilling to seek chow and water, were euthanized.

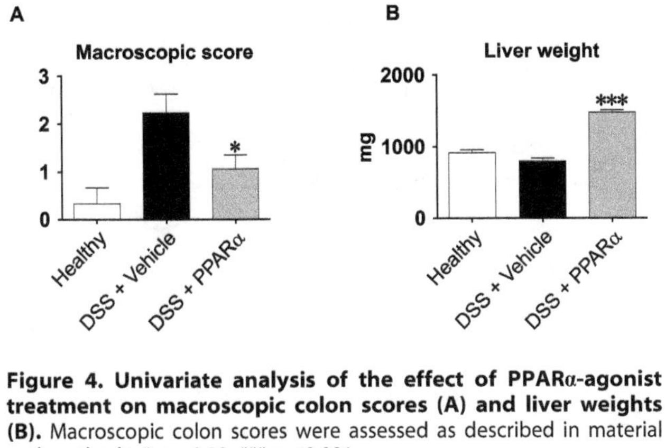

Figure 4. Univariate analysis of the effect of PPARα-agonist treatment on macroscopic colon scores (A) and liver weights (B). Macroscopic colon scores were assessed as described in material and methods. * p = 0.02; *** p<0.001.

Mice, induction of colitis and tissue sampling

Specific pathogen-free female BALB/cOlaHsD or C57BL/6OlaHsD mice obtained from Harlan (Netherlands) were used. The mice were housed in groups of up to 8 mice per cage and acclimatised for two weeks before the start of the experiment. The mice were fed R3 pellet chow (Lactamin) and tap water *ad lib*. Addition of DSS to the drinking water was used to induce colitis as previously described [9,18]. Briefly, a 3% (w/v) solution of 45 kD DSS (TdB consultancy, Uppsala, Sweden) was given for 5 days to C57BL/6 mice or 5% DSS for the indicated number of days to BALB/c mice. Fresh DSS was prepared daily to avoid bacterial growth in the solution. Healthy controls received normal tap water. Throughout the study, mice were monitored for symptoms (body weight, hunched posture, piloerection, and blood in the anus). During termination of the study, blood was taken by retroorbital puncture under isofluran anaesthesia and collected in EDTA-containing tubes, after which the mice were killed by cervical dislocation. The blood samples were centrifuged 3000 rpm for 10 minutes at 4°C, and plasma aliquoted and frozen at −80°C. The colon was dissected out, cut open, carefully rinsed and scored for macroscopical signs of inflammation (rigidity, thickness, ulcerations and oedema), yielding a maximal score of 10 [19], after which the distal 3 cm was divided and either frozen in liquid nitrogen (for cytokine analysis) or fixed in Zinc formaldehyde (for histology analyses) [9].

Biomarker analyses

As a marker for systemic inflammation, the plasma levels of the acute phase protein haptoglobin were measured using a Cobas Bio centrifugal analyser with a haptoglobin reagent kit (TP801, Tridelta development). In the strain comparison shown in Figure 1, plasma was also analysed for the levels of IL-6, IL-12p40, TNF and CXCL1/KC using the xMAP technology developed by Luminex Corporation (Austin, Texas) as previously described [9].

To analyse local levels of inflammatory mediators, colon tissue was homogenised in PBS (Gibco, Invitrogen Corp UK) supplemented with 10% foetal calf serum and a protease inhibitor cocktail (Complete Mini, Roche Molecular Biochemicals), using a Homogenizer (Ultra Turrax T8, Tamro, Sweden). The homogenised material was centrifuged, 18000 rpm for 10 min, at +4°C, after which the supernatant was aliquoted and frozen at −80°C. To generate the data shown in Figure 1, the colonic levels of IL-1β, IL-12p40, IL-18, IFNγ, CXCL1/mouse KC, CXCL2/3-MIP-2, CXCL9/MIG, CXCL10/IP-10, CCL2/mouse JE/MCP-1, CCL4/MIP-1β, CCL5/RANTES and PGE_2 were determined by ELISA according to the manufacturer's instructions (R&D Systems, UK and Cayman Chemical Company, MI (PGE_2)). All cytokine data are expressed as pg/100 mg colon tissue.

Treatment with nuclear hormone receptor agonists

BALB/c mice were exposed to 5% DSS in the drinking water for 6 days. The mice were orally treated by gavage with either

30 μmol/kg of the Liver X receptor (LXR)-agonist AZ-37328, 1 μmol/kg of the peroxisome proliferation activating receptor (PPAR)α-agonist AZ-63233 or 30 μmol/kg of the PPARγ-agonist AZ-15188, each group containing 12 mice. The compounds were suspended in hydroxypropylmethyl cellulose (Kleptose, Roquette) and administered at 10 ml/kg bodyweight. All treatments were performed once daily, starting one day before the addition of DSS and continued until the day before the termination of the experiment. Biomarkers in these experiments were colon levels of cytokines (IL-12p40, IL-6, MCP1 and KC determined by xMAP technology), and plasma levels of haptoglobin, triglycerides (Diagnostics GMBH, Mannheim Germany) and adiponectin (Linco Research Inc Missouri, USA). In addition, colon and liver weights were recorded and colons macroscopically scored for inflammation as described above.

Data analysis and statistics

Data analyses were performed using PCA as implemented in the SIMCA-P software v. 11.0 and 12.0 (Umetrics, Umea, Sweden, see www.umetrics.com). PCA bilinearise a data matrix into scores and loading vectors, representing the objects and variables respectively [20]. Each endpoint (i.e. variable with its related loading) was, through-out all principal component analyses in the present study, given equal leverage to the ensuing model by the unit variance normalization procedure (according to the SIMCA P+ software default implementation) First the variance (i.e. the squared standard deviation SD) was calculated for each biomarker's data column and thereafter each individual datum value was divided by its biomarker variance value rendering a unit variance scaling. Thus the full data-set became re-scaled to comprise the standard deviation equal to 1, for each normalized biomarker data column, which in practise means an a priori equal chance of influence for each included biomarker measure independent on the initial raw data scale.

The relevant number of principal components (PC) was decided from the R^2, Eigen value and loading structure, related to the respective component. Furthermore, cross-validation [21] was used as an additional measure for model judgement of proper model complexity.

Statistical significance shown in Figure 4 was calculated using the Mann-Whitney U-test in the software GraphPad Prism 4.0.

Acknowledgments

We are grateful to Agneta Karlsson for excellent technical assistance with the DSS-studies, to Lise Hallengren and crew for excellent care of mice and to Anders Elmgren and his team for help with biomarker analyses.

Author Contributions

Conceived and designed the experiments: JG SM EM. Performed the experiments: JG SM EM. Analyzed the data: JG SM EM. Contributed reagents/materials/analysis tools: JG SM EM. Wrote the paper: JG SM EM.

References

1. Saccenti E, Westerhuis JA, Smilde AK, van der Werf MJ, Hageman JA, et al. (2011) Simplivariate models: uncovering the underlying biology in functional genomics data. PLoS One 6: e20747.
2. Gottfries J, Blennow K, Lehmann MW, Regland B, Gottfries CG (2001) One-carbon metabolism and other biochemical correlates of cognitive impairment as visualized by principal component analysis. J Geriatr Psychiatry Neurol 14: 109–114.
3. Gottfries J, Sjogren M, Holmberg B, Rosengren L, Davidsson P, et al. (2004) Proteomics for drug target discovery. Chemometrics and Intelligent Laboratory Systems 73: 47–53.
4. van der Greef J, Adourian A, Muntendam P, McBurney RN (2006) Lost in translation? Role of metabolomics in solving translational problems in drug discovery and development. Drug Discovery Today: Technologies 3: 205–211.
5. Byrne FR, Viney JL (2006) Mouse models of inflammatory bowel disease. Curr Opin Drug Discov Devel 9: 207–217.
6. Koboziev I, Karlsson F, Zhang S, Grisham MB (2011) Pharmacological intervention studies using mouse models of the inflammatory bowel diseases: translating preclinical data into new drug therapies. Inflamm Bowel Dis 17: 1229–1245.
7. Modigliani R, Mary JY, Simon JF, Cortot A, Soule JC, et al. (1990) Clinical, biological, and endoscopic picture of attacks of Crohn's disease. Evolution on prednisolone. Groupe d'Etude Therapeutique des Affections Inflammatoires Digestives. Gastroenterology 98: 811–818.
8. Roth-Cline MD (2006) Clinical trials in the wake of Vioxx: requiring statistically extreme evidence of benefit to ensure the safety of new drugs. Circulation 113: 2253–2259.
9. Melgar S, Karlsson A, Michaelsson E (2005) Acute colitis induced by dextran sulfate sodium progresses to chronicity in C57BL/6 but not in BALB/c mice: correlation between symptoms and inflammation. Am J Physiol Gastrointest Liver Physiol 288: G1328–1338.
10. Kelly D, Campbell JI, King TP, Grant G, Jansson EA, et al. (2004) Commensal anaerobic gut bacteria attenuate inflammation by regulating nuclear-cytoplasmic shuttling of PPAR-gamma and RelA. Nat Immunol 5: 104–112.
11. Tanaka T, Kohno H, Yoshitani S, Takashima S, Okumura A, et al. (2001) Ligands for peroxisome proliferator-activated receptors alpha and gamma inhibit chemically induced colitis and formation of aberrant crypt foci in rats. Cancer Res 61: 2424–2428.
12. Oprea TI, Gottfries J (2001) Chemography: the art of navigating in chemical space. J Comb Chem 3: 157–166.
13. Navarro V, Fernandez-Quintela A, Churruca I, Portillo MP (2006) The body fat-lowering effect of conjugated linoleic acid: a comparison between animal and human studies. J Physiol Biochem 62: 137–147.
14. Gottfries CG, Häger O, Gottfries J, Zachrisson O (2009) Immunotherapy of Fibromyalgia and Chronic Fatigue Syndrome by a Staphylococcus Toxoid Vaccine. Bulletin of the IACFS/ME 17: 168–183.
15. Chalmers I (2006) From optimism to disillusion about commitment to transparency in the medico-industrial complex. J R Soc Med 99: 337–341.
16. Vanhoutte K, de Asmundis C, Francesconi A, Figysl J, Steurs G, et al. (2009) Leaving out control groups: an internal contrast analysis of gene expression profiles in atrial fibrillation patients–a systems biology approach to clinical categorization. Bioinformation 3: 275–278.
17. Calciano MA, Zhou W, Snyder PJ, Einstein R (2010) Drug treatment of Alzheimer's disease patients leads to expression changes in peripheral blood cells. Alzheimers Dement 6: 386–393.
18. Okayasu I, Hatakeyama S, Yamada M, Ohkusa T, Inagaki Y, et al. (1990) A novel method in the induction of reliable experimental acute and chronic ulcerative colitis in mice. Gastroenterology 98: 694–702.
19. Larsson AE, Melgar S, Rehnstrom E, Michaelsson E, Svensson L, et al. (2006) Magnetic resonance imaging of experimental mouse colitis and association with inflammatory activity. Inflamm Bowel Dis 12: 478–485.
20. Jackson EJ A user's guide to principal components: John Wiley and sons, Inc.
21. Wold S (1978) Cross-Validatory Estimation of the Number of Components in Factor and Principal Component Models. Technometrics 20: 397–405.

9

Confocal Laser Endomicroscopy for *In Vivo* Diagnosis of *Clostridium difficile* Associated Colitis

Helmut Neumann[1]*, Claudia Günther[1], Michael Vieth[2], Martin Grauer[1], Nadine Wittkopf[1], Jonas Mudter[1], Christoph Becker[1], Christoph Schoerner[3], Raja Atreya[1], Markus F. Neurath[1]

1 Department of Medicine I, University of Erlangen-Nuremberg, Erlangen, Germany, **2** Institute of Pathology, Klinikum Bayreuth, Bayreuth, Germany, **3** Institute of Microbiology, Immunology and Hygiene, University of Erlangen-Nuremberg, Erlangen, Germany

Abstract

Background: *Clostridium difficile* infection (CDI) is one of the most dreaded causes of hospital-acquired diarrhea. Main objective was to investigate whether confocal laser endomicroscopy (CLE) has the capability for *in vivo* diagnosis of *C. difficile* associated histological changes. Second objective was to prove the presence of intramucosal bacteria using CLE.

Methods: 80 patients were prospectively included, 10 patients were diagnosed with CDI based on toxigenic culture. To validate the presence of intramucosal bacteria *ex vivo*, CLE was performed in pure *C. difficile* culture; additionally fluorescence *in situ* hybridization (FISH) was performed. Finally, CLE with fluorescence labelled oligonucleotide probe specific for *C. difficile* was performed *ex vivo* in order to prove the presence of bacteria.

Results: CLE identified CDI-associated histological changes *in vivo* (sensitivity and accuracy of 88.9% and 96.3%). In addition, intramucosal bacteria were visualized. The presence of these bacteria could be proven by CLE with labeled, specific molecular *C. difficile* probe and FISH-technique. Based on comparison between CLE and FISH analyses, sensitivity and specificity for the presence of intramucosal bacteria were 100%.

Conclusion: CLE has the potential for *in vivo* diagnosis of CDI associated colitis. In addition, CLE allowed the detection of intramucosal bacteria *in vivo*.

Editor: Markus M. Heimesaat, Charité, Campus Benjamin Franklin, Germany

Funding: The authors have no funding or support to report.

Competing Interests: The authors have declared that no competing interests exist.

* E-mail: helmut.neumann@uk-erlangen.de

Introduction

Clostridium difficile infection has emerged as one of the most clinically significant causes of hospital-acquired diarrhea and is associated with significant morbidity and mortality. *C. difficile* infection is often accompanied by fever and leukocytosis and frequently affects older and immunocompromised patients. Nevertheless, recent data suggest that even young and healthy persons who have previously not been exposed to a health care environment or antimicrobial therapy are at risk as well [1,2].

C. difficile can colonize the large bowel and, in the presence of antibiotic therapy that limits the growth of naturally residing microorganisms, produce endotoxins and cytotoxins that can cause severe mucosal damage, resulting in colitis that may have a pseudomembranous appearance at endoscopy [1]. It has been estimated that *C. difficile* causes approximately 25% of the antibiotic-associated diarrhea (AAD) and most cases of pseudomembranous colitis. In the United States, there are about 300,000 cases of *C. difficile*-associated diarrhea and colitis per year, resulting in an annual economic burden of more than one billion dollars to the health care system [2].

Since a new epidemic strain of *C. difficile* associated with more severe disease, mortality and frequent relapses has been identified in 2003, *C. difficile* infection has becoming increasingly difficult to control and eradicate [3]. Accordingly, *C. difficile* infection now rivals methicillin-resistant *Staphylococcus aureus* (MRSA) as the most common cause for hospital-acquired infections in the United States.

Therefore, rapid and accurate diagnosis of *C. difficile* infection is of crucial importance, not only for individual patient management but also for prevention of nosocomial transmission. Currently, diagnosis of *C. difficile* infection is based on patients' clinical history and laboratory tests, including toxigenic culture, which still remains the gold standard for diagnosis [4].

Recently, confocal laser endomicroscopy has been introduced as a new endoscopic imaging technique enabling real time *in vivo* histology of the cellular and subcellular mucosal layer at a magnification of 1000 fold. Previously it was shown that endomicroscopy has the capability to facilitate histopathological diagnosis of different gastrointestinal diseases including Barrett's esophagus, celiac disease, microscopic colitis and inflammatory bowel diseases [5–11].

Our main study objective was to prospectively investigate whether CLE has the capability for the *in vivo* diagnosis of *C. difficile* associated histological changes. Second objective of our study was to prove the presence of *C. difficile* bacteria using CLE.

Patients and Methods

Patients

Consecutive patients, including both, in-patients and out-patients with diarrhea who underwent colonoscopy for the evaluation of their symptoms were prospectively included between October 2009 and September 2010. All patients signed informt consent to participate in this study after the endoscopist and attending physician had explained the procedure in detail to them. Subjects were enrolled if they met the following inclusion criteria: more than 18 years of age, ability to provide written informt consent, diarrhea. Patients with one or more of the following criteria were excluded from the study: inability to provide written informt consent, severe uncontrolled coagulopathy, impaired renal function, pregnancy or breast feeding, active gastrointestinal bleeding, known allergy to fluorescein or acriflavine and residing in institutions (e.g. prison).

The study was approved by the local ethical committee and government authorities (IRB approval of the University of Erlangen-Nuremberg; http://www.ethik.med.uni-erlangen.de/) and was conducted according to the declaration of Helsinki. The UMIN Clinical Trials Registry identification number for this study was NCT01072110. Written informt consent was obtained from all participants. Clinical data, including patients' history and laboratory data were recorded. Final diagnosis of *C. difficile* infection was based on toxigenic culture. Two endoscopists and one experienced gastrointestinal pathologist read the images. Endoscopists and pathologist were blinded to all microbiological results.

In vivo confocal laser endomicroscopy in *C. difficile* patients

Patients underwent a standard bowel preparation using either oral sodium phosphate or polyethylene glycol-electrolyte lavage solution. All endomicroscopy procedures were performed under conscious sedation with constant monitoring of vital signs using either integrated-endomicroscopy (iCLE; EC-3870CILK, Pentax, Tokyo, Japan) or probe-based endomicroscopy (pCLE; Cellvizio, ColoFlex^{UHD}, Mauna Kea Technologies, Paris, France). Both systems use an incident 488 nm wavelength laser (blue laser light) and enable the detection of fluorescence between 205 – 585 nm wavelengths [9]. Randomization was performed as followed: Patients were randomized into both groups by using a computer-aided system. The results of the randomization were kept in sealed envelopes that were opened just before the endoscopic procedure. Authors were blinded to diagnosis of *C. difficile* infection. In every patient, 10 localisations were analysed. In case of mucosal abnormalities, like erythema or ulcers, CLE was performed at these places. In case of macroscopically normal appearing mucosa, CLE was performed in the rectum (proximal and distal part), sigmoid colon (proximal and distal part), descending colon (proximal and distal part), transverse colon (proximal and distal part), ascending colon und caecum. During CLE *in vivo* diagnosis of CDI was either made or excluded. Therefore, 100 lesions were examined in CDI patients and 700 in control patients which were not affected with CDI. iCLE images were collected at a frame rate of 0.8/s at 1024×1024 pixels or 1.6/s at 1024×512 pixels. Intravenous fluorescein was used in every patient to optimize tissue contrast. Additionally, in some patients topical acriflavine hydrochloride (0.05%; Sigma-Aldrich, Steinheim, Germany) or topical cresyl violet (0.13%; Alcon Laboratories, Texas, USA) was applied after intravenous injection of fluorescein using standard spraying catheters (Olympus, Tokyo, Japan). First, confocal images were analyzed in real time. Subsequently, images were reviewed offline to digitally zoom in on details (iCLE), allowing a higher magnification of the mucosa (approximately 10,000 fold) or by using the Cellvizio Viewer (Mauna Kea Technologies, Paris, France) for virtual staining of mucosal structures to enhance tissue contrast.

Normal mucosa and pathological lesions were evaluated according to the Mainz confocal pattern classification for iCLE and according to the modified Miami classification for pCLE [12,13].

After endomicroscopy, biopsies were taken from macroscopically normal and altered mucosa and specimens were fixed in 4% buffered formalin for subsequent histopathological analysis. In case of macroscopically normal mucosa random biopsies were performed from all evaluated colon segments (e.g. terminal ileum, caecum, ascending colon, transverse colon, descending colon, sigmoid colon, and rectum). In case of macroscopically visible lesions targeted biopsies were performed from these areas.

In order to reach total concordance between *in vivo* iCLE-imaging and biopsy acquisition, mild suctioning was applied to the mucosa for confocal imaging. Technically, the resulting mucosal hemorrhage was located 5 mm to the right from the area which had been evaluated using iCLE. After performing pCLE, the probe was gently pushed against the mucosal wall, thereby marking the area. Thus, the exact correlation between *in vivo* imaging and biopsy acquisition was determined.

Ex-vivo endomicroscopy of C. difficile

First, the *C. difficile* strain was cultured on *C. difficile* selective agar and harvested. Subsequently, the pure *C. difficile* culture was resuspended in physiological NaCl. Afterwards, a diluted solution of 0.05% acriflavine hydrochloride or fluorescein sodium was added and the solution was subsequently imaged using the integrated confocal laser endomicroscopy system.

In addition, biopsy samples were obtained from two patients with *C. difficile*-infection and subsequently incubated with phosphate buffered saline (PBS). Afterwards, a 5% solution of fluorescein-labelled *C. difficile* specific probe was added and the biopsy specimens were subsequently imaged using the integrated confocal laser endomicroscopy system (Five 1, Optiscan, Notting Hill, Australia).

Endomicroscopy images were collected at a frame rate of 0.8/s at 1024×1024 pixels and digitally magnified after image acquisition at 10,000 fold to further zoom in on details.

Fluorescence *in Situ* Hybridization (FISH) of *C. difficile*

FISH was performed on biopsies from different areas of the sigmoid colon of four patients, two control patients and two patients infected with *C. difficile*. FISH staining of bacterial rRNA on glass slides was performed as previously described [14–16]. In short, FISH hybridization of bacterial rRNA was performed on 3 µm cross sections of formalin fixed paraffin embedded biopsies on glass slides. Slides were dewaxed and rehydrated by incubating them for 30 minutes at 60°C and additional 3 cycles of xylol (each 5 minutes), 2 cycles of 100% ethanol (each 3 minutes), 1 cycle of 96% ethanol (3 minutes), 1 cycle of 70% ethanol and 1 cycle of distilled water (3 minutes). Afterwards, paraffin cross sections on glass slides were shortly washed with PBS and preincubated using hybridization buffer containing 20% formamide for 10 minutes. For the detection of bacterial rRNA, samples were incubated with 47.5 ng of a Cy3-labeled *C. difficile* specific probe in 50 µl of hybridization buffer containing 20% formamide for 90 minutes at 46 °C. Finally, the paraffin cross sections were washed with incubation buffer for 15 minutes at 46°C and afterwards shortly with PBS. Nuclear counterstaining was performed using Hoechst dye 3342. The *C. difficile* specific probe (Cd-198 m; 5′ CAT CCT GTA CTG GCT CAC) was previously designed in a study by Bloedt and coworkers [17]. We also refer to this study regarding the evaluation of the FISH probe for *C. difficile* and the phylogenetical analysis.

Statistical Analysis

The statistical software program PASW Statistics 18 (SPSS, Inc., Chicago, USA) was used for all data analysis. Final statistical analysis for *in vivo* histology was based on the results of *in vivo* CLE and the results of the toxigenic culture based on a per-patient analysis. The *t*-test was used for all continues variables to determine whether differences between any two groups existed. A two-sided P value <0.05 was considered to be significant. To evaluate the impact of image interpretation for diagnosis of CDI we calculated the positive and negative predictive values. In addition, the sensitivity, specificity and accuracy of the endomicroscopy findings were also calculated. The median in this study is presented for non-normally distributed variables, and the mean for normally distributed variables. The range indicated the range between the minimum and maximum values. Correlation between endomicroscopy diagnosis and histopathology was determined using kappa statistics, which assesses agreement beyond chance among investigators. Therefore, the strength of rater agreement was categorized according to the definition proposed by Landis and Koch for kappa values [18]: 0 – 0.20, slight; 0.21 – 0.40, fair; 0.41 – 0.60, moderate; 0.61 – 0.80, substantial; 0.81 – 1.00, almost perfect.

Results

During the study period, a total of eighty patients with diarrhea were prospectively included. In ten (4 female, 6 male; mean age 72.5 years, range 37 – 96 years) out of these eighty patients *C. difficile* infection (CDI) was diagnosed as the constitutive cause for diarrhea based on toxigenic culture as the gold standard. Remaining causes for diarrhea included infectious pathogens other than CDI and inflammatory bowel diseases.

High-resolution endoscopy

On high-resolution white-light endoscopy (EC 3840FK2, Pentax, Tokyo, Japan) the colonic mucosa was covered with confluent pseudomembranes and showed linear ulcers in two out of ten patients with CDI. In three patients, discrete cream to yellowish coloured plaques, varying in size between 2 to 30 mm were visualized [Figure 1]. The plaques were only loosely attached to the colon wall and the underlying mucosa was hyperaemic. In five patients, only a slightly erythematous mucosa without any plaques was visible.

In vivo confocal laser endomicroscopy

Overall, 100 lesions were examined using CLE in CDI patients and the results were compared to 700 locations of control patients as mentioned in the "Patients and Methods" section. According to disease manifestation, different characteristics of *C. difficile* infection were found. Following intravenous injection of fluorescein, at early disease stages without macroscopically visible pseudomembranes, small surface erosions of the superficial colonic crypts were visualized. Additionally, an increased cellular infiltrate within the lamina propria was visible. Microvessels within the lamina propria were slightly dilated but showed no leakage [Figure 1]. The average distance between colonic crypts was weakly augmented, indicating mucosal edema. On the luminal side, endomicroscopy demonstrated mucus, fibrin and epithelial cells. These areas were surrounded by normal appearing mucosa.

In advanced disease stages of CDI with macroscopically visible pseudomembranes, confocal laser endomicroscopy demonstrated massively dense cellular infiltrates within the lamina propria. Colonic crypts were variously shaped and irregular in arrangement. Normal colonic appearance was nearly completely abolished. According to the degree of inflammation, fragile vessels and leakage demonstrated by extravasation of fluorescein became visible [Figure 1]. Furthermore, a plaque of loosely cells, fibrin and debris covered the mucosal surface.

Sensitivity, specificity, and accuracy of endomicroscopy to determine CDI-associated histological changes *in vivo* were 88.9%, 97.2%, and 96.25%, respectively. Positive and negative predictive values were calculated as being 80.0% and 98.6%, respectively. Correlation between endomicroscopy and histopathology was good (kappa 0.8209; 95% confidence interval 0.6221 – 1.00).

Fluorescein-based CLE has recently been described as a new technique to identify translocating bacteria in the mucosa of patients with inflammatory bowel diseases suggesting that this approach has the capacity to identify mucosal bacteria [19]. Surprisingly, in this study no specific bacteria translocating into the mucosa could be identified in CDI using fluorescein-aided CLE. However, in contrast to fluorescein-aided CLE, white focal spots in the colonic mucosa and the pericryptal space could be identified after topical application of acriflavine hydrochloride [Figure 2]. Image review of confocal images at 10,000 fold digital magnification revealed a rod like appearance of the white focal spots suggesting the presence of *C. difficile* bacteria [Figure 2]. In contrast to acriflavine, the topical application of cresyl violet did not add any additional information compared to single fluorescein staining. No adverse events regarding the procedure or the use of the different dye agents were observed.

Ex vivo confocal laser endomicroscopy

Consistent with the above *in vivo* findings, fluorescein-aided *ex vivo* endomicroscopy of pure *C. difficile* culture revealed no noticeable structures [Figure 2] suggesting that these bacteria lack the potential for fluorescein uptake. In contrast, *ex vivo* endomicroscopy of pure *C. difficile* culture after application of acriflavine hydrochloride revealed white focal spots comparable to the *in vivo* confocal imaging. In addition, image review at 10,000 fold digital magnification confirmed the rod like appearance of the white focal lesions in the presence of *C. difficile* [Figure 2].

To prove the potential of CLE for the identification of *C. difficile* bacteria, we performed a final series of studies with *ex vivo* CLE of colonic biopsies with a labeled specific probe for *C. difficile* [17]. Interestingly, *ex vivo* CLE with a fluorescein-labelled *C. difficile* specific probe visualized intramucosal bacteria within the colonic epithelium similar to *in vivo* endomicroscopy and FISH-technique [Figure 3] indicating that CLE with molecular probes could potentially be used to specifically identify *C. difficile* bacteria.

Fluorescence in Situ Hybridization (FISH) of intramucosal bacteria

To provide additional validation for the identification of intramucosal *C. difficile* bacteria at endomicroscopy, we performed FISH of intestinal biopsies which were taken from areas previously evaluated using endomicroscopy. In all biopsies from CDI patients, FISH confirmed the presence of intramucosal bacteria in the colonic mucosa and the pericryptal space [Figure 3]. These bacteria corresponded to the focal spots which were previously imaged by *in vivo* and *ex vivo* endomicroscopy. Sensitivity and

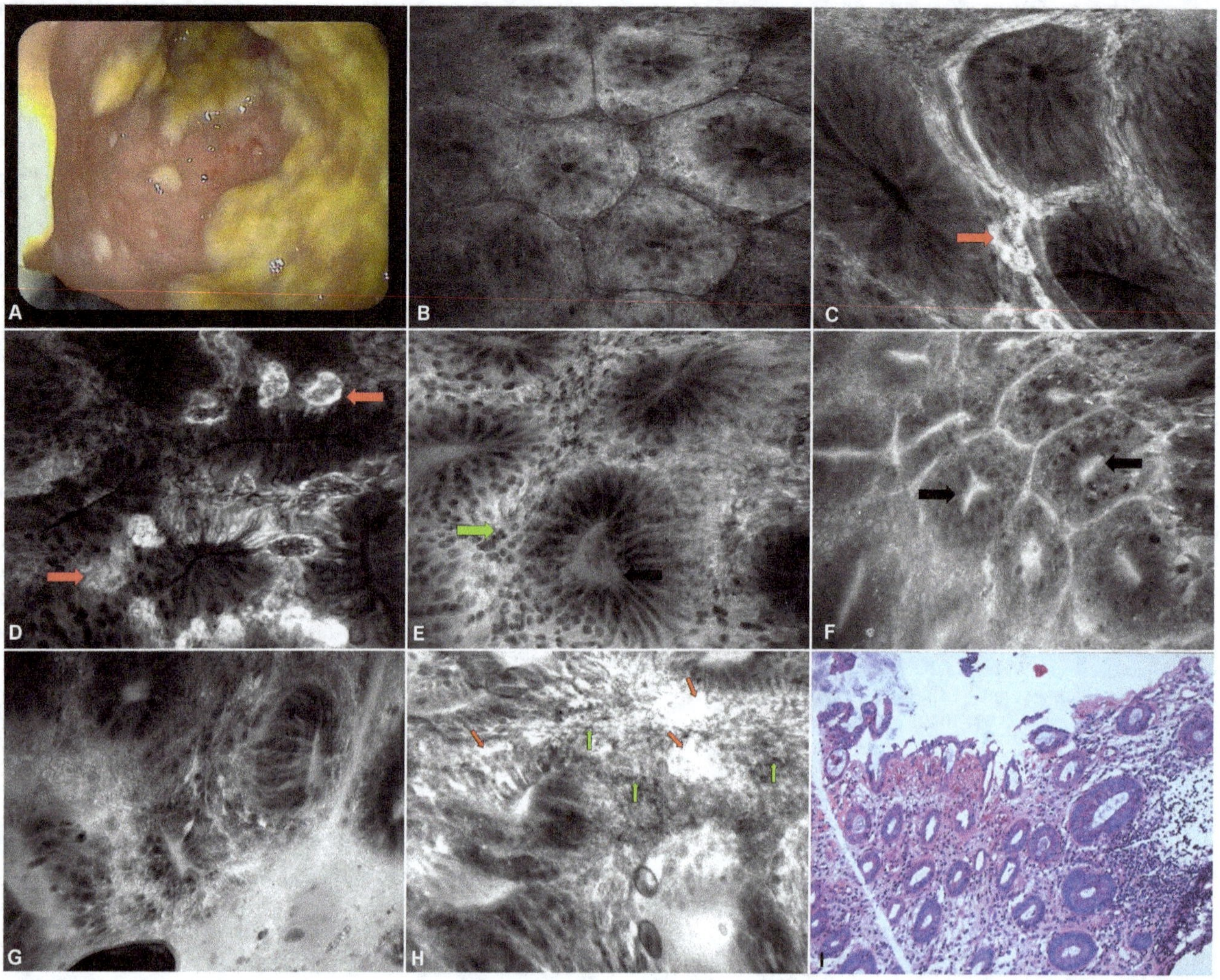

Figure 1. Endoscopic and endomicroscopic appearance of C. difficile infection. Panel A highlights the macroscopic appearance of advanced *C. difficile* infection using high-resolution endoscopy. Confluent cream to yellow coloured plaques varying in size, which were only loosely attached to the colon wall, were seen. The underlying mucosa was hyperaemic. Note the confocal lens of the integrated-endomicroscopy system at the 7 o'clock position. Panel B shows normal colonic architecture in disease-free mucosa as control (×1000). Dependent on the extent of disease manifestation, colonic crypts in *C. difficile* colitis were variously shaped (black arrows) (Panels C-F; ×1000). Furthermore, microvessels (red arrows) were dilated but showed no signs of leakage in milder forms of colitis (Panel C-F; ×1000). Furthermore, an increased cellular infiltrate (green arrows) within the lamina propria became visible in *C. difficile* colitis (Panel E; ×1000). Fluorescein-aided endomicroscopy of advanced *C. difficile*-infection (Panel G, H; ×1000) showed fragile vessels with fluorescein leakage (red arrows) and dense cellular infiltrates (green arrows) in the lamina propria. In these cases, the normal colonic architecture was nearly completely abolished. Histopathological assessment of mild *C. difficile* infection is shown in panel I (×200).

specificity for the presence of intramucosal bacteria detected by CLE were 100% when compared to FISH findings.

Discussion

In this pilot study, we have identified confocal laser endomicroscopy (CLE) as a potential novel technique for the diagnosis of *C. difficile* infection (CDI). CLE enabled real time, *in vivo* diagnosis of CDI associated histological changes regardless from the disease stage. Additionally, acriflavine-aided endomicroscopy was able to visualize intramucosal *C. difficile* bacteria within the lamina propria. The presence of intramucosal *C. difficile* bacteria was additionally proven using *ex vivo* CLE with specific molecular probe and FISH technique. The finding of intramucosal bacteria in our study did not correlate to the clinical symptoms of the patients.

Endomicroscopy is a new, emerging endoscopic imaging modality enabling real time *in vivo* histology during ongoing endoscopy. Currently, two FDA approved devices for endomicroscopy are available [9]. While one device is integrated into the distal tip of a high-resolution endoscope (iCLE, Pentax, Tokyo, Japan), the other device represents a stand-alone confocal miniprobe which is capable of passage through the accessory channel of a standard endoscope (pCLE, Cellvizio, Mauna Kea Technologies, Paris, France). In our study, we used both systems for confocal diagnosis. Although it was not the purpose of this study to compare both techniques, both confocal imaging systems could readily identify architectural changes in *C. difficile* infection without obvious differences. Nevertheless, for the first time both endomicroscopy systems were evaluated in one study.

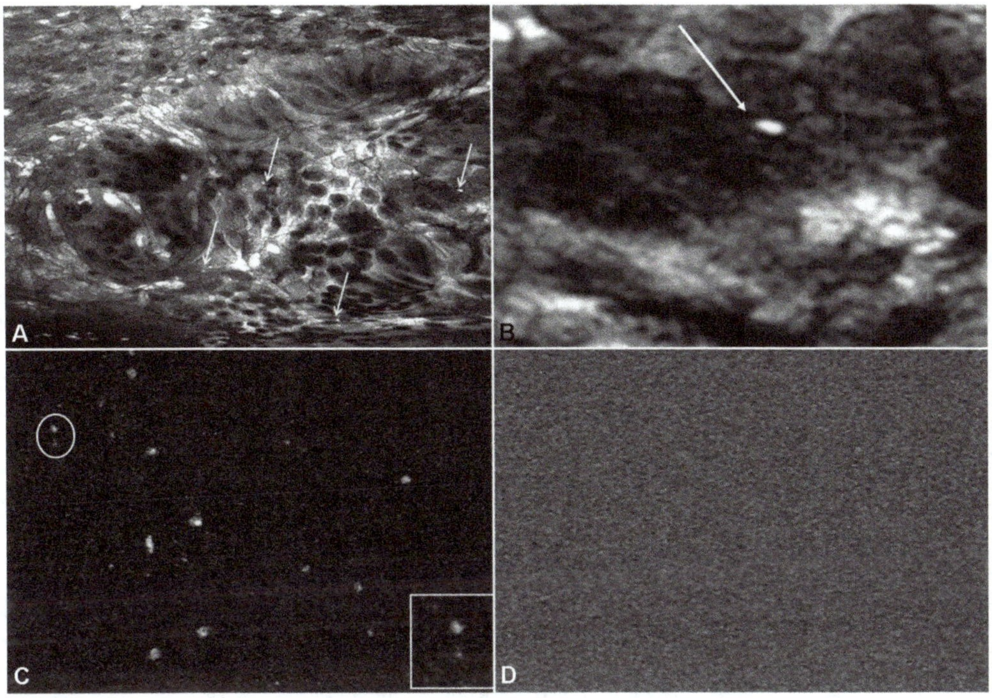

Figure 2. ***In vivo*** **visualization of intramucosal bacteria within the colonic mucosa in** ***C. difficile*** **colitis by confocal laser endomicroscopy.** Fluorescence confocal image below the surface of the colonic mucosa after topical application of acriflavine hydrochloride identified single bacteria (Panel A, arrows). At 10,000 fold digital magnification the rod-like appearance of bacteria (arrow) in the colonic mucosa became visible (Panel B). Panel C shows *ex vivo* imaging of pure cultured *C. difficile* at 1000-fold magnification and 10,000 fold magnification (insert in lower right quadrant) after staining with acriflavine hydrochloride. In contrast, after application of fluorescein no bacteria were visible by confocal imaging (Panel D).

C. difficile associated colitis is known to lead to a superficial inflammation and is therefore ideally suited for CLE based analysis [20]. In fact, we were able to observe similar changes by CLE as compared to standard histopathology with high sensitivity, specificity and accuracy. In fact, the correlation between real time *in vivo* histology and *ex vivo* histology in predicting CDI-associated histological changes was good. In comparison, assessment of toxins A and B by ELISA has a sensitivity of 63–99% and a specificity of 93–100% with a PPV of 73% and a NPV of 96% [21]. As CLE allows on demand *in vivo* diagnosis of cellular and subcellular structures in real time during ongoing endoscopy CLE may have the potential to provide a faster diagnosis of CDI as compared to conventional culture. However, our approach needs further validation by a prospective multicenter study with a respective sample size calculation.

Our study has potential limitations. First, although the investigators had long experience in performing and interpreting endomicroscopy, this may not have been sufficient to reliably obtain and interpret endomicroscopy images in CDI. Second, endomicroscopy images do not represent typical histological images, as they illustrate a horizontal field of view. Therefore, it is possible that additional new criteria for CDI-associated colitis on horizontal sections have to be defined. Third, infectious colitis caused by other pathogens may also mimic CDI-associated endoscopic and histologic changes [22]. Finally, although a large number of patients were included in our study, CDI was only

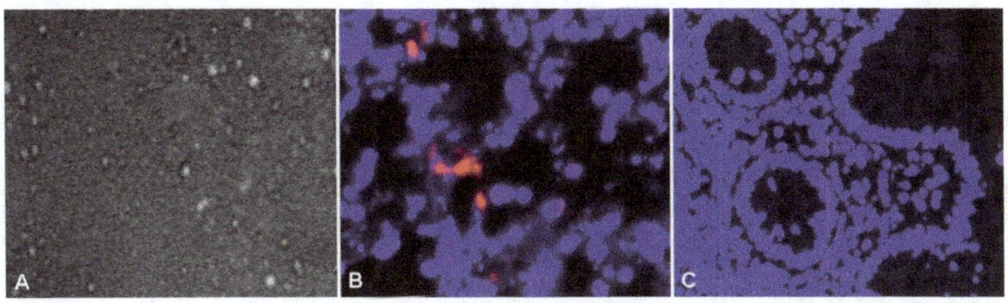

Figure 3. ***Ex vivo*** **verification of** ***C. difficile*** **using a fluorescence labelled** ***C. difficile*** **specific probe in CDI.** Panel A shows a characteristic endomicroscopic image of a patient with *C. difficile*-infection after exposure of the biopsy to the labelled probe and subsequent CLE analysis. Intramucosal bacteria were clearly visible (white spots). Fluorescence in situ hybridization (FISH) confirmed the presence of intramucosal bacteria in this patient due to the bright red fluorescence. Nuclei and DNA are displayed in blue (Panel B). Panel C shows FISH in a control patient without *C. difficile* infection. No bacteria could be visualized.

proven in a subset of patients, thereby potentially affecting statistical analysis. A future prospective multicenter study with a respective sample size calculation addressing these points is thus highly warranted.

Interestingly, CLE allowed the identification of bacteria in the mucosa of patients with CDI *in vivo*. Previously, it was shown by Kiesslich and coworkers that endomicroscopy with topically applied acriflavine could readily identify *Helicobacter pylori* infection *in vivo* [23]. Very recently, the same group demonstrated that endomicroscopy was able to identify intramucosal enteric bacteria *in vivo* in the colon and ileum of patients with ulcerative colitis and Crohn's disease using fluorescein-aided endomicroscopy [19]. It was shown that intramucosal bacteria were more frequently and with a wider distribution found in patients with inflammatory bowel disease than in patients with a normal intestine. However, in our study no bacteria in the colonic mucosa could be identified by fluorescein-aided CLE. Importantly, we were only able to visualize bacteria after application of acriflavine which is a cationic dye that can be detected by its intrinsic fluorescence and accumulates in the endosomal/lysosomal compartment of cells [24]. Thus, our findings suggest that topical administration of acriflavine results in translocation of the dye in the mucosa via epithelial gaps or epithelial erosions followed by its uptake in *C. difficile* bacteria [25]. The fact that these bacteria are negative by fluorescein staining but positive upon acriflavine use is striking and discriminates this bacterial strain from other bacteria previously identified in the colonic mucosa [19]. To our knowledge, this is the first report on a fluorescein-negative bacterial strain in the colonic mucosa by CLE analysis. Thus, your finding of staining patterns is very interesting and may aid in the further classification of different bacteria. Therefore, we suggest that in the future CLE should be evaluated to analyze bacterial cultures of various gram-negative and gram-positive pathogens.

In order to validate the presence of intramucosal *C. difficile* bacteria in patients with CDI, we performed several *ex vivo* studies. Intramucosal bacteria imaged by endomicroscopy *in vivo* looked similar to *C. difficile* in an *ex vivo* cell suspension of pure *C. difficile* culture when analyzed by CLE. Again, only acriflavine-aided endomicroscopy was feasible to detect *C. difficile* by *ex vivo* CLE, while fluorescein-aided endomicroscopy revealed no bacteria. This finding underlines our *in vivo* results where we could only identify bacteria after topical application of acriflavine.

High-magnification of *C. difficile* bacteria, both *in* and *ex vivo* revealed a rod like appearance of these microorganisms. Additionally, there was a strong concordance between the presence of intramucosal bacteria identified *in vivo* and bacteria identified by FISH in biopsies of areas which were previously investigated using endomicroscopy. In order to further highlight the potential of CLE for detection of specific bacteria in CDI, additional *ex vivo* studies on endomicroscopy with previously validated specific molecular probe for *C. difficile* were performed and the results were compared to those of the FISH analysis. By using this approach, we could identify the presence of specific intramucosal *C. difficile* bacteria within the colon in CDI. These findings underline the potential of endomicroscopy for molecular imaging of CDI and specific detection of *C. difficile* bacteria. By using *ex vivo* CLE with the *C. difficile* specific probe we have shown that the probe seems to be able to penetrate the cells without the use of previous fixation. Our hypothesis is that the mucosal structure of the inflamed tissue (according to *C. difficile* colitis) allows penetration of the probe. This speculation is underlined by recent studies evaluating *in vivo* confocal imaging in patients with inflammatory bowel diseases. These studies suggested that patients with colitis has an increased number of epithelial gaps in human small and large intestine and that these gaps must be considered as a component of the intestinal barrier and may therefore have potential implications for intestinal barrier dysfunction in human diseases [25,26].

Our findings could have a substantial clinical impact, as endomicroscopy has the potential to diagnose *C. difficile* infection *in vivo*, thus potentially enabling an accelerated diagnosis and an improved patient management. Therefore, endomicroscopy might have the potential to refine our understanding of *C. difficile* diagnosis and may help to prevent nosocomial transmission of this life-threatening disease. Moreover, we were able to describe intramucosal bacteria *in vivo*. The clinical significance of our findings should be elucidated in future prospective studies.

Author Contributions

Conceived and designed the experiments: HN MV MG CG NW CB CS. Performed the experiments: HN MV MG CG NW CB CS. Analyzed the data: HN MV CB MFN. Contributed reagents/materials/analysis tools: HN MV MG CG NW JM CB CS RA MFN. Wrote the paper: HN MV MG CG NW JM CB CS RA MFN.

References

1. Kelly CP, LaMont JT (2008) Clostridium difficile--more difficult than ever. N Engl J Med 359: 1932–1940.
2. Centers for Disease Control and Prevention (CDC) (2005) Severe Clostridium difficile-associated disease in populations previously at low risk. MMWR Morb Mortal Wkly Rep 54: 1201–1205.
3. Huang H, Weintraub A, Fang H, Nord CE (2009) Antimicrobial resistance in Clostridium difficile. Int J Antimicrob Agents 34: 516–522.
4. Crobach MJ, Dekkers OM, Wilcox MH, Kuijper EJ (2009) European Society of Clinical Microbiology and Infectious Diseases (ESCMID): data review and recommendations for diagnosing Clostridium difficile-infection (CDI). Clin Microbiol Infect 15: 1053–1566.
5. Kiesslich R, Gossner L, Goetz M, Dahlmann A, Vieth M, et al. (2006) In vivo histology of Barrett's esophagus and associated neoplasia by confocal laser endomicroscopy. Clin Gastroenterol Hepatol 4: 979–987.
6. Leong RW, Nguyen NQ, Meredith CG, Al-Sohaily S, Kukic D, et al. (2008) In vivo confocal endomicroscopy in the diagnosis and evaluation of celiac disease. Gastroenterology 135: 1870–1876.
7. Buchner AM, Shahid MW, Heckman MG, Krishna M, Ghabril M, et al. (2010) Comparison of probe-based confocal laser endomicroscopy with virtual chromoendoscopy for classification of colon polyps. Gastroenterology 138: 834–842.
8. Neumann H, Grauer M, Vieth M, Neurath MF (2013) In vivo diagnosis of lymphocytic colitis by confocal laser endomicroscopy. Gut 62: 333–334.
9. Neumann H, Kiesslich R, Wallace MB, Neurath MF (2010) Confocal laser endomicroscopy: technical advances and clinical applications. Gastroenterology 139: 388–392.
10. Günther U, Epple HJ, Heller F, Loddenkemper C, Grünbaum M, et al. (2008) In vivo diagnosis of intestinal spirochaetosis by confocal endomicroscopy. Gut 57: 1331–1333.
11. Neumann H, Vieth M, Atreya R, Grauer M, Siebler J, et al. (2012) Assessment of Crohn's disease activity by confocal laser endomicroscopy. Inflamm Bowel Dis. 18: 2261–2269.
12. Kiesslich R, Burg J, Vieth M, Gnaendiger J, Enders M, et al. (2004) Confocal laser endoscopy for diagnosing intraepithelial neoplasias and colorectal cancer in vivo. Gastroenterology 127: 706–713.
13. Wallace M, Lauwers GY, Chen Y, Dekker E, Fockens P, et al. (2011) Miami classification for probe-based confocal laser endomicroscopy. Endoscopy 43: 882–891.
14. Becker C, Wirtz S, Blessing M, Pirhonen J, Strand D, et al. (2003) Constitutive p40 promoter activation and IL-23 production in the terminal ileum mediated by dendritic cells. J Clin Invest 112: 693–706.
15. Amann RI, Ludwig W, Schleifer KH (1995) Phylogenetic identification and in situ detection of individual microbial cells without cultivation. Microbiol Rev 59: 143–169.
16. Moter A, Göbel UB (2000) Fluorescence in situ hybridization (FISH) for direct visualization of microorganisms. J Microbiol Methods 41: 85–112.

17. Bloedt K, Riecker M, Poppert S, Wellinghausen N (2009) Evaluation of new selective culture media and a rapid fluorescence in situ hybridization assay for identification of Clostridium difficile from stool samples. J Med Microbiol 58: 874–877.
18. Landis JR, Koch GG (1977) The measurement of observer agreement for categorical data. Biometrics 33: 159–174.
19. Moussata D, Goetz M, Gloeckner A, Kerner M, Campbell B, et al. (2011) Confocal laser endomicroscopy is a new imaging modality for recognition of intramucosal bacteria in inflammatory bowel disease in vivo. Gut 60: 26–33.
20. Monaghan T, Boswell T, Mahida YR (2008) Recent advances in Clostridium difficile-associated disease. Gut 57: 850–860.
21. Bartlett JG, Gerding DN (2008) Clinical recognition and diagnosis of Clostridium difficile infection. Clin Infect Dis 46: 12–18.
22. Mönkemüller K, Patasiūte I, Walther F, Peitz U, Fry LC, et al. (2006) Pseudomembranous colitis due to Salmonella enterica serotype infantis. Endoscopy 38: 546.
23. Kiesslich R, Goetz M, Burg J, Stolte M, Siegel E, et al. (2005) Diagnosing Helicobacter pylori in vivo by confocal laser endoscopy. Gastroenterology 128: 2119–2123.
24. Davies JP, Chen FW, Ioannou YA (2000) Transmembrane molecular pump activity of Niemann-Pick C1 protein. Science 290:2295–2298.
25. Kiesslich R, Goetz M, Angus EM, Hu Q, Guan Y, et al. (2007) Identification of epithelial gaps in human small and large intestine by confocal endomicroscopy. Gastroenterology 133: 1769–1778.
26. Liu JJ, Wong K, Thiesen AL, Mah SJ, Dieleman LA, et al. (2011) Increased epithelial gaps in the small intestines of patients with inflammatory bowel disease: density matters. Gastrointest Endosc 73: 1174–1180.

10

BTZO-15, an ARE-Activator, Ameliorates DSS- and TNBS-Induced Colitis in Rats

Hiroshi Yukitake[1], Haruhide Kimura[1]*, Hirobumi Suzuki[1], Yasukazu Tajima[1], Yoshimi Sato[1], Toshihiro Imaeda[1], Masahiro Kajino[2], Masayuki Takizawa[1]

1 Pharmaceutical Research Division, Takeda Pharmaceutical Company Limited, Fujisawa, Japan, **2** Chemistry, Manufacturing and Controls, Takeda Pharmaceutical Company Limited, Osaka, Japan

Abstract

Inflammatory bowel disease (IBD) is a group of chronic inflammatory disorders that are primarily represented by ulcerative colitis and Crohn's disease. The etiology of IBD is not well understood; however, oxidative stress is considered a potential etiological and/or triggering factor for IBD. We have recently reported the identification of BTZO-1, an activator of antioxidant response element (ARE)-mediated gene expression, which protects cardiomyocytes from oxidative stress-induced insults. Here we describe the potential of BTZO-15, an active BTZO-1 derivative for ARE-activation with a favorable ADME-Tox profile, for the treatment of IBD. BTZO-15 induced expression of heme oxygenase-1 (HO-1), an ARE-regulated cytoprotective protein, and inhibited NO-induced cell death in IEC-18 cells. Large intestine shortening, rectum weight gain, diarrhea, intestinal bleeding, and an increase in rectal myeloperoxidase (MPO) activity were observed in a dextran sulfate sodium (DSS)-induced colitis rat model. Oral administration of BTZO-15 induced HO-1 expression in the rectum and attenuated DSS-induced changes. Furthermore BTZO-15 reduced the ulcerated area and rectal MPO activity in 2,4,6-trinitrobenzene sulfonic acid (TNBS)-induced colitis rats without affecting rectal TNF-α levels. These results suggest that BTZO-15 is a promising compound for a novel IBD therapeutic drug with ARE activation properties.

Editor: Stefan Bereswill, Charité-University Medicine Berlin, Germany

Funding: This study was funded by Takeda Pharmaceutical Company Limited. All authors were employees of Takeda Pharmaceutical Company Limited and were paid as such, therefore Takeda Pharmaceutical Company Limited had a role in the study design, data collection and analysis, and decision to publish.

Competing Interests: The authors are/were employees of Takeda Pharmaceutical Company Limited.

* E-mail: kimura_haruhide@takeda.co.jp

Introduction

Ulcerative colitis (UC) and Crohn's disease (CD) are human inflammatory bowel diseases (IBD) of unknown etiology characterized by chronic relapses of hyperinflammation of the gastrointestinal tract and a dysregulated mucosal immune response [1]. Many factors participate in the pathology of IBD such as oxidative stress, neutrophil infiltration, overproduction of proinflammatory mediators including cytokines, dysfunction of immune systems, and imbalance of microflora [1,2]. Among these factors, oxidative stress appears to be a major factor in the pathogenesis of IBD and may be the mainstay of disease initiation and perpetuation [3–6]. Heme oxygenase-1 (HO-1), an enzyme that degrades heme to carbon monoxide, ferrous iron, and biliverdin, participates in the cellular defense against oxidative stress. Interestingly, up-regulation of HO-1 shows promise as a clinical intervention of IBD [3,7].

In a previous study, we reported the identification of BTZO-1, 2-pyridin-2-yl-4H-1,3-benzothiazin-4-one, which inhibits the apoptosis of cardiomyocytes by inducing cytoprotective factors, such as glutathione S-transferase (GST) Ya and HO-1 via activation of antioxidant response elements (ARE) [8]. BTZO-2, an active BTZO-1 derivative, protected heart tissues during ischemia/reperfusion injury in rats [8]. BTZO-1 selectively bound macrophage migration inhibitory factor (MIF), and reduction of cellular MIF protein levels by siRNA suppressed BTZO-1-induced GST Ya expression. Therefore, MIF may be a target protein of BTZO-1.

ARE is a cis-acting DNA regulatory element located in the regulatory regions of multiple genes encoding phase II detoxifying enzymes and cytoprotective proteins including GSTs, HO-1, reduced nicotinamide adenine dinucleotide phosphate (NAD(P)H), quinone oxidoreductases (NQOs), UDP-glucuronosyl transferase (UDP-GT), epoxide hydrase, γ-glutamylcystein synthetase (γ-GCS), and peroxiredoxin 1 [9–11]. In mammalian cells, activation of the ARE is of critical importance to cellular protection against oxidative stress [10–12]. In fact, t-BHQ, which up-regulates a battery of ARE-regulated genes, reportedly protects cells from oxidative damage *in vitro* [13]. There is also a growing body of evidence suggesting that modulation of these cytoprotective genes has profound effects on immune and inflammatory responses. Activation of cytoprotective ARE-regulated genes can suppress inflammatory responses, whereas decreased expression of these genes results in autoimmune disease and enhances inflammatory responses to oxidant insults. For instance, it has been reported that 15-Deoxy-$\Delta^{12,\ 14}$-Prostaglandin J_2 (15d-PGJ_2), which exerts its anti-inflammatory activity through activation of ARE, suppresses carrageenan induced pleurisy [14]. Thus, coordinate induction of cytoprotective genes via activation of AREs may represent a novel therapeutic approach for the treatment of immune and inflammatory diseases [8,10,15].

Here we show the cytoprotective effects of BTZO-15, a BTZO-1 derivative with favorable absorption-distribution-metabolism-elimination-toxicity (ADME-tox). BTZO-15 suppressed NO-onduced cell death in IEC-18 cell line derived from rat intestinal epithelial cells. BTZO-15 also showed protective effects against dextran sulfate sodium (DSS)-induced colitis and 2,4,6-trinitrobenzene sulfonic acid (TNBS)-induced colitis in rats. To date, no ARE activator have been used as therapeutic drugs for IBD. The results suggest that ARE activation can be an attractive and novel approach to IBD therapy.

Results

BTZO-15 interacts with MIF

The binding of BTZO-15 (Fig. 1A) to purified recombinant human MIF (hMIF) was analyzed using a surface plasmon resonance (SPR) biosensor. hMIF was immobilized on the active sensor chip CM5 with a surface density of 12,080 resonance units (RU) (MIF sensor chip). Analysis of the BTZO-15 solution revealed dose-dependent binding signals to the MIF sensor chip (Fig. 1B).

Next, binding of BTZO-15 to purified recombinant rat MIF with a 6His-tag to C terminus (rMIF-His) was measured by a scintillation proximity assay (SPA) which measured the competitive inhibition of the radio-labeled [^{3}H]-BTZO-1 binding to rMIF-His [8]. BTZO-15 inhibited the binding of [^{3}H]-BTZO-1 to rMIF-His in a dose-dependent manner (Fig. 1C). These results, and those of the SPR biosensor analysis, suggested that BTZO-15 directly interacts with MIF.

BTZO-15 activates ARE-mediated transcriptional induction

The effect of BTZO-15 on ARE activation was investigated using a luciferase reporter assay in H9c2 cells. The pGL3-ARE-Luc reporter plasmid, which expresses luciferase under the control of a rat GST Ya ARE (Fig. 1D), and the pGL3-mARE-Luc reporter plasmid, in which a point mutation (A to G) was introduced into the core sequence (TGACAAAGC) to almost completely abolish its activity, were used in this assay (Fig. 1D) [8,16]. When H9c2 cells transfected with pGL3-ARE-Luc, but not pGL3-mARE-Luc, were treated with BTZO-15, luciferase activity was induced in a dose dependent manner (Fig. 1E). Thus, increment values of luciferase activity in cells transfected with pGL3-ARE-Luc are ARE-dependent. Accordingly, BTZO-15 induced expression of ARE-regulated genes, such as HO-1 and GST Ya, in H9c2 cells; BTZO-15 increased both HO-1 and GST Ya mRNA expression in a dose dependent manner (Fig. 1F).

Reduction in cellular MIF levels decreases BTZO-15-induced GST Ya mRNA expression

The effects of reducing the cellular MIF protein level on BTZO-15-induced GST Ya mRNA expression were investigated by lowering the MIF mRNA level with small interfering RNA (siRNA). A reduction of MIF mRNA level was attained by MIF siRNA transfection into H9c2 cells (Fig. 1G). Under these conditions, induction of GST Ya mRNA expression by BTZO-15 was significantly reduced (Fig. 1G).

BTZO-15 induces HO-1 mRNA levels and suppresses NO-induced cell death in IEC-18 cells

The effect of BTZO-15 on expression of HO-1 was evaluated using IEC-18 cells. BTZO-15 increased HO-1 mRNA levels in a dose dependent manner (Fig. 2A). GST Ya mRNA could not be measured, probably due to its low level of expression in IEC-18 cells. The effect of BTZO-15 on NO-induced cell death was also examined in IEC-18 cells with Cell Counting Kit-8. Stimulation of IEC-18 cells with 130 µM of NOR3, a NO-generator, reduced cell viability. BTZO-15 treatment suppressed the NO-induced cell death in a dose-dependent manner (Fig. 2B).

BTZO-15 ameliorates DSS-induced colitis in rats

The effect of BTZO-15 on DSS-induced colitis rats was assessed in a double blinded study; body weight, stool consistency/diarrhea score, bleeding score, large intestine length, and rectum weight were evaluated. The addition of 2.3% DSS to drinking water for 7 days caused colitis with a reduction in body weight and large intestine length, and an increase in the rectum weight, stool consistency/diarrhea score, bleeding score, and rectal MPO activity (Fig. 3A–G). Oral administration of BTZO-15 for 4 days from experimental day 3 to 6 improved all parameters in a dose-dependent manner (Fig. 3B–G).

BTZO-15 increases HO-1and GST Ya protein levels in the rectum of DSS induced colitis rats

The effect of BTZO-15 on the expression of rectal HO-1 and GST Ya was studied in rats with DSS-induced colitis. DSS treatment for 7 days resulted in an increase in the level of rectal HO-1 protein (Fig. 4A). Oral administration of BTZO-15 (10 mg/kg) tended to increase HO-1 protein levels (Fig. 4A). Decreased rectal levels of GST Ya protein were significantly recovered by oral administration of BTZO-15 (10 mg/kg) (Fig. 4B).

BTZO-15 ameliorates TNBS induced colitis in rats

We next evaluated the effects of BTZO-15 on TNBS-induced colitis in rats (Fig. 5A). TNBS administration led to ulcers in the rectum, increased rectal MPO activity, and up-regulated TNF-α levels (Fig. 5B–D). Oral administration of BTZO-15 significantly decreased the ulcerated area and rectal MPO activity (Fig. 5B, C) without affecting rectal TNF-α levels (Fig. 5D).

Discussion

The etiology of IBD is still unclear, although there is evidence that oxidative stress plays a role in the pathogenesis of IBD and could be the mainstay of disease initiation and perpetuation [3–5]. Many agents, such as 5-amino salicylic acid (5-ASA), antibiotics, steroids, immunosuppressive agents, and anti tumor necrosis factor (TNF)-α, infliximab, are available for IBD therapy; however, they have problems of lower efficacy and/or side effects. For example 5-ASA, a pharmacological standard therapy for UC, [2,17], does not exhibit adequate efficacy in maintenance and remission and produces side-effects, such as interstitial nephritis [2,17]. Antibiotics, steroids, and immunosuppressive agents, including cyclosporine, are powerful therapeutic approaches to avoid sepsis or life-threatening complications in IBD in an acute setting; however, their routine use has been hindered by side-effects that include infectious complications [2,17]. Although infliximab has attracted attention for its curative effect on moderate/severe UC and CD, there are problems of resistance and side effects upon long term dosage [2,17,18]. Thus, novel therapeutic drugs with better efficacy and side effects profiles are needed.

Both DSS- and TNBS-induced colitis are considered useful experimental models for IBD [19]. DSS is toxic to colonic epithelial cells in the basal crypts, and elicits an inflammatory response that causes colitis similar to human UC [19,20]. BTZO-15 significantly suppressed the typical symptoms of DSS-induced colitis in rats: large intestine shortening, rectum weight gain,

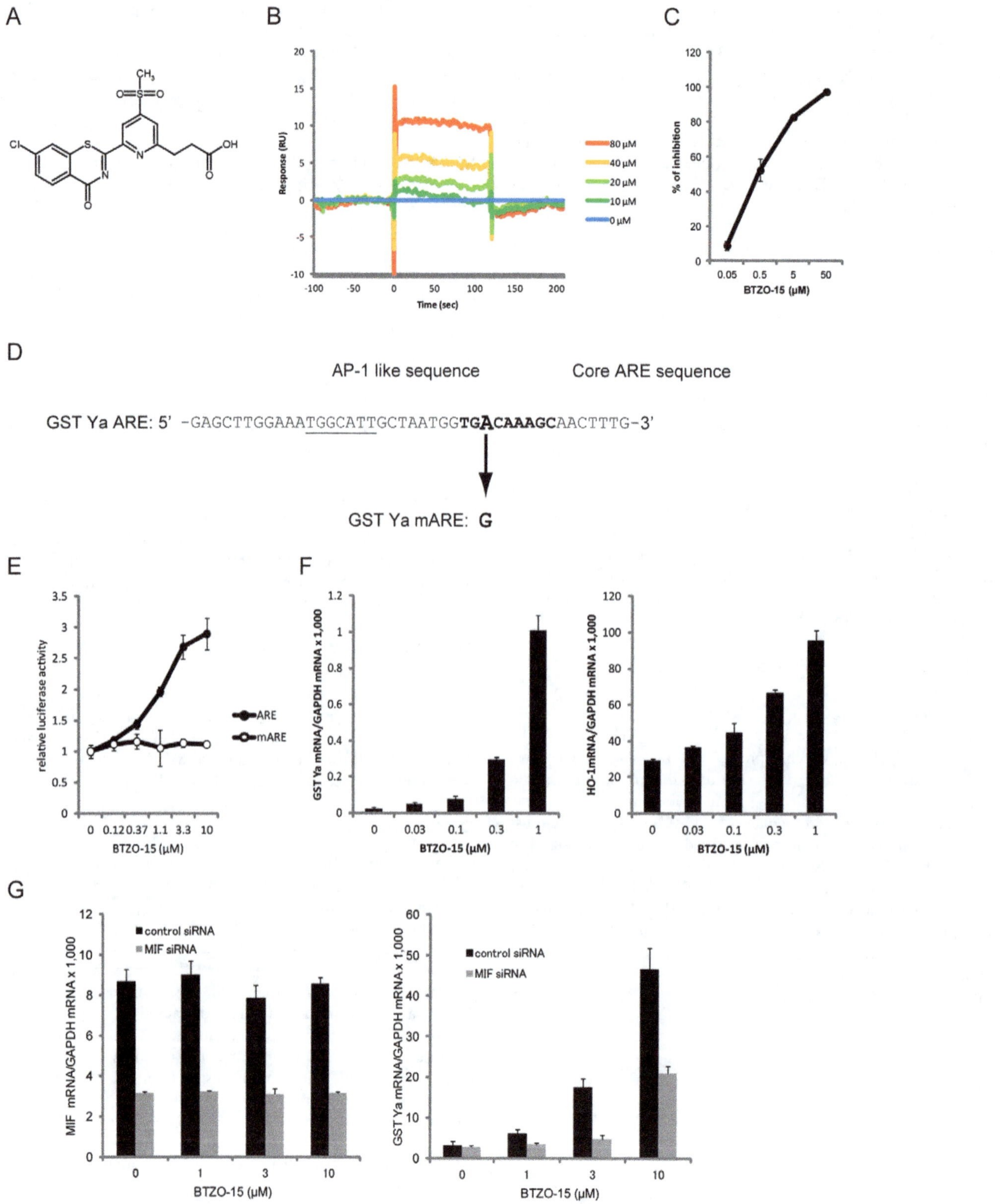

Figure 1. BTZO-15 activates the GST Ya ARE by interacting with MIF. (A) Chemical structures of BTZO-15. (B) Sensorgram showing binding of BTZO-15 to immobilized hMIF on a CM5 sensor chip using an SPR biosensor. (C) Displacement studies with BTZO-15 by the SPA showing inhibition of BTZO-1 binding to captured rMIF on SPA beads. Results shown are the mean ± SD, n = 3. (D) Nucleotide sequence of the rat GST Ya ARE. The core ARE sequence is indicated by the nucleotides in boldface type. (E) Reporter gene assays showing the effect of BTZO-15 on ARE activity. H9c2 cells transiently transfected with either pGL3-ARE-Luc or pGL3-mARE-Luc reporter plasmids were treated with the indicated concentrations of BTZO-15 for 24 h and luciferase activities were measured. Results shown are the mean ± SD, n = 3. (F) BTZO-15 induced ARE-regulated cytoprotective proteins in H9c2 cells. The cells were treated with the indicated concentrations of BTZO-15 for 6 h (HO-1) or 21 h (GST Ya). HO-1 mRNA levels were measured by real-time PCR and normalized by GAPDH mRNA. Results shown are the mean ± SD, n = 3. (G) Effects of reducing the cellular MIF protein level on BTZO-15-induced GST Ya and HO-1 gene expression in H9c2 cells. H9c2 cells transfected with control siRNA (control siRNA) or siRNAs directed against

rMIF (MIF siRNA) were treated with 3 μM BTZO-15 with or without 0.8 μM rMIF for 24 h. Messenger RNA levels of MIF, GST Ya, and HO-1 were measured by real-time PCR. MIF protein level in cell lysates was measured by ELISA.

diarrhea, and bleeding. BTZO-15 also suppressed an increase in rectal MPO activity, which is an index of tissue-associated neutrophil accumulation. In contrast, TNBS-induced colitis is believed to induce a T-cell-mediated response against hapten-modified autologous proteins/luminal antigens similar to a Th1 immune response and comparable to the inflammatory processes present in human CD [21,22]. BTZO-15 significantly decreased the ulcer-affected area with suppression of rectal MPO activity in rats with TNBS-induced colitis. Interestingly, BTZO-15 did not affect the rectal TNF-α level. These results indicate that BTZO-15 has potential as a novel therapeutic drug for both UC and CD.

BTZO-15 induced expression of HO-1 and suppressed NO-induced cell death in a rat intestinal epithelial cell line (IEC-18). Reactive oxygen species (ROS), such as NO, play an important role in the pathogenesis of various inflammatory diseases, including IBD [4–6], and ARE is an important countermeasure against oxidative stress in mammalian cells [10–12]. Thus, ARE activation could be an attractive strategy for IBD therapy. Here we show that DSS treatment increased HO-1 protein levels in the rectum and BTZO-15 further increased HO-1 protein levels. This HO-1 up-regulation by DSS may be an intrinsic defense mechanism against oxidative stress [23]. GST-Ya levels in the rectum decreased by DSS treatment. This GST-Ya down-regulation by DSS is in accord with a previous report that GSTs levels and GSTs activities are reduced by DSS treatment [24,25]. BTZO-15 significantly recovered GST-Ya levels in the rectum. These results are in accord with a previous report that GSTs levels and GSTs activities are reduced by DSS treatment [24,25]. Serum TNF-α was up-regulated in rats with TNBS-induced colitis, and BTZO-15 did not affect TNF-α levels. These results, and those of the *in vitro* experiments, suggest that the therapeutic effects of BTZO-15 in animal models of IBD are based on increases in HO-1 and GST Ya levels via ARE activation in rectum, not suppression of cytokine production, although further studies will be needed to clarify the precise mechanisms of action.

It is evident that activation of ARE-regulated genes contributes to the regulation of cellular antioxidant defense systems, and pharmacological activation of endogenous cytoprotective proteins through ARE activation is predicted to serve as a novel strategy for the treatment of cardiovascular and inflammatory diseases [10,15]. Thus, BTZO-1 derivatives appear to have therapeutic potential for a broad range of diseases caused by oxidative stress. In fact, BTZO-2, an active BTZO-1 derivative of ARE activation, confers protection to heart tissues during ischemia/reperfusion injury in rats [8]. Evaluation of the effects of BTZO-1 derivatives on other oxidative stress-related disease models is worthy of additional investigation.

A forward chemical genetics approach has been used to show that BTZO-1 derivatives may activate AREs via binding to MIF [8,26]. Here we show that BTZO-15 directly interacts with MIF and induces ARE-mediated expression of cytoprotective genes, such as GST-Ya and HO-1. This induction of GST Ya mRNA expression by BTZO-15 was decreased in MIF siRNA-transfected H9c2 cells. These results, and those of our previous report [8], suggest that BTZO-15 activates AREs by binding to MIF. MIF reportedly contributes to the symptoms of IBD, and inhibition of MIF could be a potential treatment [27–29]. However, our results suggest that activation of MIF by BTZO-15 induces ARE

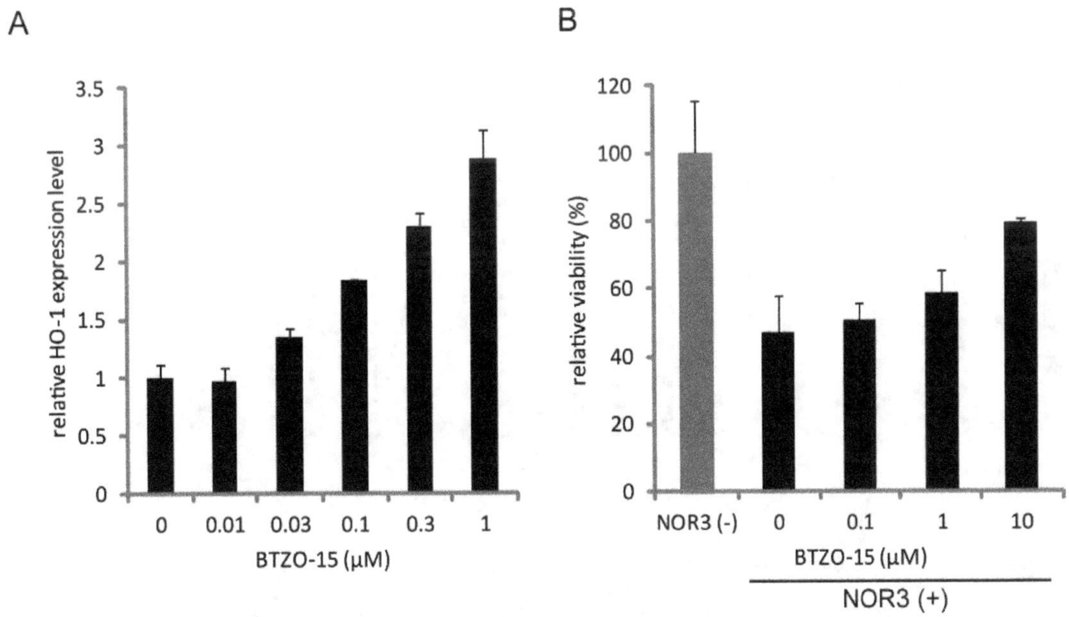

Figure 2. BTZO-15 increases HO-1 mRNA levels and suppresses NO-induced cell death in IEC-18 cells. (A) Real-time PCR expression analysis showing the effects of BTZO-15 on the induction of HO-1 mRNA in IEC-18 cells. The cells were treated with the indicated concentrations of BTZO-15 for 24 h. HO-1 mRNA levels were measured by real-time PCR and normalized by GAPDH mRNA. Results shown are the mean ± SD, n = 3. (B) Cell death inhibitory activity of BTZO-15 in IEC-18 cells. The cells were cultured in the presence of either vehicle or the indicated concentrations of BTZO-15 in serum free medium for 1 h. The cells were then treated with 130 μM NOR3 and cultured for 24 h. Cell viability was determined using the WST-8 cell respiratory assay. The experimental value for cell death inhibitory activities is expressed as relative viability and is the mean ± SD, n = 3.

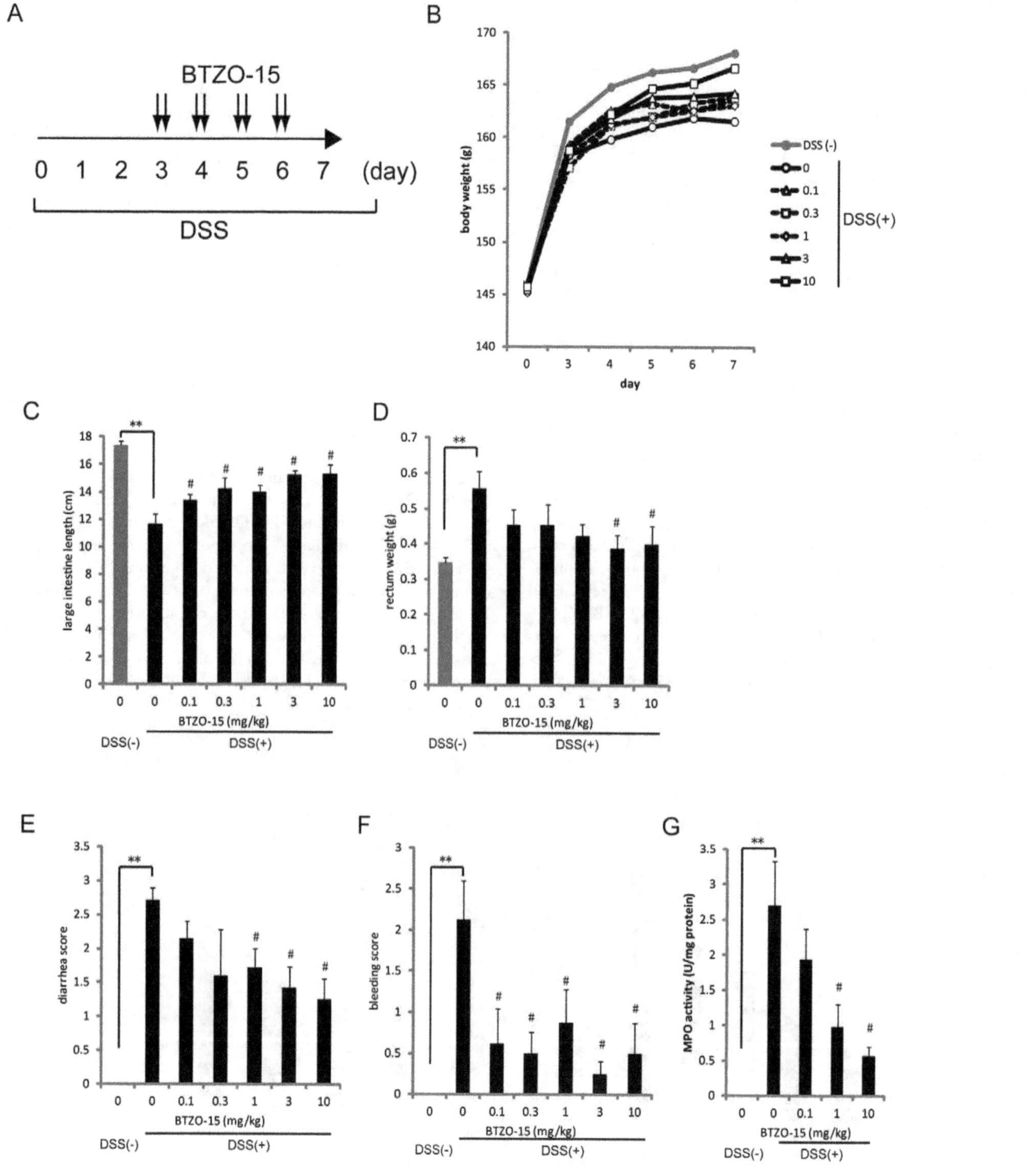

Figure 3. BTZO-15 ameliorates DSS-induced colitis in rats. Colitis was induced in male F344/Du rats by daily treatment with 2.3% DSS solution in drinking water for 7 days. BTZO-15 was orally administered to rats at the indicated doses of 0.1, 0.3, 1, 3, and 10 mg/kg (b.i.d.) for 4 days from experimental day 3 to 6 (A). Body weight (B) was measured every day. At experimental day 7, the rats were sacrificed, and large intestine length (C), rectum weight (D), diarrhea score (E), bleeding score (F), and MPO activity (G) underwent a double blind evaluation. All data except body weight shown are mean ± S.E.M. Body weight data shown are means, n = 8. ** P≤0.01: compared the DSS (−) vehicle control group with DSS (+) vehicle control group using Student's t test, and # P≤0.025: compared the DSS (+) vehicle control group with DSS (+) + BTZO-15 treated groups by one-tailed Williams's test (C and D). **P≤0.01: compared the DSS (−) vehicle control group with DSS (+) vehicle control group using Wilcoxon test, and # P≤0.025: compared the DSS (+) vehicle control group with DSS (+) + BTZO-15 treated groups by one-tailed Shirley-Williams test (E and F). ** P≤0.01: compared the DSS (−) vehicle control group with DSS (+) vehicle control group with Aspin-Welch test, and # P≤0.025: compared the DSS (+) vehicle control group with DSS (+) + BTZO-15 treated groups with one-tailed Williams's test (G).

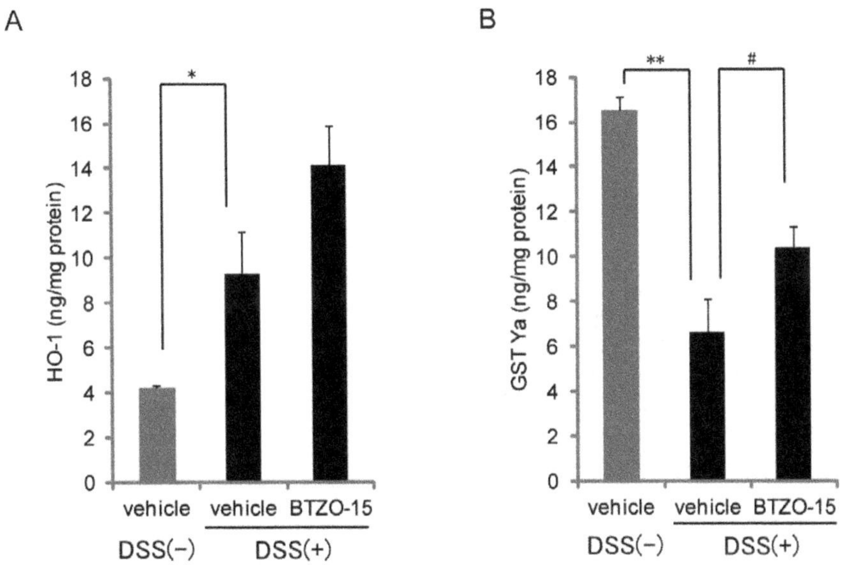

Figure 4. BTZO-15 induces HO-1 and GST Ya protein expression in the rectum of rats with DSS-induced colitis. Colitis was induced in rats by daily treatment with 2.3% DSS solution in drinking water for 7 days. During this period, the rats were orally administered BTZO-15 (3 mg/kg, b.i.d.) or vehicle (0.5% MC). Rectal HO-1 (A) and GST-Ya (B) protein expression was assessed after excision and homogenization in PBS supplemented with 0.1% NP-40. The amount of GST Ya and HO-1 protein was quantified using ELISA. Results shown are the mean ± S.E.M, n = 8. * $P \le 0.05$: compared the DSS (−) vehicle control group with DSS (+) vehicle control group using Aspin-Welch test. # $P \le 0.05$: compared the DSS (+) vehicle control group with DSS (+) + BTZO-15 treated groups with Student's t test.

activation, leading to the therapeutic effects in IBD models. Further studies are needed to reveal how MIF participates in IBD and how BTZO-15 works in this system.

In summary, we demonstrate that BTZO-15 activates ARE-mediated gene expression and suppresses NO-induced cell death *in vitro*. In addition, BTZO-15 ameliorates both DSS- and TNBS-induced colitis in rats. Since no ARE activator have been used as therapeutic drugs for IBD, BTZO-15 could be a novel drug for IBD with potent therapeutic activity and a low side effects profile. Our studies further demonstrate that ARE activation can be an attractive and novel approach to IBD therapy.

Materials and Methods

Experimental animals

Ethics statement. The care and use of the animals and experimental protocol were approved by the Experimental Animal Care and Use Committee at Takeda Pharmaceutical Company (Approval ID: TEACUC-1822, TEACUC-1824, and TEACUC-2414).

Seven-week-old male F344/Du rats were obtained from Charles River Laboratories Japan Inc. (Yokohama). The rats were housed 4 per cage in specific pathogen-free and standard controlled environmental conditions with a 12-h light/dark cycle and with food (MF; Clea Japan Inc., Tokyo) and water provided ad libitum.

Materials

BTZO-15 was synthesized at Takeda Pharmaceutical Company Limited. Detailed methods for the synthesis of BTZO-15 will be described elsewhere. Recombinant human MIF-His (hMIF) and recombinant rat MIF (rMIF) were prepared as described previously [8].

Surface plasmon resonance (SPR) analysis

The interaction of MIF with BTZO-15 was examined using the BIACORE 3000 System (GE Healthcare UK Limited) at 25°C. Human MIF (hMIF) was immobilized with a surface density of 12,080 resonance units (RU) on an activated sensor chip CM5 according to the manufacturer's instructions. A reference surface was prepared without hMIF in flow cell 1. The interaction of BTZO-15 with hMIF was tested in PBS containing 3% DMSO under a 30 μM/min continuous flow at 25°C. Sixty microliters of sample containing the indicated concentrations of compounds were injected onto the sensor chip. The sensor surfaces were regenerated to remove all bound analyte between binding cycles by serial injections of 5 μL of 10 mM NaOH at a flow rate of 60 μL/min. Binding data were analyzed using the BIACORE 3000 control software and BIAevaluation Software (GE Healthcare UK Limited).

Scintillation proximity assay (SPA)

The [^{3}H]-BTZO-1/rMIF-His SPA assay was conducted as described previously [8]. In the SPA measuring the competitive inhibition of [^{3}H]-BTZO-1 binding to rMIF-His, 62.5 μg of Ysi (2–5 μm) copper His-tag SPA beads and 0.25 μg of rMIF-His protein were incubated in PBS containing 0.025% Triton X-100 at 4°C overnight. Subsequently, the indicated concentrations of BTZO-15 and 20 nM of [^{3}H]-BTZO-1 were added to each well to give a final volume of 100 μL. After a 3-h-incubation, radioactivity derived from the bound [^{3}H]-BTZO-1 was measured using a microplate scintillation counter. The final concentration of solvent was kept to 0.5% DMF.

ARE-Luc reporter assays

The ARE-Luc reporter assay used the reporter plasmids pGL3-ARE-Luc and pGL3-mARE-Luc [8]. In brief, H9c2 (ATCC, Manassas, VA, USA) cells were cultured in D-MEM supplemented with 10% FBS and 1% penicillin and streptomycin (PS) for about 16 h before they were transfected with pGL3-ARE-Luc or pGL3-mARE-Luc using FuGENE6 transfection reagent (Roche, Indianapolis, IN, USA) according to the manufacturer's instructions. After a 7-h-incubation, the cells were harvested in a trypsin-EDTA solution, suspended in D-MEM supplemented with

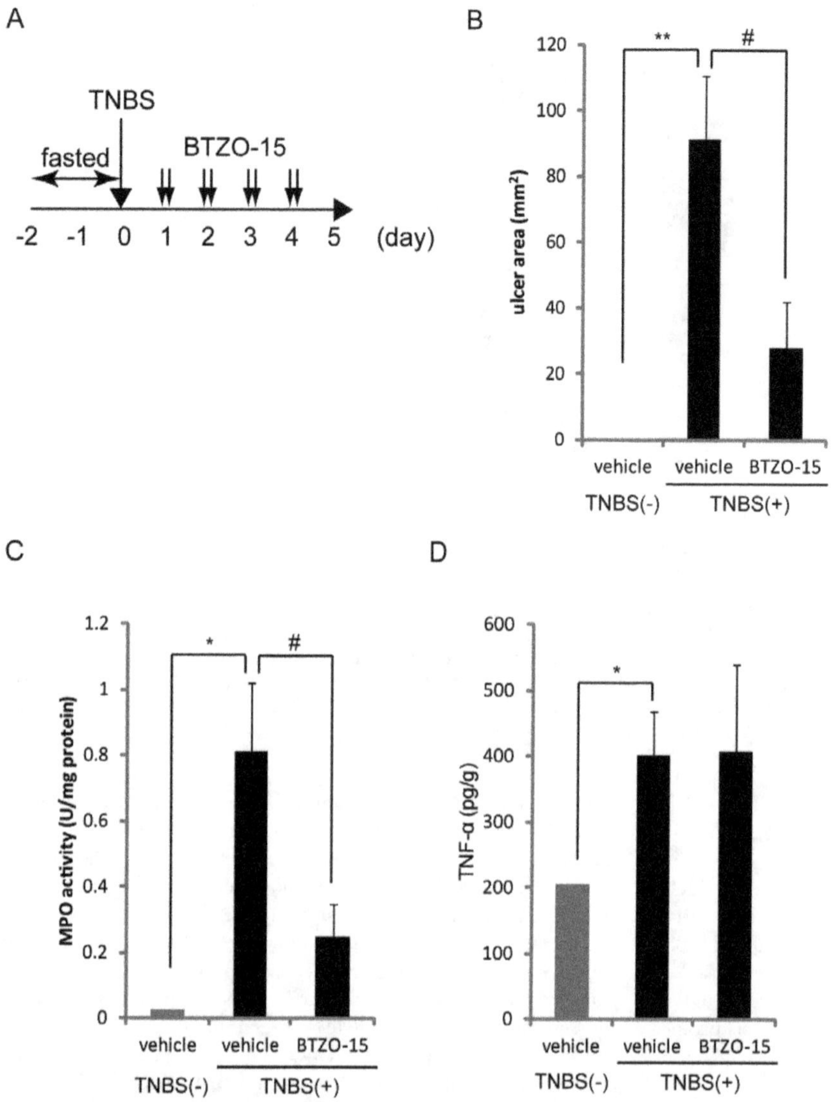

Figure 5. BTZO-15 ameliorates TNBS-induced colitis in rats. Colitis was induced in male F344/Du rats by topical intracolonic application of a TNBS solution. BTZO-15 was orally administered to rats at the indicated doses of 10 mg/kg (b.i.d.) for 4 days from experimental day 1 to 4 (A). The efficacy of BTZO-15 was evaluated using the size of the rectal ulcer (B), MPO activity (C), and TNF-α level in rectum. Results shown are the mean ± S.E.M. TNBS-treated group, n = 6; TNBS untreated group, n = 2. ** P≤0.01: compared the DSS (−) vehicle control group with DSS (+) vehicle control group by Aspin-Welch test, and # P≤0.05 compared the DSS (+) vehicle control group with DSS (+) + BTZO-15 treated groups with Student's t test (B). * P≤0.05: compared the DSS (−) vehicle control group with DSS (+) vehicle control group using Aspin-Welch test, and # P≤0.05 compared the DSS (+) vehicle control group with DSS (+) + BTZO-15 treated groups by Aspin-Welch test (C and D).

10% FBS and 1% PS, and cultured in 96-well plates (Becton Dickinson, San Jose, CA, USA) for 17 h at a density of 1×10^4 cells/well. The cells were washed three times with DMEM supplemented with 1% PS and further cultured with various concentrations of BTZO-15 for about 24 h. Cell lysates were prepared using the Steady-Glo Luciferase Assay System (Promega, Madison WI, USA) and luciferase activity was measured with the WALLAC ARVO SX (GE Healthcare UK Limited, Buckinghamshire, UK). All samples were dissolved in DMF, with the final concentration of DMF at 0.1%.

Real-time PCR analysis of HO-1 and GST Ya mRNA expression in H9c2 cells

H9c2 cells were suspended in DMEM including 10% FBS, 2 mM glutamine, and 1% PS at a density of 3.0×10^4 cells/well and cultured in 12-well plates at 37°C in 5% CO2/95% humidified air for 1 day. The cell were washed three times with DMEM supplemented with 2 mM glutamine and 1% PS. After medium change with DMEM supplemented with 2 mM glutamine and 1% PS, the indicated concentrations of BTZO-15 were added to the culture medium and incubated for 6 h or 21 h for expression analysis of HO-1 or GST Ya, respectively. For quantitative PCR, total RNA was extracted with RNeasy 96 Kit (QIAGEN GmbH, Hilden, Germany) following the manufacturer's instructions and further purified by DNase digestion using MessageClean (GenHunter Corporation, Nashville, TN, USA). Real-time PCR was carried out with an ABI PRISM 7900HT sequence detection system (Life Technologies, Carlsbad, CA, USA) using TaqMan reagents (Life Technologies). RNA was normalized using glyceraldehyde-3-phosphate dehydrogenase (GAPDH) TaqMan probes according to the manufacturer's instructions. The following primers and probe were used for

HO-1 analysis: forward primer (rHO-1F2), 5′-CCGCCTT-CCTGCTCAACA-3′; reverse primer (rHO-1R2), 5′-AAGAAA-CTCTGTCTGTGAGGGACTCT-3′; TaqMan probe (rHO-1-2), 5′-FAM-CAGGCACTGCTGACAGAGGAACACAAAG-T-AMRA-3′. The FAM (6-carboxyfluorescein) reporter is covalently linked to the 5′ end of the probe; TAMRA (6-carboxy-N, N, N′, N′-tetramethyl-rhodamine), located at the 3′ end of the probe, is used for quenching. The following primers and probes were used for GST Ya analysis: forward primer (rGSTYaF1), 5′-TGC-CAGCCTTCTGACCTCTTT-3′; reverse primer (rGSTYaR1), 5′-CTGCAGGAACTTCTTCACATTGG-3′; TaqMan probe (rGSTYa-1), 5′-FAM-AAGGCCTTCAAGAGCAGAATCAGC-AGC-TAMRA-3′. The following primers and probe were used for GAPDH analysis: forward primer (rGAPDHF2), 5′-TGCCAAG-TATGATGACATCAAGAAG-3′; reverse primer (rGAPDHR2), 5′-AGCCCAGGATGCCCTTTAGT-3′; TaqMan probe (rGAP-DH-2), 5′-VIC-TGGTGAAGCAGGCGGCCGAG-TAMRA-3′.

RNA interference

RNA interference was carried out as described previously [8]. H9c2 cells were suspended in DMEM supplemented with 10% FBS and 1% PS at a density of 1×10^5 cells/mL and cultured for 1 day. After washing three times with DMEM supplemented with 3% FBS, the cells were transfected with MIF siRNA (5′-G-CUCAUGACUUUUAGUGGC-3′) (Life Technologies) or control siRNA (4611, Life Technologies) (100 nM), using Opti-MEM (Life Technologies) and Oligofectamine (Life Technologies), and cultured for 1 day. The cells were then washed three times with DMEM supplemented with 3% FBS and cultured for 3 days. The cells were harvested with a trypsin-EDTA solution, suspended in DMEM supplemented with 3% FBS at a density of 5×10^4 cells/mL and cultured for 1 day. The cells were again transfected with either MIF siRNA or control siRNA (100 nM) using Opti-MEM and Oligofectamine, cultured for 2 days, washed three times with DMEM, and then incubated with the indicated concentrations of BTZO-15 for 24 h. Total RNA was extracted using an RNeasy 96 Kit (QIAGEN GmbH) following the manufacturer's instructions.

Real-time PCR analysis of HO-1 and GST Ya mRNA expression in IEC-18 cells

IEC-18 cells were suspended in MEM including 10% FBS and 1% PS at a density of 1.5×10^4 cells/well and cultured in 48-well plates at 37°C in 5% CO2/95% humidified air for 1 day. After a medium change with MEM supplemented with 1% PS, the cells were pretreated with various concentrations of BTZO-15 for 7.5 h. Quantitative PCR was carried out as described above.

Cell survival assays for the evaluation of NO-induced cell death

IEC-18 cells were suspended in MEM supplemented with 10% FBS and 1% PS at a density of 1.5×10^4 cells/well and cultured in 96-well plates at 37°C in 5% CO_2/95% humidified air for 1 day. After a medium change with MEM plus 1% PS, cells were pretreated with various concentrations of BTZO-15 for 1 h. Cell death was induced by treatment with 130 µM of (±)-(E)-4-Ethyl-2-[(E)-hydroxyimino]-5-nitro-3-hexenamide (NOR3; Dojindo, Makishi), which generates nitric oxide (NO), for 1 day. Afterwards, cell viability was evaluated with the Cell Counting Kit-8 (Dojindo).

Induction and treatment of DSS-induced colitis

F344 DuCrj rats, except the normal group, received drinking water with 2.3% (wt/vol.) DSS (molecular weight 5,000 Da; Wako Pure Chemical Industries Co., Ltd., Osaka) for 7 days, from experimental day 0 (starting day) to experimental day 7. Control rats received drinking water without DSS.

BTZO-15 was suspended in a 0.5% methylcellulose solution and administered orally twice per day at an interval of 4 h in a volume of 5 mL/kg from experimental day 3 to day 6 (n = 8 rats in each group). The rats were sacrificed under ether anesthesia by decapitation. The efficacy of BTZO-15 in this model was evaluated in a double-blind fashion using the following parameters; body weight, stool consistency/diarrhea score (0 points = normal and formed, 1 points = pasty and formed, 2 points = pasty to soft and unformed, 3 points = diarrhea), bleeding score (0 points = no bleeding, 1 points = slight bleeding, 2 points = obvious bleeding, 3 points = mostly bleeding) [30], large intestine length from appendix subjacency to anus, rectum weight from anus to 5 cm, and myeloperoxidase (MPO) activity.

MPO activity

MPO activity was measured to monitor the degree of neutrophil infiltration in the rectum. Rats were sacrificed under ether anesthesia by decapitation and rectums were removed and gently cleared of feces and rinsed with chilled PBS. The specimens were weighed, cut into small pieces in 0.5% hexadecyl trimethyl-ammonium bromide (HTAB) (Sigma-Aldrich, St. Louis, MO, USA)/50 mM KH_2PO_4 and Na_2PO_4 buffer (pH 6.0), and homogenized with a Physcotron (Microtec Co., Ltd., Funabashi). The homogenates were subjected to two sonication and freeze-thaw cycles. The suspensions were centrifuged at 3,000 rpm for 10 min at 4°C and the supernatants were reacted with a Peroxidase Colorimetric Kit (Sumitomo Bakelite Company Limited, Tokyo). Myeloperoxidase Polymorphonuclear Leukocytes (Merck KGaA, Darmstadt, Germany) were used as a standard and the data were presented as units per milligram of protein.

Rat GST-Ya ELISA

The rat GST Ya protein was prepared using a pET system (Merck KGaA) as described previously [8]. Anti-GST serum was generated by immunizing SPF Japanese white rabbits with recombinant GST Ya protein (MBL, Nagoya). Anti-GST Ya IgG was purified from the serum using protein-G affinity chromatography (GE Healthcare UK Limited) following the manufacturer's instructions. Rectal concentrations of GST Ya were quantified with a sandwich ELISA using polyclonal rabbit anti-GST Ya detector, a biotin-labeled polyclonal rabbit anti-GST Ys detector, and purified recombinant rat GST Ys protein.

Analysis of rectal GST-Ya and HO-1 protein levels

Rats were anesthetized with ether and sacrificed by decapitation. Rectums were quickly removed and gently cleared of feces and rinsed with chilled PBS. The specimens were excised in 4 volumes of PBS supplemented with nonidet P-40 (NP-40) and homogenized with a Teflon homogenizer. The homogenates were centrifuged at 1,000× g for 5 min and the supernatants were retained. Protein content was determined with a BCA Protein Assay Kit (Thermo Fisher Scientific Inc., Rockford, IL, USA) and equal protein levels of the supernatants were used to evaluate the concentrations of GST-Ya and HO-1 using rat GST-Ya ELISA and rat Heme Oxygenase-1 EIA Kit (Takara Bio Inc., Ohtsu), respectively.

Induction and assessment of TNBS-induced colitis

Seven-week-old male F344/Du rats were given water but no food for 48 h. After fasting, at experimental day 0, the rats were anesthetized with 30 mg/kg pentobarbital, and colitis was induced by topical intracolonic application of 0.4 mL of a solution containing 4 mg of TNBS (Wako Pure Chemical Industries Co., Ltd.) in 50% ethanol (Wako Pure Chemical Industries Co., Ltd.) with a rubber cannula. The rats received 10 mg/kg of BTZO-15 orally twice per day at an interval of 4 h from experimental day 1 to day 4 (n = 8 rats in each group). On experimental day 5, the rats were sacrificed under ether anesthesia by decapitation and their rectums were dissected. The efficacy of the BTZO-15 in this model was evaluated based on the size of the ulcerated area on the rectum, which was quantified by MacScope, MPO activity, and TNFα contents.

Statistical analysis

In Figure 3, the statistical significance of the difference between the vehicle- and DSS-treated groups on diarrhea and bleeding scores were determined by Wilcoxon's test. Statistical significance between two groups was also determined using the Student's t test for homogenous data or Aspin-Welch test for non-homogenous data. In the experiments that examine the effect of multiple doses of test compounds, the statistical significance was determined by a one-tailed Williams test for homogenous data or a one-tailed Shirley-Williams test for non-homogenous data.

Acknowledgments

We wish to express our sincere thanks to Drs. Tetsuo Miwa, Hideaki Nagaya, Kaneyoshi Kato, Keisuke Hirai, Akihiro Tasaka, Nobuhiro Inatomi, Noboru Tsuchimori, Yasuhiro Tsukimi, and Shogo Marui for their helpful discussions. We also thank Dr. Takeshi Watanabe for toxicological studies, Hisashi Fujita for pharmacokinetic studies, and Shikiko Shiki for her technical assistance.

Author Contributions

Conceived and designed the experiments: HY HK MT. Performed the experiments: HY HK HS YT YS MT. Analyzed the data: HY HK YS MT. Contributed reagents/materials/analysis tools: TI MK. Wrote the paper: HY HK.

References

1. Sands BE (2007) Inflammatory bowel disease: past, present, and future. J Gastroenterol 42: 16–25.
2. Rosenberg LN, Peppercorn MA (2010) Efficacy and safety of drugs for ulcerative colitis. Expert Opin Drug Saf 9: 573–592.
3. Vijayan V, Mueller S, Baumgart-Vogt E, Immenschuh S (2010) Heme oxygenase-1 as a therapeutic target in inflammatory disorders of the gastrointestinal tract. World J Gastroenterol 16: 3112–3119.
4. Damiani CR, Benetton CA, Stoffel C, Bardini KC, Cardoso VH, et al. (2007) Oxidative stress and metabolism in animal model of colitis induced by dextran sulfate sodium. J Gastroenterol Hepatol 22: 1846–1851.
5. Dryden GW, Jr., Deaciuc I, Arteel G, McClain CJ (2005) Clinical implications of oxidative stress and antioxidant therapy. Curr Gastroenterol Rep 7: 308–316.
6. Rezaie A, Parker RD, Abdollahi M (2007) Oxidative stress and pathogenesis of inflammatory bowel disease: an epiphenomenon or the cause? Dig Dis Sci 52: 2015–2021.
7. Varga C, Laszlo F, Fritz P, Cavicchi M, Lamarque D, et al. (2007) Modulation be heme and zinc protoporphyrin of colonic heme oxygenase-1 and experimental inflammatory bowel disease in the rat. Eur J Pharmacol 561: 164–171.
8. Kimura H, Sato Y, Tajima Y, Suzuki H, Yukitake H, et al. (2010) BTZO-1, a Cardioprotective Agent, Reveals that Macrophage Migration Inhibitory Factor Regulates ARE-mediated Gene Expression. Chem Biol 17: 1282–1294.
9. Nguyen T, Sherratt PJ, Pickett CB (2003) Regulatory mechanisms controlling gene expression mediated by the antioxidant response element. Annu Rev Pharmacol Toxicol 43: 233–260.
10. Chen XL, Kusch C (2004) Induction of cytoprotective genes through Nrf2/ antioxidant response element pathway: a new therapeutic approach for the treatment of inflammatory diseases. Curr Pharm Des 10: 879–891.
11. Kasper JW, Niture SK, Jaiswal AK (2009) Nrf2:INrf2 (Keap1) signaling in oxidative stress. Free Radic Biol Med 47: 1304–1309.
12. de Vries HE, Witte M, Hondius D, Rozemuller AJM, Drukarch B, et al. (2008) Nrf2-induced antioxidant protection: a promising target to counteract ROS-mediated damage in neurodegenerative disease? Free Radic Biol Med 45: 1375–1383.
13. Hara H, Ohta M, Ohta K, Kuno S, Adachi T (2003) Increase of antioxidative potential by tert-butylhydroquinone protects against cell death associated with 6-hudroxydopamine-induced oxidative stress in neuroblastoma SH-SY5Y cells. Brain Res Mol Brain Res 119: 125–131.
14. Itoh K, Mochizuki M, Ishii Y, Ishii T, Shibata T, et al. (2004) Transcription factor Nrf2 regulates inflammation by mediating the effect of 15-Deoxy-$\Delta^{12,14}$-Prostaglandin J_2. Mol Cell Biol 24: 36–45.
15. Ishii T, Itoh K, Takahashi S, Sato H, Yanagawa T, et al. (2000) Transcription factor Nrf2 coordinately regulates a group of oxidative stress-inducible genes in macrophages. J Biol Chem 275: 16023–160-29.
16. Rushmore TH, Morton MR, Pickett CB (1991) The antioxidant responsive element. J Biol Chem 266: 11632–11639.
17. Xu CT, Meng SY, Pan BR (2004) Drug therapy for ulcerative colitis. World J Gastroenterol 10: 2311–2317.
18. Blonski W, Lichtenstein GR (2007) Safety of biologic therapy. Inflamm Bowel Dis 13: 769–796.
19. Wirtz S, Neufert C, Weigmann B, Neurath MF (2007) Chemically induced mouse models of intestinal inflammation. Nat Protoc 2: 541–546.
20. Dieleman LA, Ridwan BU, Tennyson GS, Beagley KW, Bucy RP, et al. (1994) Dextran sulfate sodium-induced colitis occurs in severe combined immunodeficient mice. Gastroenterology 107: 1643–1652.
21. Foligne B, Nutten S, Steidler L, Dennin V, Goudercourt D, et al. (2006) Recommendations for improved use of the murine TNBS-induced colitis model in evaluating anti-inflammatory properties of lactic acid bacteria: technical and microbiological aspects. Dig Dis Sci 51: 390–400.
22. Elson CO, Sartor RB, Tennyson GS, Riddell RH (1995) Experimental models of inflammatory bowel disease. Gastroenterology 109: 1344–1367.
23. Zhong W, Xia Z, Hinrichs D, Rosenbaum JT, Wegmann KW, et al. (2010) Hemin exerts multiple protective mechanisms and attenuates dextran sulfate sodium-induced colitis. J Pediatr Gastroenterol Nurt 50: 132–139.
24. Clapper ML, Adrian RH, Pfeiffer GR, Kido K, Everley L, et al. (1999) Depletion of colonic detoxication enzyme activity ain mice with dextran sulphate sodium-induced colitis. Aliment Pharmacol Ther 13: 389–396.
25. Arafa HMM, Hemeida RA, EI-Bahrawy AIM, Hamada FMA (2009) Prophylactic role of curcumin in dextran sulfate sodium (DSS)-induced ulcerative colitis murine model. Food Chem Toxicol 47: 1311–1317.
26. Kimura H, Yukitake H, Tajima Y, Suzuki H, Chikatsu T, et al. (2010) ITZ-1, a client-selective Hsp90 inhibitor, efficiently induces heat shock factor 1 activation. Chem Biol 17: 18–27.
27. Ohkawara T, Nishihira J, Takeda H, Hide S, Kato M, et al. (2002) Amelioration of dextran sulfate dosium-induced colitis by anti-macrophage migration inhibitory factor antibody in mice. Gastroenterology 123: 256–270.
28. Ohkawara T, Nishihira J, Ishiguro Y, Otsubo E, Nagai K, et al. (2006) Resistance to experimental colitis depends on cytoprotective heat chock proteins in macrophage migration inhibitory factor null mice. Immunol Lett 107: 148–154.
29. Nishihira J, Mitsuyama K (2009) Overview of the role of macrophage migration inhibitory factor (MIF) in inflammatory bowel disease. Curr Pharm Des 15: 2104–2109.
30. Alex P, Zachos NC, Nguyen T, Gonzales L, Chen TE, et al. (2009) Distinct Cytokine Patterns Identified from multiplex profiles of murine DSS and TNBS-induced Colitis. Inflamm Bowel Dis 15: 341–352.

11

Fetal Exposure to Maternal Inflammation does not Affect Postnatal Development of Genetically-Driven Ileitis and Colitis

Jana Hemmerling[1,2], Katharina Heller[1,2], Gabriele Hörmannsperger[1,2], Monika Bazanella[1,2], Thomas Clavel[1,2], George Kollias[3], Dirk Haller[1,2]*

1 Chair of Nutrition and Immunology, Technische Universität München, Freising- Weihenstephan, Bavaria, Germany, **2** ZIEL - Research Center for Nutrition and Food Sciences, Freising-Weihenstephan, Bavaria, Germany, **3** Biomedical Sciences Research Centre, Institute for Immunology, Alexander Fleming, Vari, Athens, Greece

Abstract

Background: Chronic inflammatory disorders have been increasing in incidence over the past decades following geographical patterns of industrialization. Fetal exposure to maternal inflammation may alter organ functions and the offspring's disease risk. We studied the development of genetically-driven ileitis and colitis in response to maternal inflammation using mouse models.

Methods: Disease susceptible ($Tnf^{\Delta ARE/+}$ and $IL10^{-/-}$) and disease-free ($Tnf^{+/+}$ and $IL10^{-/+}$) offspring were raised in inflamed and non-inflamed dams. Ileal, caecal and colonic pathology was evaluated in the offspring at 8 or 12 weeks of age. Ly6G-positive cells in inflamed sections from the distal ileum and distal colon were analysed by immunofluorescence microscopy. Gene expression of pro-inflammatory cytokines was measured in whole tissue specimens by quantitative PCR. Microarray analyses were performed on laser microdissected intestinal epithelium. Caecal bacterial communities were assessed by Illumina sequencing of 16S rRNA amplicons.

Results: Disease severity, the number of infiltrated neutrophils as well as *Tnf* and *Il12p40* mRNA expression were independent of maternal inflammation in the offspring of mouse models for ileitis ($Tnf^{\Delta ARE/+}$) and colitis ($IL10^{-/-}$). Although TNF-driven maternal inflammation regulated 2,174 (wild type) and 3,345 ($Tnf^{\Delta ARE/+}$) genes in the fetal epithelium, prenatal gene expression patterns were completely overwritten after birth. In addition, co-housing experiments revealed no change in phylogenetic diversity of the offspring's caecal microbiota in response to maternal inflammation. This is independent of the offspring's genotype before and after the onset of tissue pathology.

Conclusions: Disease risk and activity in mouse models of chronic ileitis and colitis was independent of the fetal exposure to maternal inflammation. Likewise, maternal inflammation did not alter the diversity and composition of offspring's caecal microbiota, clearly demonstrating that changes of the gene expression program in the fetal gut epithelium were not relevant for the development of chronic inflammatory disorders in the gut.

Editor: Mathias Chamaillard, INSERM, France

Funding: This work was supported by the 'Nutritional Adaptation and Epigenetic Mechanisms' program of ZIEL - Research Center for Nutrition and Food Sciences. The funders had no role in study design, data collection and analysis, decision to publish, or preparation of the manuscript.

Competing Interests: The authors have declared that no competing interests exist.

* E-mail: Dirk.Haller@tum.de.

Introduction

Lifestyle changes in industrialized countries are associated with a sharp increase in the incidence of immune-mediated chronic pathologies such as inflammatory bowel diseases (IBD), multiple sclerosis or type-1 diabetes. Th1-driven inflammatory processes are key mechanisms in the pathogenesis of these chronic pathologies[1]. IBD are spontaneously relapsing, immunologically mediated disorders of the gastrointestinal tract[2]. Although the pathogenesis of these multifactorial diseases is still not fully understood, the combination of genetic predisposition[3] and environmental factors (microbiota, diet and lifestyle)[4] drives disease development. Apart from the major impact of IBD on life quality of the affected patients, epidemiological studies link Crohn's disease (CD) activity during pregnancy to adverse outcomes such as preterm birth, spontaneous abortion and labor complications[5,6].This is not clear in the context of ulcerative colitis.

Despite the fact that alterations of the cytokine milieu during CD-associated pregnancy lead to peri- and postnatal complications[6–8], the transmission of maternal inflammation to the offspring with consequences for later disease susceptibility, severity or phenotype is completely unknown. A potential impact of inflammatory processes during pregnancy on fetal organ functions was recently shown for endotoxin-induced chorioamnionitis[9]. In this context, the maturation of the fetal gut barrier was prevented [10]. Furthermore, maternal exposure to high-fat diet was recently reported to induce intestinal inflammation in fetal sheep, suggesting that even low grade maternal inflammation might affect intestinal functions and IBD susceptibility in the offspring[11]. Maternally transmitted compositional changes of the microbiota might be an important factor that contributes to this influence on disease susceptibility in the offspring [12].

In this context, we asked the question whether chronic maternal inflammation is a risk factor for postnatal disease susceptibility in the normal and genetically susceptible host. We applied sophisticated breeding systems with heterozygous $Tnf^{\Delta ARE/+}$ and homozygous $IL10^{-/-}$ mice to generate genetically-driven inflammatory disease environments *in utero* in two well-established models of chronic ileitis and colitis, enabling us to study the role of maternal inflammation on postnatal disease onset. Exemplarily, we took also advantage of the $Tnf^{\Delta ARE/+}$ model with ileitis to assess transcriptional profiling of fetal and postnatal intestinal epithelial cells (IEC) obtained by laser microdissection in order to provide high resolution of cellular specificity at this disease relevant interface. This second objective fits with the hypothesis that the pathogenesis of CD is characterized by a failure of innate immune mechanisms to recognize microbial triggers at the early stage of disease development[4]. Selective overexpression of TNF in the intestinal epithelium seems to be sufficient to trigger CD-like ileitis[13], suggesting an important role of the epithelium in the pathogenesis of chronic intestinal inflammation in $Tnf^{\Delta ARE/+}$ mice[14].

Thus, the aim of the present study was to characterize the role of genetically-driven maternal inflammation in programming the fetal epithelium towards postnatal development of intestinal inflammation.

Materials and Methods

Ethics Statement

Mouse experiments were performed between 2009 and 2011 in accordance to the German guidelines for animal care (Regierung von Oberbayern, Bavaria, Germany). No animal approval was obtained, because no intervention was performed with living mice. All mice were reported as mice "sacrificed for research purposes" at the Regierung von Oberbayern.

Animals and Experimental Design

All mice were conventionally housed in groups of 3–5 mice per cage at a 12 h light/dark cycle at 24–26°C. They received fresh tap water and breeding diet (Ssniff Chow) ad libitum and were sacrificed by neck dislocation. $Tnf^{\Delta ARE/+}$(ARE) dams were bred with $Tnf^{+/+}$ wildtype (WT) sires (C57BL/6N genetic background) and vice versa (n = 5–10 breeding pairs), generating offspring from healthy WT dams (WT and ARE) and inflamed ARE dams (iWT and iARE) (Figure 1A) (n = 5 each). The period of conception was set from 8–12 weeks in order to avoid suffering in genetically susceptible ARE dams. Dams were sacrificed at an average age of 13 weeks +/− 5 d (WT dams) and 11 weeks +/− 1 d (ARE dams) for the prenatal time point and at 17 weeks +/− 1 d (WT dams) and 14 weeks +/− 3 d (ARE dams) for the weaning time point (3 weeks after giving birth). Offspring were sacrificed at the age of 17.5 days post conception (dpc), 3 (weaning) and 8 weeks by neck dislocation. Morphological criteria of fetuses at 17.5 dpc were evaluated according to Theiler stage 25 (TS25) based on the onset of skin wrinkling, whiskers and eyelid closure. Placentas and offspring's gut were embedded in Optimal Cutting Temperature (O.C.T.) matrix (Sakura Finetek, Torrance, USA) and stored at −80°C until laser microdissection of intestinal epithelial cells and subsequent microarray experiments.

For co-housing experiments, ARE and WT dams were kept together in one cage to generate mixed beddings from the age of 4 weeks. From week 8 on, dams were mated with WT males overnight only until pregnancy was observed. During the day, dams were co-housed again. After giving birth, beddings of ARE and WT dams and litters were exchanged to create a synchronized environment independent of the dam's genotype, so as to be able to analyse only the effect of inflammation *in utero* on shaping gut bacterial colonization. Dams and offspring were sacrificed before weaning, *i.e.*, 3 weeks after birth.

Female $IL10^{-/-}$ were bred with male $IL10^{+/-}$ (both on the 129Sv/Ev genetic background) and vice versa (n = 5–6 each), generating offspring (n = 5–15 each) from healthy $IL10^{+/-}$ dams ($IL10^{+/-}$, $IL10^{-/-}$) or inflamed $IL10^{-/-}$ dams (i$IL10^{+/-}$, i$IL10^{-/-}$) (Figure 1B). The breeding period was set between 15–21 weeks. Dams were sacrificed at weaning at an average age of 25 +/− 2 weeks ($IL10^{-/-}$ dams) and 27 +/− 4 weeks ($IL10^{+/-}$ dams). $IL10^{-/-}$ dams showing a total colitis score of at least 2 (0–12) (Figure 1 D) were considered as inflamed and the offspring was included in the analysis. Offspring were sacrificed at the age of 12 weeks by neck dislocation in order to blindly determine histological colitis scores.

Histopathology

Scoring was performed on 10% formalin-fixed paraffin-embedded or cryo-fixed tissue for the postnatal or prenatal time point, respectively. The histological score was ascertained in a blinded fashion on H&E-stained transversal sections of the terminal ileum (WT, iWT, ARE, iARE) or of the cecum tip, proximal colon and distal colon ($IL10^{+/-}$, $IL10^{-/-}$, i$IL10^{+/-}$, $IL10^{-/-}$), resulting in a score from 0 (non-inflamed) to 12 (highly inflamed) per section as previously described[15]. The total colitis score per mouse was determined by calculating the mean of all three colonic compartments.

Plasma Measurements of Maternal Tumor Necrosis Factor

Plasma TNF was measured using Mouse TNF alpha ELISA Ready –SET-Go! ELISA, according to the manufacturer's instructions (eBioscience, San Diego, USA). A volume of 100 µl total plasma was incubated on a pre-coated plate for 2 h at RT (room temperature), followed by incubation of anti-TNF detection antibody linked with Avidin/Biotin. HRP-conjugated antibody was incubated for 30 min and substrate conversion was stopped after 15 min with 2N H_2SO_4. The product absorbance of standard dilutions and plasma sample was measured at 405 nm to the reference wavelength of 570 nm. Quantification was performed using the linear equation of the standard dilutions.

Immunofluorescence Staining of Ly6G and REG3B in the Intestine

Transversal sections (5 µm thick) were cut from either formalin-fixed paraffin embedded (FFPE) or from frozen distal ileum or colon and transferred onto Superfrost Plus slides (Thermo Scientific, Braunschweig, Germany). After deparaffinization of FFPE tissue (Leica ST5020 Multistainer system), antigen demasking was performed by boiling in 1× sodium citrate buffer (pH 6, 900 W, 23 min). After cool down to RT, slides were washed 3 times in dH2O for 5 min, followed by 5 min in PBS. Frozen sections were equilibrated to room temperature (30 min), fixed in ice cold acetone (−20°C) for 10 min, followed by 30 min air drying at RT and 3 times 5 min washing in PBS. Sections were blocked with 50 µl blocking buffer raised against the species of the secondary antibody for 60 min at RT in a humidified chamber.

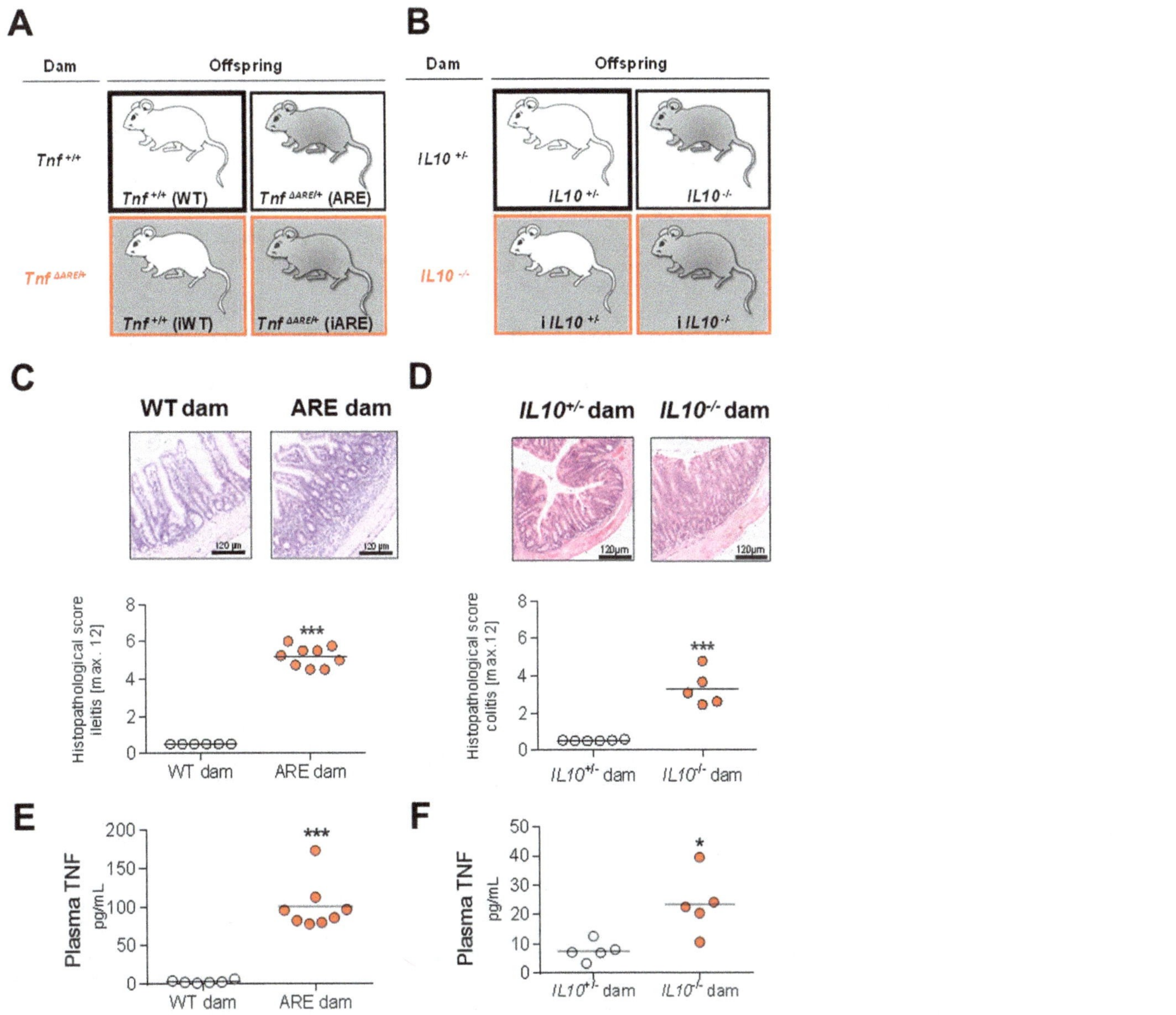

Figure 1. Breeding schemes and the maternal inflammatory environment. Breeding schemes of TNF- (A) and IL10-driven (B) maternal inflammation. Offspring developed under non inflamed conditions (white background: white mouse = WT or IL10+/−; grey mouse = ARE or IL10−/−) and under maternal inflammation (grey background: white mouse = iWTor iIL10+/−; grey mouse = iARE or iIL10−/−). (C) Representative H&E-stained transversal sections of the distal ileum and individual plots of ileitis score in WT (n = 6) and ARE (n = 8) dams. (D) Total colitis score in IL10+/− (n = 6) and IL10−/− dams (n = 8) and representative H&E-stained sections of distal colon from non-inflamed IL10+/− and inflamed IL10−/− dams. Scores [0, not inflamed, to 12, highly inflamed] were determined using tissue sections from dams sacrificed 3 weeks after giving birth. TNF in maternal plasma indicates that the inflammation is also systemically relevant in both the ileitis (E) and colitis (F) models. Individual data and means are shown; t-test, $^{*}p<0.05$, $^{***}p<0.001$.

Primary antibody against Ly6G (rat-anti-Ly6G, BD Pharmingen, 1:500) was incubated overnight at 4°C. Primary antibody against REG3B (sheep- anti-REG3B, R&D Systems, 1:100 dilution) was incubated at RT for 1–3 hours in a humidified chamber. Fluorochrome-conjugated secondary antibodies, namely goat anti-rat IgG (H+L) Alexa Fluor 546 (Invitrogen) or donkey anti-sheep IgG (H+L) DyLight 488 (Jackson ImmunoResearch), were diluted 1:200 and incubated for 1 h at RT. Nuclei were counterstained using DAPI (1:2000) in secondary antibody solution. Sections were visualized using a confocal microscope (Olympus Fluoview 1000 using the FV10-ASW software). The amount of Ly6G positive cells per area was counted using the Volocity 5.51 software (Perkin Elmer) defining the lamina propria as region of interest. For each individual mouse, 3 microscopic fields at a 600-fold magnification were quantified for mean Ly6G-positive cells per mm^2. Immunofluorescence intensity of REG3B was quantified with Volocity Demo 5.5 software (Perkin Elmer) defining epithelial cells as region of interest. For each individual mouse 3 different areas were quantified as mean intensity of the fluorescence signal per μm^2.

Gene Expression Analysis of Whole Gut Tissue and Laser Microdissected IEC

RNA from cryosections of distal ileum (3 sections of 10 µm each) and colonic swiss rolls (2 sections of 10 µm each) was isolated using the RNA isolation kit according to the manufacturer's instructions (Macherey & Nagel). Reverse transcription was performed using SuperScript III Reverse Transcriptase (Invitrogen). RNA of laser microdissected IEC (10 ng) was preamplified with the QuantiTect Whole Transcriptome Kit (Oiagen, Hilden, Germany) according to the manufacturer's instructions. Gene-specific nucleotide sequences and accession numbers were obtained from the National Center for Biotechnology Information (NCBI) website (http://www.ncbi.nlm.nih.gov/gene). Primer pairs (Table 1) were designed using the Universal ProbeLibrary (UPL) design center (Roche Diagnostics, Mannheim, Germany). Quantitative real-time PCR was performed on 10 ng cDNA using the LightCycler 480 System (Roche Diagnostics, Mannheim, Germany). Crossing points (Cp) were determined using the second derivative maximum method by the LightCycler 480 software release 1.5.0. Data were normalized to the Cp mean of reference genes (*Gapdh* for whole gut tissue and *18s*, *Rpl13a* and *Gapdh* for pre-amplified cDNA of IEC) and expressed as $2^{-\Delta Ct}$ values in order to compare expression levels among all groups.

Laser Microdissection (LMD) Microscopy of Intestinal Epithelial Cells

Ileal cryo-sections (Microm, Walldorf, Germany) were generated at −20°C. PET frame slides (MicroDissect, Herborn, Germany) were treated with RNase ZAP (Sigma-Aldrich, Steinheim, Germany) before use and dried at RT. Transversal sections (10 µm) were mounted on slides, air-dried and stored at −80°C for short periods of time (<7 d) until use. Each slide was stained directly before LMD microscopy. Briefly, after equilibration to RT (2 min), slides were fixed for 1 min with 70%(v/v) EtOH, rinsed with Diethylpyrocarbonate (DEPC) water for 30 sec, stained with Harris hematoxylin for 1 min and rinsed with DEPC water for 30 sec. After bluing with 0.1% (v/v) NH_4OH for 30 sec, slides were counterstained with 2.5% Eosin for 2 min. Finally, sections were dehydrated in ascending EtOH series (96%, 100%) for 30 sec each and air dried at RT for 5 min. Ileal IEC were cut at a magnification of 630× using the UV laser-cutting system LMD 6000 and the Leica Application Suite software (Leica, Wetzlar, Germany). Lysis buffer (100 µl) supplied in the AllPrep DNA/RNA Micro Kit (Qiagen, Hilden, Germany) was added to epithelial pieces directly after dissection. Samples were kept frozen at −80°C until DNA/RNA isolation. In total, a mean area of $1.330 \pm 0.024 \times 10^6$ µm^2 IECs was collected per sample (Figure S1).

RNA Isolation and Quality Control

Total RNA was isolated using the column-based AllPrep DNA/RNA Micro Kit (Qiagen, Hilden, Germany). RNA concentration was measured using the Quant-iT RiboGreen RNA Assay Kit (Invitrogen, Eugene, USA). RNA integrity was determined using the RNA 6000 Pico Kit and the Bioanalyzer 2100 (Agilent, Waldbronn, Germany). An amount of 50 ng total RNA (3 µl sample volume adjusted by vacuum centrifugation) was used for microarray analysis.

Microarray-based Gene Expression Analysis

Microarray analysis was performed with ileal IEC from 17.5 *dpc* and 8-week-old mice (n = 20 in total). All samples from one time point were run together. RNA preparation, reverse-transcription, amplification and biotin labeling were performed using the GeneChip 3′ IVT Express kit (Affymetrix, Santa Clara, USA). Hybridization, washing and staining were performed using the GeneChip Hybridization, Wash and Stain (Affymetrix) and the GeneChip Fluidics Station 450 (Affymetrix). Labeled RNA samples were hybridized to customized murine genome NuGO_Mm1a520177 microarrays containing 23,865 probe sets (covering 15,313 genes, Affymetrix). Gene chips were visually inspected for irregularities and scanned with GeneChip Scanner 3000. Data were analyzed using the Affymetrix GCOS Manager software and the R- and Bioconductor-based MADMAX interface (Management and Analysis Database for Multi-platform micro-Array eXperiments, https://madmax.bioinformatics.nl), including R version 2.11.1, Bioconductor version 2.6 and AnnotationDbi version 1.10.2. Data were normalized using the gc Robust Multichip Average (slow) algorithm. Probe sets were annotated to the transcripts with Custom Chip Definition files version 13.0.0. (nugomm1a520177mmentrezg.cdf). No previous filtering was applied to the datasets. MADMAX calculated Fold Changes (FCs), *p*-values, FDR-values and q-values to the study groups with the LIMMA procedure. The LIMMA (log2 based) FCs were calculated comparing iWT, ARE and iARE groups to the WT control group (n = 5 each). Genes were considered to be significantly regulated according to the raw *p*-value of LIMMA with $p<0.05$ and a threshold FC of ±1.5. Heatmaps were generated using the MultiExperiment Viewer (TigrMEV) software. Gene Ontology (GO) terms were computed using the GeneRanker program (Genomatix, München, Germany). Over-representation of biological terms were calculated and listed in the output together with respective *p*-values.

Table 1. Primer sequences and UPL probe IDs for qPCR analysis.

Gene	Forward primer	Reverse primer	Probe	Amplicon
Gapdh	5′-tcc act cat ggc aaa ttc aa	5′-ttt gat gtt agt ggg gtc tcg	#9	108 nt
Rpl13a	5′-atc cct cca ccc tat gac aa	5′-gcc cca ggt aag caa act t	#108	97 nt
18s	5′-aaa tca gtt atg gtt cct ttg gtc	5′-gct cta gaa tta cca cag tta tcc aa	#55	67 nt
C3	5′-acc tta cct cgg caa gtt tct	5′-ttg tag agc tgc tgg tca gg	#76	75 nt
Il12p40	5′-atc gtt ttg ctg gtg tct cc	5′-gga gtc cag tcc acc tct aca	#78	80 nt
Tnf	5′-tgc cta tgt ctc agc ctc ttc	5′-gag gcc att tgg gaa ctt ct	#49	117 nt

Housekeeping genes are underlined.

Illumina Sequencing of 16S rRNA Gene Amplicons from Caecal Contents

Bacterial DNA was obtained after bead beating and ethanol precipitation [16] from directly frozen caecal contents (co-housing experiment) or from ceacal contents embedded in O.C.T. Amplicons of the V4 region of 16S rRNA genes were obtained after 25 PCR cycles as described previously[17]. They were sequenced in paired-end modus (PE200) using the MiSeq system (Illumina Inc., San Diego, USA). Sequences were analyzed using in-house developed pipelines partly based on UPARSE [18], the open source software package QIIME[19] and the Ribosomal Database Project[20]. Sequences were filtered at a base call accuracy of 99%. Sequences containing any ambiguous nucleotide (N character) were discarded. The presence of chimeras was checked after dereplication using UCHIME [21]. Operational taxonomic units (OTUs) were picked at a threshold of 97%. Only those OTUs occurring in at least one sample at abundances >0.5% total sequences were included in the analysis. Sequence proportions of bacterial taxa were analyzed for significant differences using F-Test followed by Benjamini-Hochberg correction for multiple testing in the R programing environment (2008, ISBN 3-900051-07-0).

Statistics

Statistical analyses were performed with SigmaPlot 11.0 using unpaired t-test, Kruskal-Wallis test followed by Dunn's multiple comparison or ANOVA followed by pairwise comparisons testing (Holm-Sidak test). Data were expressed as mean ± SD. Differences between groups were considered significantly if *p*-values were <0.05 (*), <0.01 (**), <0.001 (***). Graphics were created using GraphPad Prism version 5.00 (GraphPad software, San Diego, USA).

Results

Maternal Inflammation does not Influence Postnatal Development of Intestinal Inflammation

Conventionally raised $Tnf^{\Delta ARE/+}$ (ARE) and $IL10^{-/-}$ mice were used to study the impact of maternal inflammation on the intestine in healthy and genetically susceptible offspring. As expected, all ARE dams were affected by moderate inflammation in the distal ileum (score 5.2 ± 0.5) (Figure 1C). $IL10^{-/-}$ dams showed a more heterogeneous inflammation in the large intestine and an inflammation score of 2 was set as minimal value to discriminate inflamed dams, resulting in a mean inflammatory score of 3.3 ± 0.8 for the dams that were included in the study (Figure 1D). The local inflammation in the intestine of dams was reflected systemically by significantly elevated TNF levels in the plasma of both inflamed $Tnf^{\Delta ARE/+}$ (2.9 ± 1.9 pg/mL vs. 100.0± 31.6 pg/mL) and $IL10^{-/-}$ mice (7.6 ± 3.3 pg/mL vs. 23.5 ± 10.4 pg/mL) (Figures 1E and F). The abundance of plasma TNF significantly correlated with the inflammation grade in the intestine (data not shown). The intestinal inflammation of healthy and genetically susceptible offspring was found to be unaffected by maternal inflammation in both models at the age of 8 weeks (ileitis) and 12 weeks (colitis) (Figure 2A and B). Both, ARE and iARE mice developed moderate ileitis with comparable histological scores (4.4 ± 0.9 and 4.0 ± 0.7). Likewise, $IL10^{-/-}$ and i$IL10^{-/-}$ offspring showed similar histological grades of colitis (3.0 ± 1.1 and 2.7 ± 1.1). There was no correlation between maternal and offspring's intestinal inflammation (data not shown). Additionally, the number of infiltrated Ly6G-positive cells into inflamed tissue of the distal ileum of $Tnf^{\Delta ARE/+}$ offspring or the distal colon of $IL10^{-/-}$ offspring was unaffected by maternal inflammation (ARE vs. iARE: 473 ± 262 cells/mm^2 vs. 621 ± 434 cells/mm^2; $IL10^{-/-}$ vs. i$IL10^{-/-}$: 521 ± 454 cells/mm^2 vs.497 ± 441 cells/mm^2) (Figures 2C and D). The variation of neutrophil numbers in the distal colon of $IL10^{-/-}$ was strongly associated (r = 0.82, p<0.0001) with histological scores in the distal colon, which showed high heterogeneity (total colitis score from 0.6 to 8.8). The fact that histological scores were not affected by maternal inflammation was supported by unchanged mRNA expression of pro-inflammatory cytokines in whole gut sections from the distal ileum ($Tnf^{\Delta ARE/+}$) and colonic swiss rolls ($IL10^{-/-}$) between the different offspring groups (Figures 2E and F). In other words, *Tnf* and *Il12p40* mRNA levels were not altered between ARE and iARE or $IL10^{-/-}$ and i$IL10^{-/-}$, but were significantly increased between WT and ARE or $IL10^{+/-}$ and $IL10^{-/-}$ offspring. All these data consistently show that maternal inflammation does not impact genetically-driven disease phenotypes in both mouse models of intestinal inflammation. In addition, these results raised the question of whether there is any early transcriptional programming effect on the offspring's epithelium that is induced by maternal inflammation.

Transcriptional Fingerprints of the Fetal Epithelium in Response to Maternal Inflammation do not Persist in Grownup Mice

Selective overexpression of TNF in the intestinal epithelium is sufficient to trigger CD-like ileitis[13], suggesting an important role of the epithelium in the pathogenesis of chronic intestinal inflammation in $Tnf^{\Delta ARE/+}$ mice. Furthermore, TNF plays a pivotal role in the development of CD, which has been effectively treated with anti-TNF agents[22]. To further characterize the role of maternal inflammation on the offspring's intestinal homeostasis, we focused on the impact of maternal inflammation on IEC. Since $IL10^{-/-}$ dams and offspring showed variable degrees of disease severity along the large intestine, we focused on offspring from $Tnf^{\Delta ARE/+}$ and $Tnf^{+/+}$ mice to perform this more detailed cell-specific analysis. Therefore, we measured gene expression profiles in IEC at pre- (17.5 *dpc*) and postnatal (8 weeks) time points using laser dissected ileal epithelium. Randomly selected fetuses of different stages (15–19 *dpc*) are shown in Figure 3A. At 17.5 *dpc*, fetuses had comparable sizes, but body weight was decreased in iARE compared to ARE fetuses (Figure 3B). Equivalent surface areas of laser microdissected IEC were collected in all groups (Figure S1A). RNA integrity numbers (RIN) were 5.0 ± 0.8 and 5.5 ± 1.2 for fetal and postnatal RNA, respectively.

Gene expression profiles showed two distinct patterns according to maternal and postnatal inflammation (GEO data base accession number GSE44433). In fetal IEC, gene expression was highly influenced by maternal inflammation with 2,174 and 3,345 significantly regulated genes in iWT and iARE progeny, respectively (Figure 3C). Heatmap comparisons showed similar patterns in iWT and iARE, indicating that similar genes were regulated under conditions of maternal inflammation (1,614 common genes) (Figure 3D, Table 2). The 5 most up- and down-regulated genes at pre- and postnatal time points are shown in Table 3. *Reg3b* (*regenerating islet-derived 3 beta*) and *Fabp6* (*fatty acid binding protein 6*) were identified among the top-regulated genes under maternal inflammation. The fetal ARE genotype was apparently not relevant at this early gut developmental stage (only 117 regulated genes). In contrast to the fetal stage, gene expression profiles in postnatal IEC were highly influenced by the ARE genotype with 1,154 and 1,197 significantly regulated genes under ARE and iARE conditions, respectively (Figure 3A). Only 229 genes were significantly regulated in iWT compared to WT mice, indicating that the postnatal environment and the disease

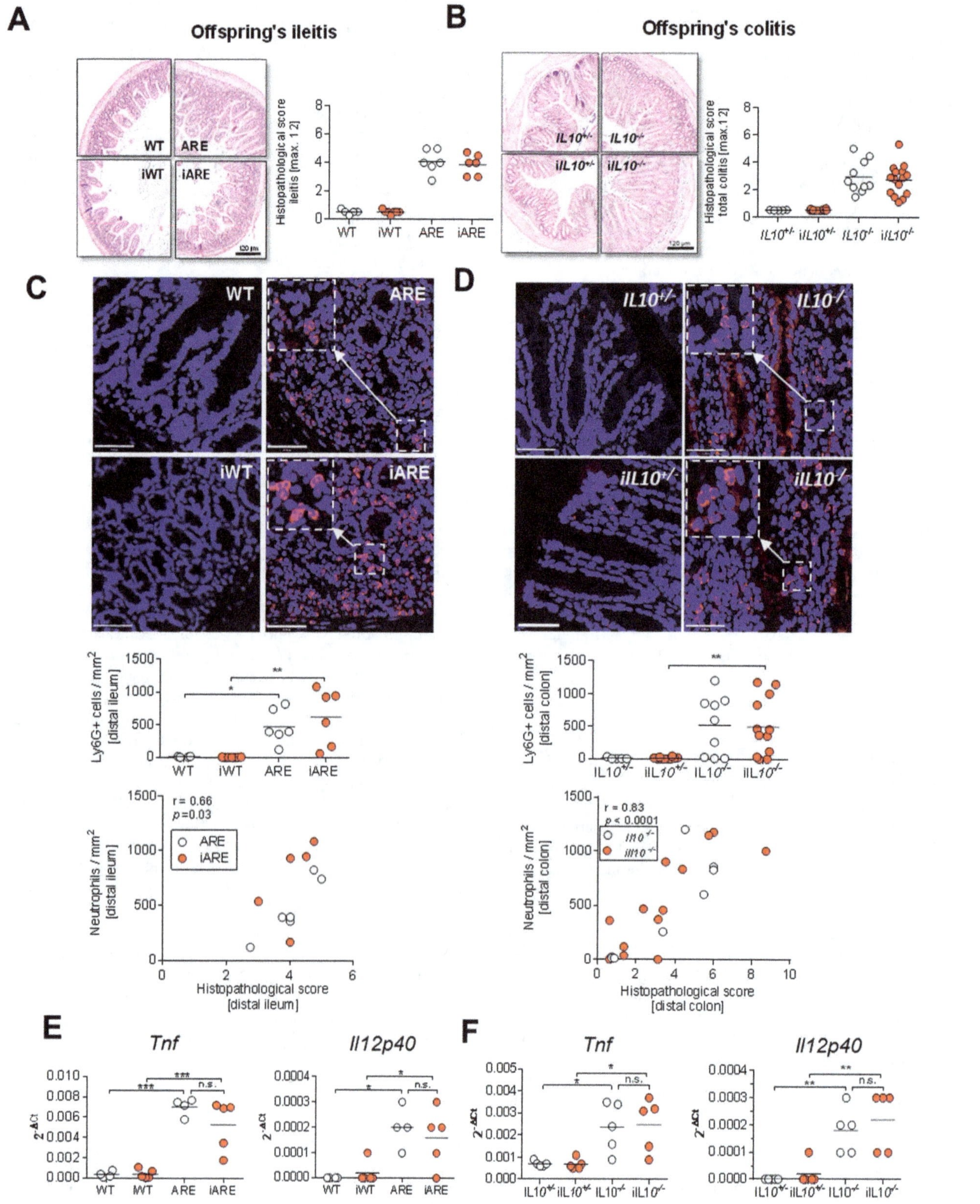

Figure 2. Postnatal tissue inflammation in *Tnf*$^{\Delta ARE/+}$ and *IL10*$^{-/-}$ mice is not affected by maternal inflammation. (A) Ileitis scores from WT, iWT, ARE and iARE (each n = 5–7) offspring sacrificed at 8 weeks of age with representative H&E stained sections of the distal ileum. (B) Total colitis scores from *IL10*$^{+/-}$, *iIL10*$^{+/-}$, *IL10*$^{-/-}$ and i*IL10*$^{-/-}$ offspring at 12 weeks of age (n = 5–15) with representative H&E-stained sections of the distal colon. Individual data and means are shown, *p<0.05, *** p<0.001 Kruskal-Wallis Test with Dunn's multiple comparisons. (C+D) Representative microscopic pictures (600× magnification) of confocal laser microscopy for Ly6G-immunofluorescence (red) from distal ileum in WT, iWT, ARE and iARE offspring and from distal colon in *IL10*$^{+/-}$, i*IL10*$^{+/-}$, *IL10*$^{-/-}$ and i*IL10*$^{-/-}$ offspring. Nuclei are counterstained with DAPI (blue). Three pictures per mouse were analyzed. Lamina propria and submucosa were defined as regions of interest. The numbers of Ly6G-positive cells per mm^2 from all 3

pictures per mouse were counted. Individual data and means are shown (Two-Way ANOVA, *$p<0.05$, **$p<0.01$). Correlation analysis in *Tnf*$^{\Delta ARE/+}$ and *IL10*$^{-/-}$ offspring indicated strong associations between histopathological scores and infiltration of Ly6G-positive neutrophils. (E+F) Whole tissue specimens were analyzed for *Tnf* and *Il12p40* gene expression in offspring from ileitis and colitis mouse models as described in the method section. RNA was isolated from distal ileal cryosections (3×10 μm) of WT, iWT, ARE and iARE offspring and from colonic swiss rolls of *IL10*$^{+/-}$, i*IL10*$^{+/-}$, *IL10*$^{-/-}$ and i*IL10*$^{-/-}$ offspring (n = 5 each). Single values and means are indicated as $2^{-\Delta Ct}$. Two Way ANOVA, *$p<0.05$, **$p<0.001$, ***$p<0.0001$.

susceptible genotype of the offspring almost completely overwrote the gene expression program in the fetal gut. Heatmap analysis confirmed these different patterns and showed that postnatal tissue inflammation (ARE and iARE) most strikingly triggered *C3* and *S100a8* gene expression. The majority of regulated genes were shared according to postnatal tissue inflammation (830 commonly regulated genes between ARE and iARE mice).

The two distinct gene expression patterns (pre- and postnatal) were reflected as well in the Gene Ontology (GO) terms for 'biological processes' (GO_BP) (Figure 3F). 'Metabolic' (GO:0008152) and 'cellular processes' (GO:0009987) were predominantly overrepresented according to maternal inflammation in the prenatal state and according to postnatal inflammation in adult mice, respectively. For example, among 'metabolic processes', 989 (iWT) and 1,501 (iARE) genes were significantly regulated in the fetal stage. *Fabp6* was highly up-regulated due to maternal inflammation and is part of both 'metabolic' and 'cellular processes'. In the absence of maternal inflammation, fetal IEC from ARE mice were characterized by only 47 significant genes involved in 'metabolic processes' (Figure 3F, red bars). In contrast, the transcriptional profile of postnatal IEC revealed a lower significance of association (log10 *p*-value) for 'biological processes', highly influenced by postnatal but not maternal inflammation. In ARE mice, 507 and 695 genes were significantly regulated in 'metabolic' and 'cellular processes', respectively, whereas in iWT mice only 105 and 124 genes were responsible for overrepresentation (Figure 3F, grey bars). At this postnatal stage, *C3* encoding complement component 3 had the strongest impact on 'metabolic' and 'cellular processes' in ARE and iARE groups, but not in iWT mice.

Microarray Validation of *Tnf* and *C3* mRNA Expression by qPCR

In order to validate the microarray data, we performed targeted gene expression analysis of two candidate genes via qPCR. Our first target was *Tnf* mRNA, which is stabilized in the genetically engineered *Tnf*$^{\Delta ARE/+}$ mouse model and therefore served as control. We observed a very high correlation between microarray fluorescence data and $2^{-\Delta Ct}$ values (Figure 3E). In the prenatal stage, *Tnf* was not expressed and not regulated in both microarrays and qPCR. At 8 weeks of age, when the inflammation in the offspring was fully established, *Tnf* was highly up-regulated in *Tnf*$^{\Delta ARE/+}$ mice in both datasets. These data mirror the increased *Tnf* transcript levels in whole distal ileal tissues from *Tnf*$^{\Delta ARE/+}$ offspring seen in Figure 2E. We further analyzed *complement component C3* (*C3*), which was identified by microarray analysis as the top up-regulated gene between WT and ARE offspring (FC 39.04). We again observed a high correlation between the microarray fluorescence intensities and qPCR results (Figure 3E). *Reg3b* was identified as the strongest induced gene under maternal inflammation at 17.5 *dpc*, albeit at low gene expression levels (GEO data base accession number GSE44433). In essence, the success of microarray validation is fragile as many factors can influence both methodologies [23]. For instance, low array spot intensities for *Reg3b* ranged from ~ 10–300 (prenatal stage) and might have resulted in a discrepancy of results indicated by a low correlation between microarray fluorescence intensities and $2^{-\Delta Ct}$ values (r = 0.51, p = 0.0007). Therefore, we investigated the intestinal expression of REG3B at the level of proteins.

Maternal Inflammation Influences REG3B Protein Expression in Adult WT Offspring, but has no Influence on the Intestinal Inflammation in *Tnf*$^{\Delta ARE/+}$ Offspring

Immunofluorescence analysis of REG3B expression overtime was performed in ileal gut sections from WT and *Tnf*$^{\Delta ARE/+}$ offspring at 17.5 *dpc*, 3 and 8 weeks of age. In all groups, REG3B protein was not detectable in the prenatal gut, but protein expression was clearly detectable in the epithelium of 8-week-old mice (Figure 4A–C). REG3B protein expression appeared earliest in the ileal epithelium at weaning (3 weeks of age) and further increased at 8 weeks. Quantification of REG3B proteins in IEC of 8-week-old mice revealed significant reduction in iWT mice compared to WT control ($p = 0.008$), suggesting that maternal inflammation slightly affects postnatal protein expression in the absence of any tissue pathology. But, under intestinal inflammation, both ARE and iARE mice showed almost a complete loss of REG3B protein expression when compared with WT ($p<0.0001$). The loss of REG3B protein suggests that postnatal tissue inflammation profoundly impacts the expression of REG3B protein (Figure 4C and D). Tissue pathology of the distal ileum in *Tnf*$^{\Delta ARE/+}$ offspring was not detectable in the pre- and perinatal period (until 3 weeks of age), but was moderate in 8-week-old-offspring, the age where an inflammation-driven loss of epithelial REG3B occurs. With the finding that maternal and postnatal inflammation was associated with decreased REG3B expression in the epithelium, we measured REG3B in aqueous and bacterial fractions of caecal contents from 8-week-old mice in order to evaluate an alteration in luminal secreted REG3B. Representative blots revealed the presence of REG3B in bacterial fractions (Figure 4E). Large amounts of REG3B were detected in bacterial fractions of WT mice, whereas moderate and low amounts were found in WT and inflamed ARE/iARE mice, respectively.

Caecal Bacterial Communities are not Altered in Response to Maternal Inflammation

Down-regulation of REG3B expression in healthy WT offspring suggested that maternal inflammation has a priming effect on the offspring's gut bacterial ecosystem. We were preferentially interested in early development of the microbiota due to maternal inflammation independently of postnatal inflammation and REG3B regulation. Therefore, we analyzed 16S-based diversity and composition in the caecal content from offspring at 3 weeks of age (pre-weaning). At this stage, we circumvented possible effects of postnatal diet on gut bacteria. We followed two different breeding strategies. Our first strategy was to co-house WT and *Tnf*$^{\Delta ARE/+}$ dams in order to synchronize the dam's microbiota prior to colonization of the pups at birth. We obtained a total of 1,755,593 quality-checked sequences (28,633 to 86,232 per sample) representing a total of 263 OTUs with an average of 122 ± 33 molecular species per sample. Members of the phyla *Firmicutes*, *Bacteroidetes* and *Proteobacteria* were dominant, with abundances of 70.9%, 21.3% and 4.6% total sequences, respectively. *Lachnospiraceae* (59.3%) and *Porphyromonadaceae* (8%) were the most abundant families. We observed no effect of maternal

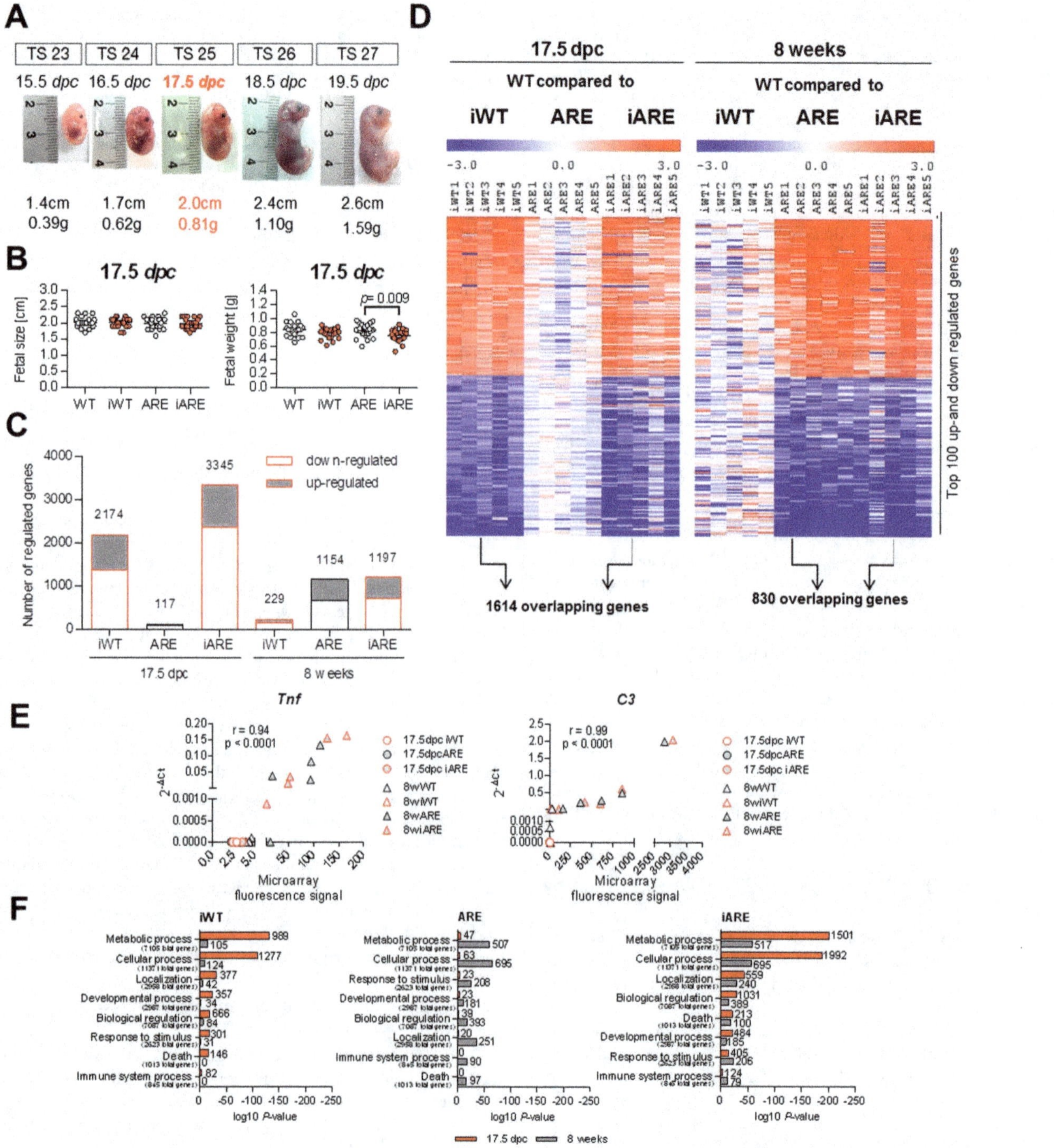

Figure 3. Fetal gene expression profiles in the ileal epithelium are overwritten by postnatal inflammation. (A) Randomly selected fetuses of the last 5 Theiler stages (TS) (15–19 *dpc*). (B) 17.5 *dpc* fetus genotypes plotted against fetal size and weight (total of 98 fetuses); Two-Way ANOVA followed by Holm-Sidak test, $^{*}p<0.05$, $^{***}p<0.001$. (C) Number of regulated genes in iWT, ARE and iARE mice at 17.5 *dpc* and 8 weeks of age when compared to WT considering a threshold fold change of $\pm$ 1.5, $p<0.05$ (each group and time point n = 5). (D) Heat map of top-100 up- and down-regulated genes in iWT, ARE and iARE mice plotted as signal log ratios from −3 to 3. Two distinct gene clusters are shown between maternal (fetal iWT and iARE) and postnatal inflammation (ARE and iARE). Data are based on corresponding WT control mice according to MADMAX statistical analysis. (E) Microarray validation of the *Tnf* and *C3* genes by plotting individual microarray fluorescence intensities against $2^{-\Delta Ct}$ values obtained by qPCR from both prenatal and postnatal mice. Correlation coefficient (r) and significance levels are indicated in the respective plots. (F) Significantly overrepresented GO_BP of prenatal (red bars) and postnatal (grey bars) iWT, ARE and iARE mice. Numbers below the GO terms indicate total genes for the particular process. Numbers next to the bars indicate observed numbers of significantly regulated genes belonging to the respective process.

Table 2. Top 10 up- and down-regulated overlapping genes between prenatal WT/iWT and WT/iARE gene expression patterns (effect of maternal inflammation) and between postnatal WT/ARE and WT/iARE gene expression patterns (effect of offspring genotype/disease).

Overlapping genes between WT/iWTand WT/iARE at 17.5 dpc				Overlapping genes between WT/ARE and WT/iARE at 8 weeks			
ID	**Gene**	**FC iWT**	**FC iARE**	**ID**	**Gene**	**FC ARE**	**FC iARE**
18489	*Reg3b*	22.45	15.53	12266	*C3*	39.04	37.53
16204	*Fabp6*	15.61	30.29	20201	*S100a8*	38.08	21.38
58861	*Cysltr1*	6.69	4.20	17105	*Lyz2*	25.47	21.82
319636	*Fsd1l*	6.66	8.17	68891	*Cd177*	18.34	16.52
17967	*Ncam1*	5.58	4.72	17388	*Mmp15*	16.11	16.31
12843	*Col1a2*	5.29	3.04	70045	*2610528A11Rik*	15.46	14.98
12660	*Chka*	5.17	5.74	20202	*S100a9*	15.46	8.83
12552	*Cdh11*	4.82	2.04	22418	*Wnt5a*	14.78	15.00
77700	*9130208D14Rik*	4.68	3.47	14990	*H2-M2*	14.42	17.06
19876	*Robo1*	4.54	4.22	13419	*Dnase1*	11.42	16.73
208677	*Creb3l3*	−4.44	−1.66	105387	*Akr1c14*	−8.71	−12.00
18605	*Enpp1*	−5.13	−5.35	70564	*5730469M10Rik*	−8.82	−5.89
68979	*Nol11*	−5.54	−8.16	13487	*Slc26a3*	−8.96	−7.01
381259	*Als2cr4*	−5.62	−4.79	14344	*Fut2*	−9.18	−8.35
667373	*Gm14446*	−5.81	−2.39	109731	*Maob*	−9.59	−8.39
100647	*Upk3b*	−6.01	−7.90	17161	*Maoa*	−12.93	−15.73
66350	*Pla2g12a*	−7.53	−6.07	170752	*Bco2*	−16.1	−19.65
19336	*Rab24*	−8.62	−6.47	432720	*Akr1c19*	−17.17	−10.11
107272	*Psat1*	−9.03	−11.71	12116	*Bhmt*	−22.04	−23.73
12696	*Cirbp*	−10.18	−7.56	16173	*Il18*	−25.04	−24.48

FC = log 2 based fold change, $p<0.05$.

Table 3. Top 5 up- and down-regulated genes in iWT, ARE and iARE mice pre- and postnatally.

5 most up- and down- regulated genes								
17.5 dpc					**8 weeks**			
	ID	**Gene**	**Description**	**FC**	**ID**	**Gene**	**Description**	**FC**
iWT	18489	Reg3b	regenerating islet-derived 3 beta	22.45	14170	Fgf15	fibroblast growth factor 15	4.50
	16204	Fabp6	fatty acid binding protein 6, ileal (gastrotropin)	15.61	56485	Slc2a5	solute carrier family 2, member 5	4.15
	58861	Cysltr1	cysteinyl leukotriene receptor 1	6.69	224093	Fam43a	family with sequence similarity 43, member A	2.87
	319636	Fsd1l	fibronectin type III and SPRY domain containing 1-like	6.66	64452	Slc5a4a	solute carrier family 5, member 4a	2.73
	17967	Ncam1	neural cell adhesion molecule 1	5.58	17388	Mmp15	matrix metallopeptidase 15	2.48
	12696	Cirbp	cold inducible RNA binding protein	−10.18	20753	Sprr1a	small proline-rich protein 1A	−3.88
	107272	Psat1	phosphoserine aminotransferase 1	−9.03	14583	Gfpt1	glutamine fructose-6-phosphate transaminase 1	−3.03
	19336	Rab24	RAB24, member RAS oncogene family	−8.62	625599	Gml	GPI anchored molecule like protein	−2.97
	66350	Pla2g12a	phospholipase A2, group XIIA	−7.53	71578	Sval1	seminal vesicle antigen-like 1	−2.80
	14607	Gip	gastric inhibitory polypeptide	−6.38	20210	Saa3	serum amyloid A 3	−2.73
ARE	18489	Reg3b	regenerating islet-derived 3 beta	3.73	12266	C3	complement component 3	39.04
	69814	Prss32	protease, serine, 32	3.41	20201	S100a8	S100 calcium binding protein A8 (calgranulin A)	38.08
	16204	Fabp6	fatty acid binding protein 6, ileal (gastrotropin)	3.23	17105	Lyz2	lysozyme 2	25.47
	19662	Rbp4	retinol binding protein 4, plasma	2.37	68891	Cd177	CD177 antigen	18.34
	56312	Nupr1	nuclear protein 1	2.02	17388	Mmp15	matrix metallopeptidase 15	16.11
	259301	Leap2	liver-expressed antimicrobial peptide 2	−3.60	16173	Il18	interleukin 18	−25.04
	56012	Pgam2	phosphoglycerate mutase 2	−2.69	12116	Bhmt	betaine-homocysteine methyltransferase	−22.04
	106861	Abhd3	abhydrolase domain containing 3	−2.66	432720	Akr1c19	aldo-keto reductase family 1, member C19	−17.17
	23958	Nr2e3	nuclear receptor subfamily 2, group E, member 3	−2.51	170752	Bco2	beta-carotene oxygenase 2	−16.10
	14058	F10	coagulation factor X	−2.28	17161	Maoa	monoamine oxidase A	−12.93
iARE	16204	Fabp6	fatty acid binding protein 6, ileal (gastrotropin)	30.29	12266	C3	complement component 3	37.53
	14963	H2-Bl	histocompatibility 2, blastocyst	26.14	17105	Lyz2	lysozyme 2	21.82
	18489	Reg3b	regenerating islet-derived 3 beta	15.53	20201	S100a8	S100 calcium binding protein A8 (calgranulin A)	21.38
	67092	Gatm	glycine amidinotransferase	12.39	14990	H2-M2	histocompatibility 2, M region locus 2	17.06
	319636	Fsd1l	fibronectin type III and SPRY domain containing 1-like	8.17	13419	Dnase1	deoxyribonuclease I	16.73
	545369	Gm5835	predicted gene 5835	−12.81	16173	Il18	interleukin 18	−24.48
	107272	Psat1	phosphoserine aminotransferase 1	−11.71	12116	Bhmt	betaine-homocysteine methyltransferase	−23.73
	665146	Gm7517	predicted gene 7517	−11.21	170752	Bco2	beta-carotene oxygenase 2	−19.65
	68979	Nol11	nucleolar protein 11	−8.16	17161	Maoa	monoamine oxidase A	−15.73
	12466	Cct6a	chaperonin containing Tcp1, subunit 6a (zeta)	−7.92	105387	Akr1c14	aldo-keto reductase family 1, member C14	−12.00

Fold changes refer to WT control mice according to MADMAX statistical analysis (n = 5 per group, $p<0.05$; FC = log 2 based fold change).

inflammation on the phylogenetic make-up of caecal bacterial communities between WT and iWT offspring at the age of 3 weeks, *i.e.*, there was no clustering of samples according to dam genotypes based on the analysis of weighted Unifrac distances (Figure 4F). Our second strategy was to assess whether there is a general effect of $Tnf^{\Delta ARE/+}$ dams on the offspring's microbiota compared to WT dams. Therefore, we performed a second breeding of WT and $Tnf^{\Delta ARE/+}$ dams that were housed separately. We obtained in this case a total of 1,940,009 quality-checked sequences (16,865 to 61,102 per sample) representing a total of 286 OTUs. Again, we found no influence of the maternal $Tnf^{\Delta ARE/+}$ genotype on the phylogenetic make-up of bacterial communities in caecal contents in both WT and $Tnf^{\Delta ARE/+}$ offspring (n = 4 to 6 mice per group) (Figure 4G). The number of phylotypes was also not influenced by maternal inflammation and offspring's genotype (Table S1). These data demonstrate that overall bacterial diversity is not affected by maternal inflammation or offspring's genotype before the onset of postnatal inflammation. Interestingly, analysis of the caecal microbiota at 8 weeks of age, when inflammation of the distal ileum is established (n = 4 to 6 mice per group), revealed that REG3B does not affect bacterial diversity and composition of Chow diet-fed offspring (Figure S2). Taxonomic assignment revealed no statistically significant differences in sequence abundances due to maternal or postnatal inflammation after adjustment for multiple testing (Tables S2A and S2B). However, feeding offspring a well-defined semisynthetic

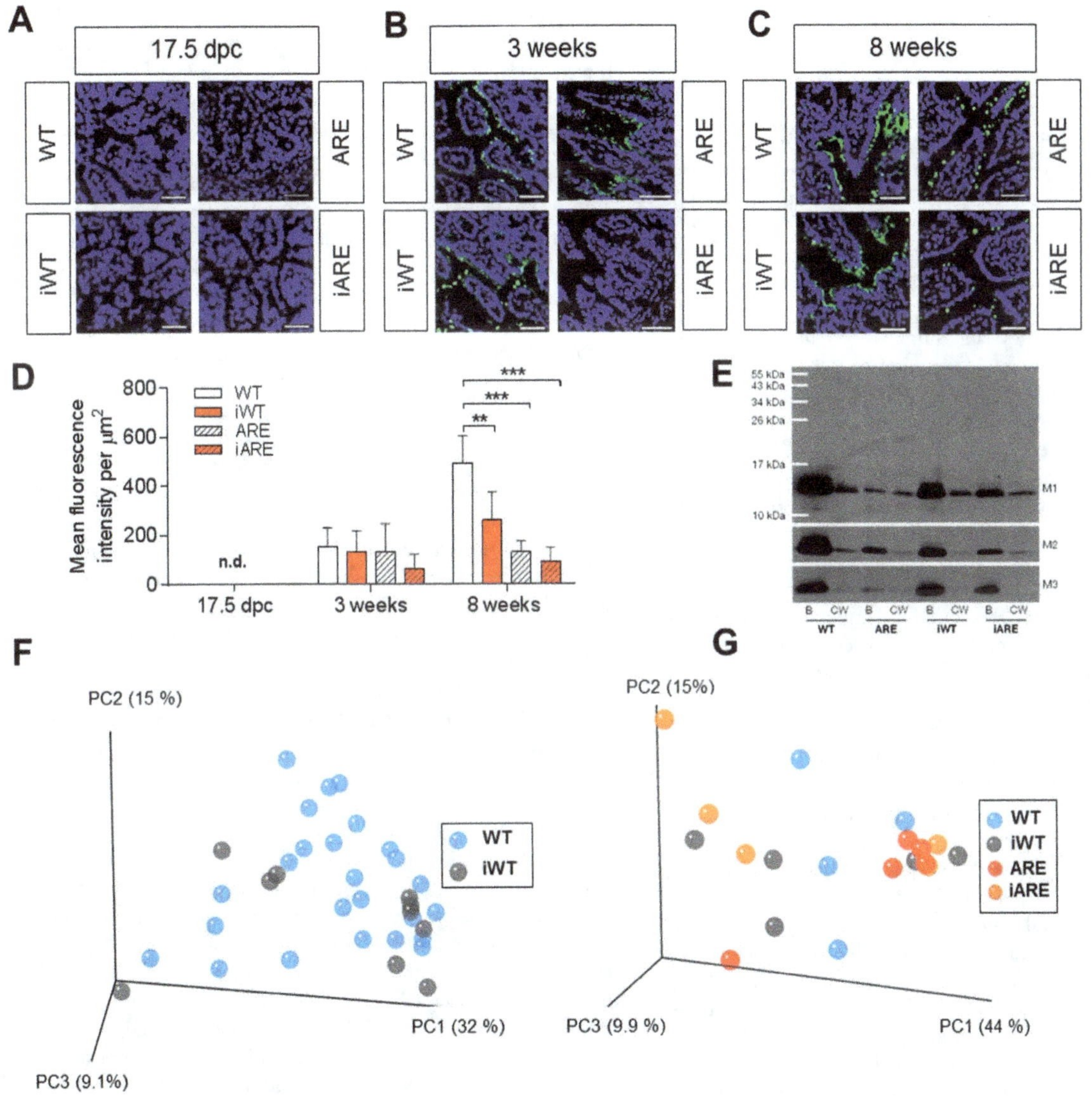

Figure 4. Pre- and postnatal REG3B protein expression in the distal ileum and offspring's caecal bacterial diversity are unaffected by maternal inflammation. (A–C) Immunofluorescence analysis overtime (17.5 dpc, 3 and 8 weeks) of REG3B (green) from distal ileal sections of WT, iWT, ARE, iARE mice. Nuclei were counterstained with DAPI (blue). (D) Data represent mean fluorescence intensity of REG3B signal per μm^2 ±SD from 5 mice per group (3 regions per mouse were evaluated). Significant differences in comparison to WT mice were assessed by Two-Way ANOVA followed by Holm-Sidak method; ***p*<0.01, ****p*<0.001, n.d. = not detectable. (E) Western blot analysis of REG3B in cecal content (B = bacterial fraction, CW = cecal water fraction, M1–M3 = 3 individual mice of each group). (F+G) PCoA analysis of weighted UniFrac distances indicated no change in phylogenetic diversity at 3 weeks of age after cohousing (F) of WT and $Tnf^{\Delta ARE/+}$ dams and litters (n = 10–25 offspring per group) (left panel; even sampling of 28,633 sequences) or without co-housing (G) (n = 4–6 offspring per group) (right panel; even sampling of 16,865 sequences). 16S ribosomal RNA gene amplicons of the V4 region (233 bp) in caecal contents were sequenced using a MiSeq platform and analyzed as described in the methods section.

experimental diet revealed clear differences in bacterial diversity according to the offspring's genotype, i.e., PCoA analysis indicated a change in beta-diversity between WT and *Tnf*$^{\Delta ARE/+}$ offspring (n = 4–5 mice each). Statistical analysis on mean phylogenetic distances between groups (inter-group distances) clearly indicated significance (Figure S2). Besides inflammation-associated alterations driven by the offspring genotype, we did not observe any shifts in diversity in response to maternal inflammation (Fig S2D and S2F). When comparing chow-fed mice at the age of 3 and 8 weeks, we observed age-dependent shifts in *beta*-diversity independently of dam and offspring genotype (Figure S3A). Major age-dependent effects on bacterial taxa included an increase in members of the *Lactobacillaceae*, and *Prevotellaceae* as well as decreased proportions of *Lachnospiraceae* and *Deferribacteriaceae* (Figure S3B and Table S3).

Discussion

In the present work, we provide clear experimental evidence that maternal inflammation has no impact on the offspring's risk to develop genetically-driven ileitis and colitis, despite the fact that TNF-driven maternal ileitis extensively modulates transcriptional responses in the fetal epithelium. This clearly suggests that effects of maternal inflammation are overwritten in genetically-driven models for intestinal inflammation, indicating that the disease end point might be independent of fetal exposure to inflammation[24].

CD-associated pregnancy in humans is characterized by alterations of the cytokine milieu leading to peri- and postnatal complications including preterm labor and low birth weights [6,7]. Most importantly, we showed that 8-week-old ARE and iARE mice developed similar levels of ileal inflammation. This effect was confirmed in a second mouse model for colitis, clearly supporting the hypothesis that maternal inflammation does not affect the onset or severity of disease in the genetically susceptible offspring. Nevertheless, our experiments demonstrate for the first time that TNF-driven maternal inflammation substantially modulates the transcriptional profile in the fetal intestinal epithelium, supporting the hypothesis that not only infection-driven acute but also chronic maternal inflammation impacts on the progeny[25,26]. We identified two clearly distinct clusters of genes that were strongly associated with fetal exposure to maternal inflammation (1,614 genes) or postnatal development of TNF-mediated tissue pathology (830 genes). In fetuses, similar patterns were observed in iWT and iARE with 1,614 common genes in both groups (around 70% overlap). The fetal ARE genotype however seemed not to be relevant at the early developmental stage (117 regulated genes), suggesting that the disease-susceptible genotype does not have a major influence on fetal gut programing. In contrast, gene expression profiles in postnatal IEC were highly influenced by the genetically-driven disease phenotype with 1,154 and 1,197 significantly regulated genes under ARE and iARE conditions, respectively. Heat map analysis confirmed the substantial overlap of similarly regulated genes (around 70%; 830 genes) in these two groups of ARE mice, implying that transcriptional fingerprints in the fetal gut were completely overwritten by signals derived from the postnatal environment independently of the disease-susceptible genotype. These findings may suggest that genetically-driven ileitis in mice is largely induced by the postnatal environment.

Gene ontology analysis identified 'metabolic and cellular' processes as being significantly linked to maternal inflammation to a higher extent in the fetal than in the postnatal stage. Consistent with the over representation of 'metabolic processes', *Fabp6* was strongly up-regulated in the fetal gut in response to maternal inflammation. FABP6 facilitates efficient transepithelial transport of both bile and fatty acids [27]. Although other biological processes such as 'localization' and 'death' were not influenced to the same extent as 'metabolic and cellular processes', they included top-regulated genes such as *C3*, *S100a8* and *Lyz2* in both ARE and iARE offspring. This reflects a disease-associated inflammatory program[28,29] as well as bacterial defense mechanisms[30,31]. Additionally, the strong down-regulation of *Il18* by approximately 25-fold, hints at the relevance of missing immune tolerance in the *Tnf*$^{\Delta ARE/+}$ model for CD[32].

Both the fetal and postnatal stage revealed a significant changes within the GO category 'response to stimulus', albeit with lower number of observed genes when compared with top-categories like 'metabolic and cellular processes'. Interestingly, this category comprises *Reg3b* as top-regulated gene under maternal inflammation at 17.5dpc. The *Reg*3 gene family belongs to a group of C-type lectins, based on their carbohydrate recognition domains[33]. Interestingly, REG3B protein was not detectable in the prenatal gut, but was clearly visible in the epithelium of mice at 8 weeks of age. Immunofluorescence analysis of REG3B expression over time showed appearance earliest at weaning (3 weeks). This observation is consistent with a previously published *Reg3g* expression analysis from Matsumoto *et al.*[34]. The closely related lectin REG3G is known to drive host-bacterial segregation[35], preferentially targeting Gram-positive bacteria[36]. Thus, loss of REG3B seems to be associated with inflammatory signals at postnatal stages and may contribute to the development of genetically-driven ileitis through mechanisms that involve the intestinal microbiota of *Tnf*$^{\Delta ARE/+}$ mice[16,37]. Quantification of REG3B protein levels in IEC of 8-week-old mice revealed significant reduction in iWT, suggesting that maternal inflammation can slightly affect postnatal protein expression. However, ARE and iARE mice almost completely lost REG3B, suggesting that postnatal tissue inflammation profoundly impacts REG3B expression independently of earlier gene transcriptional up-regulation by maternal inflammation. This is supported by the fact that, fetal epithelial programming is completely overwritten in adult offspring, clearly suggesting that postnatal disease-relevant signals initialize genetically-driven ileal pathogenesis.

Interestingly, loss of REG3B in the epithelium was linked to lower REG3B levels preferably bound to bacterial fractions in the caecal content, clearly suggests that the postnatal microbiota harbors disease-relevant signals that show stronger potential to initialize the genetically-driven ileal pathogenesis compared to maternal stimuli. This is supported by the fact that maternally-induced changes in the fetal epithelium did not cause any shifts in diversity and composition of caecal bacterial communities at 3 weeks of age before weaning. This was shown in two different breeding strategies, with and without co-housing of WT and *Tnf*$^{\Delta ARE/+}$ dams. However, at 8 weeks of age, we observed an inflammation-driven loss of REG3B in IEC and bacterial fractions of the caecal content that is not additionally affected by maternal inflammation. The fact that the microbial composition and diversity was not affected by maternal or offspring's inflammation indicates that REG3B expression in the epithelium has no influence on the overall phylogenetic make-up of caecal bacterial communities in the *Tnf*$^{\Delta ARE/+}$ mouse model. We cannot fully explain this absence of any major signs of maternal or inflammation-driven dysbiosis in the offspring's microbiota despite changes in REG3B expression. Diet might be one main confounding factor, since wheat-based Ssniff Chow diets are characterized by highly varying quality due to heterogeneity of raw products used during production. This suggestion was supported by clear inflammation-driven shifts in *beta*-diversity between WT and ARE mice when fed a well-defined semisynthetic experimental diet based on corn starch.

Taking all these findings together, we summarize that neither maternal nor genetically-driven inflammation impact the overall phylogenetic diversity of caecal bacterial communities in the offspring under conventional conditions. The observation of age-dependent shifts in bacterial diversity and composition between 3 and 8 weeks of age goes in line with a previously published work by Garrett et al. [12]. But, unlike their findings that a colitogenic microbiota is transmitted from mothers to offspring under SPF conditions, we could not observe any changes through maternal inflammation in our experiments. Altogether, we conclude from our studies that maternal inflammation impacts the ileal transcriptome in fetuses, but these effects do not persist in grownup mice and are therefore not relevant for the modulation of intestinal inflammation in the genetically susceptible $Tnf^{\Delta ARE/+}$ mouse. Consistent with these findings is the occurrence of age- and diet- but not maternal-dependent shifts in bacterial diversity and composition, indicating that postnatal factors largely overwrite a possible maternal influence on the offspring's microbial ecosystem in both non-disease and disease susceptible offspring. This is also in line with the fact that the host immune response at the site of inflammation is consistently unaffected by maternal inflammation in two different mouse models for genetically-driven ileitis and colitis inflammation. Consequently, maternal inflammation during gestation in mouse models did not alter the genetically-driven risk to develop chronic inflammation in the intestine.

Supporting Information

Figure S1 Fetal environment and laser microdissection of fetal intestinal epithelial cells. (**A**) Randomly selected fetuses of the last 5 Theiler stages (TS) (15–19 *dpc*). (**B**) Macroscopic view of a 17.5 *dpc* gut and subsequent laser microdissection procedure of fetal ileal epithelium. Epithelial areas of $1.33 \pm 0.024 \times 10^6$ μm^2 (mean ± SD) were cut for microarray analysis.

Figure S2 Experimental diet clearly influences changes in caecal bacterial diversity in response to postnatal but not maternal inflammation. Histological scores of terminal ileum from WT, iWT, ARE and iARE offspring on (**A**) chow diet (experiment from Figure 2A, n = 5–7 mice each), or (**B**) experimental diet (n = 6–16 mice each). With both diets, there was no difference in inflammatory scores relative to maternal inflammation. (**C+E**) Analysis of phylogenetic distances indicated no significant change in *beta*-diversity between offspring fed the Ssniff chow diet. Comparisons of mean phylogenetic distances (weighted UniFrac) between individual mice (WT, iWT, ARE, iARE) within groups (intra-group distances, e.g. all WT) and between mice from different groups (inter-group distances, e.g. WT vs. iWT) revealed no significant differences related to the offspring's genotype or maternal inflammation. (**D+F**) PCoA analysis indicated an inflammation-driven change in *beta*-diversity between 8-week-old WT and $Tnf^{\Delta ARE/+}$ offspring fed an experimental diet (n = 4–5 mice each). Statistical comparisons of phylogenetic distances indicated significant separation between WT and ARE or iWT and iARE but not between WT and iWT or ARE and iARE (Two-Way ANOVA, ***p>0.0001).
(TIF)

Figure S3 Age-dependent shifts in bacterial diversity and composition. (**A**) PCoA analysis indicated a change in diversity between mice at the age of 3 and 8 weeks (n = 18–19). (**B**) Major bacterial taxa that were characterized by significantly different sequence proportions at 3 and 8 weeks of age are shown in box plots (F-test followed by Benjamini-Hochberg adjustment). Individual data for all taxa are given in Table S3.
(TIF)

Table S1 Observed phylotype numbers in caecal contents of WT, iWT, ARE and iARE offspring at 3 and 8 weeks of age. Indicated are means ±SD (n = 4–5 per group). Three Way ANOVA.
(XLSX)

Table S2 Sequence proportions of bacterial taxa in ceacal contents from offspring (n = 4–5) at (A) 3 or (B) 8 weeks of age. OTUs occurring in less than 2 mice and <0.05% total sequences per sample were excluded from the analysis. Sequence proportions were analyzed for significant differences using F-Test followed by Benjamini-Hochberg correction for multiple testing in the R programing environment after adjustment for multiple testing.
(XLSX)

Table S3 Sequence proportions of bacterial taxa in ceacal contents from 3- and 8-week old offspring (n = 4–6) show age differences. OTUs occurring in less than 2 mice and <0.05% total sequences per sample were excluded from the analysis. Sequence proportions were analyzed for significant age-differences using F-Test followed by Benjamini-Hochberg correction for multiple testing in the R programing environment after adjustment for multiple testing.
(XLSX)

Acknowledgments

We thank Melanie Manyet for helping with immunofluorescence analysis. None of the material has been published or is under consideration elsewhere, including the internet. The animal experiments were performed according to the German guidelines for animal care. Raw microarray data are available on the GEO database (?http://www.ncbi.nlm.nih.gov/geo/query/acc.cgi?token = hrqhlcqmccoishc&acc = GSE44433).

Author Contributions

Conceived and designed the experiments: DH. Performed the experiments: JH KH GH MB. Analyzed the data: JH KH TC. Wrote the paper: JH DH. Provided the $TNF^{\Delta ARE/+}$ mouse: GK. Critically revised the manuscript: TC GH.

References

1. Renz H, von Mutius E, Brandtzaeg P, Cookson WO, Autenrieth IB, et al. (2011) Gene-environment interactions in chronic inflammatory disease. Nature immunology 12: 273–7.
2. Khor B, Gardet A, Xavier RJ (2011) Genetics and pathogenesis of inflammatory bowel disease. Nature 474: 307–17.
3. Franke A, McGovern DP, Barrett JC, Wang K, Radford-Smith GL, et al. (2010) Genome-wide meta-analysis increases to 71 the number of confirmed Crohn's disease susceptibility loci. Nature genetics 42: 1118–25.
4. Kaser A, Zeissig S, Blumberg RS (2010) Inflammatory bowel disease. Annual review of immunology 28: 573–621.
5. Morales M, Berney T, Jenny A, Morel P, Extermann P (2000) Crohn's disease as a risk factor for the outcome of pregnancy. Hepato-gastroenterology 47: 1595–8.
6. Dominitz JA, Young JC, Boyko EJ (2002) Outcomes of infants born to mothers with inflammatory bowel disease: a population-based cohort study. The American journal of gastroenterology 97: 641–8.
7. Malek A, Sager R, Schneider H (2001) Effect of hypoxia, oxidative stress and lipopolysaccharides on the release of prostaglandins and cytokines from human term placental explants. Placenta 22 Suppl A:S45–50.
8. Challis JR, Lockwood CJ, Myatt L, Norman JE, Strauss JF 3rd, et al. (2009) Inflammation and pregnancy. Reprod Sci 16: 206–15.

9. Wolfs TG, Buurman WA, Zoer B, Moonen RM, Derikx JP, et al. (2009) Endotoxin induced chorioamnionitis prevents intestinal development during gestation in fetal sheep. PloS one 4:e5837.
10. Renz H, Brandtzaeg P, Hornef M (2012) The impact of perinatal immune development on mucosal homeostasis and chronic inflammation. Nat Rev Immunol 12: 9–23.
11. Yan X, Huang Y, Wang H, Du M, Hess BW, et al. (2011) Maternal obesity induces sustained inflammation in both fetal and offspring large intestine of sheep. Inflamm Bowel Dis 17: 1513–22.
12. Garrett WS, Gallini CA, Yatsunenko T, Michaud M, DuBois A, et al. (2010) Enterobacteriaceae act in concert with the gut microbiota to induce spontaneous and maternally transmitted colitis. Cell host & microbe 8: 292–300.
13. Roulis M, Armaka M, Manoloukos M, Apostolaki M, Kollias G (2011) Intestinal epithelial cells as producers but not targets of chronic TNF suffice to cause murine Crohn-like pathology. Proceedings of the National Academy of Sciences of the United States of America 108: 5396–401.
14. Swamy M, Jamora C, Havran W, Hayday A (2010) Epithelial decision makers: in search of the 'epimmunome'. Nature immunology 11: 656–65.
15. Katakura K, Lee J, Rachmilewitz D, Li G, Eckmann L, et al. (2005) Toll-like receptor 9-induced type I IFN protects mice from experimental colitis. J Clin Invest 115: 695–702.
16. Werner T, Wagner SJ, Martinez I, Walter J, Chang JS, et al. (2011) Depletion of luminal iron alters the gut microbiota and prevents Crohn's disease-like ileitis. Gut 60: 325-33.
17. Caporaso JG, Lauber CL, Walters WA, Berg-Lyons D, Lozupone CA, et al. (2011) Global patterns of 16S rRNA diversity at a depth of millions of sequences per sample. Proceedings of the National Academy of Sciences of the United States of America 108 Suppl 1: 4516–22.
18. Edgar RC (2013) UPARSE: highly accurate OTU sequences from microbial amplicon reads. Nature methods 10: 996–8.
19. Caporaso JG, Kuczynski J, Stombaugh J, Bittinger K, Bushman FD, et al. (2010) QIIME allows analysis of high-throughput community sequencing data. Nature methods 7: 335–6.
20. Cole JR, Chai B, Marsh TL, Farris RJ, Wang Q, et al. (2003) The Ribosomal Database Project (RDP-II): previewing a new autoaligner that allows regular updates and the new prokaryotic taxonomy. Nucleic acids research 31: 442–3.
21. Edgar RC, Haas BJ, Clemente JC, Quince C, Knight R (2011) UCHIME improves sensitivity and speed of chimera detection. Bioinformatics 27: 2194–200.
22. Behm BW, Bickston SJ (2008) Tumor necrosis factor-alpha antibody for maintenance of remission in Crohn's disease. The Cochrane database of systematic reviews:CD006893.
23. Morey JS, Ryan JC, Van Dolah FM (2006) Microarray validation: factors influencing correlation between oligonucleotide microarrays and real-time PCR. Biological procedures online 8: 175–93.
24. Wagner SJ, Schmidt A, Effenberger MJ, Gruber L, Danier J, et al. (2013) Semisynthetic diet ameliorates Crohn's disease-like ileitis in TNFDeltaARE/WT mice through antigen-independent mechanisms of gluten. Inflamm Bowel Dis 19: 1285–94.
25. Cardenas I, Mulla MJ, Myrtolli K, Sfakianaki AK, Norwitz ER, et al. (2011) Nod1 activation by bacterial iE-DAP induces maternal-fetal inflammation and preterm labor. J Immunol 187: 980–6.
26. Urakubo A, Jarskog LF, Lieberman JA, Gilmore JH (2001) Prenatal exposure to maternal infection alters cytokine expression in the placenta, amniotic fluid, and fetal brain. Schizophrenia research 47: 27–36.
27. Labonte ED, Li Q, Kay CM, Agellon LB (2003) The relative ligand binding preference of the murine ileal lipid binding protein. Protein expression and purification 28: 25–33.
28. Yuan Y, Ren J, Cao S, Zhang W, Li J (2012) Exogenous C3 protein enhances the adaptive immune response to polymicrobial sepsis through down-regulation of regulatory T cells. International immunopharmacology 12: 271–7.
29. Vogl T, Gharibyan AL, Morozova-Roche LA (2012) Pro-Inflammatory S100A8 and S100A9 Proteins: Self-Assembly into Multifunctional Native and Amyloid Complexes. International journal of molecular sciences 13: 2893–917.
30. Salzman NH, Hung K, Haribhai D, Chu H, Karlsson-Sjoberg J, et al. (2010) Enteric defensins are essential regulators of intestinal microbial ecology. Nature immunology 11: 76–83.
31. Cadwell K, Liu JY, Brown SL, Miyoshi H, Loh J, et al. (2008) A key role for autophagy and the autophagy gene Atg16l1 in mouse and human intestinal Paneth cells. Nature 456: 259–63.
32. Oertli M, Sundquist M, Hitzler I, Engler DB, Arnold IC, et al. (2012) DC-derived IL-18 drives Treg differentiation, murine Helicobacter pylori-specific immune tolerance, and asthma protection. J Clin Invest 122: 1082–96.
33. Gallo RL, Hooper LV (2012) Epithelial antimicrobial defence of the skin and intestine. Nat Rev Immunol 12: 503–16.
34. Matsumoto S, Konishi H, Maeda R, Kiryu-Seo S, Kiyama H (2012) Expression analysis of the regenerating gene (Reg) family members Reg-IIIbeta and Reg-IIIgamma in the mouse during development. The Journal of comparative neurology 520: 479–94.
35. Vaishnava S, Yamamoto M, Severson KM, Ruhn KA, Yu X, et al. (2011) The antibacterial lectin RegIIIgamma promotes the spatial segregation of microbiota and host in the intestine. Science 334: 255–8.
36. Cash HL, Whitham CV, Behrendt CL, Hooper LV (2006) Symbiotic bacteria direct expression of an intestinal bactericidal lectin. Science 313: 1126–30.
37. von Schillde MA, Hormannsperger G, Weiher M, Alpert CA, Hahne H, et al. (2012) Lactocepin secreted by Lactobacillus exerts anti-inflammatory effects by selectively degrading proinflammatory chemokines. Cell host & microbe 11: 387–96.

12

Rac2-Deficiency Leads to Exacerbated and Protracted Colitis in Response to *Citrobacter rodentium* Infection

Ramzi Fattouh[1], Cong-Hui Guo[1], Grace Y. Lam[1], Melanie G. Gareau[1], Bo-Yee Ngan[2], Michael Glogauer[3], Aleixo M. Muise[1,4,5,6]⁹, John H. Brumell[1,5,6,7]*⁹

1 Cell Biology Program, Hospital for Sick Children, Toronto, Ontario, Canada, 2 Department of Pathology, Hospital for Sick Children, Toronto, Ontario, Canada, 3 Faculty of Dentistry, University of Toronto, Toronto, Ontario, Canada, 4 Division of Gastroenterology, Hepatology, and Nutrition, Department of Pediatrics, Hospital for Sick Children, University of Toronto, Toronto, Ontario, Canada, 5 Institute of Medical Science, University of Toronto, Toronto, Ontario, Canada, 6 Sickkids IBD Centre, Hospital for Sick Children, Toronto, Ontario, Canada, 7 Department of Molecular Genetics, University of Toronto, Toronto, Ontario, Canada

Abstract

Recent genetic-based studies have implicated a number of immune-related genes in the pathogenesis of inflammatory bowel disease (IBD). Our recent genetic studies showed that *RAC2* is associated with human IBD; however, its role in disease pathogenesis is unclear. Given Rac2's importance in various fundamental immune cell processes, we investigated whether a defect in Rac2 may impair host immune responses in the intestine and promote disease in the context of an infection-based (*Citrobacter rodentium*) model of colitis. In response to infection, $Rac2^{-/-}$ mice showed i) worsened clinical symptoms (days 13–18), ii) increased crypt hyperplasia at days 11 and 22 (a time when crypt hyperplasia was largely resolved in wild-type mice; WT), and iii) marked mononuclear cell infiltration characterized by higher numbers of T ($CD3^+$) cells (day 22), compared to WT-infected mice. Moreover, splenocytes harvested from infected $Rac2^{-/-}$ mice and stimulated *in vitro* with *C. rodentium* lysate produced considerably higher levels of interferon-γ and interleukin-17A. The augmented responses observed in $Rac2^{-/-}$ mice did not appear to stem from Rac2's role in NADPH oxidase-driven reactive oxygen species production as no differences in crypt hyperplasia, nor inflammation, were observed in infected $NOX2^{-/-}$ mice compared to WT. Collectively, our findings demonstrate that $Rac2^{-/-}$ mice develop more severe disease when subjected to a *C. rodentium*-induced model of infectious colitis, and suggest that impaired Rac2 function may promote the development of IBD in humans.

Editor: Jörg Hermann Fritz, McGill University, Canada

Funding: This work was supported by an operating grant from the Canadian Institutes of Health Research (MOP#97756) to JHB and AM and by a Trainee Start-up Fund Award from the Hospital for Sick Children to RF. AMM is supported by an Early Researcher Award from the Ontario Ministry of Research and Innovation and a CDHNF/NASPGHAN George Ferry young Investigator Development Award, and funded by a CIHR Operating Grant (MOP119457). RF is currently supported by a post-doctoral fellowship award from the CIHR in partnership with the Canadian Association of Gastroenterology and the Crohn's and Colitis Foundation of Canada. The funders had no role in study design, data collection and analysis, decision to publish, or preparation of the manuscript.

Competing Interests: The authors have declared that no competing interests exist.

* E-mail: john.brumell@sickkids.ca

⁹ These authors contributed equally to this work.

Introduction

Inflammatory bowel disease (IBD) is a family of chronic, relapsing and remitting, inflammatory disorders of the gastrointestinal tract [1,2]. The available evidence suggests that IBD develops as a result of an exaggerated immune response directed against the host microbiota. Despite considerable research the precise etiology of these diseases remains largely uncertain [3]. As there is no cure, and treatments are geared primarily at alleviating intestinal inflammation and symptoms, there is an urgent need to identify the determinants that predispose the development of IBD. Improved understanding of the causes of IBD will undoubtedly aid in the development of more effective treatment strategies.

In addition to various environmental factors it is clear that genetic factors also influence susceptibility to IBD. Recent genetic based studies have identified greater than 100 genetic loci as being associated with the development of IBD [2,4,5]. Of the numerous genes implicated by these studies, many are known to be integrally involved in various aspects of the immune response including, pathogen recognition, cytokine/growth factor signalling, intestinal epithelial barrier function and defense, and lymphocyte activation, among others.

We have recently identified several single nucleotide polymorphisms (SNPs) in the gene encoding RAC2, a small guanosine triphosphatase (GTPase) that is almost exclusively expressed in leukocytes [6]. RAC2 is one of four regulatory cytosolic subunits (the other three being $p40^{phox}$, $p47^{phox}$, $p67^{phox}$) that together with two transmembrane components $gp91^{phox}$ (Nox2) and $p22^{phox}$ constitute the predominant nicotinamide adenine dinucleotide phosphate (NADPH) oxidase (Nox) complex in leukocytes [7,8]. The functional requirement for RAC2 in various immune cell-related processes has been explored in several *in vitro*-based studies using, primarily, macrophages and neutrophils; two cell types of the innate immune response that are critically required for protection against microbes. Collectively, previous findings demonstrate that in the absence of Rac2, macrophages and/or neutrophils display suppressed reactive oxygen species (ROS) production, defective chemotaxis, impaired phagocytosis, and

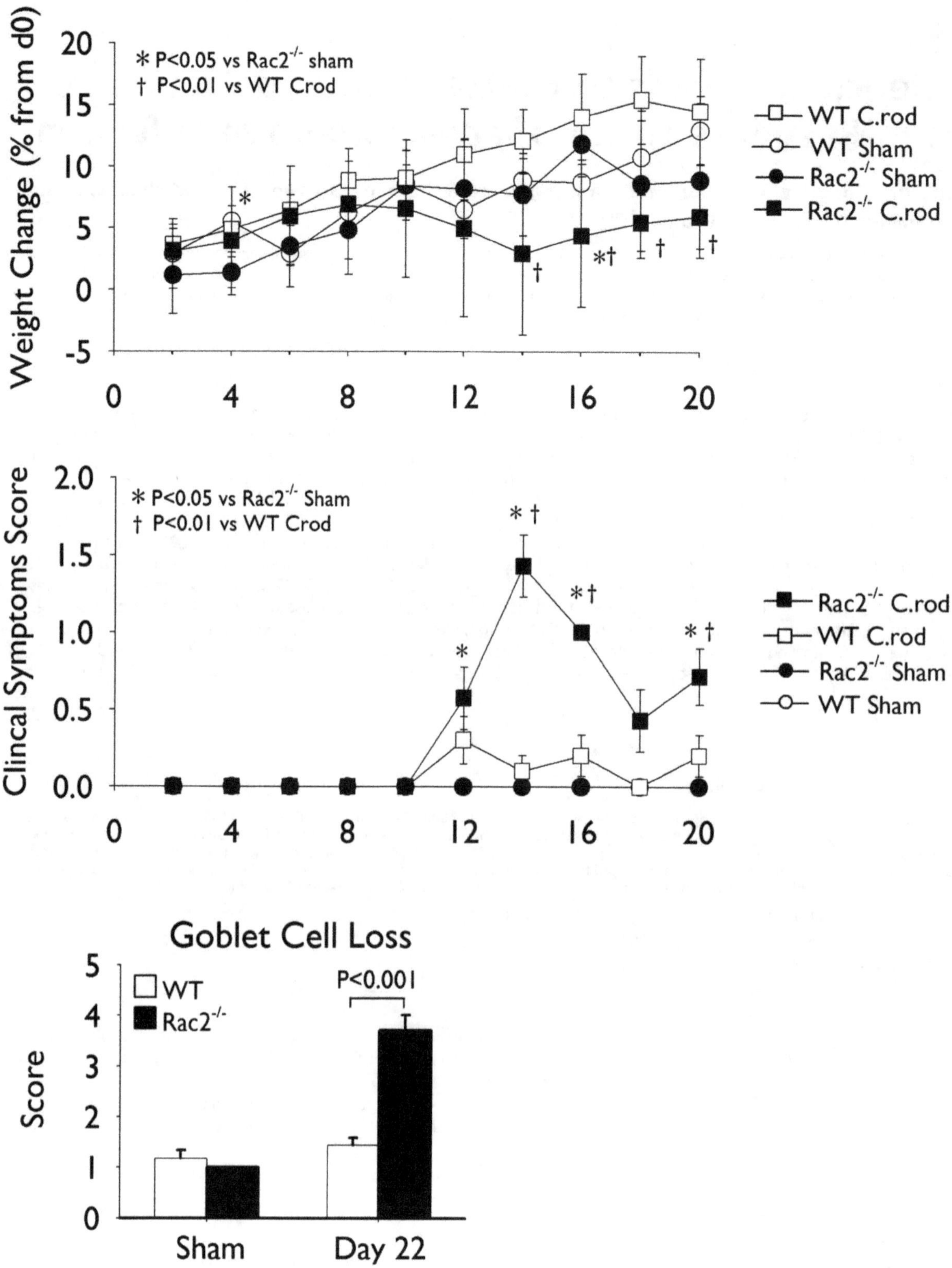

Figure 1. Rac2$^{-/-}$ mice infected with Citrobacter rodentium display worsened signs of disease. Separate groups of wild-type (WT; *white bars/symbols*) and Rac2$^{-/-}$ (*black bars/symbols*) mice were infected with *C. rodentium* or given vehicle control (sham) by orogastric gavage. (A) Percent weight change (relative to day 0) and (B) clinical symptoms score in WT and Rac2$^{-/-}$ uninfected (*circles*) and infected (*squares*) mice. (C) Scoring of goblet cell loss at day 22 of infection. n = 4–11/group. Data are expressed as mean ± SEM and are from one of three independent experiments. Statistical analysis was performed using two-way ANOVA with Tukey's post hoc test.

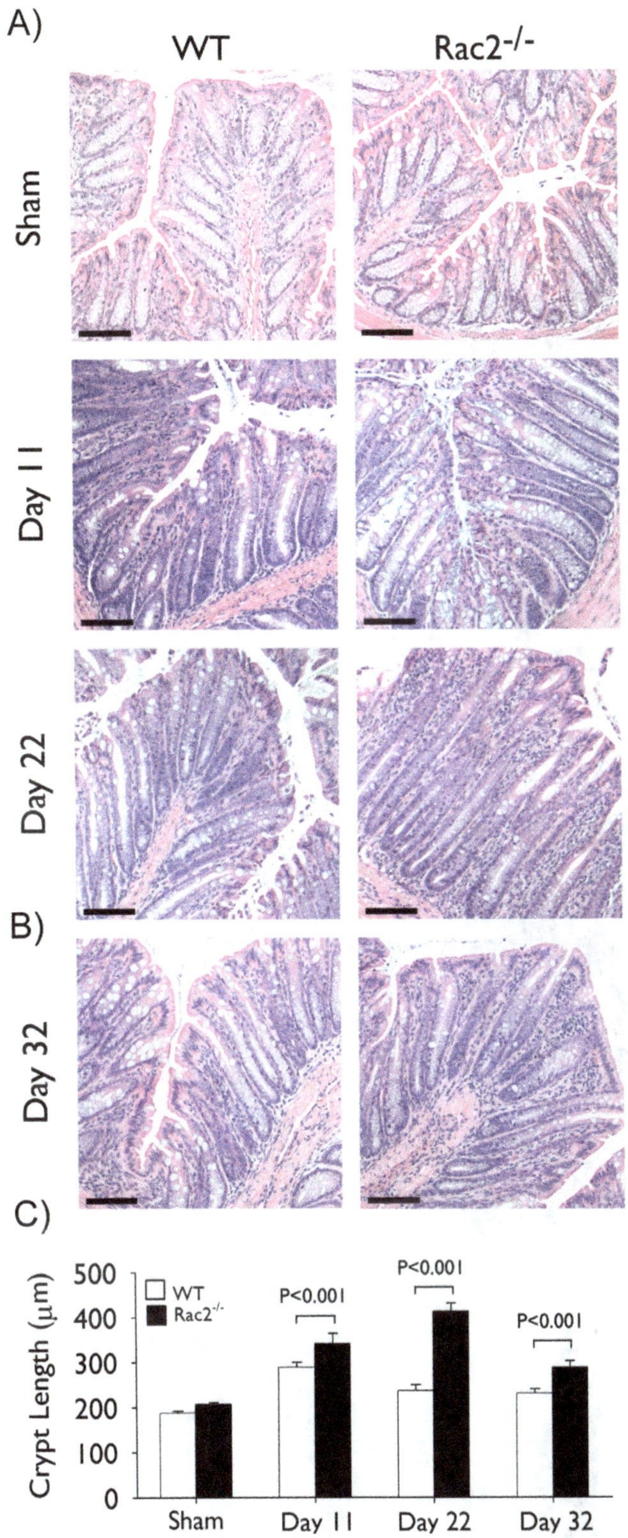

Figure 2. Kinetic analysis of Citrobacter rodentium-induced colonic hyperplasia in Rac2$^{-/-}$ and WT mice. Separate groups of wild-type (WT; *white bars*) and Rac2$^{-/-}$ (*black bars*) mice were infected with *C. rodentium* or given vehicle control (sham) by orogastric gavage. (A-B) Pictures show representative light photomicrographs of hematoxylin and eosin stained paraffin-embedded cross-sections of colon tissue obtained at the indicated time points of infection. Scale bar 100 μm. (C) Morphometric analysis of colonic hyperplasia; data represent average crypt length. All pictures were taken at 10× original magnification. n = 4–10/group. Data are expressed as mean ± SEM and are from one of three (in *A*) or two (in *B*) independent experiments. Statistical analysis was performed using two-way ANOVA with Tukey's post hoc test.

decreased microbial killing [9,10,11,12,13,14,15,16,17,18]. Importantly, the involvement of Rac2 in immunity is not limited to cells of the innate arm. Indeed, Rac2-deficiency has also been shown to impact B- and T-cell migration, activation, development (to a lesser extent in T-cells) [19,20,21,22,23], and, in some reports, T-cell differentiation into T-helper type 1 (Th1) cells [21,24]. The contribution of Rac2 to host defense responses *in vivo* has been less well studied. Rac2$^{-/-}$ mice infected intradermally with *Leishmania major* displayed little to no impaired ability to clear infection [21]. However, in a separate report Rac2$^{-/-}$ mice challenged intravenously with the opportunistic pathogen *Aspergillus fumigatus*, showed marked increases in mortality, decreased survival time to death, and increased pathogen loads, compared to infected wild-type (WT) mice [13]. Interestingly, a dominant-negative mutation in RAC2 (D57N) has been described in two case reports of infants less than eight-weeks of age [25,26,27,28]. Both patients suffered from repeated life-threatening bacterial infections necessitating stem cell transplantation. Together, the evidence from these *in vivo* reports further support the notion that impairments in RAC2 may compromise host defenses against, at least some, pathogens.

Whether defects in RAC2 impact the intestinal immune response, *in vivo*, and influence the development of IBD is unknown. Given the putative importance of RAC2 to immunity and the strong connection between altered immune functioning and IBD pathogenesis, we investigated the impact of defective Rac2 function on the intestinal immune response and the development of disease using a model of *Citrobacter rodentium*-induced colitis. Our findings show that Rac2$^{-/-}$ mice infected with *C. rodentium* develop worsened symptoms, augmented and protracted colonic epithelial hyperplasia, and marked colitis associated with heightened T-cell responsiveness.

Materials and Methods

Ethics Statement

Experiments described in this study were carried out in accordance with the Guide for the Humane Use and Care of Laboratory Animals and were approved by the University of Toronto (Toronto, ON, Canada; #9558) and The Hospital for Sick Children's Animal Care Committees (Toronto, ON, Canada; # 13639).

Animals

Previously generated and characterized Rac2$^{-/-}$ and wild-type (WT) mice (on a Balb/c.129Sv background) were bred as previously described at the University of Toronto Animal Care Facility [14], and maintained as separate lines. The genotypes of WT and Rac2$^{-/-}$ mice were confirmed by PCR analysis on tail DNA as previously described [13]. C57BL/6 and gp91$^{phox-/-}$ (Cybb/tm1d; Stock#2365) mice were purchased from The Jackson Laboratory (Bar Harbor, ME). All experiments were performed with 7–9 week old male mice that were maintained on a 12-hour light-dark cycle, with food and water available *ad libitum*.

Infection

C. rodentium, strain DBS100 (ATCC #51459), was kindly provided by Dr. Philip Sherman (The Hospital for Sick Children in Toronto; originally from David Schauer, Massachusetts In-

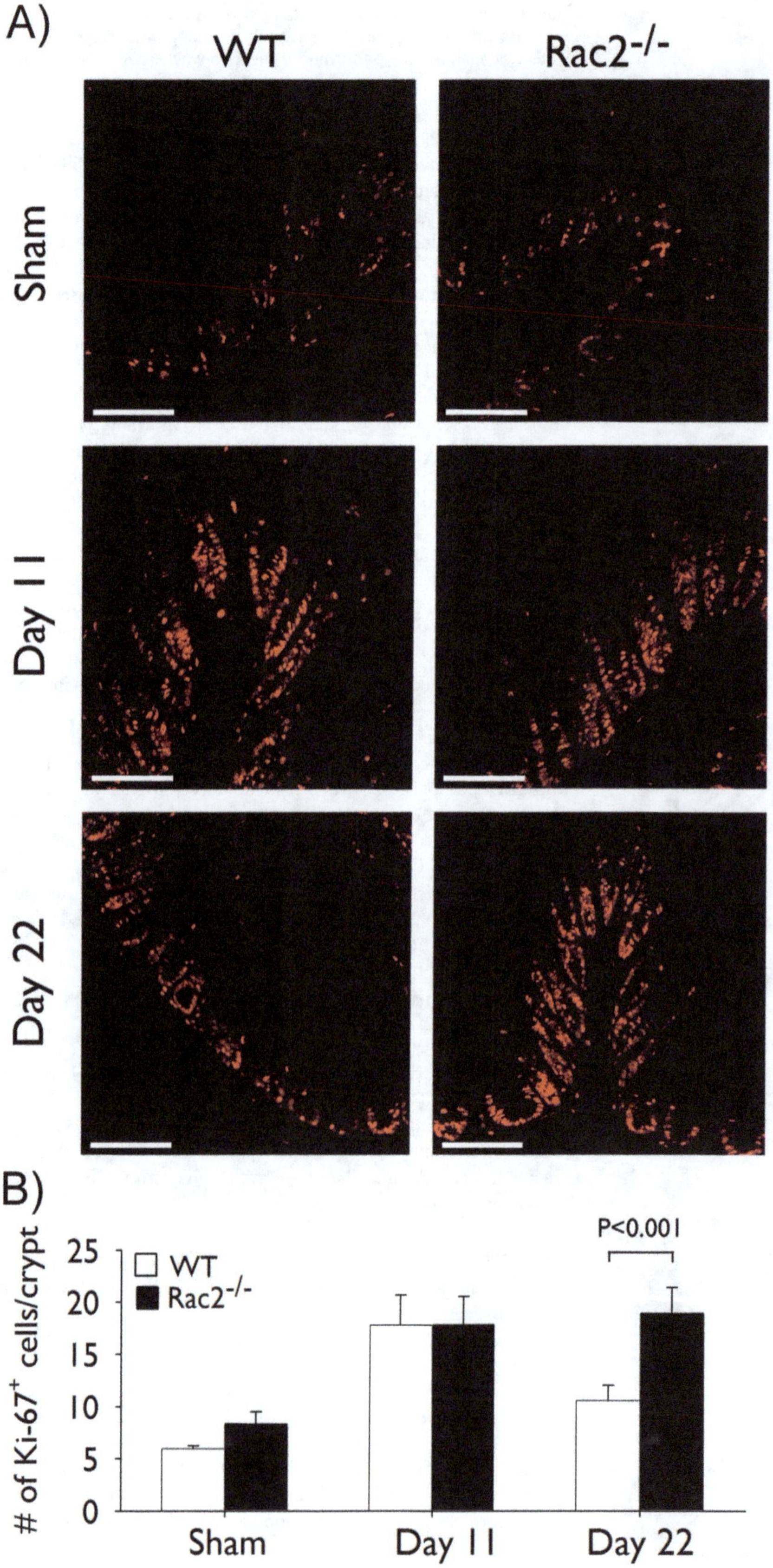

Figure 3. Prolonged colonic hyperplasia in Rac2$^{-/-}$ mice develops due to continued epithelial cell proliferation. Separate groups of wild-type (WT; *white bars*) and Rac2$^{-/-}$ (*black bars*) mice were infected with *Citrobacter rodentium* or given vehicle control (sham) by orogastric gavage. (A) Immunofluorescence for Ki-67. Pictures show representative images of Ki-67 stained paraffin-embedded cross-sections of colon tissue

obtained at the indicated time points of infection. Scale bar 100 μm. (B) Morphometric analysis of Ki-67 staining; data represent the average number of Ki-67$^+$ cells/crypt. All pictures were taken at 20× original magnification. n = 5–7/group. Data are expressed as mean ± SEM and are from one of two independent experiments. Statistical analysis was performed using two-way ANOVA with Tukey's post hoc test.

stitute of Technology). Bacteria were grown on Luria broth (LB) plates overnight at 37°C, followed by overnight culture in LB broth at 37°C without shaking. *C. rodentium* (3×10^8 cfu) was administered to mice by orogastric gavage in 200 μl of LB broth. Vehicle control mice were given an equal volume of sterile LB broth.

Collection and Measurement of Specimens

Mice were monitored every other day for weight change, stool consistency, rectal bleeding, and general appearance. At the indicated time points, colon (terminal 3 cm starting from ~0.5 cm away from the anus) and spleen were collected. Following dissection, the lumen of the colon was washed, gently, with sterile PBS using a feeding needle. The terminal 0.75 cm of the colon was cut and fixed in 10% formalin for 24 hours for histochemical and morphometric analysis. Where applicable, the remaining ~2.25 cm were collected in PBS for leukocyte isolation and flow cytometric analysis. Harvested spleens were placed in sterile tubes containing sterile Hank's Balanced Salt Solution (HBSS) for splenocyte culture.

Histological and Clinical Symptoms Scoring

Inflammatory infiltrate and goblet cell loss were scored by a pathologist blinded to the experimental conditions based on the scoring system used in [29] and shown in Table S1. The clinical symptoms score was adapted from [29] and calculated as shown in Table S2.

Histology and Immunohistochemistry

After formalin fixation, the colon was cut cross-sectionally in half, yielding two pieces of tissue. Tissues were embedded in paraffin, and two separate 3-μm-thick cross-sections (>100 μm apart) were cut and stained with hematoxylin and eosin (H&E). Immunohistochemistry for Ki-67, *C. rodentium*, and CD3 were performed using the protocol previously described in detail [30], with the following changes: tissues were not incubated in permeabilization buffer, heat-induced epitope retrieval was performed using a vegetable steamer and slides were boiled (95–100°C) in sodium citrate buffer for 25–30 minutes, and tissues were incubated in block solution for 45–60 minutes. The following antibodies were used: rat anti-mouse Ki-67 (TEC-3; Dako; 1:250), rabbit anti-*C. rodentium* (generated by the Sherman Lab, The Hospital for Sick Children, 1:250), rabbit anti-CD3 (polyclonal, Sigma, 1:2000), goat anti-rabbit AlexaFluor 488 and 568 (Molecular Probes, 1:200) and donkey anti-rat Cy3 (Jackson ImmunoResearch Laboratories Inc, 1:200).

Morphometric Analysis

H&E stained sections were visualized using a Leica DMI 6000B microscope, Leica DFC420 camera and Leica Application Suite Advanced Fluorescence software (Leica, Toronto, ON). Crypt length was assessed by microscopy on coded sections by a single blinded observer. A minimum of 15, non-adjacent and well-orientated, crypts were measured per sample and used to determine the average crypt length/mouse. Images and morphometric analysis of Ki-67, *C. rodentium*, and CD3 were captured and analyzed using Volocity (v6.0; Perkin Elmer, Billerica, Massachusetts) via a Hamamatsu Orca R2 camera and Nikon Ti-E microscope. Multiple images were taken of the colon cross-section of each individual mouse (~5–10 at 20× magnification, encompassing 95% of each section). For quantification of Ki-67$^+$ cells in the crypts, the number of Ki-67$^+$ cells/crypt was counted manually by a blinded observer; a minimum of 15 crypts were counted per sample. For quantification of colonic epithelial-associated *C. rodentium*, a 'region of interest' was drawn to encompass all of the colon tissue observable in a given image, being careful to exclude luminal contents. Within this 'region of interest', a colour intensity was selected that best captured the stain of interest and minimized or eliminated background staining. The total areas of both the 'region of interest' and the stained area were quantified and weighted averages were calculated for each individual mouse. The data shown represent the average percentage of the area of interest that is stained with *C. rodentium.* Similarly for CD3, a 'region of interest' was identified, the total area quantified, and Volocity used to determine the number of cells stained positive for CD3 (on the basis on signal intensity) within this region. The data shown represent the average number of CD3$^+$ cells per unit of area.

Colonic Cell Isolation and Flow Cytometric Analysis

Leukocytes of the lamina propria were isolated from the colon by mechanical digestion, using a method similar to that described in [31] with modification. Colon pieces (~2.25 cm) were, first, cut longitudinally, and then cross-sectionally in pieces of ~0.5 cm in length. Tissues were then incubated in 5 ml Ca^{2+}/Mg^{2+} free HBSS supplemented with 10 mM Hepes, 5 mM ethylenediamine tetra-acetic acid, and 1 mM dithiothreitol, pH 7.4 for 20 minutes at 37°C in a shaker. Tissues were then vortexed vigorously for ~5 s and dissociated cells in the supernatant (predominantly epithelial) were separated by pouring the mixture through a 100 μm cell strainer (BD PharMingen, Mississauga, ON). Tissue pieces were returned to a fresh 5 ml aliquot of HBSS solution and the process was repeated for a total of four times. Tissues were then washed with FACS buffer (0.5% bovine serum albumin in PBS) to remove traces of EDTA, chopped into 1–2 mm pieces and incubated in RPMI supplemented with 25 mM Hepes and 0.125 Wunsch units/ml Liberase-TM (Roche, Laval, Quebec) for approximately 50–60 minutes at 37°C with shaking. The resulting tissue fragments and supernatant were poured through a 40 μm cell strainer, crushed with the plunger of a 3 ml syringe and rinsed with FACS Buffer. Cells were subsequently pelleted (1400 rpm for 10 minutes at 4°C), washed once with FACS buffer, and resuspended in a final volume of 0.5–1 ml. Total cell counts were then performed by trypan blue counting. Each sample was filtered again through a 40 μm cell strainer prior to surface marker staining. For staining, cells were first incubated with FcBlock (anti-CD16/CD32; BD PharMingen, Mississauga, ON, Canada) in FACS buffer for 15 minutes at 4°C (to minimize nonspecific binding). Antibodies were titrated to determine optimal concentration. For each antibody combination, 2×10^6 cells were incubated with mAbs on ice for 30 minutes. Cells were then washed twice with FACS buffer, fixed in 2.5% paraformaldehyde for 20 minutes on ice, and washed once more. Data were collected using a LSRII^{TM} (BD) flow cytometer and analyzed using FlowJo^{TM} software (Tree Star Inc., Ashland, OR, USA). The following antibodies were used: anti-CD4 (fluoresceine-isothiocyanate-conjugated RM4-5 clone), anti-CD45 (Alexa-Fluor 700-conjugated 30-F11 clone), purchased from BD PharMingen;

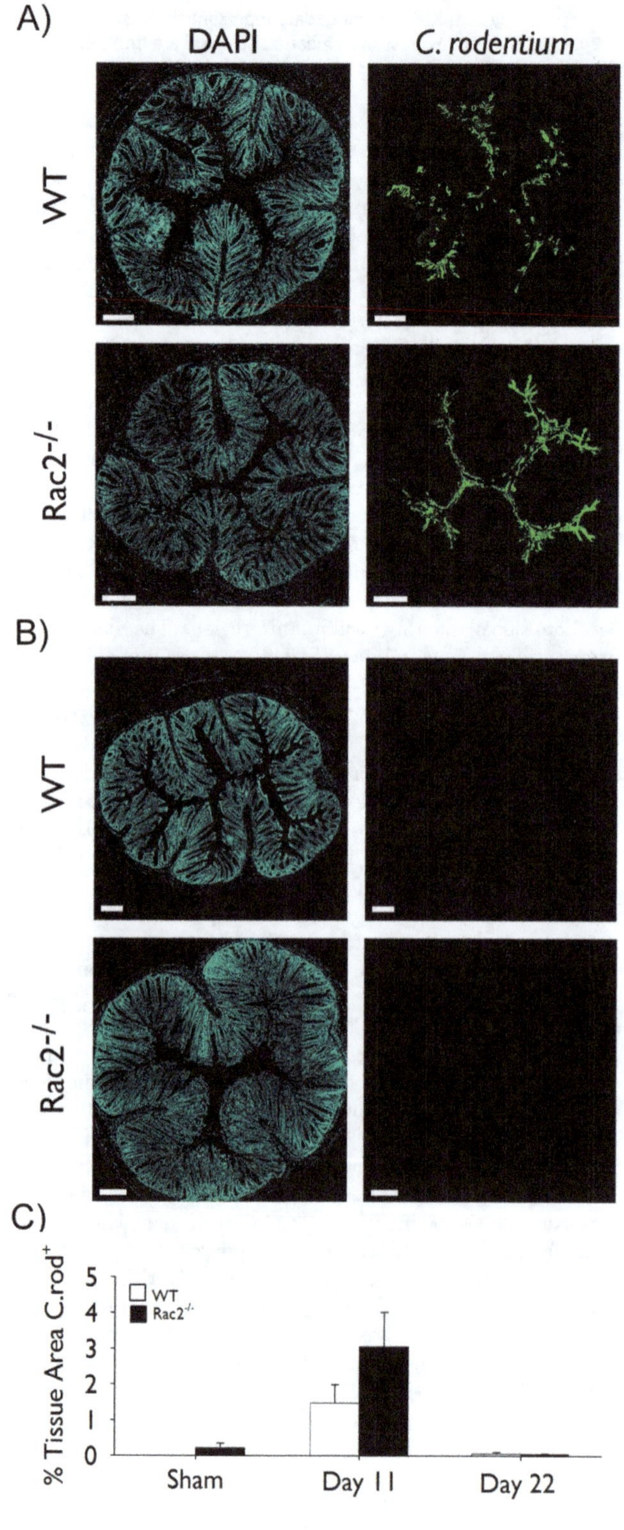

Figure 4. Epithelial-associated Citrobacter rodentium is cleared by WT and Rac2$^{-/-}$ mice at day 22 of infection. Separate groups of wild-type (WT; *white bars*) and Rac2$^{-/-}$ (*black bars*) mice were infected with *C. rodentium* or given vehicle control (sham) by orogastric gavage. (A-B) Immunofluorescence for epithelial cell-associated *C. rodentium*. Pictures show representative stitched images of DAPI and *C. rodentium* co-stained paraffin-embedded cross-sections of colon tissue obtained at days 11 *(A)* and 22 *(B)* of infection. Scale bar 200 µm. (C) Morphometric analysis of *C. rodentium* staining; data represent the percentage of the total tissue area that is stained positive for *C. rodentium*. Individual images were taken at 10× and stitched together using image analysis software to create a composite cross-section. n = 6–8/group. Data are expressed as mean ± SEM and are from one of two independent experiments. Statistical analysis was performed using two-way ANOVA with Tukey's post hoc test.

anti-CD3 (eFluor450-conjugated 500A2 clone), purchased from ebioscience (San Diego, CA, USA). The following gating strategy was used: whole leukocytes were first selected on the basis of CD45 expression, then 'singlets' were identified using FSC-W vs. FSC-A. CD4$^+$ and CD8$^+$ T cells were then identified by gating on the lymphocyte area on a graph of SSC vs FSC-A, and subsequently gating on CD4$^+$ or CD8$^+$ cells within the CD3$^+$ population of the lymphocyte region. The 'absolute cell numbers' were calculated by multiplying the appropriate population percentages by the total cell count for each sample.

Splenocyte Culture

Splenocytes were isolated by triturating whole spleens through a 40 µm cell strainer (BD), using the plunger from a 3 ml syringe, into HBSS. Cells were then centrifuged at 1200 rpm for 10 minutes at 4°C and red blood cells were lysed using ACK lysis buffer. HBSS was used to stop lysis after 1 minute (1:10 volume ratio). Splenocytes were then washed in complete RPMI (RPMI supplemented with 10% FBS – Sigma Aldrich; 1% L-glutamine; 1% penicillin/streptomycin – Invitrogen, Grand Island, NY, USA; and 0.1% β-mercaptoethanol – Invitrogen). Splenocytes were then resuspended in complete RPMI at a concentration of 6×10^6 cells/ml and cultured in medium alone, or with medium supplemented with a *C. rodentium* lysate (7.5 µg/ml; prepared by repeated rounds of freeze-thaw and sonication of live *C. rodentium*) in a round-bottom, 96-well plate (BD), in triplicate; 100 µl of medium ± lysate +100 µl of cell suspension per well. After 3 days of culture, supernatants were harvested and triplicates were pooled and stored at −20°C for cytokine measurements.

Cytokine Measurements by ELISA

Levels of mouse interleukin (IL)-4, -17A and interferon (IFN)-γ were measured by ELISA using DuoSet kits purchased from R&D Systems (Minneapolis, MN, USA) and performed according to the manufacturer's instructions. Each of these assays has a threshold of detection between 2–10 pg/ml.

Data Analysis

Data were analyzed using SigmaStat v3.0 (SPSS Inc., Chicago, IL). Data are expressed as mean ± SEM. Results were analyzed using two-way analysis of variance (ANOVA) with Tukey's post hoc test. Differences were considered statistically significant at $P<0.05$.

Results

C. rodentium Infection Induces Increased and Prolonged Colonic Hyperplasia in Rac2$^{-/-}$ Mice

To investigate the impact of a Rac2-deficiency on intestinal immune responses and the development of colitis, we subjected WT and Rac2$^{-/-}$ mice to a model of *C. rodentium* induced colitis. Separate groups of mice were infected (day1) with *C. rodentium* by oral gavage and sacrificed on days 11 and 22 of infection, time points that represent peak and resolution stages of infection, respectively. In response to infection, Rac2$^{-/-}$ mice displayed weight loss, a worsened clinical symptoms score (days 12–18), and considerable goblet cell loss (day 22; Figure 1) compared to infected WT mice. As expected, we observed that colonic

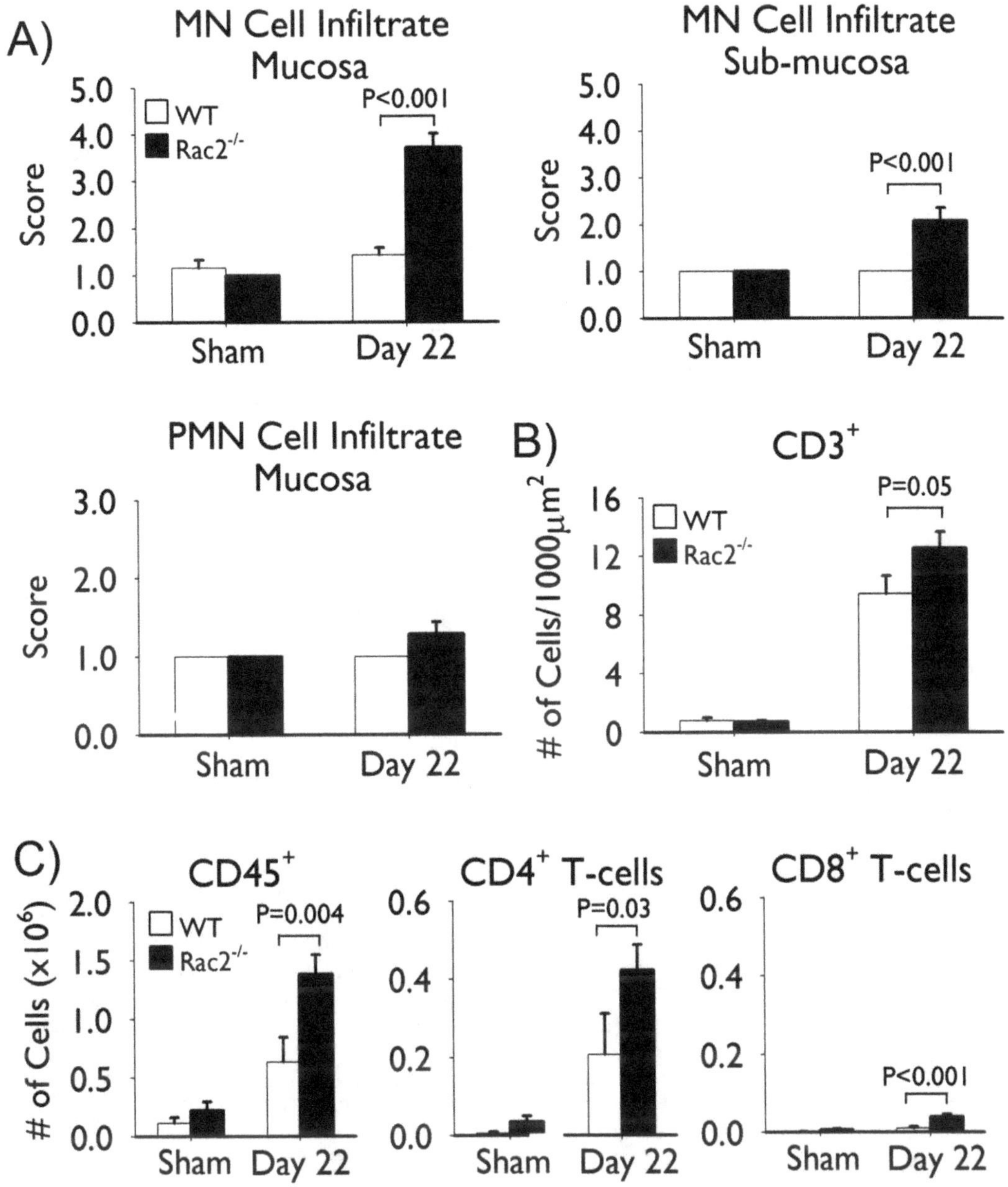

Figure 5. Rac2$^{-/-}$ mice infected with Citrobacter rodentium develop marked mononuclear cell infiltration at day 22 of infection. Separate groups of wild-type (WT; *white bars*) and Rac2$^{-/-}$ (*black bars*) mice were infected with *C. rodentium* or given vehicle control (sham) by orogastric gavage. (A) Scoring of mononuclear and polymorphonuclear cell infiltration into the submucosa and/or mucosa at day 22 of infection. (B) Average number of CD3^{+} cells per crypt in colon tissues obtained at day 22 of infection. (C) Flow cytometric analysis of colon digests showing the number of total leukocytes (CD45^{+} cells), T-helper (CD45^{+} CD3^{+} CD4^{+}), and cytotoxic (CD45^{+} CD3^{+} CD8^{+}) T-cells. n = 3–8/group in (*A-B*) and n = 3–4/group in (*C*). Data are expressed as mean ± SEM and are from one of two independent experiments. Statistical analysis was performed using two-way ANOVA with Tukey's post hoc test.

hyperplasia was significantly increased in WT infected mice compared to uninfected (sham) controls at day 11, and that this response had largely resolved by day 22 (Figures 2A and C). Interestingly, Rac2$^{-/-}$ infected mice developed significantly elevated hyperplasia at day 11 compared to WT mice that was considerably increased at day 22 (Figures 2A and C). To examine whether the colonic hyperplasia would continue to increase in Rac2$^{-/-}$ mice we infected an independent cohort of mice and measured colonic hyperplasia at day 32 of infection. Although colonic hyperplasia remained significantly elevated over uninfected and WT infected mice at day 32, this response was decreased relative to day 22, indicating that the hyperplasia was resolving (Figures 2B and C).

Colonic Hyperplasia is Driven by Enhanced Epithelial Cell Proliferation

To determine if the increase in colonic hyperplasia observed at day 22 in Rac2$^{-/-}$ mice was mediated by active epithelial cell proliferation we quantified Ki-67 staining, a marker of proliferating cells, in the colon. We observed significant increases in the number of Ki-67^{+} epithelial cells/crypt that were similar between WT and Rac2$^{-/-}$ infected mice at day 11 of infection

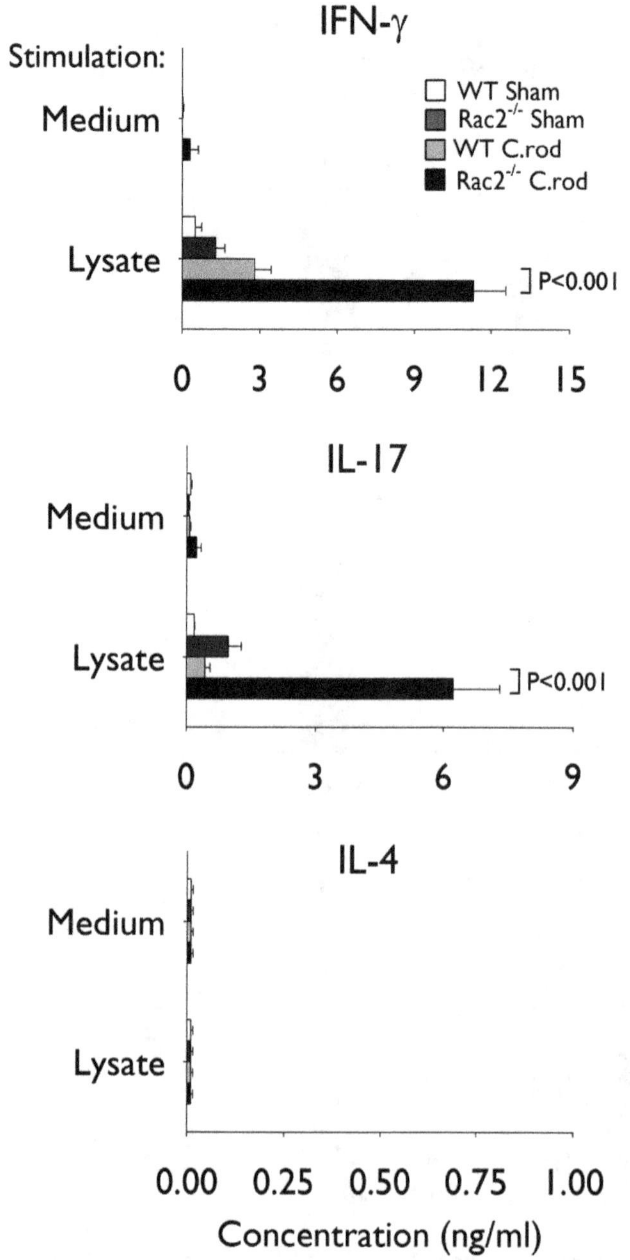

Figure 6. Heightened Th1- and Th17-associated cytokine production by splenocytes from Rac2$^{-/-}$ mice at day 22 of infection. Separate groups of wild-type (WT) and Rac2$^{-/-}$ mice were infected with *Citrobacter rodentium* or given vehicle control (sham) by orogastric gavage. Graphs show interferon-γ (IFN-γ), interleukin (IL)-17A and IL-4 production by splenocytes. Splenocytes from individual mice were harvested at day 22 of infection and cultured in medium alone or stimulated with *C. rodentium* lysate *in vitro*. n = 3–5/group. Statistical analysis was performed using two-way ANOVA with Tukey's post hoc test. WT uninfected (*white bars*), WT *C. rodentium*-infected (*light grey bars*), Rac2$^{-/-}$ uninfected (*dark grey bars*), and Rac2$^{-/-}$ *C. rodentium*-infected (*black bars*).

(Figure 3). At day 22, the number of Ki-67^{+} cells had decreased substantially in WT infected mice but remained elevated in Rac2$^{-/-}$ infected with *C. rodentium* (Figure 3), demonstrating that the increase in colonic hyperplasia in Rac2$^{-/-}$ mice at day 22 is, at least in part, being driven by increased epithelial cell proliferation.

Epithelial-associated *C. rodentium* is Cleared by day 22 of Infection in WT and Rac2$^{-/-}$ Mice

Given the putative importance of Rac2 in various immune cell-related functions and our observations of increased colonic hyperplasia, we questioned whether a deficiency in Rac2 negatively impacted bacterial clearance *in vivo*. To this end, we stained colon sections for the presence of *C. rodentium* and quantified the amount of bacteria associated with the colonic epithelium. Immunofluorescence analysis revealed a trend towards increased *C. rodentium* presence in Rac2$^{-/-}$ infected mice compared to WT controls at day 11, but this difference was not statistically significant (Figures 4A and C). Moreover, no *C. rodentium* could be detected in either strain at day 22 of infection (Figures 4B and C). No *C. rodentium* was ever detected in uninfected mice (Figure 4C). These results suggest that Rac2$^{-/-}$ mice are able to control and clear the infection.

C. rodentium Infection Induces Marked Colitis in Rac2$^{-/-}$ Mice

Histopathological analysis revealed marked inflammation in the colons of Rac2$^{-/-}$, but not WT, mice at day 22 of infection. Scoring of the inflammatory infiltrate by a pathologist blinded to the experimental conditions indicated that the inflammation was mononuclear cell in nature, with few if any polymorphonuclear cells observable at this stage of infection (Figure 5A). Immunofluorescence staining for CD3 demonstrated that a large number of these infiltrating cells were CD3^{+} (Figure 5B). To better quantify the extent of T-cell infiltrate we isolated cells from the colon and performed flow cytometric analysis to determine the number of, Th (CD45^{+} CD3^{+} CD4^{+}) and cytotoxic T-cells (CD45^{+} CD3^{+} CD8^{+}). In agreement with the histopathology, we isolated considerably higher numbers of total leukocytes (CD45^{+}) and detected significantly more T-cells in the colons of infected Rac2$^{-/-}$ mice compared to WT-infected mice (Figure 5C). The T-cell profile consisted predominantly of CD4^{+} T-cells with a limited number of CD8^{+} T-cells observed (Figure 5C).

Rac2$^{-/-}$ Mice Infected with *C. rodentium* Develop Heightened Th1 and Th17-associated Cytokine Responses

To evaluate the impact of Rac2 deficiency on the T cell response against *C. rodentium* we harvested splenocytes from Rac2$^{-/-}$ and WT-infected mice and measured the production of T cell-associated cytokines by ELISA following *in vitro* stimulation with a *C. rodentium* lysate. Splenocytes from infected Rac2$^{-/-}$ mice produced considerably more of the Th1- and Th17-associated cytokines IFN-γ and IL-17A in response to *C. rodentium* than WT mice (Figure 6). No differences in IL-4 production (a Th2-associated cytokine) were observed between WT- and Rac2$^{-/-}$infected mice. The proportion of Th cells in the spleen were similar between WT and Rac2$^{-/-}$ mice, indicating that the differences in IFN-γ and IL-17A production observed were not due, simply, to an aberrant, overall, increase in baseline Th cell number resulting from genetic ablation of Rac2 (data not shown).

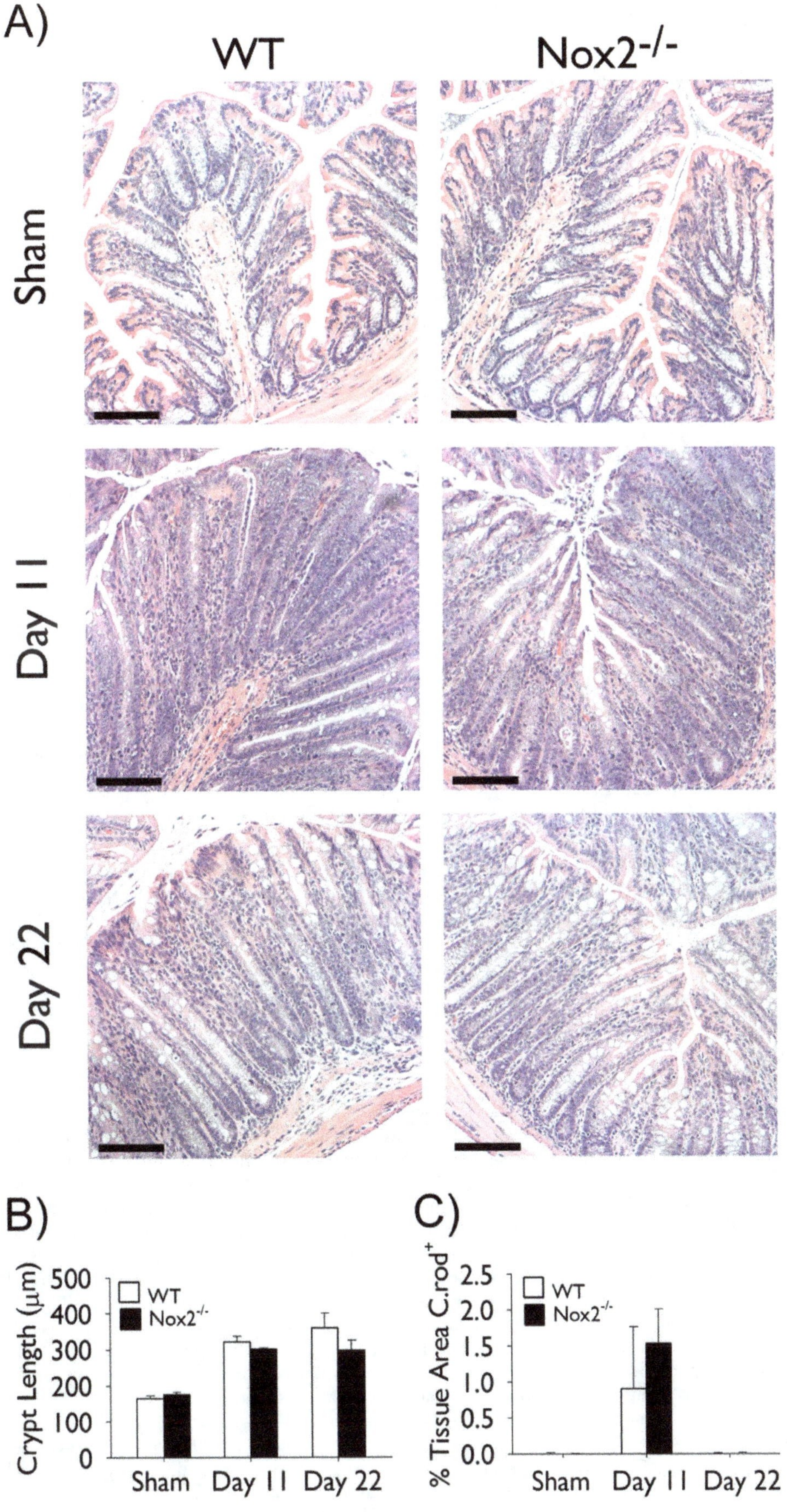
A)
WT
Nox2-/-
Sham
Day 11
Day 22
B)
Crypt Length (μm)
500
400
300
200
100
0
WT
Nox2-/-
Sham
Day 11
Day 22
C)
% Tissue Area C.rod+
2.5
2.0
1.5
1.0
0.5
0.0
WT
Nox2-/-
Sham
Day 11
Day 22

Figure 7. Nox2$^{-/-}$ mice infected with Citrobacter rodentium do not develop exaggerated colonic hyperplasia or colitis. Separate groups of wild-type (WT; *white bars*) and Nox2$^{-/-}$ (*black bars*) mice were infected with *C. rodentium* or given vehicle control (sham) by orogastric gavage. (A) Pictures show representative light photomicrographs of hematoxylin and eosin stained paraffin-embedded cross-sections of colon tissue obtained at the indicated time points of infection. Scale bar 100 µm. (B) Morphometric analysis of colonic hyperplasia at the indicated time points; data represent average crypt length. (C) Morphometric analysis of *C. rodentium* staining at the indicated time points of infection; data represent the percentage of the total tissue area that is stained positive for *C. rodentium*. All pictures were taken at 10× original magnification. n = 5–6/group. Data are expressed as mean ± SEM. Statistical analysis was performed using two-way ANOVA with Tukey's post hoc test.

Nox2$^{-/-}$ Mice do not Develop Exaggerated Colonic Hyperplasia or Colitis following Infection with *C. rodentium*

In light of the importance of Rac2 in NADPH oxidase-driven ROS production in leukocytes [7,8], we questioned the extent to which the enhanced responses observed in infected Rac2$^{-/-}$ mice were related to defects in leukocyte-derived ROS production. To address this, Nox2$^{-/-}$ mice were infected with *C. rodentium* and colonic hyperplasia was examined at days 11 and 22 of infection. We observed that crypt hyperplasia developed to a similar extent in infected WT and Nox2$^{-/-}$ mice (Figure 7A and B). Moreover, no significant differences were observed in the extent of *C. rodentium* colonization at day 11 of infection and bacteria were cleared from WT and Nox2$^{-/-}$ mice at day 22 of infection (Figure 7C).

Discussion

Our findings demonstrate that a genetic deficiency in Rac2 leads to worsened disease in mice infected with *C. rodentium* as evidenced by increased clinical symptoms score, colonic epithelial hyperplasia and colitis. However, the infection was not severe and all Rac2$^{-/-}$ mice recovered from infection. In addition, Rac2$^{-/-}$ mice did not appear to suffer from major innate immune defects as might have been predicted on the basis of the findings from previous *in vitro*-based studies [9,10,11,12,13,14,15,16,17,18]. We noted that *C. rodentium* colonization was controlled and that all bacteria were cleared at day 22. Moreover, there was no evidence of systemic bacterial dissemination and no signs of colonic hemorrhaging. A previous study examining the impact of Rac2-deficiency on susceptibility to *L. major* infection reported that intradermally-infected Rac2$^{-/-}$ mice displayed no differences in disease (i.e. lesion score and pathogen burden) compared to WT-infected mice [21]. Yet, in another report, Rac2$^{-/-}$ mice were found to be more susceptible to systemic challenge with *A. fumigatus*, showing increased pathogen burden and mortality [13]. These findings, in conjunction with our own, suggest that the requirement for Rac2 in the host defense response against pathogens may depend heavily on the pathogen itself and the mode of infection.

How can our findings be reconciled with the findings from human and *in vitro* studies that suggest that the absence of Rac2 may exert a crippling effect on several aspects of the innate immune response, in particular, on immune phagocyte function? With respect to the findings of the two human case reports, interpretation of those results, as it pertains to RAC2, is somewhat confounded by the knowledge that the mutation identified therein is known to impart dominant-negative activity on RAC2 [26]. Thus, the observed defects in host defense responses in those patients may have developed, in part, from consequences unrelated to impaired RAC2 function per se. For example, the acquisition of dominant negative activity may result in the sequestration of guanine nucleotide exchange factors (GEFs) that activate other Rho GTPases potentially involved in distinct immune-related signalling pathways [32]. Furthermore, it is worth noting that in humans, RAC2 constitutes 75–95% of the total Rac content, whereas Rac1 and Rac2 are present in roughly equal proportions in murine neutrophils [12,33,34]. Regarding the *in vitro*-based studies, we argue that the findings of these reports may overestimate the absolute requirement for Rac2 in various innate immune cell functions. While neutrophils and macrophages isolated from the peripheral blood and bone marrow of Rac2$^{-/-}$ mice display significant defects in phagocytosis, chemotaxis and/or ROS production, we and others propose that these cells may not exhibit such severe deficiencies when present in the setting of an active immune-inflammatory environment. In this regard, neutrophils isolated from the peritoneum of Rac2$^{-/-}$ mice following thioglycollate injection showed only marginal defects in ROS production and, similarly, bone marrow-derived Rac2$^{-/-}$ neutrophils stimulated with tumour necrosis factor (TNF)-α showed only a modest impairment in ROS production following secondary stimulation [13]. Thus, in the context of activating conditions (be they cytokine stimulation, inflammation, etc.), the loss of Rac2 may be partially compensated for by, presumably, other Rac isoforms. It is important to acknowledge that studies have consistently observed marked, albeit incomplete, defects in neutrophil chemotaxis and migration both *in vitro* and *in vivo*, in mice and humans [11,13,14,25]. Neutrophils are known to be a significant contributing cell type in the response mounted against *C. rodentium* [35,36], although perhaps not as essential as some other immune cells. In the studies presented here, whatever impact the loss of Rac2 had on neutrophil migration was not sufficient enough to impair bacterial control/clearance.

Interestingly, despite the absence of *C. rodentium* in Rac2$^{-/-}$ infected mice at day 22, we observed augmented colonic epithelial cell hyperplasia and exaggerated inflammation in the colon. These findings suggest that Rac2 may play a role, either directly or indirectly, in pathways related to the regulation and/or resolution of inflammation. That we documented dramatic increases in the production of IFN-γ and IL-17 from Rac2$^{-/-}$ splenocytes recalled *in vitro* with *C. rodentium* lysate, further suggests that the regulatory defects may lie in the processes that influence T-cell responses.

Previous reports have demonstrated that Rac2 is involved in various T-cell processes including migration, differentiation and apoptosis [21,24,37,38], and defects in any of these could have contributed to the heightened responses we observed in infected Rac2$^{-/-}$ mice. The loss of Rac2 in T-cells may have affected development of regulatory T-cells and, hence, resulted in at least a partial loss of inflammatory regulation. The involvement of Rac2 in T-cell differentiation is not without precedent as some, although not all, studies have shown that Rac2 plays a role in Th1 cell differentiation [21,24]. Although our results (i.e. IFN-γ production by splenocytes) do not support the idea of impaired Th1 development in infected Rac2$^{-/-}$ mice, they do not rule out the possibility that defects may exist in the differentiation pathways of other T-cell phenotypes such as T regulatory cells. Although somewhat unlikely, it is possible that the exaggerated immune-responsiveness we report here is related to impaired T-cell migration to or within the colon. Rac2$^{-/-}$ T-cells do exhibit chemotactic defects *in vitro* and Rac2$^{-/-}$ mice have been reported to display abnormal peripheral T-cell distribution [21]. However, we did not observe any overt aggregations or limitations in overall T-cell distribution (sub-mucosa vs. mucosa) in the colons of infected $Rac2^{-/-}$ mice. Alternatively, Rac2-deficiency may have impacted resolution mechanisms via some detriment to apoptosis. Along these lines, Rac2 has been shown to be a key signalling component of restimulation-induced cell death (RICD) [37]; a process that is thought to be an essential self-limiting negative feedback mechanism for controlling T-cell expansion during ongoing immune responses [39]. T-cells from $Rac2^{-/-}$ mice and Rac2-siRNA treated human primary $CD4^{+}$ T-cells displayed significantly impaired TCR-induced cell death [37]. Importantly, as RICD is thought to limit immunopathology that may arise from excessive effector T-cell expansion [39], it is plausible that defects in Rac2-mediated RICD may account for the exaggerated T-cell responses and associated inflammatory and hyperplasia we report here.

Our observations regarding *C. rodentium* infection in $Nox2^{-/-}$ mice suggest that at least some of the heightened immunoresponsiveness we found in infected $Rac2^{-/-}$ mice may not be a result of Rac2's role in NADPH-derived ROS production. Interestingly, previous studies that have investigated the contribution of the Nox2 complex to host defense responses in the intestine have reported mixed results. Mice deficient in $p47^{phox}$ displayed no overt differences compared to their WT controls in response to dextran sulphate sodium (DSS)-induced disease [40] and, interestingly, $gp91^{-/-}$ mice were partially protected from DSS-induced responses [41]. On the other hand, a recent study reported that $p40^{phox-/-}$ mice have increased inflammation and more severe colonic tissue injury in both DSS and $Rag1^{-/-}$ mouse models of colitis [42]. The differences in these findings are somewhat difficult to reconcile strictly in terms of the role of Nox2-derived ROS in models of colitis, however, they may derive, in part, from the participation of 'Nox' components (i.e. $p40^{phox}$, $p47^{phox}$, gp91) in other, Nox2-independent, processes/signalling pathways.

A considerable body of research supports the notion that impairments in host immunity, be they related to inflammatory- or regulatory-associated networks, contribute to the pathogenesis of IBD. In the studies presented here, we sought to investigate whether a defect in RAC2, a well-recognized mediator of various fundamental innate and adaptive immune cell processes, may impact host immune responses in the intestine and the development of disease. Our findings demonstrate that Rac2-deficient mice subjected to an infection-based model of colitis develop worsened disease characterized by increased and protracted colonic epithelial cell hyperplasia and exacerbated colonic inflammation. Importantly, the findings presented here speak to the possible contribution of variants in the *RAC2* gene, which may affect RAC2 expression and/or function, on the development of intestinal disease in humans. The issue is of relevance as population-based genetic studies continue to implicate an increasing number of genes whose roles in the pathogenesis of IBD are not well understood. While many of these genes are thought to, individually, contribute only modestly to IBD risk, their identification will, at the very least, form the basis for more detailed analyses into the influence of gene pathways/ networks. Coupled with detailed functional studies in both experimental models and patients, the knowledge gained is sure to furnish a foundation that not only inspires novel development but also guides the implementation of treatment strategies on a patient-by-patient basis.

Acknowledgments

We thank members of the Brumell lab for critical reading of the manuscript. We also thank Mike Woodside and Paul Paroutis for their support with microscopy, Ziad Al Adham and Sandeep Dhillon for technical help with experiments, Dr. Chun Sun for help with genotyping, and Drs. Manel Jordana and Susanna Goncharova for reagents and assistance with ELISA.

Author Contributions

Conceived and designed the experiments: RF AMM JHB. Performed the experiments: RF CHG GYL MGG BYN. Analyzed the data: RF. Contributed reagents/materials/analysis tools: MG. Wrote the paper: RF AMM JHB.

References

1. Cosnes J, Gower-Rousseau C, Seksik P, Cortot A (2011) Epidemiology and natural history of inflammatory bowel diseases. Gastroenterology 140: 1785–1794.
2. Vermeire S, Van Assche G, Rutgeerts P (2011) Inflammatory bowel disease and colitis: new concepts from the bench and the clinic. Curr Opin Gastroenterol 27: 32–37.
3. Cho JH, Brant SR (2011) Recent insights into the genetics of inflammatory bowel disease. Gastroenterology 140: 1704–1712.
4. Franke A, McGovern DP, Barrett JC, Wang K, Radford-Smith GL, et al. (2010) Genome-wide meta-analysis increases to 71 the number of confirmed Crohn's disease susceptibility loci. Nat Genet 42: 1118–1125.
5. Anderson CA, Boucher G, Lees CW, Franke A, D'Amato M, et al. (2011) Meta-analysis identifies 29 additional ulcerative colitis risk loci, increasing the number of confirmed associations to 47. Nat Genet 43: 246–252.
6. Muise AM, Xu W, Guo CH, Walters TD, Wolters VM, et al. (2011) NADPH oxidase complex and IBD candidate gene studies: identification of a rare variant in NCF2 that results in reduced binding to RAC2. Gut.
7. Bokoch GM (1995) Regulation of the phagocyte respiratory burst by small GTP-binding proteins. Trends Cell Biol 5: 109–113.
8. Knaus UG, Heyworth PG, Evans T, Curnutte JT, Bokoch GM (1991) Regulation of phagocyte oxygen radical production by the GTP-binding protein Rac 2. Science 254: 1512–1515.
9. Filippi MD, Harris CE, Meller J, Gu Y, Zheng Y, et al. (2004) Localization of Rac2 via the C terminus and aspartic acid 150 specifies superoxide generation, actin polarity and chemotaxis in neutrophils. Nat Immunol 5: 744–751.
10. Gu Y, Filippi MD, Cancelas JA, Siefring JE, Williams EP, et al. (2003) Hematopoietic cell regulation by Rac1 and Rac2 guanosine triphosphatases. Science 302: 445–449.
11. Koh AL, Sun CX, Zhu F, Glogauer M (2005) The role of Rac1 and Rac2 in bacterial killing. Cell Immunol 235: 92–97.
12. Li S, Yamauchi A, Marchal CC, Molitoris JK, Quilliam LA, et al. (2002) Chemoattractant-stimulated Rac activation in wild-type and Rac2-deficient murine neutrophils: preferential activation of Rac2 and Rac2 gene dosage effect on neutrophil functions. J Immunol 169: 5043–5051.
13. Roberts AW, Kim C, Zhen L, Lowe JB, Kapur R, et al. (1999) Deficiency of the hematopoietic cell-specific Rho family GTPase Rac2 is characterized by abnormalities in neutrophil function and host defense. Immunity 10: 183–196.
14. Sun CX, Downey GP, Zhu F, Koh AL, Thang H, et al. (2004) Rac1 is the small GTPase responsible for regulating the neutrophil chemotaxis compass. Blood 104: 3758–3765.
15. Yamauchi A, Marchal CC, Molitoris J, Pech N, Knaus U, et al. (2005) Rac GTPase isoform-specific regulation of NADPH oxidase and chemotaxis in murine neutrophils in vivo. Role of the C-terminal polybasic domain. J Biol Chem 280: 953–964.
16. Zhang H, Sun C, Glogauer M, Bokoch GM (2009) Human neutrophils coordinate chemotaxis by differential activation of Rac1 and Rac2. J Immunol 183: 2718–2728.
17. Wheeler AP, Wells CM, Smith SD, Vega FM, Henderson RB, et al. (2006) Rac1 and Rac2 regulate macrophage morphology but are not essential for migration. J Cell Sci 119: 2749–2757.

18. Yamauchi A, Kim C, Li S, Marchal CC, Towe J, et al. (2004) Rac2-deficient murine macrophages have selective defects in superoxide production and phagocytosis of opsonized particles. J Immunol 173: 5971–5979.
19. Walmsley MJ, Ooi SK, Reynolds LF, Smith SH, Ruf S, et al. (2003) Critical roles for Rac1 and Rac2 GTPases in B cell development and signaling. Science 302: 459–462.
20. Croker BA, Tarlinton DM, Cluse LA, Tuxen AJ, Light A, et al. (2002) The Rac2 guanosine triphosphatase regulates B lymphocyte antigen receptor responses and chemotaxis and is required for establishment of B-1a and marginal zone B lymphocytes. J Immunol 168: 3376–3386.
21. Croker BA, Handman E, Hayball JD, Baldwin TM, Voigt V, et al. (2002) Rac2-deficient mice display perturbed T-cell distribution and chemotaxis, but only minor abnormalities in T(H)1 responses. Immunol Cell Biol 80: 231–240.
22. Yu H, Leitenberg D, Li B, Flavell RA (2001) Deficiency of small GTPase Rac2 affects T cell activation. J Exp Med 194: 915–926.
23. Dumont C, Corsoni-Tadrzak A, Ruf S, de Boer J, Williams A, et al. (2009) Rac GTPases play critical roles in early T-cell development. Blood 113: 3990–3998.
24. Li B, Yu H, Zheng W, Voll R, Na S, et al. (2000) Role of the guanosine triphosphatase Rac2 in T helper 1 cell differentiation. Science 288: 2219–2222.
25. Ambruso DR, Knall C, Abell AN, Panepinto J, Kurkchubasche A, et al. (2000) Human neutrophil immunodeficiency syndrome is associated with an inhibitory Rac2 mutation. Proc Natl Acad Sci U S A 97: 4654–4659.
26. Williams DA, Tao W, Yang F, Kim C, Gu Y, et al. (2000) Dominant negative mutation of the hematopoietic-specific Rho GTPase, Rac2, is associated with a human phagocyte immunodeficiency. Blood 96: 1646–1654.
27. Kurkchubasche AG, Panepinto JA, Tracy TF, Jr., Thurman GW, Ambruso DR (2001) Clinical features of a human Rac2 mutation: a complex neutrophil dysfunction disease. J Pediatr 139: 141–147.
28. Routes JM, Grossman WJ, Verbsky J, Laessig RH, Hoffman GL, et al. (2009) Statewide newborn screening for severe T-cell lymphopenia. JAMA 302: 2465–2470.
29. Muise AM, Walters T, Wine E, Griffiths AM, Turner D, et al. (2007) Protein-tyrosine phosphatase sigma is associated with ulcerative colitis. Curr Biol 17: 1212–1218.
30. Kaniuk NA, Brumell JH (2010) Examining ubiquitinated protein aggregates in tissue sections. Methods Mol Biol 648: 175–182.
31. Lefrancois L, Lycke N (2001) Isolation of mouse small intestinal intraepithelial lymphocytes, Peyer's patch, and lamina propria cells. Curr Protoc Immunol Chapter 3: Unit 3 19.
32. Bokoch GM (2005) Regulation of innate immunity by Rho GTPases. Trends Cell Biol 15: 163–171.
33. Quinn MT, Evans T, Loetterle LR, Jesaitis AJ, Bokoch GM (1993) Translocation of Rac correlates with NADPH oxidase activation. Evidence for equimolar translocation of oxidase components. J Biol Chem 268: 20983–20987.
34. Heyworth PG, Bohl BP, Bokoch GM, Curnutte JT (1994) Rac translocates independently of the neutrophil NADPH oxidase components p47phox and p67phox. Evidence for its interaction with flavocytochrome b558. J Biol Chem 269: 30749–30752.
35. Spehlmann ME, Dann SM, Hruz P, Hanson E, McCole DF, et al. (2009) CXCR2-dependent mucosal neutrophil influx protects against colitis-associated diarrhea caused by an attaching/effacing lesion-forming bacterial pathogen. J Immunol 183: 3332–3343.
36. Lebeis SL, Bommarius B, Parkos CA, Sherman MA, Kalman D (2007) TLR signaling mediated by MyD88 is required for a protective innate immune response by neutrophils to Citrobacter rodentium. J Immunol 179: 566–577.
37. Ramaswamy M, Dumont C, Cruz AC, Muppidi JR, Gomez TS, et al. (2007) Cutting edge: Rac GTPases sensitize activated T cells to die via Fas. J Immunol 179: 6384–6388.
38. Lores P, Morin L, Luna R, Gacon G (1997) Enhanced apoptosis in the thymus of transgenic mice expressing constitutively activated forms of human Rac2GTPase. Oncogene 15: 601–605.
39. Snow AL, Pandiyan P, Zheng L, Krummey SM, Lenardo MJ (2010) The power and the promise of restimulation-induced cell death in human immune diseases. Immunol Rev 236: 68–82.
40. Krieglstein CF, Cerwinka WH, Laroux FS, Salter JW, Russell JM, et al. (2001) Regulation of murine intestinal inflammation by reactive metabolites of oxygen and nitrogen: divergent roles of superoxide and nitric oxide. J Exp Med 194: 1207–1218.
41. Bao S, Carr ED, Xu YH, Hunt NH (2011) Gp91(phox) contributes to the development of experimental inflammatory bowel disease. Immunol Cell Biol 89: 853–860.
42. Conway KL, Goel G, Sokol H, Manocha M, Mizoguchi E, et al. (2012) p40phox Expression Regulates Neutrophil Recruitment and Function during the Resolution Phase of Intestinal Inflammation. J Immunol 189: 3631–3640.

13

Therapeutic Effects of Novel Sphingosine-1-Phosphate Receptor Agonist W-061 in Murine DSS Colitis

Yasuaki Sanada[1,2], Tsunekazu Mizushima[3], Yasuyuki Kai[3], Junichi Nishimura[3], Hiroshi Hagiya[4], Haruto Kurata[4], Hirotaka Mizuno[5], Etsuko Uejima[2], Toshinori Ito[1]*

1 Departments of Complementary and Alternative Medicine, Graduate School of Medicine, Osaka University, Osaka, Japan, **2** Department of Hospital Pharmacy Education, Graduate School of Pharmaceutical Science, Osaka University, Osaka, Japan, **3** Department of Surgery, Gastroenterological Surgery, Graduate School of Medicine, Osaka University, Osaka, Japan, **4** Minase Research Institute, Ono Pharmaceutical Co., Ltd, Osaka, Japan, **5** Tsukuba Research Institute, Ono Pharmaceutical Co., Ltd, Ibaraki, Japan

Abstract

Although IL-17 is a pro-inflammatory cytokine reportedly involved in various autoimmune inflammatory disorders, its role remains unclear in murine models of colitis. Acute colitis was induced by 2.5% dextran sodium sulfate (DSS) treatment for 5 days. A novel sphingosine-1-phosphate receptor agonist W-061, a prototype of ONO-4641, was orally administered daily, and histopathological analysis was performed on the colon. The number of lymphocytes and their cytokine production were also evaluated in spleen, mesenteric lymph node, Peyer's patch and lamina propria of the colon. Daily administration of W-061 resulted in improvement of DSS-induced colitis, and significantly reduced the number of CD4+ T cells in the colonic lamina propria. Numbers of both Th17 and Th1 cells were reduced by W-061 treatment. W-061, however, had no influence on the number of Treg cells in lamina propria. Thus, Th17 and Th1 cells in lamina propria were thought to be the key subsets in the pathogenesis of DSS-induced colitis. In conclusion, W-061 may be a novel therapeutic strategy to ameliorate acute aggravation of inflammatory bowel diseases.

Editor: Jan-Hendrik Niess, Ulm University, Germany

Funding: The authors have no support or funding to report.

Competing Interests: YS, TM, YK, JN, EU and TI have declared that no competing interests exist. HH, HK, and HM are employers of Ono Pharmaceutical Co., Ltd. This company did not provide direct financial support, it can be considered to be as an indirect funder for this study. This company provided us a base powder of W-061 free of charge and some in vitro pharmacological data. There are no patents, products in development or marketed products to declare.

* E-mail: juki@cam.med.osaka-u.ac.jp

Introduction

Inflammatory bowel diseases (IBDs), such as Crohn's disease (CD) and ulcerative colitis (UC), are chronic relapsing disorders of the gastrointestinal tract [1]. In humans, CD is generally characterized by elevated production of helper T (Th) 1 cytokines, such as interferon (IFN)-γ [2], while UC is characterized by the enhanced expression of Th2 cytokines, such as interleukin (IL)-4 and IL-13 [3]. Recent clinical data have indicated that treatment with infliximab, a chimeric anti-tumor necrosis factor (TNF)-α antibody, was further effective as compared to azathioprine therapy in patients with CD [4]. Despite its efficacy, infliximab therapy for patients with rheumatoid arthritis (RA) was associated with the risk of malignancies and serious infections, such as tuberculosis [5]. Therefore, novel therapeutic strategies with different mechanisms are required.

In recent years, Th17, a third subset of inflammatory helper T cells that produce IL-17A, IL-17F, IL-22 and IL-23, was discovered [6]. Th17 has been reported to be associated with aggravation of various autoimmune inflammatory diseases, such as rheumatoid arthritis and multiple sclerosis [7-9]. Although IL-17 expression in the mucosa and its serum levels were increased in active IBD patients [10], treatment strategies for the regulation of Th17 functions has not yet been established.

It has been reported that serum IL-17 concentration is elevated in the acute phase in a dextran sodium sulfate (DSS)-induced colitis model [11], however, the role of IL-17 remains unclear in animal models of colitis. For example, controversial data have been obtained in the DSS-induced colitis model [12,13] and $CD4^+$ $CD45RB^{high}$ adoptive cell transfer model [14,15].

In contrast, regulatory T (Treg) cells are a distinct subset in suppressing excessive immune responses [16]. This subset is characterized by the presence of a surface marker, CD25, and a transcription factor, Foxp3. In a $CD4^+$ $CD45RB^{high}$ cell-transfer colitis model, the development of colitis was suppressed by concomitant transfer of $CD4^+$ $CD25^+$ T cells [17].

It was recently reported that sphingosine-1-phosphate (S1P) receptor agonists, such as FTY720 (fingolimod), exhibited immunodulatory function through induction of $CD4^+$ T cell migration into secondary lymphoid tissues and sequestration of these cells [18] and that FTY720, which has a particular binding affinity for $S1P_1$, was clinically effective in the treatment of multiple sclerosis [19]. FTY720 was also reported to be effective for the treatment of colitis in IL-10-deficient mice [20], DSS-induced colitis and $CD4^+CD62L^+$ cell-transfer model [21]. Another S1P receptor agonist, KRP-203, was also useful for colitis in IL-10 deficient mice [22]. However, the effects of these agents on Th17 and Treg in colitis mice have not been examined and reported to date.

W-061, a prototype of ONO-4641 [23], has recently been developed to target S1P receptors. In the present study, we evaluated the activity of W-061 on S1P receptors and the effects of this agent on specific T cells, such as Th17 and Treg, in a mouse model of DSS-induced colitis.

Results

W-061 has specific agonistic activity on $hS1P_1$

Compared to FTY720 phosphate, binding affinity of S1P receptors and agonistic activity of W-061 was evaluated in CHO-K1 cells. W-061 bound to human S1P receptors except for $hS1P_2$ (Table 1). Its binding affinity of S1P receptors was lower than that of FTY720 phosphate, however, W-061 had higher agonistic activity on $S1P_1$ compared to $S1P_3$ (Table 2), while FTY720 phosphate had agonistic activity on $S1P_3$ as well as $S1P_1$.

Body weight and colon length were improved by treatment of W-061

No change of body weight was observed in mice treated with W-061 (3 mg/kg) alone (Figure S1). After 5-day DSS treatment, body weight in each group was reduced by approximately 20% (Figure 1A). After day 7, however, a significant body weight increase was observed in W-061-treated mice (95.8±5.6% vs. 80.0±7.2% on day 10). DSS treatment induced a reduction in colon length in each group; however, colon length in W-061 treated mice was significantly longer than in control mice on day 10 (10.8±0.6 cm vs. 9.1±1.6 cm, $p<0.05$).

Daily W-061 administration significantly promoted recovery from acute DSS-induced colitis

Histological analysis indicated that cellular infiltration in the lamina propria, mucin depletion and thickness of the mucosa were severe in control mice when compared with W-061 treated mice (Figure 1B). Mean histologic score in mice treated with W-061 was significantly lower than in control mice (Figure 1C: 3.7±0.6 vs. 10.8±4.5).

Daily W-061 administration induced homing of lymphocytes to secondary lymphoid tissues

The number of lymphocytes in LP was sequentially increased by DSS treatment. However, W-061 administration suppressed lymphocyte migration to SP and LP, and promoted their homing to secondary lymphoid tissues, such as MLN and PP (Figure 2A–D). Specifically, W-061 inhibited $CD4^+$ T cell migration to LP on day 3, 6 and 10 (Figure 2D).

Daily W-061 administration inhibited migration of Th17 and Th1 to lamina propria

In the control group, an increase in the number of Th1 cells in LP was observed following the increase in the number of Th17 cells. On the other hand, W-061 treatment inhibited the increase in Th17 cells on days 6 and 10 (Figure 3D). In addition, W-061 also inhibited the increase in Th1 cells on day 10 (Figure 4D).

Table 1. Binding affinity of W-061 on S1P receptors.

	$hS1P_1$	$hS1P_2$	$hS1P_3$	$hS1P_4$	$hS1P_5$
S1P	0.131	0.439	0.0782	7.60	0.372
FTY720-P	0.160	4090	3.74	2.16	1.09
W-061	4.11	>43800	1710	65.4	10.1

Data were shown as Ki value. FTY720-P; FTY720-phosphate.

Table 2. Agonistic activity of W-061 on $S1P_1$ and $S1P_3$.

	$hS1P_1$	$hS1P_3$
S1P	4.7	30
FTY720-P	0.23	20
W-061	10	>30000

Instead, Th17 cells increased in PP on day 6, and Th1 cells increased in MLN and PP on day 10. The number of Treg cells in both groups increased on day 6 (Figure 5D); however, there was no difference in the change in Treg cells. Changes in the number of Th1, Th17 and Treg cells were also confirmed in SP, MLN and PP (Figure 5A–C). In PP, the number of Th17 cells was significantly higher in the W-061 group on day 6, and the numbers of Th1 and Treg cells were significantly higher on day 10 (Figure 4C, 5C). Similarly, in MLN, the numbers of Th1 and Treg cells were also significantly higher in W-061 group on day 10 (Figure 4B, 5B).

Discussion

In the clinical course of IBD, patients occasionally become immunocompromised due to treatment with immunosuppressive reagents, such as infliximab, steroids, antimetabolites and calcineurin inhibitors. It has been reported that RA patients receiving infliximab can develop serious opportunistic infections, such as tuberculosis [5]. In terms of the potent properties in anti-opportunistic infections [24] and anti-tumor effects [25,26], we have been investigating the efficacy of S1P receptor agonists in promoting lymphocyte homing and sequestrating lymphocytes into secondary lymphoid organs. We previously reported the usefulness of FTY720 and KRP-203 in IL-10-deficient mice as a CD-like colitis model [20,22]. In this study, a novel and potent S1P receptor agonist, W-061, which is structurally different from sphingosine, was examined. In contrast to conventional S1P receptor agonists, W-061, which is biologically active *in vivo* without undergoing phosphorylation, is more specific to lymphocytes than FTY720.

We first evaluated the membrane binding activity of W-061 to S1P receptors, which has five subtypes ($S1P_{1-5}$) [18]. The specific roles of S1P receptor subtypes have been reported, with $S1P_1$ and $S1P_4$ being strongly expressed in T cells [27]. $S1P_1$ is particularly associated with lymphocyte migration. In some clinical reports of FTY720, symptomatic bradycardia was noted as an adverse event [28], and this is related to agonistic activity of $S1P_3$ [29]. W-061 was found to have a lower affinity for $S1P_1$, but to have a much lower affinity for and $S1P_3$ than FTY720 phosphate (Table 1). Thus, it could be considered that W-061 had a higher selectivity for $S1P_1$ than FTY720 phosphate. In addition, W-061 had little agonistic activity on $S1P_3$ (Table 2). Taken together, these properties may be helpful not only for adjusting lymphocyte trafficking with less adverse events such as symptomatic bradycardia.

The recent advances in our knowledge of the immunopathologic basis of IBD have been approaching the elucidation of the inflammatory cytokines driving the two main components of IBD, CD and UC. CD patients, but not UC patients, exhibit elevated amounts of IFN-γ in the inflamed LP, suggesting the presence of a Th1-mediated inflammatory process. Recently, a novel helper T cell, Th17, was identified, and was reported to be a proin-

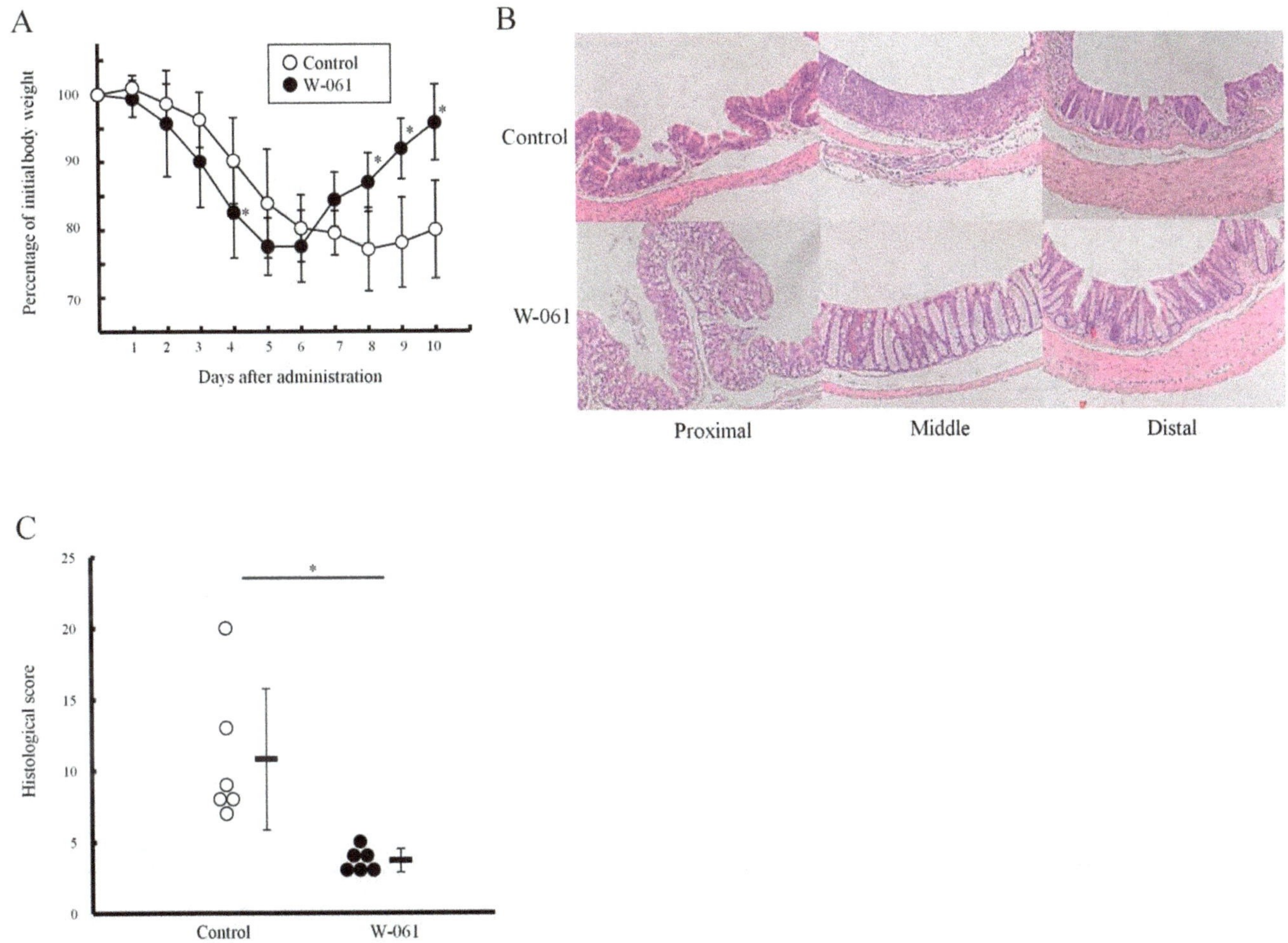

Figure 1. DSS-induced colitis was ameliorated by W-061 treatment. (A) Change in body weight of W-061-treated and control mice with the DSS-induced colitis (n = 6 mice for each group, *p<0.05). (B) Pathological evaluation of the DSS-induced colitis on day 10. (C) Histological score of the DSS-induced colitis on day 10. Data represent absolute values (means ± SD, n = 6 mice for each group, *p<0.05).

flammatory subset in several autoimmune diseases [7–9]. In the case of 2,4,6-trinitrobenzenesulfonic acid (TNBS)-induced colitis, it was also shown to be driven by a cytokine including IL-12p40 and to be reversed by anti-IL-12p40 mAb [30]. Furthermore, it was found that a novel cytokine, IL-23, shared the common p40 chain with IL-12 [31]. It is generally recognized that Th17 cells are induced by IL-23 together with TGFβ, while Th1 cells are induced by IL-12 or IL-23 without TGFβ [6]. Therefore, anti-IL-12p40 mAb inhibits Th17 as well as Th1.

Although the role of Th1 is reported to be an indispensable subset [32], the role of Th17 remains controversial in DSS-induced colitis or the $CD4^{+}$ $CD45RB^{high}$ lymphocyte transfer model. In the case of DSS-induced colitis, inflammation is improved in IL-17-deficient mice [12], but is aggravated by neutralization of IL-17 due to anti-IL-17 mAb [13]. In the adoptive transfer model, transfer of RORγ-null T cells do not induce colitis [14]; however, lymphocytes from IL-17A-deficient mice induced severe colitis [15]. Thus, the type of colitis model or the time of inflammation may influence whether Th1 or Th17 cells contribute the pathogenesis of colitis.

In the previous reports, however, we did not evaluate the effects of S1P receptor agonists on the new T cell subsets, such as Th17 and Treg. In order to investigate the effect of W-061 on these T cells, we utilized a DSS-induced mice colitis model which does not exhibit any immune disorder, in contrast to IL-10 deficient mice. Treg cells cannot be evaluated in IL-10-deficient mice because IL-10 is necessary for the effector function of the regulatory T cell population [32]. We showed that the number of Th17 cells in LP was markedly higher after the initiation of colitis, and then decreased significantly, which appears to be due to the induction of Treg cells. After downregulation of Th17 cells, it is likely that IFN-γ-producing Th1 cells prolong the inflammation in LP.

In contrast, when W-061 was administered, the number of Th1 and Th17 cells was markedly decreased in the acute phase of inflammation. Interestingly, W-061 did not influence the migration of Treg cells. These data suggest that W-061 promotes the migration of Th17 and Th1 cells, but not Treg cells into secondary lymphoid tissues. It is generally known that S1P receptor agonists do not affect migration of memory T and B cells into secondary lymphoid tissues, resulting in the maintenance of the anti-opportunistic infections or anti-tumor effects [24-26]. The chemokine receptor CCR7 is reported to be a major homing receptor in T cells [33]. Although CCR7 is expressed in Treg cells, as well as other T cell subsets, its effects differ between naïve-like Treg and effector/memory-like Treg [34]. Namely, naïve like Treg can enter themelves into lymph node via CCR7 to control the priming phase of immune responses. On the other hand, CCR7 on effector/memory Treg is associated to emigrate

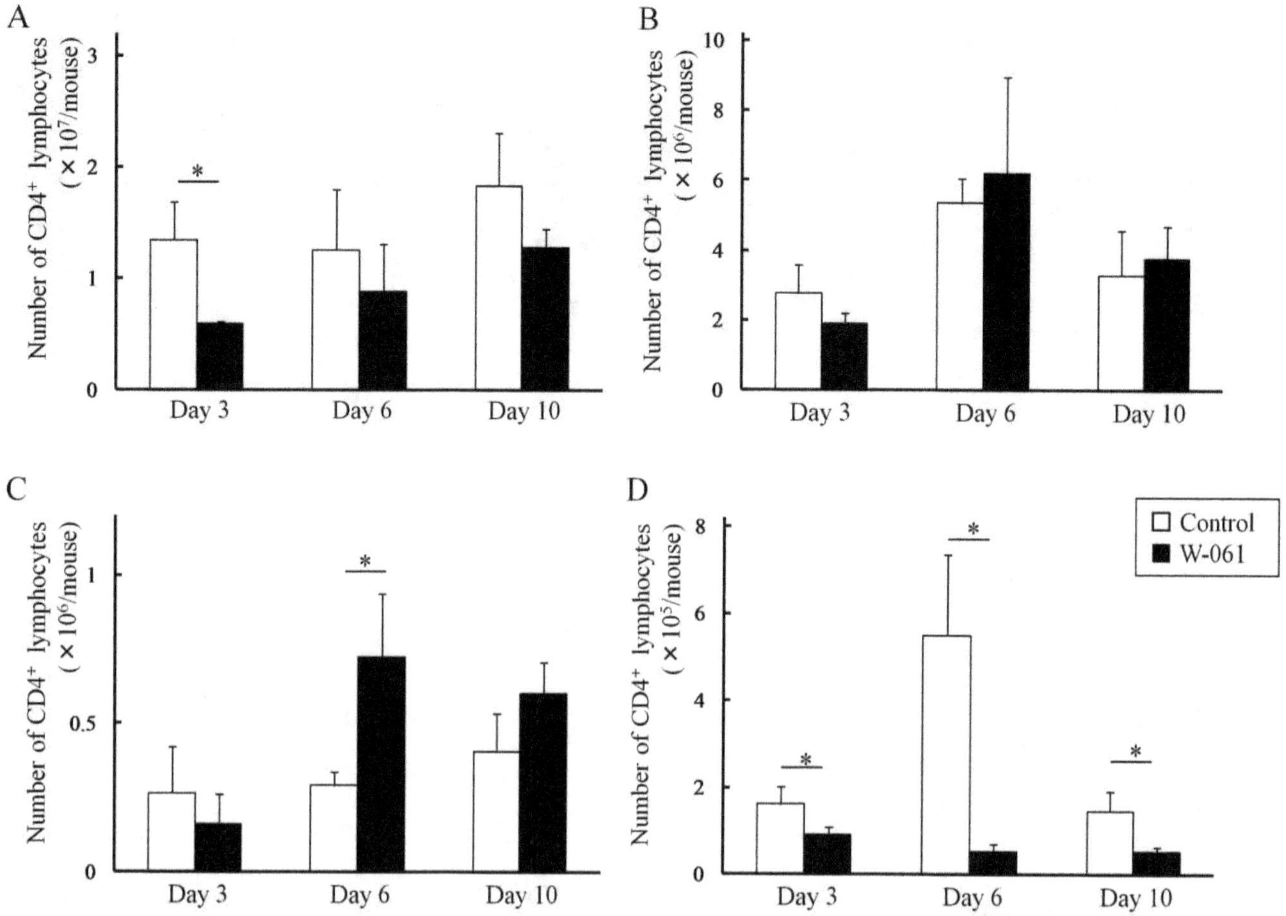

Figure 2. Change of the numbers of CD4$^+$ T cells in (A) SP, (B) MLN, (C) PP and (D) LP. Data represent absolute values (means ± SD, n = 4 per group on days 3 and 6, n = 6 per group on day 10, * $p<0.05$).

themselves from the inflamed site. In terms of lymphocyte homing, W-061 is likely to have some selectivity. Considering that accumulation of effector/memory-like Treg at inflamed sites was induced by CCR7 deficiency [34], W-061 may affect CCR7 expression. Further study is thus needed to clarify whether migration of Treg via $S1P_1$ receptor is different from that of other T cell subsets.

In summary, we herein demonstrate that a novel S1P receptor agonist W-061 is effective in the treatment of acute colitis induced by DSS. This effect is attributed to the suppression of increases in Th17 and Th1 in LP by the sequestration of these cells into the secondary lymphoid tissues. Thus, Th17 and Th1 in LP are a key subset in the pathogenesis of DSS-induced colitis. S1P receptor agonists, including W-061, may therefore represent a novel therapeutic strategy for ameliorating acute aggravation of IBDs.

Materials and Methods

Cell Culture

CHO-K1 cells stably expressing human $S1P_1$ ($hS1P_1$), human $S1P_2$ ($hS1P_2$), human $S1P_3$ ($hS1P_3$), human $S1P_4$ ($hS1P_4$) or human $S1P_5$ ($hS1P_5$) were cultured in Ham's F12 medium supplemented with 10% bovine serum (Sigma-Aldrich, St Louis, MO) and 0.25 mg/mL G418 sulfate (Invitrogen, Carlsbad, CA) in 5% CO_2/95% air at 37°C.

Membrane binding assay

Membranes were prepared from CHO-K1 cells stably expressing human S1P receptors based on the methods of Mandala *et al.* [35]. Briefly, cells were washed in PBS, suspended in 10 mM Tris-HCl (pH 7.5), 5 mM EDTA, and 1x Complete protease inhibitor cocktail (Roche Diagnostics, Mannheim, Germany), and were disrupted on ice using a polytron homogenizer. Following centrifugation at 80,000 × *g* for 40 min at 4°C, the pellet was suspended in 10 mM Tris-HCl (pH 7.5), 10% glycerol, and 1x Complete protease inhibitor cocktail and stored at −80°C. [^{33}P]-S1P (American Radiolabeled Chemicals, St. Louis, MO) were used as radio-labeled ligands. Test compounds in assay buffer 1 (for $S1P_1$, $S1P_2$, $S1P_3$, and $S1P_5$; 50 mM Tris-HCl, pH 7.5, 5 mM $MgCl_2$, 0.5% fatty acid-free BSA, and 1x Complete protease inhibitor cocktail) or assay buffer 2 (for $S1P_4$ 50 mM Tris-HCl, pH 7.5, 100 mM NaCl, 15 mM NaF, 0.5% fatty acid-free BSA, and 1x Complete protease inhibitor cocktail) were added to a 96-well plate. Radio-labeled ligands and membranes were added to give a final volume of 200 μL. Binding was performed for 60 min at room temperature and was terminated by collecting the membranes onto unifilter GF/B plates (Perkin Elmer, Boston, MA) with a UniFilter96 Harvester (Perkin Elmer). After drying the filter plates for 30 min, filter-bound radionuclides were measured on a TopCount NXT microplate scintillation counter (Perkin Elmer). Specific binding was calculated by subtracting the radioactivity that remained in the presence of a 1000-fold excess of unlabeled S1P.

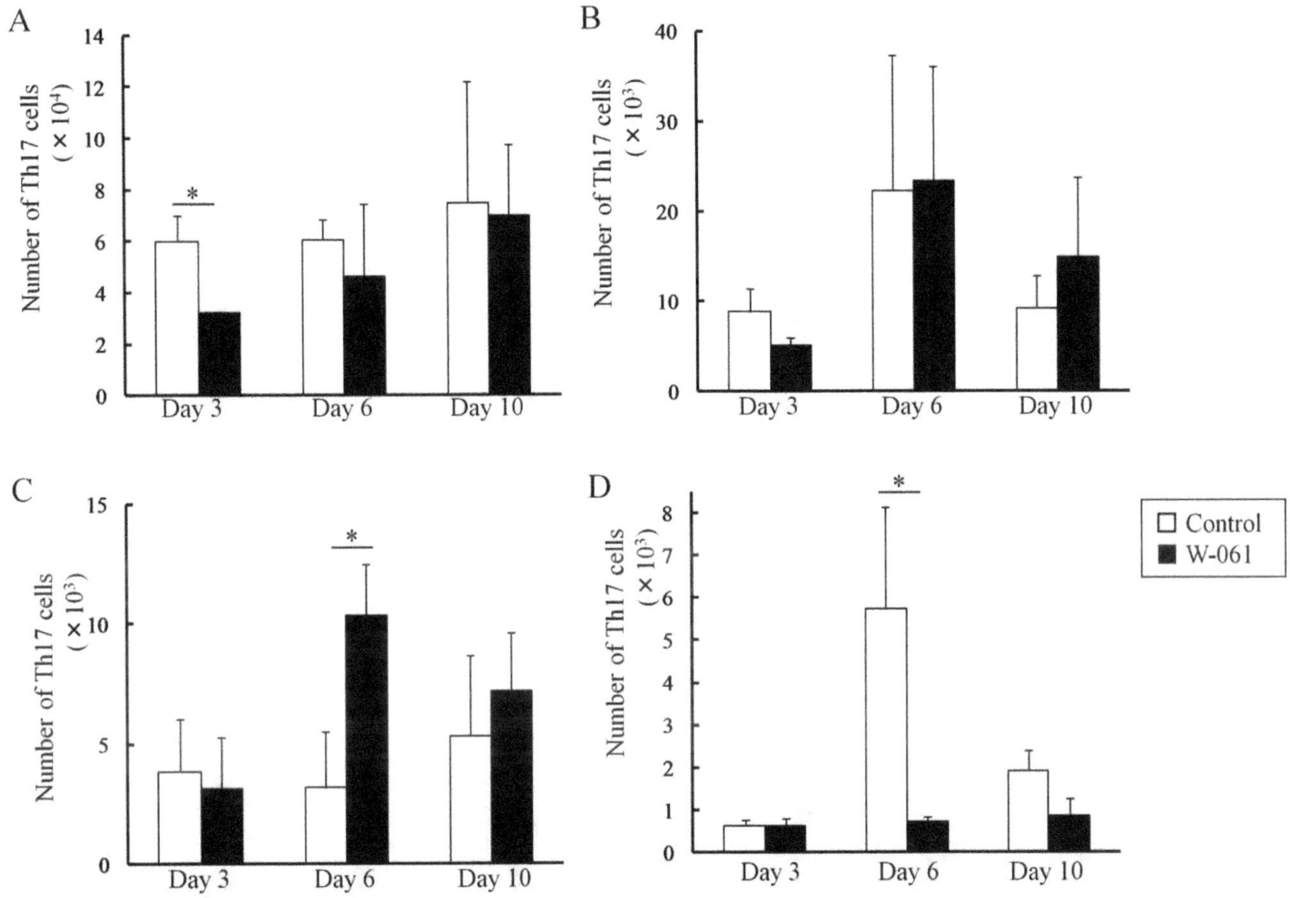

Figure 3. Change of the numbers of Th17 cells in (A) SP, (B) MLN, (C) PP and (D) LP. Data represent absolute values (means ± SD, n = 4 per group on days 3 and 6, n = 6 per group on day 10, * $p<0.05$).

Intracellular calcium measurement

CHO-K1 cells stably expressing $hS1P_1$ or $hS1P_3$ were plated at 2×10^4 cells/well in 96-well plate and incubated for 2 days at 37°C in 5% CO_2/95% air. Cells were loaded with Ham's F12 medium containing 5 μM Fura2-AM and 20 mM HEPES (pH 7.4) at 37°C for 1 h. After loading, cells were washed with Hanks solution containing 20 mM HEPES (pH 7.4), and stimulated with test compounds. Fluorescence intensity was measured by the ratio of emission fluorescence at 500 nm by excitation at 340 and 380 nm using a Fluorescence Drug Screening System (FDSS-6000, Hamamatsu Photonics K.K., Shizuoka, Japan).

Mice

Six- to 7-week-old male Balb/c mice were purchased from Charles River Japan, Inc. (Kanagawa, Japan). Before use, mice were maintained in a specific pathogen-free animal facility Fat the Institute of Experimental Animal Sciences, Osaka University Graduate School of Medicine, and were kept in a room maintained at 25°C with a 12 h light/dark cycle and free access to food and water. All experiments were performed in accordance with the Guidelines for Animal Experiments of Osaka University. The protocol was approved by the Committee on the Ethics of Animal Experiments of Osaka University (approval ID: J003549-009). All surgery was performed under sevoflurane anesthesia, and all efforts were made to minimize suffering.

Drug Treatment

Colitis was induced by 2.5% w/v DSS (MW: 5000, Wako, Osaka, Japan) in drinking water for 5 days. W-061 (Ono Pharmaceutical, Osaka, Japan) was dissolved in 0.5% w/v methylcellulose solution. The drug was administered orally at a dose of 3 mg/kg/day. After induction of colitis, daily clinical assessment of colitis was performed by measuring body weight and food intake, and observing fecal properties. Mice were sacrificed on day 3, 6 or 10.

Isolation of lymphocytes

Lymphocytes were isolated from spleen (SP), mesenteric lymph nodes (MLN), Peyer's patches (PP) and lamina propria (LP) using a modification of the method reported by Atarashi *et al.* [36]. Briefly, single-cell suspensions were obtained by gently pressing the SP and MLN, filtered through 70-μm nylon meshes and suspended in HBSS (Wako) supplemented with 2% fetal bovine serum (FBS). Cells from lymphocytes were treated with RBC lysis buffer (eBioscience, San Diego, CA) before suspension. To prepare single-cell suspensions from PP, tissues were treated with RPMI 1640 (Sigma-Aldrich) containing 2% FBS and 1 mg/mL collagenase type II (Invitrogen) for 20 min at 37°C. For isolation from LP lymphocytes, intestines were opened longitudinally, washed with ice-cold PBS to remove fecal content, and were shaken in HBSS supplemented with 2% FBS and 5 mM EDTA for 20 min at 37°C. Intestines were then cut into small pieces and

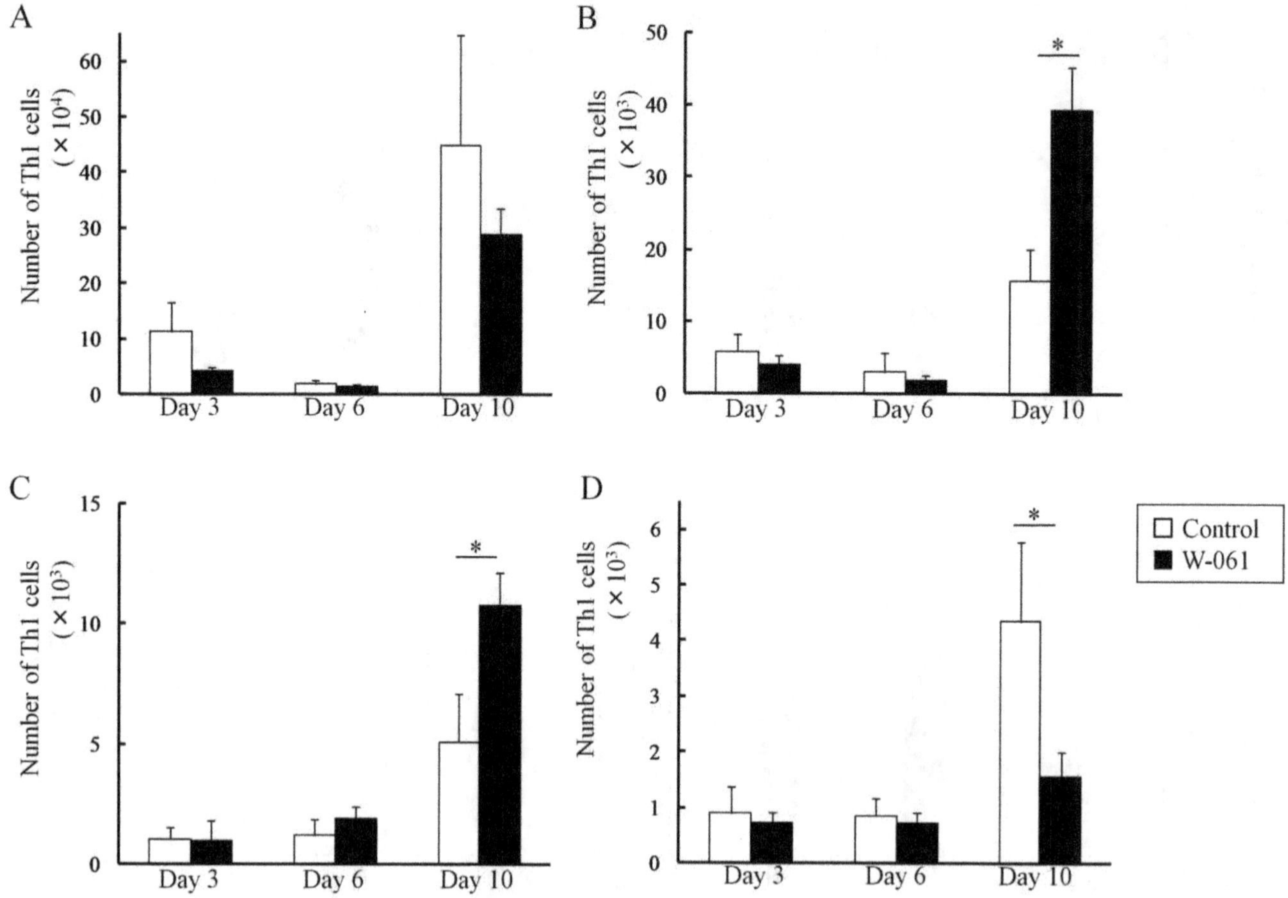

Figure 4. Change of the numbers of Th1 cells in (A) SP, (B) MLN, (C) PP and (D) LP. Data represent absolute values (means ± SD, n = 4 per group on days 3 and 6, n = 6 per group on day 10, * $p<0.05$).

shaken with RPMI 1640 containing 2% FBS and 1 mg/mL collagenase type II for 25 min at 37°C. Digested tissues were resuspended with 8 mL of 40% Percoll (GE Healthcare, Waukesha, WI) and overlaid on 4 mL of 75% Percoll. Gradient separation was performed by centrifugation at 760 × g for 20 min at 37°C. Lymphocytes were collected at the interface of the Percoll gradient, washed and suspended in RPMI 1640 containing 2% FBS.

Flow Cytometric Analysis

Anti-CD4 monoclonal antibody (mAb) (RM4-5), anti-IL-17A mAb (TC11-18H10.1), anti-IFN-γ mAb (XMG1.2) and anti-CD25 mAb (PC61) were purchased from Becton Dickinson, and anti-Foxp3 mAb (FJK-16s) was purchased from eBioscience.

Intracellular expression of IL-17, IFN-γ or Foxp3 in $CD4^+$ T cells were analyzed using a Cytofix/Cytoperm Kit (Becton Dickinson) according to the manufacturer's instructions. Briefly, lymphocytes from SP, MLN, PP or LP were incubated with 50 ng/mL phorbol myristate acetate (Sigma), 5 μM calcium ionophore (Sigma) and Golgistop (Becton Dickinson) at 37°C for 4 h.

For Th17 and Th1 determination, surface staining for lymphocytes were performed with a cocktail of fluorescently labeled anti-CD4 mAb for 30 min at 4°C. Subsequently, cells were permeabilized with Cytofix/Cytoperm for 20 min at 4°C, and intracellular cytokine staining was performed with fluorescently labeled anti-cytokine antibodies for 30 min at 4°C. Similarly, for Treg determination, lymphocytes were stained with a cocktail of fluorescently labeled anti-CD4 mAb and anti-CD25 mAb. After Cytofix/Cytoperm treatment, cells were stained with fluorescently labeled anti-Foxp3 mAb. Stained lymphocytes were analyzed on a FACSCalibur Flow Cytometer (Becton Dickinson) using Cell Quest software. Among lymphocytes, $CD4^+$ IL-17^+ cells were considered to be Th17. Similarly, $CD4^+$ IFN-γ^+ lymphocytes were considered to be Th1, and $CD4^+$ $CD25^+$ $Foxp3^+$ lymphocytes were considered to be Treg.

Histological Analysis of Colon

Histological analysis was performed on colon divided into three areas; proximal, medial and distal. Tissue was fixed in 4% paraformaldehyde in PBS and embedded in paraffin. Sections (2 μm) were prepared and stained with hematoxylin and eosin. Histopathologic changes in the colonic mucosa were semi-quantified according to a modified scoring system [18]: (a) cellular infiltration in the lamina propria (scored from 0 to 3); (b) mucin depletion (scored from 0 to 2); (c) crypt abcesses (scored from 0 to 2); (d) epithelial erosion (scored from 0 to 2); (e) hyperemia (scored from 0 to 3); and (f) thickness of mucosa (scored from 1 to 3).

Statistical analysis

All data are expressed as means ± SD. Data were analyzed by two-tailed Student's *t* test. Values of $p<0.05$ were considered to be significant.

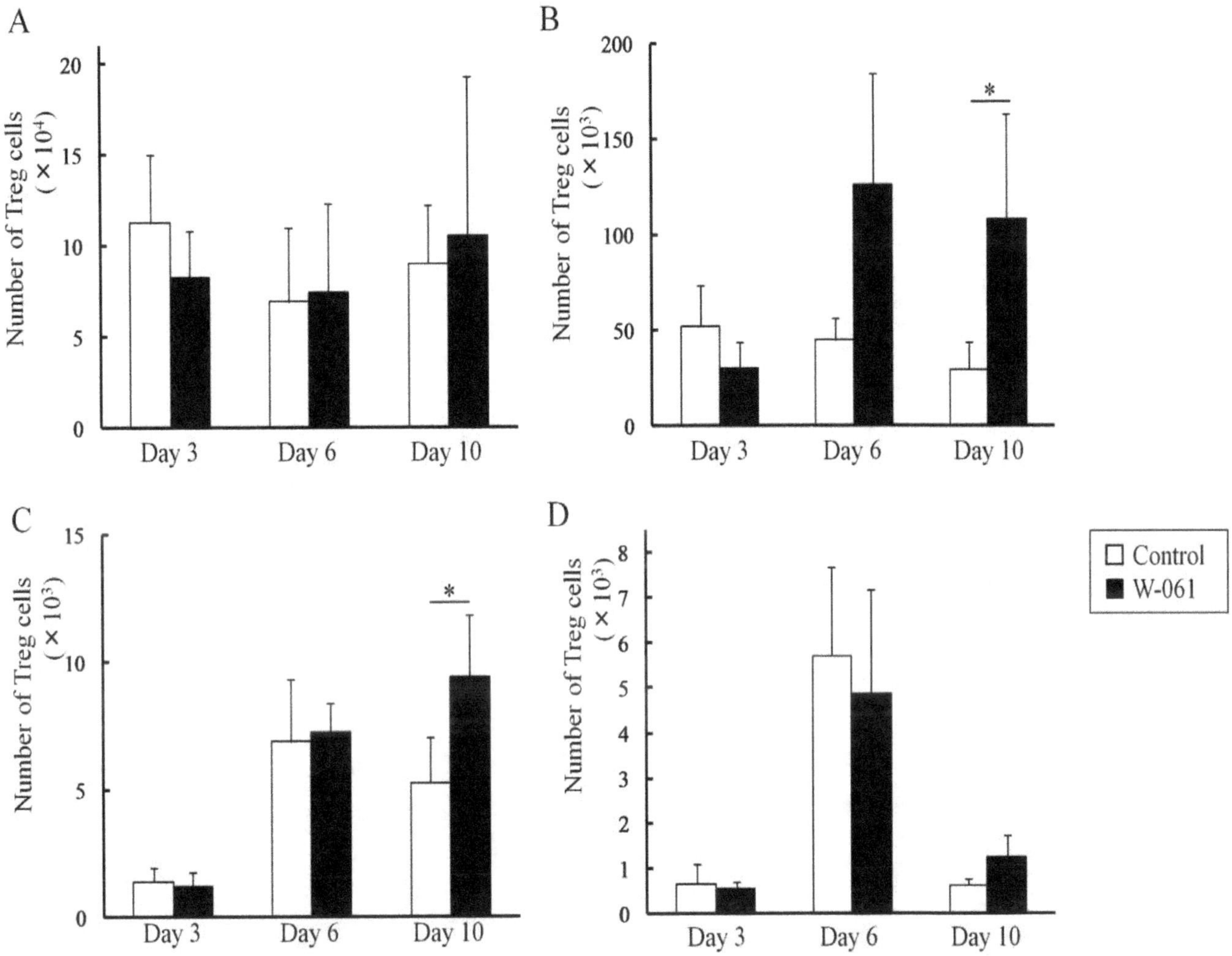

Figure 5. Change of the numbers of Treg cells in (A) SP, (B) MLN, (C) PP and (D) LP. Data represent absolute values (means ± SD, n = 4 per group on days 3 and 6, n = 6 per group on day 10, * $p<0.05$).

Acknowledgments

The authors would like to thank Satomi Yamane (Osaka University) for her technical assistance.

Author Contributions

Conceived and designed the experiments: TM YK JN TI. Performed the experiments: YS JN HH HK HM. Analyzed the data: YS TM YK JN EU TI. Contributed reagents/materials/analysis tools: HH HK HM. Wrote the paper: YS TI.

References

1. Baumgart DC (2007) Carding SR. Inflammatory bowel disease: cause and immunobiology. Lancet 369: 1627–1640.
2. Fuss IJ, Neurath M, Boirivant M, Klein JS, de la Motte C, et al. (1996) Disparate CD4+ lamina propria (LP) lymphokine secretion profiles in inflammatory bowel disease. Crohn's disease LP cells manifest increased secretion of IFN-gamma, whereas ulcerative colitis LP cells manifest increased secretion of IL-5. J Immunol 157: 1261–1270.
3. Inoue S, Matsumoto T, Iida M, Mizuno M, Kuroki F, et al. (1999) Characterization of cytokine expression in the rectal mucosa of ulcerative colitis: correlation with disease activity. Am J Gastroenterol 94: 2441–2446.
4. Colombel JF, Sandborn WJ, Reinisch W, Mantzaris GJ, Kornbluth A, et al. (2010) Infliximab, azathioprine, or combination therapy for Crohn's disease. N Engl J Med 362: 1383–1395.
5. Bongartz T, Sutton AJ, Sweeting MJ, Buchan I, Matteson EL, et al. (2006) Anti-TNF antibody therapy in rheumatoid arthritis and the risk of serious infections and malignancies: systematic review and meta-analysis of rare harmful effects in randomized controlled trials. JAMA 295: 2275–2285.
6. McGeachy MJ, Cua DJ (2008) Th17 cell differentiation: the long and winding road. Immunity 28: 445–453.
7. Tesmer LA, Lundy SK, Sarkar S, Fox DA (2008) Th17 cells in human disease. Immunol Rev 223: 87–113.
8. van den Berg WB, Miossec P (2009) IL-17 as a future therapeutic target for rheumatoid arthritis. Nat Rev Rheumatol 5: 549–553.
9. Goverman J (2009) Autoimmune T cell responses in the central nervous system. Nat Rev Immunol 9: 393–407.
10. Fujino S, Andoh A, Bamba S, Ogawa A, Hata K, et al. (2003) Increased expression of interleukin 17 in inflammatory bowel disease. Gut 52: 65–70.
11. Alex P, Zachos NC, Nguyen T, Gonzales L, Chen TE, et al. (2009) Distinct cytokine patterns identified from multiplex profiles of murine DSS and TNBS-induced colitis. Inflammm Bowel Dis 15: 341–352.
12. Ito R, Kita M, Shin-Ya M, Kishida T, Urano A, et al. (2008) Involvement of IL-17A in the pathogenesis of DSS-induced colitis in mice. Biochem Biophys Res Commun 377: 12–16.

13. Ogawa A, Andoh A, Araki Y, Bamba T, Fujiyama Y (2004) Neutralization of interleukin-17 aggravates dextran sulfate sodium-induced colitis in mice. Clin Immunol 110: 55–62.
14. Leppkes M, Becker C, Ivanov II, Hirth S, Wirtz S, et al. (2009) RORgamma-expressing Th17 cells induce murine chronic intestinal inflammation via redundant effects of IL-17A and IL-17F. Gastroenterology 136: 257–267.
15. O'Connor W Jr., Kamanaka M, Booth CJ, Town T, Nakae S, et al. (2009) A protective function for interleukin 17A in T cell-mediated intestinal inflammation. Nat Immunol 10: 603–609.
16. Sakaguchi S, Yamaguchi T, Nomura T, Ono M (2008) Regulatory T cells and immune tolerance. Cell 133: 775–787.
17. Makita S, Kanai T, Nemoto Y, Totsuka T, Okamoto R, et al. (2007) Intestinal lamina propria retaining CD4+CD25+ regulatory T cells is a suppressive site of intestinal inflammation. J Immunol 178: 4937–4946.
18. Brinkmann V, Davis MD, Heise CE, Albert R, Cottens S, et al. (2002) The immune modulator FTY720 targets sphingosine 1-phosphate receptors. J Biol Chem 277: 21453–21457.
19. Kappos L, Radue EW, O'Connor P, Polman C, Hohlfeld R, et al. (2010) A placebo-controlled trial of oral fingolimod in relapsing multiple sclerosis. N Engl J Med 362: 387–401.
20. Mizushima T, Ito T, Kishi D, Kai Y, Tamagawa H, et al. (2004) Therapeutic effects of a new lymphocyte homing reagent FTY720 in interleukin-10 gene-deficient mice with colitis. Inflamm Bowel Dis 10: 182–192.
21. Deguchi Y, Andoh A, Yagi Y, Bamba S, Inatomi O, et al. (2006) The S1P receptor modulator FTY720 prevents the development of experimental colitis in mice. Oncol Rep 16: 699–703.
22. Song J, Matsuda C, Kai Y, Nishida T, Nakajima K, et al. (2007) A novel sphingosine 1-phosphate receptor agonist, 2-amino-2-propanediol hydrochloride (KRP-203), regulates chronic colitis in interleukin-10 gene-deficient mice. J Pharmacol Exp Ther 324: 276–283.
23. Ohno T, Hasegawa C, Nakade S, Kitagawa J, Honda N, et al. (2010) The prediction of human response to ONO-4641, a sphingosine 1-phosphate receptor modulator, from preclinical data based on pharmacokinetic-pharmacodynamic modeling. Biopharm Drug Dispos 31: 396–406.
24. Pinschewer DD, Ochsenbein AF, Odermatt B, Brinkmann V, Hengartner H, et al. (2000) FTY720 immunosuppression impairs effector T cell peripheral homing without affecting induction, expansion, and memory. J Immunol 164: 5761–5770.
25. Lee TK, Man K, Ho JW, Sun CK, Ng KT, et al. (2004) FTY720 induces apoptosis of human hepatoma cell lines through PI3-K-mediated Akt dephosphorylation. Carcinogenesis 25: 2397–2405.
26. Lee TK, Man K, Ho JW, Wang XH, Poon RT, et al. (2005) Significance of the Rac signaling pathway in HCC cell motility: implications for a new therapeutic target. Carcinogenesis 26: 681–687.
27. Matloubian M, Lo CG, Cinamon G, Lesneski MJ, Xu Y, et al. (2004) Lymphocyte egress from thymus and peripheral lymphoid organs is dependent on S1P receptor 1. Nature 427: 355–360.
28. Kappos L, Antel J, Comi G, Montalban X, O'Connor P, et al. (2006) Oral fingolimod (FTY720) for relapsing multiple sclerosis. N Engl J Med 355: 1124–1140.
29. Sanna MG, Liao J, Jo E, Alfonso C, Ahn MY, et al. (2004) Sphingosine 1-phosphate (S1P) receptor subtypes S1P1 and S1P3, respectively, regulate lymphocyte recirculation and heart rate. J Biol Chem 279: 13839–13848.
30. Neurath MF, Fuss I, Kelsall BL, Presky DH, Waegell W, et al. (1996) Experimental granulomatous colitis in mice is abrogated by induction of TGF-beta-mediated oral tolerance. J Exp Med 183: 2605–2616.
31. Oppmann B, Lesley R, Blom B, Timans JC, Xu Y, et al. (2000) Novel p19 protein engages IL-12p40 to form a cytokine, IL-23, with biological activities similar as well as distinct from IL-12. Immunity 13: 715–725.
32. Asseman C, Mauze S, Leach MW, Coffman RL, Powrie F (1999) An essential role for interleukin 10 in the function of regulatory T cells that inhibit intestinal inflammation. J Exp Med 190: 995–1004.
33. Förster R, Schubel A, Breitfeld D, Kremmer E, Renner-Müller I, et al. (1999) CCR7 coordinates the primary immune response by establishing functional microenvironments in secondary lymphoid organs. Cell 99: 23–33.
34. Menning A, Höpken UE, Siegmund K, Lipp M, Hamann A, et al. (2007) Distinctive role of CCR7 in migration and functional activity of naive- and effector/memory-like Treg subsets. Eur J Immunol 37: 1575–1583.
35. Mandala S, Hajdu R, Bergstrom J, Quackenbush E, Xie J, et al. (2002) Alteration of lymphocyte trafficking by sphingosine-1-phosphate receptor agonists. Science 296: 346–349.
36. Atarashi K, Nishimura J, Shima T, Umesaki Y, Yamamoto M, et al. (2008) ATP drives lamina propria T(H)17 cell differentiation. Nature 455: 808–812.

14

Multivariate Modeling Identifies Neutrophil- and Th17-Related Factors as Differential Serum Biomarkers of Chronic Murine Colitis

Megan E. McBee[1,3]*, Yu Zeng[1], Nicola Parry[2], Cathryn R. Nagler[3], Steven R. Tannenbaum[1], David B. Schauer[1,2†]

1 Biological Engineering Department, Massachusetts Institute of Technology, Cambridge, Massachusetts, United States of America, **2** Division of Comparative Medicine, Massachusetts Institute of Technology, Cambridge, Massachusetts, United States of America, **3** Department of Pathology, The University of Chicago, Chicago, Illinois, United States of America

Abstract

Background: Diagnosis of chronic intestinal inflammation, which characterizes inflammatory bowel disease (IBD), along with prediction of disease state is hindered by the availability of predictive serum biomarker. Serum biomarkers predictive of disease state will improve trials for therapeutic intervention, and disease monitoring, particularly in genetically susceptible individuals. Chronic inflammation during IBD is considered distinct from infectious intestinal inflammation thereby requiring biomarkers to provide differential diagnosis. To address whether differential serum biomarkers could be identified in murine models of colitis, immunological profiles from both chronic spontaneous and acute infectious colitis were compared and predictive serum biomarkers identified via multivariate modeling.

Methodology/Principal Findings: Discriminatory multivariate modeling of 23 cytokines plus chlorotyrosine and nitrotyrosine (protein adducts from reactive nitrogen species and hypochlorite) in serum and tissue from two murine models of colitis was performed to identify disease-associated biomarkers. Acute *C. rodentium*-induced colitis in C57BL/6J mice and chronic spontaneous *Helicobacter*-dependent colitis in TLR4$^{-/-}$ x IL-10$^{-/-}$ mice were utilized for evaluation. Colon profiles of both colitis models were nearly identical with chemokines, neutrophil- and Th17-related factors highly associated with intestinal disease. In acute colitis, discriminatory disease-associated serum factors were not those identified in the colon. In contrast, the discriminatory predictive serum factors for chronic colitis were neutrophil- and Th17-related factors (KC, IL-12/23p40, IL-17, G-CSF, and chlorotyrosine) that were also elevated in colon tissue. Chronic colitis serum biomarkers were specific to chronic colitis as they were not discriminatory for acute colitis.

Conclusions/Significance: Immunological profiling revealed strikingly similar colon profiles, yet distinctly different serum profiles for acute and chronic colitis. Neutrophil- and Th17-related factors were identified as predictive serum biomarkers of chronic colitis, but not acute colitis, despite their presence in colitic tissue of both diseases thereby demonstrating the utility of mathematical modeling for identifying disease-associated serum biomarkers.

Editor: Aric Gregson, University of California Los Angeles, United States of America

Funding: National Institutes of Health grants P01 CA026731 (YZ, SRT, DBS), DK 55678 (CRN), and the Singapore-MIT Alliance for Research and Technology-Infectious Diseases (MEM, DBS) supported this work. Additional facilities and instrument support were provided by the United States Army Research Office through the Institute for Soldier Nanotechnologies at Massachusetts Institute of Technology (MIT), the National Institutes of Health for Environmental Health Sciences at MIT, and an equipment loan from Agilent Technologies. The funders had no role in study design, data collection and analysis, decision to publish, or preparation of the manuscript.

Competing Interests: The authors have declared that no competing interests exist.

* E-mail: mmcbee@bsd.uchicago.edu

†Deceased.

Introduction

Intestinal inflammation develops from known causes such as infection with enteropathogenic *E. coli* (EPEC) or from unknown causes as in inflammatory bowel diseases (IBD). Compared to the chronic idiopathic intestinal inflammation that occurs in IBD patients, intestinal infections cause acute colitis that is resolved by host defenses. A need for biomarkers that predict the presence and severity of intestinal disease remains despite the individual association of several non-disease related proteins (such as C-reactive protein or antibodies against *E. coli* OmpC and glycans) with chronic intestinal disease [1–6]. Identification of disease-relevant serum biomarkers discriminating chronic colitis from other conditions, such as acute infectious colitis, or biomarkers identifying relative disease severity allowing non-invasive monitoring of disease progression and responsiveness to therapeutic treatments remain elusive.

To examine immunological factors associated with both acute and chronic intestinal disease, two murine models, one of acute infectious colitis and the other of chronic spontaneous colitis, were studied. *Citrobacter rodentium*, a murine pathogen that recapitulates much of the pathology seen in human EPEC infection, causes acute infectious colitis. *C. rodentium*-induced colitis is characterized by epithelial hyperplasia, erosion and destruction of the epithelial brush border, edema, and inflammation [7]. In C57BL/6 mice, *C. rodentium* infection is self-resolving with pathology peaking at 2 weeks post-infection (WPI) and disease resolution by 4-6 WPI [8]. Immune mediators in *C. rodentium*-induced colitis have been extensively studied in mice with targeted knockouts of innate and adaptive cells, as well as cytokines, cytokine receptors, and pattern recognition receptors. These studies have shown that bacterial clearance and disease resolution require both protective antibodies and an IFN-γ mediated T effector cell response [9–12] whereas other immunological mediators prevent early mortality through maintenance of epithelial barrier function [13–16]. Th17 cells are generated in abundance during infection, with IL-17 production peaking with maximal disease; however IL-17 is not required for survival or bacterial clearance and its role in disease pathogenesis is still not well understood [8,13,17]. The common finding of these studies has been the identification of a robust inflammatory response in the colon characterized by the increased production of the inflammatory mediators TNF-α, IFN-γ, IL-1β, IL-17, and IL-6.

In contrast to acute *C. rodentium*-induced colitis, chronic spontaneous typhlocolitis develops in IL-$10^{-/-}$ mice colonized with *Helicobacter spp.* [18]. *Helicobacter spp.*-positive (Hsp^+) IL-$10^{-/-}$ mice also deficient in TLR4 (TLR$4^{-/-}$ x IL-$10^{-/-}$ [DKO]) exhibit earlier onset and increased severity of typhlocolitis, which is dependent upon infection with *Helicobacter spp.* [19]. Interestingly, inflammatory mediators in colonic cultures from colitic DKO mice were similar to those found in colon tissue during acute *C. rodentium*-induced colitis: TNF-α, IFN-γ, IL-1β, IL-17, and IL-6 [19]. Therefore, a comprehensive study comparing the direct ex-vivo colonic cytokine protein profile with matched serum cytokine profile from the two forms of murine colitis was conducted in order to identify predictors of intestinal disease severity, specifically potential serum biomarkers of chronic intestinal inflammation. The protein adducts nitrotyrosine (NT) and chlorotyrosine (CT) along with 23 cytokines, measured in serum and colon of wild type C57BL/6J mice with acute infectious *C. rodentium*-induced colitis and DKO mice with chronic spontaneous *Helicobacter*-dependent typhlocolitis, were evaluated for their discriminatory power and ability to predict intestinal disease severity, and thereby their potential usefulness as biomarkers.

Results

Robust, comparable colitis in acute infectious and chronic spontaneous models

Infection with *C. rodentium* was monitored for 14 days post-infection (DPI) with peak bacterial burdens of 9×10^8 CFU/g feces at 4 DPI, **Figure S1A**. Development of disease was monitored by change in body weight with *C. rodentium* infected (Cr^+) mice losing 3% of initial body weight by 14 DPI compared with uninfected mice gaining 4% ($P<0.01$, **Figure S1B**). At 14 DPI histological findings included increased inflammatory infiltrates, epithelial defects, edema, hyperplasia, and dysplasia (**Figure 1A and 1B**). These five categorical lesions were scored and summed to form the histologic activity index (HAI). Marked colitis was present in Cr^+ mice (**Figure 1A and 1B**) with a median HAI of 8.0 (range 3.5 to 9.5), compared with 0.25 (0–1.0) in uninfected mice.

The age of onset of chronic spontaneous colitis in Hsp^+ DKO mice is variable, therefore colitis was evaluated when >30% of mice have rectal prolapse [19]. Gross evaluation revealed no disease in Hsp^- DKO mice, whereas Hsp^+ DKO mice had poor body condition with colonic and cecal thickening. Histological findings were similar to acute colitis (**Figure 1C and 1D**) plus focal gland herniation into the muscularis mucosa in 3 of 10 mice.

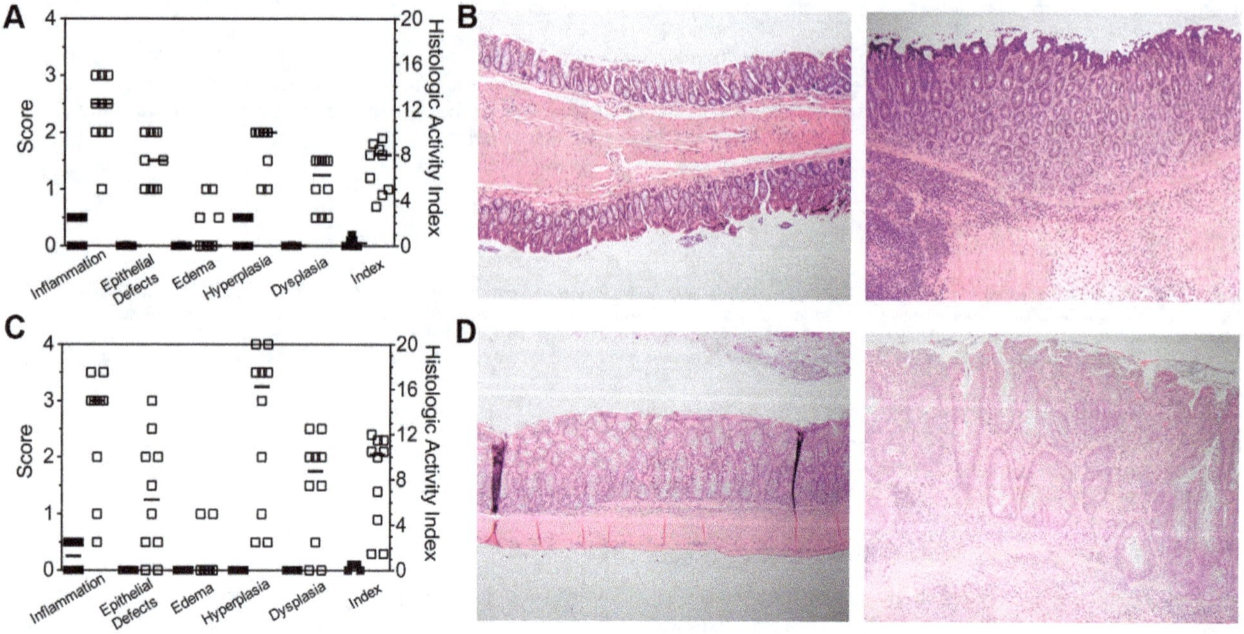

Figure 1. Marked colitis in *C. rodentium* infected and aged TLR$4^{-/-}$ x IL-$10^{-/-}$ (DKO) mice colonized with *Helicobacter* spp. Histological scores for inflammation, epithelial defects, edema, hyperplasia, and dysplasia in the colon for uninfected (Cr^-, ■) and *C. rodentium* infected (Cr^+, □) mice at 14 DPI (A) and *Helicobacter spp.* negative (Hsp^-, ■) or positive (Hsp^+, □) aged DKO mice (C). All scores were summed to form the histological activity index for individual mice. All pairings are *** $P<0.0001$ by Mann-Whitney test. (B) Representative H&E stained colon section from Cr^- (left panel) and Cr^+ (right panel) mice at 14 DPI. (D) Representative H&E stained colon section from Hsp^- (left panel) and Hsp^+ (right panel) DKO mice. Original magnification 100×.

Hsp^- mice had a median HAI of 0.5 (range 0–0.5) while Hsp^+ mice had a median HAI of 10.25 (range 1.5–12), **Figure 1C**.

Local and systemic cytokine profiles in acute colitis indicate robust inflammation

The complex colonic cytokine milieu present during peak severity of acute *C. rodentium* colitis has not previously been analyzed in detail at the protein level. To gain additional biological insight into the active disease process 23 cytokines from frozen full-thickness colon sections at 14 DPI were analyzed. Chemokines KC and MCP-1 and the cytokines IL-1β, IL-6, IL-12/23p40, and IL-17 were elevated in colon tissue of Cr^+ mice, **Figure 2A**, confirming previous studies performed at the mRNA level [8,13,14,20]. Newly identified factors induced by *C. rodentium* infection are cytokines associated with T cell and neutrophil proliferation (IL-2 and G-CSF) and chemokines (RANTES, MIP-1α, and MIP-1β), **Figure 2A and Figure S2A**. Of the 23 cytokines measured only five were significantly elevated in the serum at 14 DPI, **Figure 2B and Figure S2B**. Of note was the elevation of IFN-γ in serum indicating, perhaps, a broader systemic role for this cytokine in disease resolution. Chemotactic and proliferation promoting cytokines G-CSF, IL-2, and RANTES were elevated in serum in addition to tissue, **Figure 2B**, indicating that the presence of acute intestinal inflammation is detectable both locally and systemically.

Tissue cytokines in chronic typhlocolitis mimic acute colitis and are represented in serum

Unlike *C. rodentium* colitis where inflammation develops within 2 weeks, chronic *Helicobacter*-dependent typhlocolitis develops over several months without resolving. The gradual recruitment and activation of immune cells to the intestines in chronic colitis, as well as the lack of TLR4 and IL-10 signaling, suggests activation of immune pathways and secretion of cytokines that might differ from acute colitis. Surprisingly, the cytokines elevated in colon tissue of Hsp^+ DKO mice with chronic colitis compared with Hsp^- DKO mice mirrored those in acute colitis, **Figure 3A and Figure S3A**. This finding suggests that in chronic colitis not only is there sustained activation of acute inflammatory pathways, but also the continual presence and recruitment to the mucosa of the same cell types observed in acute colitis. In contrast to acute colitis, serum cytokines elevated in mice with chronic colitis were representative of those elevated in tissue: IL-6, IL-12/23p40, IL-17, G-CSF, and KC, **Figure 3B**. The combined elevation of these neutrophil- and Th17-associated factors in serum and tissue imply functional roles for these cells in chronic intestinal disease.

Elevation of protein adducts from reactive nitrogen species and hypochlorite in colitic mice

Upon microbial activation, numerous reactive chemical species are produced by innate immune cells (including macrophages, neutrophils, and epithelial cells). Nitric oxide (NO) reacts with

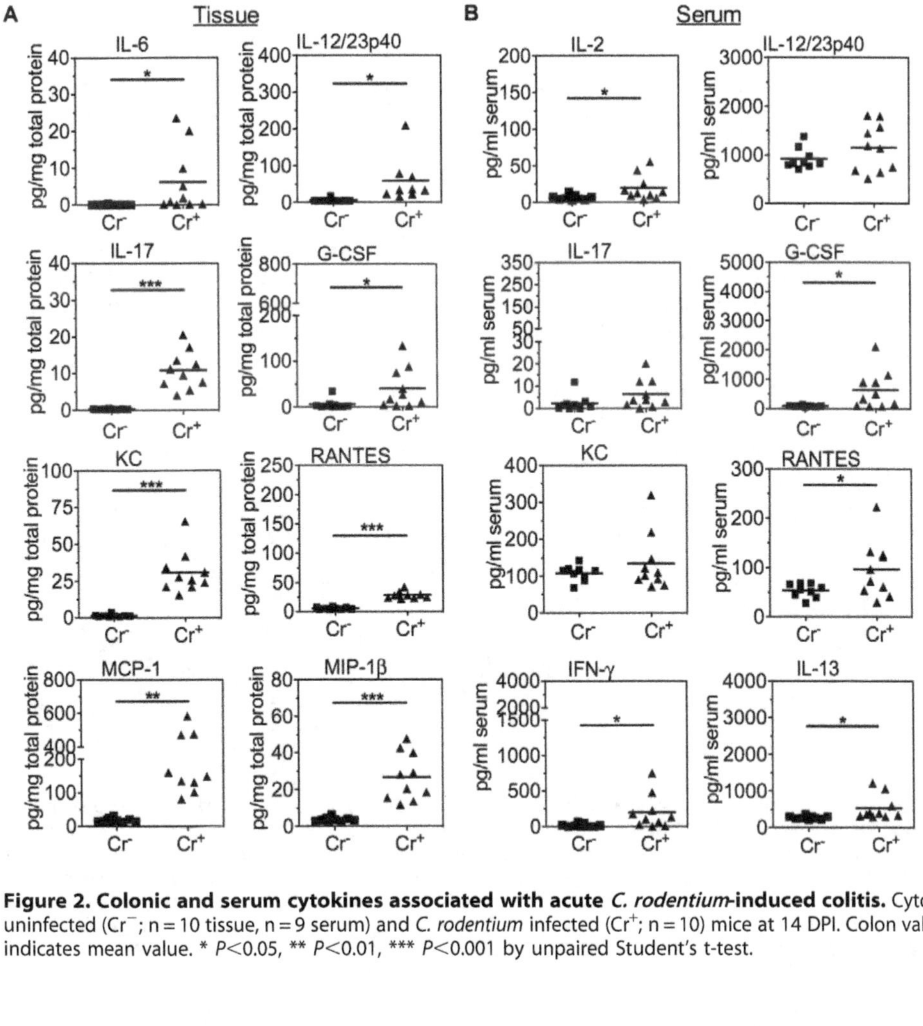

Figure 2. Colonic and serum cytokines associated with acute *C. rodentium*-induced colitis. Cytokines in colon tissue (A) and serum (B) of uninfected (Cr^-; n = 10 tissue, n = 9 serum) and *C. rodentium* infected (Cr^+; n = 10) mice at 14 DPI. Colon values were normalized to total protein. Line indicates mean value. * $P<0.05$, ** $P<0.01$, *** $P<0.001$ by unpaired Student's t-test.

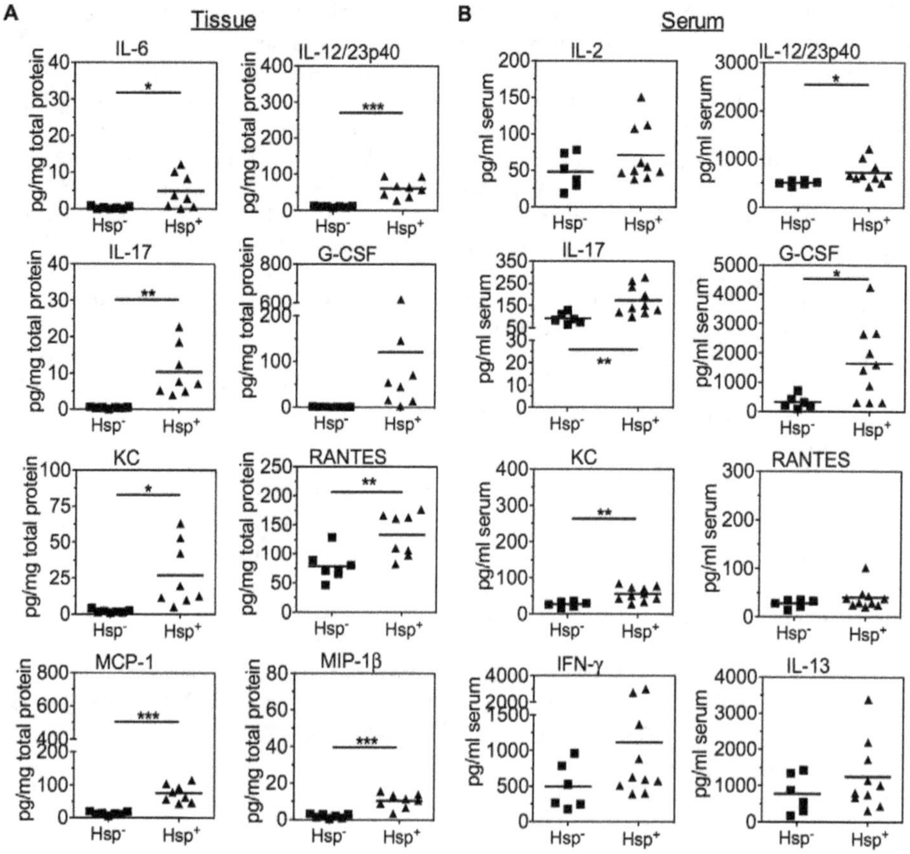

Figure 3. Colonic and serum cytokines associated with chronic *Helicobacter*-dependent colitis. Cytokines in colon tissue (A) and serum (B) in *Helicobacter*-free (Hsp$^-$; n=6) and *Helicobacter spp.*-positive (Hsp$^+$; n=8 tissue, n=10 serum) TLR4$^{-/-}$ x IL-10$^{-/-}$ mice. Colon values were normalized to total protein. Line indicates mean value. * $P<0.05$, ** $P<0.01$, *** $P<0.001$ by unpaired Student's t-test.

superoxide to form peroxynitrite, which can then react with tyrosine to form nitrotyrosine adducts (NT) [21]. Epithelial cells and colonic macrophages increase their production of NO during both acute *C. rodentium*-induced colitis and chronic *Helicobacter*-dependent colitis, although the relative contribution of NO from each cell type is unclear [22–25]. Therefore, NT was measured in colonic lysates as a marker for both macrophage infiltration and epithelial activation. NT levels in colons of Cr$^+$ mice were comparable to uninfected mice, **Figure 4A**. Despite the robust chronic inflammation in Hsp$^+$ DKO mice, there was no difference in NT levels compared with Hsp$^-$ DKO mice, **Figure 4A**. NT was also measured in serum as a biomarker for peripheral tissue inflammation. In contrast to tissue, serum NT levels were significantly elevated in Cr$^+$ mice when compared to the low levels detected in uninfected mice, **Figure 4B**. However, chronically inflamed DKO mice had no significant difference in serum NT, **Figure 4B**. Despite the presence of increased iNOS and NO during disease, protein adducts of other

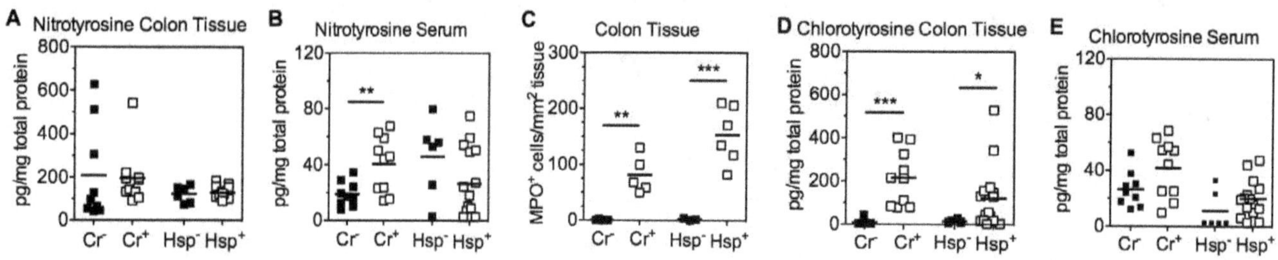

Figure 4. MPO-expressing cells in colon and level of protein adducts chlorotyrosine and nitrotyrosine in colon tissue and serum of both *C. rodentium* infected mice and Hsp$^+$ TLR4$^{-/-}$ x IL-10$^{-/-}$ (DKO) mice. Nitrotyrosine levels in colon tissue (A) and serum (B) of uninfected (Cr$^-$; n=10 for tissue, n=9 for serum) C57BL/6J mice, *C. rodentium* infected (Cr$^+$; n=10) C57BL/6J mice at 14 DPI, *Helicobacter*-negative (Hsp$^-$; n=6) DKO mice and *Helicobacter*-positive (Hsp$^+$; n=15) DKO mice at 20–35 weeks of age. (C) MPO$^+$ cells in colon tissue of Cr$^-$, Cr$^+$, Hsp$^-$, and Hsp$^+$ (n=5 per group) were counted in ten high power (40×) fields of colon tissue per mouse and averaged. Chlorotyrosine levels in colon tissue (D) and serum (E) from Cr$^-$ (n =10 for tissue, n=9 for serum), Cr$^+$ (n=10), Hsp$^-$ DKO (n=6) and Hsp$^+$ DKO (n=15). Adduct concentrations (A, B, D, E) were normalized to total protein in each sample. Line indicates mean value. * $P<0.05$, ** $P<0.01$, *** $P<0.001$ by unpaired Student's t-test.

reactive nitrogen and oxygen species may provide better markers for chronic colitis.

Myeloperoxidase (MPO), the predominant protein in neutrophils involved with reactive oxygen species, generates hypochlorous acid from chloride ions and hydrogen peroxide [26]. Hypochlorous acid, in addition to killing bacteria, reacts with tyrosyl protein residues to form the stable adduct 3-chlorotyrosine (CT) [27]. Neutrophils are required for recovery from *C. rodentium*-induced colitis with both recruitment and MPO production peaking at 2 WPI [20,28]. In the present study, MPO^+ cells were not present in colons of either uninfected C57BL/6J or Hsp^- DKO mice **Figure 4C**, whereas colon tissue from both Cr^+ C57BL/6J and Hsp^+ DKO mice had significant increases in MPO^+ cells, **Figure 4C**. As a biomarker of neutrophil presence and activity CT was measured in colon and serum. In agreement with the MPO staining, CT levels in colon from both uninfected C57BL/6J and Hsp^- DKO mice were low, **Figure 4D**, indicating minimal presence of neutrophils in non-colitic mice. A pronounced increase in CT was found in colons of both colitic Cr^+ mice and Hsp^+ DKO mice, **Figure 4D**. Serum CT was elevated in mice with either acute or chronic colitis compared with non-colitic mice, **Figure 4E**, but these increases did not reach statistical significance.

Tissue and serum factors discriminate colitic from non-colitic mice

PLS-DA (Partial Least Squares Projection to Latent Structures-Discriminant Analysis) was used to determine the variables with the highest discriminatory power for colitic and non-colitic mice. For each type of colitis (acute and chronic) two separate PLS-DA models were generated: one with factors collected non-invasively (*serum*) using serum cytokine, CT, and NT levels and a second model (*tissue*) of invasively collected factors using colon tissue cytokine, CT, and NT levels. The acute *serum* model did not discriminate colitic from non-colitic mice with only 45.7% of the class distinction explained by the model's components, and only 32.9% of the variance among samples explained by the model, **Table 1**. The most influential factors or variables of importance (VIP) in the model included: NT, CT, recruitment and proliferation cytokines IL-2, G-CSF and RANTES, and a mix of T cell cytokines (IL-4, IL-17, IL-13, and IFN-γ), **Table 2**. The chronic *serum* model was able to discriminate colitic Hsp^+ DKO mice from Hsp^- DKO mice with 84.0% of the class distinction and 69.1% of the variance explained by the model, **Table 1**. Most influential factors in the chronic *serum* model were significantly elevated and associated with both neutrophils and Th17 cells (KC, IL-17, IL-12/23p40, and G-CSF), **Table 2**.

Although discrimination of colitic from non-colitic mice by non-invasive factors is ideal, as a proof of principle for discriminatory modeling and to gain biological insight into the mucosal disease process *tissue* PLS-DA models were generated using the colon levels of the factors. Compared with the acute *serum* model, the acute *tissue* PLS-DA model was highly discriminatory with 99.1% of the class distinction and 94.8% of the variance accounted for by the components, **Table 1**. Two dominant clusters were present in the VIPs: chemokines, and neutrophil/Th17-associated factors, **Table 2**. The chemokine cluster (MCP-1, MIP-1α, MIP-1β, RANTES, and KC) agrees with the state of active, rather than resolving, acute colitis at 14 DPI in the Cr^+ mice. The other cluster, neutrophil/Th17-associated factors, included CT, KC, IL-1β, IL-6, IL-12/23p40, G-CSF and IL-17; in concordance with the influx and importance of both Th17 cells and neutrophils in the resolution of *C. rodentium* infection [13,17,20,28]. In the chronic *tissue* model 98.4% of the class distinction and 89.5% of the variance in the factors were explained by the model, demonstrating that non-colitic Hsp^- DKO mice could be distinguished from Hsp^+ DKO colitic mice, **Table 1**. The chronic *tissue* model VIPs, **Table 2**, also include a chemokine cluster (MCP-1, MIP-1β, RANTES, and KC) as well as a neutrophil/Th17-associated cluster (KC, IL-1β, IL-6, IL-12/23p40, and IL-17). The combined findings from colon tissue during acute and chronic colitis indicate that the presence of activated neutrophils and Th17 cells have a strong predictive value for the presence of both acute and chronic colitis.

Serum neutrophil- and Th17-associated factors discriminate acute from chronic colitis and predict disease severity

Although variables may discriminate between colitic and non-colitic mice, they may not be able to predict the severity of individual lesions (inflammation, epithelial defects, edema, hyperplasia, and dysplasia) in one multivariate model. By generating a PLS model with a training set of data including both X (cytokines/adducts) and Y (lesions) variables, and then using this model on another data set of X variables only (prediction set), the predictive ability of the X variables and the model to output accurate Y values can be assessed. PLS prediction models were generated using the corresponding VIPs for acute colitis *serum* or *tissue* and chronic colitis *serum* or *tissue*. For training and prediction sets, samples were randomly divided into two groups of equal size (n = 8-10) including non-colitic and colitic mice. Despite the small training set size, each of the VIP PLS models were able to accurately predict individual lesion scores and disease severity for

Table 1. PLS-DA component contributions to discrimination (R^2 Y) and variance (Q^2) of colitic and non-colitic mice.

Acute Serum					**Chronic Serum**				
Component	**R^2 Y**	**R^2 Y (cumulative)**	**Q^2**	**Q^2 (cumulative)**	**Component**	**R^2 Y**	**R^2 Y (cumulative)**	**Q^2**	**Q^2 (cumulative)**
1	0.457	**0.457**	0.329	**0.329**	1	0.415	0.415	0.246	0.246
					2	0.425	**0.840**	0.590	**0.691**
Acute Colon					**Chronic Colon**				
Component	**R^2 Y**	**R^2 Y (cumulative)**	**Q^2**	**Q^2 (cumulative)**	**Component**	**R^2 Y**	**R^2 Y (cumulative)**	**Q^2**	**Q^2 (cumulative)**
1	0.883	0.883	0.829	0.829	1	0.832	0.832	0.798	0.798
2	0.056	0.939	0.368	0.892	2	0.073	0.905	0.207	0.840
3	0.052	**0.991**	0.524	**0.948**	3	0.079	**0.984**	0.344	**0.895**

Table 2. Most influential variables in acute and chronic colitis serum and colon tissue PLS-DA models by Variable of Importance in Projection (VIP) values.

Acute Serum														
Variable	G-CSF	NT	IL-2	IFN-γ	IL-4	IL-13	RANTES	IL-17	CT					
VIP	1.82	1.64	1.59	1.5	1.41	1.33	1.29	1.24	1.17					
Acute Colon														
Variable	KC	RANTES	IL-12/23p40	IL-1β	MIP-1β	MCP-1	IL-17	MIP-1α	IL-6	CT	IL-4			
VIP	1.48	1.44	1.43	1.40	1.39	1.28	1.26	1.23	1.18	1.18	1.14			
Chronic Serum														
Variable	Eotaxin	IL-12/23p40	KC	IL-17	G-CSF	IL-6								
VIP	1.51	1.45	1.42	1.17	1.16	1.03								
Chronic Colon														
Variable	IL-17	G-CSF	KC	IL-1β	IL-12/23p40	MCP-1	MIP-1β	IL-4	IL-9	IL-13	RANTES	IL-1α	IL-2	IL-6
VIP	1.38	1.26	1.21	1.19	1.17	1.16	1.12	1.10	1.06	1.06	1.05	1.04	1.00	1.00

their complementary samples, **Figure 5A**. The false positive and false negative rates were low for each of the models: 0/5 and 2/5 in acute *serum*, 0/5 and 0/5 in acute *tissue*, 1/4 and 0/4 in chronic *serum*, and 1/4 and 0/4 in chronic *tissue*. An increased training set size could further increase the accuracy of the models, particularly for the lower range of scores.

Next, to determine whether a smaller set of serum factors were predictive biomarkers of colitis, the serum models were refined to a minimal number of input factors that retained predictive and discriminatory power for intestinal lesion scores. In addition, the models were assessed for their specificity to acute and chronic colitis. Given that colonic disease is generally not isolated to one or two lesions, predicted lesion scores were summed to form predicted HAI. The refined acute *serum* model included: RANTES, NT, G-CSF, and IFN-g. This PLS model had a false positive rate of 0% (0/4) and a false negative rate of 40% (2/5) for acute colitis samples, similar to the larger VIP model, **Figure 5B**. However, when the prediction set was chronic serum samples this acute colitis *serum* model failed to discriminate colitic from non-colitic mice or accurately predict severity, with a false positive rate of 100% (9/9) and a false negative rate of 0% (0/8), **Figure 5B**. Correlation of actual versus predicted HAI confirmed the lack of utility of the acute PLS model with Spearman r's of 0.427 and 0.389 for acute and chronic samples, respectively, and P>0.1 for both sample sets. Therefore, the acute colitis serum biomarker model did not accurately predict either acute or chronic colitis due to a high false negative rate (acute) or false positive rate (chronic).

The predictive chronic colitis *serum* model was refined to consist of G-CSF, KC, IL-17, and IL12/23p40, plus CT as an additional marker specific to neutrophils. This refined model based on chronic serum had a false negative rate of 0% (0 of 3), **Figure 5B**. One mouse with minimal disease was predicted to have moderate colitis, a false positive rate of 25% (1 of 4), however this mouse was Hsp^+ and would likely develop more severe colitis. Correlation analysis confirmed that the chronic PLS model accurately predicted disease in mice prone to chronic colitis with a Spearman r of 0.991 (P<0.001). To test the specificity of this model for chronic versus acute colitis, acute serum was input into the model. The false positive rate was 100% (4/4) with all uninfected mice predicted to have an HAI>5.0 and the false negative rate was 0% (0/10) as the HAI was over predicted for all mice with acute colitis, **Figure 5B**. Spearman correlation for the predicted HAI of acute samples using the chronic PLS model was not significant (r = 0.417, P = 0.08). This outcome demonstrates the utility of PLS modeling of serum biomarkers in predicting both presence and severity of colitis. In particular, chronic colitis was distinguished from acute colitis via five neutrophil- and Th17-related factors in serum that predict the presence of intestinal disease and severity of lesions even with a small cohort.

Discussion

Whether caused by microbes or an unknown etiology, the complex cytokine milieu of an intestinal inflammatory response provides a plethora of information about the current disease state. Comprehensive measurement and deconvolution of these potential biomarkers via multivariate analysis allows predictions of disease state and evaluation of therapeutic endpoints. In this proof of principle study immunologic parameters in serum and tissue were evaluated for their utility in modeling and predicting severity of histological lesions and colon disease severity from two forms of microbial-induced colitis: acute *C. rodentium* colitis and chronic *Helicobacter*-dependent colitis.

Tissue-specific cytokine profiling is one approach to diagnosing disease severity, however utility of identified factors as biomarkers of disease is low due to feasibility of repeated sample collection. In mice, tissue cytokine profiling of *C. rodentium*-induced colitis confirmed many previous findings at either the protein or mRNA level. Elevation of other cytokines previously reported in *C. rodentium* colitis, such as IFN-γ and TNF-α, were not detected perhaps due to normalization methods or mRNA versus translated protein abundance [8,9,13,28]. Elevated cytokines in both *C. rodentium*-induced colitis and *Helicobacter*-dependent colitis are also increased in colon tissue of chemically-induced murine colitis, as well as human IBD biopsies [29–35]. Acute infectious colitis is often considered a different disease process than chronic spontaneous colitis. This study demonstrates that intestinal inflammation from different etiologies may contain more similarities than differences. The most striking commonality is the presence of neutrophils and Th17 cells, two cell types reciprocally recruited by IL-17, G-CSF, and chemokines [36-38]. This reciprocity leads to an unending cycle that can only be disrupted by the clearance of the microbial inducer (i.e. *C. rodentium*, or *Helicobacter spp.*), which does not occur with *Helicobacter spp.* causing chronic inflammation. In both models, the anti-microbial action of neutrophils leads to breakdown of the extracellular matrix and

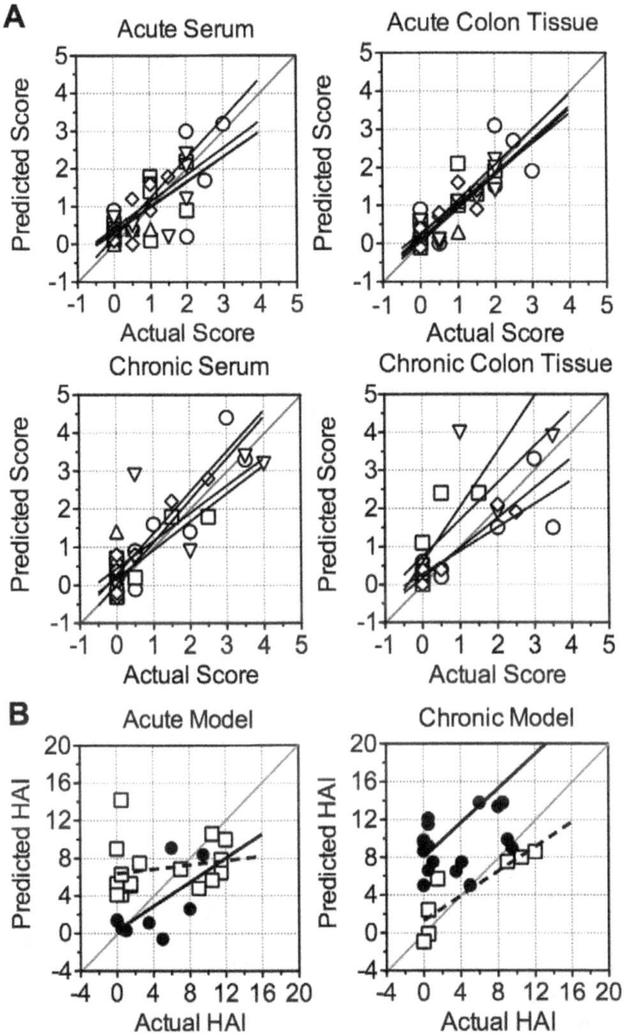

Figure 5. PLS modeling predicts histological lesion scores in colon. (A) Predicted lesion scores from *serum* or *tissue* PLS models using the VIPs of acute or chronic colitis. Lesion scores represented as: inflammation (○), epithelial defects (□), edema (△), hyperplasia (▽), dysplasia (◇). (B) Histologic activity indices (HAI, sum of individual lesion scores) for acute or chronic colitis predictions from refined acute or chronic serum PLS models using a minimal set of factors: RANTES, IFN-γ, NT, and G-CSF for acute model or IL-12/23p40, IL-17, G-CSF, CT, and KC for chronic model. Lesion scores or HAI plotted as actual versus predicted with exact predictions lying on the diagonal line (slope of 1). HAI for acute (•) and chronic (□) samples. Lines indicate linear regression of actual versus predicted lesion scores or HAI as representative visualization of Spearman correlations.

initiation of epithelial repair processes [39], whereas the role of Th17 cells, highly induced in both mucosal infections and autoimmune diseases, is not clear [40,41]. Maintenance of Th17 cells requires IL-23 that has been shown to be protective against early mortality in *C. rodentium* colitis and necessary for colitis development in *Helicobacter*-dependent colitis [17,42]. IL-23 appears to protect against early *C. rodentium* mortality via Th17 cell secretion of IL-22 rather than IL-17, which peaks during maximal colitis at 2 WPI [8,13]. In *Helicobacter*-dependent colitis IL-23 functions to regulate the IFN-γ and IL-17-producing T cell populations that lead ultimately to intestinal inflammation [42]. The precise role of IL-17 is not known in either form of colitis; however its production is associated with other Th17-related cytokines and the presence of neutrophils in the disease process. Similar to murine colitis, neutrophils, Th17 cells, and their related factors (such as IL-17, IL-8, and calprotectin, a product of neutrophil activation) are elevated in IBD patients [36,43–45]. The associative, and likely functional, relationship between neutrophils, Th17 cells, and colitis makes neutrophil- and Th17 cell-related factors reliable biomarkers of murine colitis and candidates as biomarkers for human colitis.

In addition to increased inflammatory cytokines, cell-type specific markers, such as NT and CT, provide information about the presence of macrophages or neutrophils that are commonly found among inflamed tissue in both colitic mice and IBD patients [46–49]. As demonstrated in this study stable protein adducts of nitric oxide and hypochlorous acid, NT and CT respectively, are measureable markers of cellular infiltration and activation. Previous studies have demonstrated increased macrophages, iNOS, and serum nitrate/nitrite levels in Cr^{+} mice [8,9,22] and *Helicobacter*-dependent colitis [25]. Only serum levels of NT in acute colitis were increased in this study. Interestingly, the colon had constitutively high levels of NT, which may be attributable to continual activation and surveillance of the gut microbial community by resident macrophages and epithelial cells. Unlike NT, CT was present in low levels in both the colon and serum of mice without disease. Tissue levels of chlorotyrosine mirrored many cytokines (i.e. IL-6 and IL-17) that are in low abundance except during active inflammation making it an ideal biomarker of both neutrophil activation and colitis.

Circulating cytokines represent the overall state of the host with contributions from disease sites, lymphoid organs and circulating leukocytes, as well as the liver. Given that blood draining the intestine passes through the liver before further circulation, it is likely that local responses in the liver to intestinal stimuli are a substantial source of circulating cytokines [50,51]. Serum cytokines may therefore represent the response in the intestines as well as the liver to luminal microbial stimuli and may not be identical to intestinal tissue cytokines. In this study serum cytokine profiling of two colitis models suggest circulating cytokines during acute colitis represent a broader response (perhaps that of both the intestines and liver), whereas serum cytokines during chronic colitis are predominantly those found in the intestinal tissue. Whatever the source of the cytokines, multivariate modeling of serum cytokine profiles predicted both disease presence and severity. One possible caveat is that serum cytokines may not discriminate colitis from other inflammatory diseases with similar systemic responses. Ideally, the serum profiles of multiple diseases would be compared to discriminate between a general inflammatory state and more specific sites of disease such as colitis, bronchitis, or hepatitis.

Many biomarkers in serum or feces have been identified for human IBD with some currently being evaluated for utility in clinical trials [5]. Biomarkers have predominantly been identified individually by association with either CD or UC and include antibodies against self (i.e. perinuclear anti-neutrophil cytoplasmic antibodies [pANCA]), bacterial products (i.e. ASCA, flagellin Cbir1, or *E. coli* OmpC), and glycans [1,4,6,52,53]. More general, non-antibody biomarkers of inflammation that have been applied to IBD include C-reactive protein and calprotectin [3,43]. Biomarkers specifically related to the intestinal disease process have not been extensively evaluated. Comprehensive serum profiling of cytokines followed by multivariate modeling, similar to that performed in this study of murine colitis, may identify a panel of disease-associated predictive biomarkers, particularly in individuals identified by genetic screening as having an increased risk for IBD.

Results from this study highlight immunologic similarities amongst two forms of murine colitis, particularly at the disease site. Multivariate modeling demonstrates that a limited set of in vivo measurements from serum or tissue of colitic and non-colitic mice accurately predict the severity of multiple colonic lesions and provide biological insight into factors dominating the disease process. Given that histological evaluation of disease lesions is semi-quantitative and subjective, and the small sample numbers used for predictive modeling, the accuracy of the predictions is encouraging. A larger scale study of the identified biomarkers would further improve the accuracy of the models in predicting severity. Additionally, whether the identified biomarkers are useful as accurate, quantitative markers of complex human diseases is still unknown. Further studies employing multivariate analysis and modeling of in vivo measurements will be useful for discriminating a subset of biologically relevant information from larger data sets, particularly in the setting of translational studies and evaluation of drugs for therapeutic efficacy endpoints.

Materials and Methods

Ethics statement

All animal experiments were approved by the IACUC at MIT (0207-020-10) or The University of Chicago (72039).

Mice and bacteria

For the *C. rodentium* study, female C57BL/6J (6 weeks old) mice were purchased from The Jackson Laboratory (Bar Harbor, ME) and housed at MIT. All TLR4$^{-/-}$ x IL-10$^{-/-}$ (DKO) mice on C57BL/6 background were bred and housed at The University of Chicago. The two DKO colonies originated from an specific pathogen free (SPF) colony at Massachusetts General Hospital (Boston, MA) that was *Helicobacter spp.*-positive (Hsp^{+}) by fecal PCR and from which a *Helicobacter spp.*-negative (Hsp^{-}) colony was rederived [19]. Male and female 20–35 week-old DKO mice bred and housed in Hsp^{-} or Hsp^{+} SPF facilities at The University of Chicago were utilized. All mice were fed a standard rodent diet and water *ad libitum*, housed in microisolator cages, and maintained SPF, including all known *Helicobacter* spp. (except Hsp^{+} DKO colony), in facilities approved by the Association for Assessment and Accreditation of Laboratory Animal Care. For *C. rodentium* infections, mice were gavaged $\sim 2\times 10^9$ kan^r *C. rodentium*, and fecal burdens determined as previously described [8]. Presence or absence of *Helicobacter spp.* was confirmed by genus-specific PCR on fecal DNA [54].

Tissue collection and Histopathology

Serum collected by cardiac puncture at sacrifice was stored at −80°C. For *C. rodentium* studies the colon was removed and divided longitudinally. The distal two-thirds from one section, and the distal quarter from the other were snap frozen in liquid nitrogen and stored at −80°C until protein isolation. Similarly, cecum and colon were collected from the DKO mice and divided longitudinally with one-half snap frozen for protein adduct measurements. A 1 cm piece of proximal colon (1 cm from ileocecal junction) was also collected. All remaining colon or cecum was fixed, sectioned, H&E stained, and scored by a blinded pathologist [8] or stained for MPO enumeration as previously described [25,55].

Serum and tissue cytokine measurements

For cytokines colon protein was isolated directly from frozen tissue by homogenization in cell lysis buffer containing phosphotase and protease inhibitors according to manufacturer's protocol (Bio-Rad, Hercules, CA). Cytokines were measured in serum or colon lysates using Bio-Plex Pro Mouse Cytokine 23-plex Assay according to manufacturer's instructions (Bio-Rad, Hercules, CA). Total protein in each colon sample was measured using microBCA assay (Thermo Fischer Scientific Inc., Rockford, IL). Colon cytokines were normalized to total protein concentration of each sample.

Nitrotyrosine and chlorotyrosine measurements

Nitrotyrosine and chlorotyrosine in serum and colon tissue were measured by negative-ion chemical ionization GC/MS. Briefly, serum or colon protein (2 mg) was spiked with 1 pmol internal standards (L-3-chloro-[$^{13}C_9$, ^{15}N]-tyrosine and L-3-nitro-[$^{13}C_9$, ^{15}N]-tyrosine). Protein was digested by 1 mg Pronase E (Protease from *Streptomyces griseus*, ≥4 units/mg) overnight at pH 7.4, followed by HPLC purification. The purified residue was derivatized with ethyl perfluorobutyrate and N-methyl-N-(t-butyldimethylsilyl) trifluoroacetamide + 1% trimethylchlorosilane (MtBSTFA, Regis Technologies, Morton Grove, IL). The derivatized samples were analyzed by negative-ion chemical ionization GC/MS. Separations were carried out on an Agilent 6890N GCMS system equipped with a 30 m HP-5MS capillary column (0.25 mm I.D., 0.25 μm film thickness). The ions were monitored at m/z 489 and 499 for chlorotyrosine and L-3-chloro-[$^{13}C_9$, ^{15}N]-tyrosine, and at m/z 518 and 528 for nitrotyrosine and L-3-nitro-[$^{13}C_9$, ^{15}N]-tyrosine. Quantification of protein-bound nitrotyrosine and chlorotyrosine were based on the calibration curves (5-points) constructed over the range of 0.1–5.0 pmol for both nitrotyrosine and chlorotyrosine. All analyses were carried out in triplicate.

Multivariate Analysis

SIMCA-P+ v11.5 (Umetrics Inc., Kinnelon, New Jersey) software for Partial Least Squares Projection to Latent Structures (PLS)-Discriminant Analysis (DA) was utilized to for the analysis of cytokines, chlorotyrosine and nitrotyrosine levels in colon or serum. Variables were $\log_{10}$ transformed as determined necessary by SIMCA-P+ for all analyses. Separate serum and tissue models were generated for each of the murine colitis models. Discrimination was based on assignment of each sample to class 1 (Cr^{-} or Hsp^{-}) or class 2 (Cr^{+} or Hsp^{+}) for PLS-DA models. R^2 Y, the fraction of the sum of squares of all Y variables explained by the component of the model, R^2 Y cumulative, the cumulative sum of squares of all Y variables explained by all components of the model, Q^2 the fraction of the total variation in Y variables that can be predicted by the component, and Q^2 cumulative, the cumulative Q^2 of the Y variables for all components in the model, were used to evaluate the quality of the model. R^2 cumulative and Q^2 cumulative of 1 indicate perfect fit and 100% explanation of relationship between X variables and Y variables. Variable importance in the projection (VIP) is computed from influence (weight) on Y of every term in the model. The average VIP equals 1, therefore VIPs >1 explain Y more than VIP <1. For PLS models each group was randomly divided into two sets (training or prediction). Given the small sample size, four different training/prediction sets and models were generated to ensure individual samples were not biasing the models.

Statistics

Statistical significances were determined by two-way ANOVA followed by Bonferroni post-tests or unpaired two-tailed Students' t test as appropriate. Histologic activity indices were analyzed by Mann-Whitney t test. Acute and chronic model fits of predicted to actual data were analyzed by Spearman nonparametric correlations. GraphPad Prizm Software version 5.0 (La Jolla, CA) was used for all analyses.

Supporting Information

Figure S1 Peak infection with *C. rodentium* precedes onset of weight loss and disease development. (a) Fecal burden of *C. rodentium* in uninfected (closed square) and infected (open square) mice from Day 0 to Day 14. (b) Percent change in body weight normalized to day 0 to day 14 in uninfected (closed square) and *C. rodentium*-infected (open square) mice. Data are presented as mean ± SEM. *** $P<0.001$ by two-way ANOVA with Bonferroni post-tests.

Figure S2 Cytokine measurements in C57BL/6J mice with acute infectious colitis. Colon tissue (a) and serum (b) cytokine concentrations in uninfected (Cr^-; n = 9 serum, n = 10 tissue) and *C. rodentium* infected (Cr^+; n = 10) mice at 14 DPI. Colon concentrations were normalized to total protein in sample. Bar equals mean value. * $P < 0.05$, ** $P < 0.01$, *** $P < 0.001$ by unpaired Student's T test.

Figure S3 Cytokine measurements in $TLR4^{-/-}$ x $IL10^{-/-}$ (DKO) mice with chronic spontaneous *Helicobacter*-dependent colitis. Colon tissue (a) and serum (b) cytokine concentrations in *Helicobacter* spp.-negative (Hsp^-; n = 6) and *Helicobacter* spp.-positive (Hsp^+; n = 8 tissue, n = 10 serum) DKO mice. Colon concentrations were normalized to total protein in sample. Bar equals mean value. * $P < 0.05$, ** $P < 0.01$, *** $P < 0.001$ by unpaired Student's T test.

Acknowledgments

This study is dedicated to the late Professor David B. Schauer and his lifetime of work investigating the pathogenesis of murine models of colitis. In recent years he endeavored to successfully model in vivo data using the methods derived from biological engineering.

Author Contributions

Conceived and designed the experiments: MEM DBS. Performed the experiments: MEM YZ. Analyzed the data: MEM YZ. Contributed reagents/materials/analysis tools: YZ NP CRN SRT. Wrote the paper: MEM CRN SRT.

References

1. Sendid B, Quinton JF, Charrier G, Goulet O, Cortot A, et al. (1998) Anti-Saccharomyces cerevisiae mannan antibodies in familial Crohn's disease. Am J Gastroenterol 93: 1306–1310.
2. Hanauer SB (2010) The expanding role of biologic therapy for IBD. Nat Rev Gastroenterol Hepatol 7: 63–64.
3. Langhorst J, Elsenbruch S, Koelzer J, Rueffer A, Michalsen A, et al. (2008) Noninvasive markers in the assessment of intestinal inflammation in inflammatory bowel diseases: performance of fecal lactoferrin, calprotectin, and PMN-elastase, CRP, and clinical indices. Am J Gastroenterol 103: 162–169.
4. Dotan I, Fishman S, Dgani Y, Schwartz M, Karban A, et al. (2006) Antibodies against laminaribioside and chitobioside are novel serologic markers in Crohn's disease. Gastroenterology 131: 366–378.
5. Li X, Conklin L, Alex P (2008) New serological biomarkers of inflammatory bowel disease. World J Gastroenterol 14: 5115–5124.
6. Lodes MJ, Cong Y, Elson CO, Mohamath R, Landers CJ, et al. (2004) Bacterial flagellin is a dominant antigen in Crohn disease. J Clin Invest 113: 1296–1306.
7. Borenshtein D, McBee ME, Schauer DB (2008) Utility of the Citrobacter rodentium infection model in laboratory mice. Curr Opin Gastroenterol 24: 32–37.
8. McBee ME, Zheng PZ, Rogers AB, Fox JG, Schauer DB (2008) Modulation of acute diarrheal illness by persistent bacterial infection. Infect Immun 76: 4851–4858.
9. Simmons CP, Goncalves NS, Ghaem-Maghami M, Bajaj-Elliott M, Clare S, et al. (2002) Impaired resistance and enhanced pathology during infection with a noninvasive, attaching-effacing enteric bacterial pathogen, Citrobacter rodentium, in mice lacking IL-12 or IFN-gamma. J Immunol 168: 1804–1812.
10. Yoshida M, Kobayashi K, Kuo TT, Bry L, Glickman JN, et al. (2006) Neonatal Fc receptor for IgG regulates mucosal immune responses to luminal bacteria. J Clin Invest 116: 2142–2151.
11. Masuda A, Yoshida M, Shiomi H, Ikezawa S, Takagawa T, et al. (2008) Fcgamma receptor regulation of Citrobacter rodentium infection. Infect Immun 76: 1728–1737.
12. Simmons CP, Clare S, Ghaem-Maghami M, Uren TK, Rankin J, et al. (2003) Central role for B lymphocytes and CD4+ T cells in immunity to infection by the attaching and effacing pathogen Citrobacter rodentium. Infect Immun 71: 5077–5086.
13. Zheng Y, Valdez PA, Danilenko DM, Hu Y, Sa SM, et al. (2008) Interleukin-22 mediates early host defense against attaching and effacing bacterial pathogens. Nat Med 14: 282–289.
14. Dann SM, Spehlmann ME, Hammond DC, Iimura M, Hase K, et al. (2008) IL-6-dependent mucosal protection prevents establishment of a microbial niche for attaching/effacing lesion-forming enteric bacterial pathogens. J Immunol 180: 6816–6826.
15. Gibson DL, Ma C, Rosenberger CM, Bergstrom KS, Valdez Y, et al. (2008) Toll-like receptor 2 plays a critical role in maintaining mucosal integrity during Citrobacter rodentium-induced colitis. Cell Microbiol 10: 388–403.
16. Lebeis SL, Powell KR, Merlin D, Sherman MA, Kalman D (2009) Interleukin-1 receptor signaling protects mice from lethal intestinal damage caused by the attaching and effacing pathogen Citrobacter rodentium. Infect Immun 77: 604–614.
17. Mangan PR, Harrington LE, O'Quinn DB, Helms WS, Bullard DC, et al. (2006) Transforming growth factor-beta induces development of the T(H)17 lineage. Nature 441: 231–234.
18. Kullberg MC, Ward JM, Gorelick PL, Caspar P, Hieny S, et al. (1998) Helicobacter hepaticus triggers colitis in specific-pathogen-free interleukin-10 (IL-10)-deficient mice through an IL-12- and gamma interferon-dependent mechanism. Infect Immun 66: 5157–5166.
19. Matharu KS, Mizoguchi E, Cotoner CA, Nguyen DD, Mingle B, et al. (2009) Toll-like receptor 4-mediated regulation of spontaneous Helicobacter-dependent colitis in IL-10-deficient mice. Gastroenterology 137: 1380–1390 e1381–1383.
20. Spehlmann ME, Dann SM, Hruz P, Hanson E, McCole DF, et al. (2009) CXCR2-dependent mucosal neutrophil influx protects against colitis-associated diarrhea caused by an attaching/effacing lesion-forming bacterial pathogen. J Immunol 183: 3332–3343.
21. Beckman JS, Koppenol WH (1996) Nitric oxide, superoxide, and peroxynitrite: the good, the bad, and ugly. Am J Physiol 271: C1424–1437.
22. Vallance BA, Deng W, De Grado M, Chan C, Jacobson K, et al. (2002) Modulation of inducible nitric oxide synthase expression by the attaching and effacing bacterial pathogen citrobacter rodentium in infected mice. Infect Immun 70: 6424–6435.
23. Gobert AP, Cheng Y, Akhtar M, Mersey BD, Blumberg DR, et al. (2004) Protective role of arginase in a mouse model of colitis. J Immunol 173: 2109–2117.
24. Chin MP, Schauer DB, Deen WM (2008) Prediction of nitric oxide concentrations in colonic crypts during inflammation. Nitric Oxide 19: 266–275.
25. Erdman SE, Rao VP, Poutahidis T, Rogers AB, Taylor CL, et al. (2009) Nitric oxide and TNF-alpha trigger colonic inflammation and carcinogenesis in Helicobacter hepaticus-infected, Rag2-deficient mice. Proc Natl Acad Sci U S A 106: 1027–1032.
26. Harrison JE, Schultz J (1976) Studies on the chlorinating activity of myeloperoxidase. J Biol Chem 251: 1371–1374.
27. Domigan NM, Charlton TS, Duncan MW, Winterbourn CC, Kettle AJ (1995) Chlorination of tyrosyl residues in peptides by myeloperoxidase and human neutrophils. J Biol Chem 270: 16542–16548.
28. Lebeis SL, Bommarius B, Parkos CA, Sherman MA, Kalman D (2007) TLR signaling mediated by MyD88 is required for a protective innate immune response by neutrophils to Citrobacter rodentium. J Immunol 179: 566–577.
29. Melgar S, Karlsson A, Michaelsson E (2005) Acute colitis induced by dextran sulfate sodium progresses to chronicity in C57BL/6 but not in BALB/c mice: correlation between symptoms and inflammation. Am J Physiol Gastrointest Liver Physiol 288: G1328–1338.
30. Ten Hove T, Corbaz A, Amitai H, Aloni S, Belzer I, et al. (2001) Blockade of endogenous IL-18 ameliorates TNBS-induced colitis by decreasing local TNF-alpha production in mice. Gastroenterology 121: 1372–1379.
31. Fina D, Sarra M, Fantini MC, Rizzo A, Caruso R, et al. (2008) Regulation of gut inflammation and th17 cell response by interleukin-21. Gastroenterology 134: 1038–1048.
32. Eastaff-Leung N, Mabarrack N, Barbour A, Cummins A, Barry S (2009) Foxp3(+) Regulatory T Cells, Th17 Effector Cells, and Cytokine Environment in Inflammatory Bowel Disease. J Clin Immunol.

33. Banks C, Bateman A, Payne R, Johnson P, Sheron N (2003) Chemokine expression in IBD. Mucosal chemokine expression is unselectively increased in both ulcerative colitis and Crohn's disease. J Pathol 199: 28–35.
34. Leon AJ, Gomez E, Garrote JA, Bernardo D, Barrera A, et al. (2009) High levels of proinflammatory cytokines, but not markers of tissue injury, in unaffected intestinal areas from patients with IBD. Mediators Inflamm 2009: 580450.
35. Reimund JM, Wittersheim C, Dumont S, Muller CD, Baumann R, et al. (1996) Mucosal inflammatory cytokine production by intestinal biopsies in patients with ulcerative colitis and Crohn's disease. J Clin Immunol 16: 144–150.
36. Pelletier M, Maggi L, Micheletti A, Lazzeri E, Tamassia N, et al. (2009) Evidence for a cross-talk between human neutrophils and Th17 cells. Blood.
37. Ye P, Rodriguez FH, Kanaly S, Stocking KL, Schurr J, et al. (2001) Requirement of interleukin 17 receptor signaling for lung CXC chemokine and granulocyte colony-stimulating factor expression, neutrophil recruitment, and host defense. J Exp Med 194: 519–527.
38. Wu Q, Martin RJ, Rino JG, Breed R, Torres RM, et al. (2007) IL-23-dependent IL-17 production is essential in neutrophil recruitment and activity in mouse lung defense against respiratory Mycoplasma pneumoniae infection. Microbes Infect 9: 78–86.
39. Nathan C (2006) Neutrophils and immunity: challenges and opportunities. Nat Rev Immunol 6: 173–182.
40. Steinman L (2009) Mixed results with modulation of TH-17 cells in human autoimmune diseases. Nat Immunol 11: 41–44.
41. Khader SA, Gaffen SL, Kolls JK (2009) Th17 cells at the crossroads of innate and adaptive immunity against infectious diseases at the mucosa. Mucosal Immunol 2: 403–411.
42. Kullberg MC, Jankovic D, Feng CG, Hue S, Gorelick PL, et al. (2006) IL-23 plays a key role in Helicobacter hepaticus-induced T cell-dependent colitis. J Exp Med 203: 2485–2494.
43. Costa F, Mumolo MG, Ceccarelli L, Bellini M, Romano MR, et al. (2005) Calprotectin is a stronger predictive marker of relapse in ulcerative colitis than in Crohn's disease. Gut 54: 364–368.
44. Carlson M, Raab Y, Seveus L, Xu S, Hallgren R, et al. (2002) Human neutrophil lipocalin is a unique marker of neutrophil inflammation in ulcerative colitis and proctitis. Gut 50: 501–506.
45. Fujino S, Andoh A, Bamba S, Ogawa A, Hata K, et al. (2003) Increased expression of interleukin 17 in inflammatory bowel disease. Gut 52: 65–70.
46. Grimm MC, Pavli P, Van de Pol E, Doe WF (1995) Evidence for a CD14+ population of monocytes in inflammatory bowel disease mucosa—implications for pathogenesis. Clin Exp Immunol 100: 291–297.
47. Grimm MC, Elsbury SK, Pavli P, Doe WF (1996) Interleukin 8: cells of origin in inflammatory bowel disease. Gut 38: 90–98.
48. Lampinen M, Sangfelt P, Taha Y, Carlson M (2008) Accumulation, activation, and survival of neutrophils in ulcerative colitis: regulation by locally produced factors in the colon and impact of steroid treatment. Int J Colorectal Dis 23: 939–946.
49. Mitsuyama K, Toyonaga A, Sasaki E, Watanabe K, Tateishi H, et al. (1994) IL-8 as an important chemoattractant for neutrophils in ulcerative colitis and Crohn's disease. Clin Exp Immunol 96: 432–436.
50. Chaluvadi MR, Kinloch RD, Nyagode BA, Richardson TA, Raynor MJ, et al. (2009) Regulation of hepatic cytochrome P450 expression in mice with intestinal or systemic infections of citrobacter rodentium. Drug Metab Dispos 37: 366–374.
51. Tu Z, Bozorgzadeh A, Crispe IN, Orloff MS (2007) The activation state of human intrahepatic lymphocytes. Clin Exp Immunol 149: 186–193.
52. Satsangi J, Landers CJ, Welsh KI, Koss K, Targan S, et al. (1998) The presence of anti-neutrophil antibodies reflects clinical and genetic heterogeneity within inflammatory bowel disease. Inflamm Bowel Dis 4: 18–26.
53. Joossens S, Colombel JF, Landers C, Poulain D, Geboes K, et al. (2006) Anti-outer membrane of porin C and anti-I2 antibodies in indeterminate colitis. Gut 55: 1667–1669.
54. Nagamine CM, Rogers AB, Fox JG, Schauer DB (2008) Helicobacter hepaticus promotes azoxymethane-initiated colon tumorigenesis in BALB/c-IL10-deficient mice. Int J Cancer 122: 832–838.
55. Rogers AB, Cormier KS, Fox JG (2006) Thiol-reactive compounds prevent nonspecific antibody binding in immunohistochemistry. Lab Invest 86: 526–533.

15

The Colitis-Associated Transcriptional Profile of Commensal *Bacteroides thetaiotaomicron* Enhances Adaptive Immune Responses to a Bacterial Antigen

Jonathan J. Hansen[1,2*], Yong Huang[3], Daniel A. Peterson[4], Laura Goeser[1], Ting-Jia Fan[1], Eugene B. Chang[3], R. Balfour Sartor[1,2,5]

1 Center for Gastrointestinal Biology and Disease, University of North Carolina at Chapel Hill, Chapel Hill, North Carolina, United States of America, **2** Department of Medicine, Division of Gastroenterology and Hepatology, University of North Carolina at Chapel Hill, Chapel Hill, North Carolina, United States of America, **3** Department of Medicine, Section of Gastroenterology, University of Chicago Medical Center, Chicago, Illinois, United States of America, **4** Department of Pathology, Johns Hopkins University School of Medicine, Baltimore, Maryland, United States of America, **5** Department of Microbiology and Immunology, University of North Carolina at Chapel Hill, Chapel Hill, North Carolina, United States of America

Abstract

Background: Inflammatory bowel diseases (IBD) may be caused in part by aberrant immune responses to commensal intestinal microbes including the well-characterized anaerobic gut commensal *Bacteroides thetaiotaomicron* (*B. theta*). Healthy, germ-free HLA-B27 transgenic (Tg) rats develop chronic colitis when colonized with complex gut commensal bacteria whereas non-transgenic (nTg) rats remain disease-free. However, the role of *B. theta* in causing disease in Tg rats is unknown nor is much known about how gut microbes respond to host inflammation.

Methods: Tg and nTg rats were monoassociated with a human isolate of *B. theta*. Colonic inflammation was assessed by histologic scoring and tissue pro-inflammatory cytokine measurement. Whole genome transcriptional profiling of *B. theta* recovered from ceca was performed using custom GeneChips and data analyzed using dChip, Significance Analysis of Microarrays, and Gene Set Enrichment Analysis (GSEA) software. Western Blots were used to determine adaptive immune responses to a differentially expressed *B. theta* gene.

Results: *B. theta* monoassociated Tg rats, but not nTg or germ-free controls, developed chronic colitis. Transcriptional profiles of cecal *B. theta* were significantly different in Tg vs. nTg rats. GSEA revealed that genes in KEGG canonical pathways involved in bacterial growth and metabolism were downregulated in *B. theta* from Tg rats with colitis though luminal bacterial concentrations were unaffected. Bacterial genes in the Gene Ontology molecular function "receptor activity", most of which encode nutrient binding proteins, were significantly upregulated in *B. theta* from Tg rats and include a SusC homolog that induces adaptive immune responses in Tg rats.

Conclusions: *B. theta* induces colitis in HLA-B27 Tg rats, which is associated with regulation of bacterial genes in metabolic and nutrient binding pathways that may affect host immune responses. These studies of the host-microbial dialogue may lead to the identification of novel microbial targets for IBD therapies.

Editor: Emiko Mizoguchi, Massachusetts General Hospital, United States of America

Funding: This work was supported by NIH K08 DK087896 (J.J.H.), a Career Development Award from the Crohn's and Colitis Foundation of America 2662 (J.J.H.), Center for Gastrointestinal Biology and Disease grant NIH P30 DK34987 (Robert S. Sandler, PI), NIH R01 DK53347 (R.B.S.), NIH P40 RR18803 (R.B.S.), Crohn's and Colitis Foundation of America Gnotobiotic Animal Facility (R.B.S.), University of Chicago Host-Microbe Core of the Digestive Disease Research Core Center (NIH DK42086, E.B.C.), and Helmsley Foundation (E.B.C., R.B.S.). The funders had no role in study design, data collection and analysis, decision to publish, or preparation of the manuscript.

Competing Interests: The authors have declared that no competing interests exist.

* E-mail: jjhansen@med.unc.edu

Introduction

It is becoming increasingly clear that commensal intestinal bacteria provide functions that significantly impact not only normal host physiology, but also disease pathogenesis. For example, while certain symbiotic members of the human gut microbiome supply nutrients to the host, induce protective responses in the intestinal epithelium, and influence normal mucosal immune development, other members known as pathobionts have the capacity to induce disease in susceptible hosts or specific environmental conditions [1,2]. The role of commensal bacteria in causing human disease is perhaps best illustrated by our current understanding of the pathogenesis of inflammatory bowel diseases (IBD).

IBD are a group of chronic intestinal inflammatory disorders, including Crohn's disease (CD) and ulcerative colitis, that are caused in part by dysregulated immune responses to commensal intestinal bacteria in genetically susceptible hosts. The role of host genetics in IBD is highlighted by the discovery of over 100 genes that are associated with IBD, more than 80 of which are linked to CD. NOD2, the CD susceptibility gene with the single largest effect size, and many of the other IBD susceptibility genes encode proteins that participate in host innate and adaptive immune responses to bacteria [3,4]. Thus, genetic studies indicate that defective immune responses to bacteria may contribute to the development of IBD. The pathologic role of commensal bacteria in IBD is further substantiated by clinical studies in which surgical diversion of the fecal stream reduced inflammation in bypassed intestinal segments, suggesting that luminal contents contain pro-inflammatory components such as bacteria [5].

In addition to genetic and clinical studies, profiling the composition of the intestinal microbial community has also revealed associations between CD and commensal bacteria. In general, CD is associated with decreased bacterial diversity, increased numbers of Proteobacteria, and decreased numbers of Firmicutes [6]. Specifically, compared to healthy controls, increased numbers of functionally distinct commensal *Escherichia coli* belonging to the B2+D phylotypes and commensal adherent-invasive *E. coli* strains are present in the intestinal mucosa of patients with CD affecting the colon and ileum, respectively [7,8]. Decreased numbers of the Firmicute, *Faecalibacterium prausnitzii*, are detected in intestinal mucosa from patients with post-operative recurrence of ileal CD compared to non-inflamed controls [9]. In contrast to Proteobacteria and Firmicutes, changes in the number of commensals belonging to the Bacteroidetes, one of the dominant phyla in the human gut microbiome, are variable in patients with IBD [10,11,12,13,14]. However, host immune responses to a member of the Bacteroidetes, *Bacteroides thetaiotaomicron* (*B. theta*), are elevated in colonic tissue from CD patients [15]. Together, these studies suggest that changes in the composition of the gut microbial community and aberrant immune responses to Bacteroidetes are associated with human IBD.

Studies of animal models have also provided remarkable insights into the pathogenesis of IBD. Similar to results from human studies, Proteobacteria are consistently expanded in animal models of IBD, whereas changes in Bacteroidetes are variable depending upon the model and method of detection [6]. The most direct evidence linking commensal bacteria to the development of IBD comes from gnotobiotic animal studies, in which virtually all animal models of IBD that have been tested are healthy in the germ-free (GF) state, but develop intestinal inflammation when exposed to viable commensal bacteria [16]. For example, Rag1-/- mice that are selectively colonized (monoassociated) with a human isolate of *B. theta* have increased innate immune responses in the small intestine compared to GF mice [17]. Treatment with antibiotics that eliminate certain members of the commensal microbiota abrogates spontaneous colitis in Il10R2/TGFBR2 double knockout mice, but colitis recurs when these mice are inoculated with murine isolates of *Bacteroides* spp., especially *B. theta* and *Bacteroides vulgatus*, but not *E. coli* [18]. In another model, transgenic rats harboring the human *HLA-B27* and *β2 microglobulin* genes (Tg) remain healthy when housed in germ-free conditions, but develop spontaneous multi-organ inflammation, including colitis, when colonized with commensal bacteria [19,20]. Furthermore, gnotobiotic experiments in which germ-free *HLA-B27* Tg rats are selectively colonized with defined bacteria revealed that not all commensal bacteria have equal colitogenic potential. For example, *B. vulgatus* causes worse inflammation than *B. distasonis* and *E. coli* causes no inflammation in *HLA-B27* Tg rats monoassociated with specific strains of these bacteria [20,21].

While others have shown that *B. theta* may contribute to the pathogenesis of human IBD and experimental murine colitis, relatively little is known about its role in other models of intestinal inflammation, nor is much known about how host inflammation affects *B. theta* function. Herein, we present data that a human isolate of commensal *B. theta* causes chronic colitis in mono-associated *HLA-B27* Tg rats, which in turn induces transcriptional changes in luminal bacterial genes that impact host immune responses.

Materials and Methods

Bacterial Cultures

The fully-sequenced human fecal isolate of *B. theta* (VPI-5482) was grown on Brain-Heart Infusion (BHI) agar and in BHI broth under strict anaerobic conditions using pre-reduced media. To quantify viable luminal bacteria, weighed, frozen cecal contents were thawed and diluted in PBS in an anaerobic chamber and grown on BHI agar for 3 days. For dilution calculations, we assumed that 1 g of contents has a volume of 1 mL. Results were expressed as colony forming units (CFU)/g of contents.

Animal Experiments

Four adult germ-free HLA-B27/β2 microglobulin Tg rats and five adult germ-free nTg littermate controls on the Fisher F344 background [19] were monoassociated for six weeks in gnotobiotic isolators at the National Gnotobiotic Rodent Resource Center at UNC Chapel Hill. At necropsy, serum was collected, luminal contents and intestinal tissue were snap frozen in liquid nitrogen for RNA isolation, and intestinal tissue was fixed in formalin for histologic processing. Contamination of animals with other bacteria was excluded by Gram staining and plating of cecal contents on BHI agar, which was cultured aerobically and anaerobically for seven days.

Ethics Statement

Animals were treated humanely throughout the entire experiment. All animal protocols were approved by the Institutional Animal Care and Use Committee at the University of North Carolina at Chapel Hill (Protocol 09-239.0).

Histologic Scoring

Formalin-fixed, paraffin-embedded intestinal tissue was stained with hematoxylin and eosin and inflammation was quantified using a validated blinded histological scoring system as described previously [22].

RNA Isolation

Mammalian RNA was isolated from intestinal tissue using Trizol Reagent (Invitrogen, Carlsbad, CA) according to the manufacturer's instructions. Bacterial RNA was isolated from rat cecal contents as previously described [17].

Microarray Analysis

Bacterial cDNA was synthesized and hybridized to 8 custom GeneChips (1 GeneChip per animal, 4 animals per group) as previously described [17]. The chip quality check and data normalization were processed using dChip software (http://biosun1.harvard.edu/complab/dchip/). Unsupervised hierarchical clustering of samples was also carried out by dChip software. Briefly, 6 arrays passed the established criteria for sample and chip outlier identification. We used "PM-only" background correction, "invariant set" normalization and model-based summary of gene expression levels [23]. The .cel files and normalized data were deposited in NCBI GEO database with accession number GSE34966.

We filtered the genes using criterion of coefficient of variation >0.5 and <2, resulting in 180 *B. theta* genes demonstrating large variation across all samples. Unsupervised hierarchical clustering of samples was performed based on the expression profile of these 180 genes using dChip software with "1-Pearson correlation" for distance metric and "centroid" for linkage. Three-dimensional principal components analysis was performed on normalized microarray data from the entire GeneChip using Genespring GX 11.0 software with "pruning" set at 4 eigenvectors, mean centered normalization, and scale to unit standard deviation.

Differentially expressed genes between nTg and Tg animals were identified by two-group comparison using Significance Analysis of Microarrays [24]. The criteria for identification of differentially expressed genes were fold change >1.5 and false discovery rate (FDR)<4%.

Pathways Analysis of Transcriptional Profiles

The KEGG pathways of *B. theta* were curated from NCBI BioProject Genome Project Accession No. 62913 and RefSeq NC_004663.1[25]. The *B. theta* KEGG database contains 84 metabolism and signaling pathways including 860 genes, 89% of which were covered by the approximately 5000 *B. theta* genes on the Affymetrix Human gut microbiota community GeneChip used in these experiments. The metabolism and signaling pathways significantly distinct between two experiment groups were identified using Gene Set Enrichment Analysis (GSEA) software (http://www.broadinstitute.org/gsea/index.jsp). GSEA is a computational method that determines whether an a priori defined set of genes shows statistically significant, concordant differences between two biological states [26]. Briefly, the normalized microarray data was converted into .GCT format, while the chip annotation file was converted into .CHIP format. The canonical pathways of *B. theta* were downloaded from the KEGG database (http://www.genome.jp/kegg/) and converted into .GMT format, as required by GSEA submission. The criterion for significant pathways was set at FDR<20%.

GSEA was also used to perform Gene Ontology (GO) analysis similar to KEGG analysis. GO annotation of the *B. theta* genome was performed as originally described [25,27] and was updated in the Gordon lab in 2008, http://gordonlab.wustl.edu/sonnenburg/index.html (unpublished).

Quantitative Real-time RT-PCR

Cytokine and bacterial transcripts were quantified by real-time RT-PCR using the $\Delta\Delta$Ct relative quantification method as described previously [28]. Rat β-actin and *B. theta* 16S were chosen as reference genes. Primer pairs are listed in Table S3. Mammalian primers spanned introns.

Sequence Alignment, Cloning and Purification of BT4357 Fragment

Amino acid sequence alignment between BT4357 and *Bacteroides caccae* OmpW was performed using web-based ClustalW2 software (http://www.ebi.ac.uk/Tools/msa/clustalw2/). A fragment of BT4357 corresponding to amino acid residues 160 to 741 was amplified from *B. theta* genomic DNA using PCR primers 5-attccatatgaaaggctccgccaatggtacga-3′ and 5′-cgcggatccttatacagaagggaagaaaccgaaac-3′ and subcloned into the PET15b expression vector (EMD Millipore, Billerica, MA) using standard molecular biology procedures. The cloned portion of BT4357 excludes the predicted leader peptide and a portion of the transmembrane domain in order to facilitate overexpression and purification, but includes the region that correlates to the putative epitope in *B. caccae* OmpW. The BT4357 protein fragment was overexpressed in *E. coli* BL21-DE3 (EMD Millipore, Billerica, MA) and purified using nickel agarose (Qiagen, Valencia, CA) according to the manufacturer's instructions.

Western Blots

Ten mcg of purified BT4357 fragment were separated on 10% SDS-polyacrylamide gels and transferred to nitrocellulose membranes using standard protocols. Membranes were stained with Ponceau S for five minutes and then rinsed with water to visualize protein bands. Individual membrane strips from each lane were incubated in 5% non-fat dry milk in TBST (TBST-milk) for 60 min, 1:300 rat sera in TBST-milk for 90 min, 1:4000 goat anti-rat IgG-HRP (SantaCruz Biotechnology, Santa Cruz, CA) in TBST-milk for 60 min, and ECL Prime reagent (Amersham, Piscataway, NJ) for five minutes. Immunoreactive bands were detected by exposing strips to X-ray film.

Results

Human Commensal *B. theta* Induces Chronic T-cell-mediated Inflammation in *HLA-B27* Tg Rats

Since others have previously shown that selective colonization of *HLA-B27* Tg rats with *B. vulgatus* induces variable degrees of chronic intestinal inflammation and since *B. theta* has been associated with human IBD and a model of murine colitis, we wanted to determine whether *B. theta* causes colitis in mono-associated Tg rats similar to that observed in human IBD. We therefore colonized germ-free Tg and non-transgenic (nTg) rats with the human commensal isolate of *B. theta* (VPI-5482) for 6 weeks and measured histological inflammation. We found significantly greater inflammation in the ceca and distal colons of Tg compared to nTg and germ-free rats, which was characterized primarily by increased lamina propria mononuclear cell infiltrate and mild crypt hyperplasia (Figure 1).

To determine whether the histological inflammation was associated with enhanced T-cell-mediated cytokine expression in colonic tissue from Tg rats, we performed real-time PCR of selected cytokines and found that TNFα and IFNγ transcripts were significantly higher in cecal and distal colon tissue from monoassociated Tg compared to nTg rats (Figure 2). Together, these data indicate that a human isolate of *B. theta* induces colitis in a Tg rat model of IBD and that the inflammation is characterized by upregulation of pro-inflammatory cytokines that mediate T-cell responses.

Intestinal Inflammation is Associated with Alterations in the *B. theta* Transcriptome

While much is known about the effects of commensal bacteria on host immune responses, relatively little is known about how host inflammation affects luminal bacterial function. It is plausible that chronic intestinal inflammation generates an environment that alters the function or colitogenic potential of commensal bacteria. We have previously reported that stress response genes are upregulated and tricarboxylic acid cycle genes are downregulated in commensal *E. coli* from monoassociated IL-10-/- mice with overt histologic colitis compared to *E. coli* from healthy wild-type mice [28]. Furthermore, two genes that are upregulated in luminal *E. coli* during experimental colitis may negatively impact survival and inflammatory potential of the bacteria in genetically susceptible hosts [28]. We have also shown in *B. theta* mono-

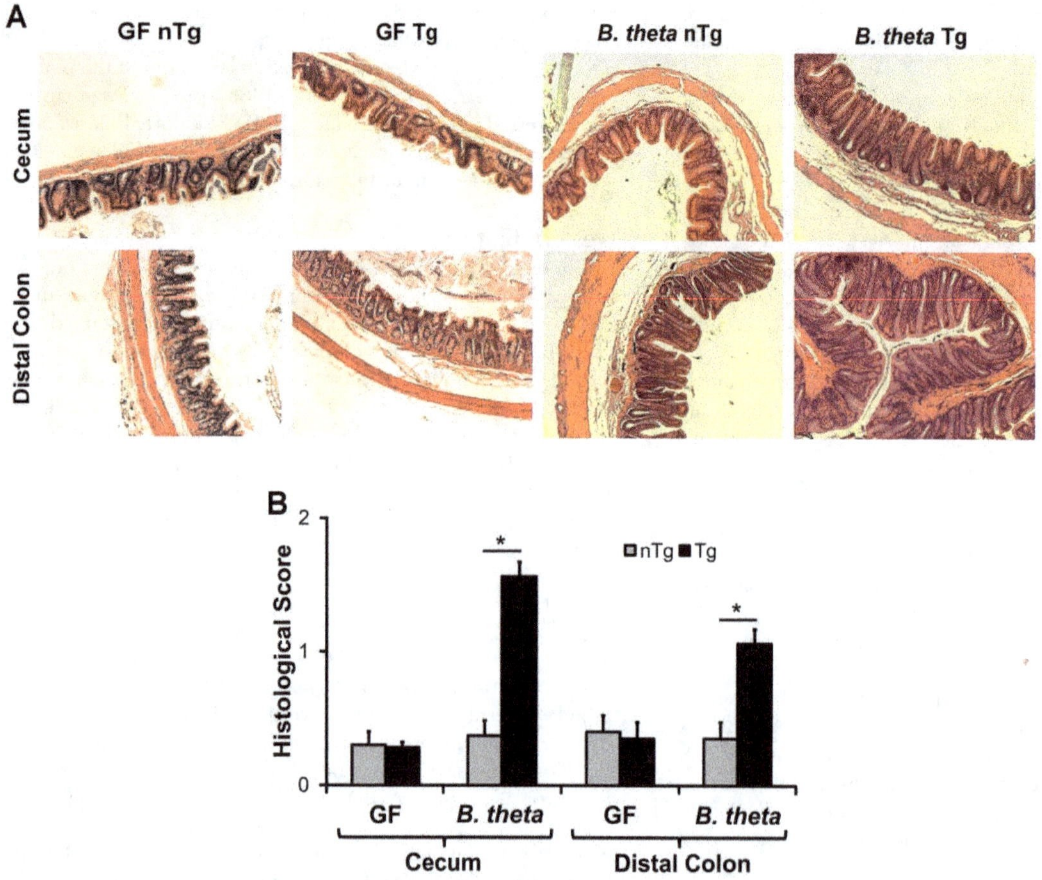

Figure 1. Colonic Inflammation in Germ-Free and *B. theta* Monoassociated Rats. (A) Representative photomicrographs of H&E stained cecum and distal colon pieces from germ-free (GF) and 6-week *B. theta*-monoassociated non-transgenic (nTg) and *HLA-B27* transgenic (Tg) rats taken using a 10× objective. (B) Blinded histological inflammation scores of cecum and distal colon tissue from GF and *B. theta*-monoassociated rats (mean+SEM, *p<0.05, n = 4–5 rats/group).

associated Rag1-/- mice, which have molecular evidence of increased innate immune responses, that luminal bacteria upregulate pathways that metabolize host innate immune effector molecules [17].

However, whether chronic, T-cell mediated inflammation affects *B. theta* gene expression is unknown. We therefore performed whole-genome transcriptional profiling with custom *B. theta* GeneChips containing probe sets that cover 98.6% of the bacterium's 4779 protein-coding genes [17,27]. Using principle component analysis and unsupervised hierarchical clustering, we found that the *B. theta* transcriptome was significantly different in cecal bacteria from Tg rats with inflammation compared to healthy nTg (Figure 3A and 3B). We detected 329 differentially expressed transcripts representing 44 Kyoto Encyclopedia of Genes and Genomes (KEGG) canonical pathways. These findings indicate that host genotype (i.e. inflammation) significantly impacts luminal bacterial gene expression in this model.

To identify the individual *B. theta* genes that are significantly affected by inflammation, we performed two-group comparison using Significance Analysis of Microarrays and a fold-change threshold of 1.5 and false discovery rate of <0.05 [24]. We identified 56 genes that were upregulated and 273 genes that were downregulated in *B. theta* from Tg rats compared to nTg rats (Tables S1 & S2). Most of the highly upregulated genes encode membrane proteins of the starch utilization system (Sus) in *B. theta*. BT_3969, the second most highly upregulated gene, encodes a cation efflux protein of the Acr family that may be involved in exporting potentially toxic molecules including bile salts, indole, and antimicrobial peptides. A larger set of genes were downregulated in bacteria from Tg rats. However, many of the most highly downregulated genes encode hypothetical proteins for which there is no known function. Of the most highly downregulated genes with known or predicted functions, many encode proteins that are involved in cell wall biosynthesis and ribosome assembly. Real-time RT-PCR confirmed microarray results of several selected genes in multiple metabolic pathways (Figure S1). These data suggest that *B. theta* responds to inflammation by upregulating genes that facilitate nutrient uptake and survival and downregulating genes that are involved in growth and metabolism.

B. theta downregulate metabolic pathways during experimental colitis

Since differential expression of individual genes does not necessarily correlate with entire pathways that are significantly affected by an experimental condition, we performed pathways analysis to test our hypothesis that *B. theta* downregulates processes of growth and cell division and upregulates processes that facilitate persistence and nutrient acquisition. We used Gene Set Enrichment Analysis (GSEA) software to analyze gene ontology (GO) molecular functions and KEGG canonical pathways that were significantly changed in *B. theta* from Tg compared to nTg rats. GSEA is a computational method that determines whether an *a*

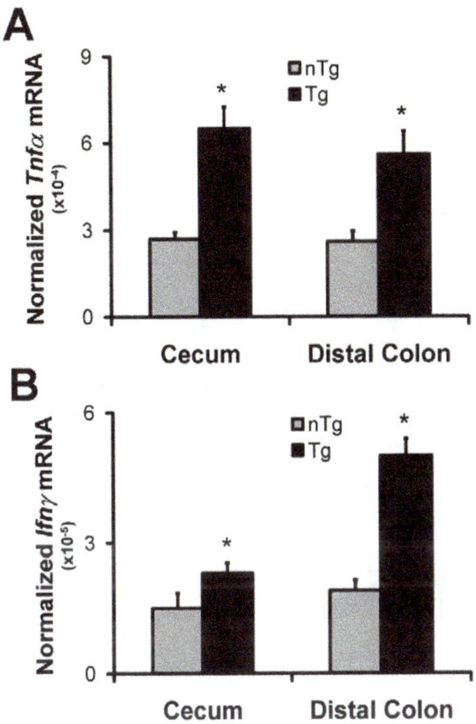

Figure 2. Expression of Pro-Inflammatory Cytokines in Colon Tissue from *B. theta* Monoassociated Rats. Abundance of TNFα (A) and IFNγ (B) mRNA normalized to β-actin as measured by real-time RT-PCR in cecum and distal colon tissue from 6-week monoassociated non-transgenic (nTg) and *HLA-B27* transgenic (Tg) rats (mean+SEM, $*p<0.05$, n = 4 rats/group).

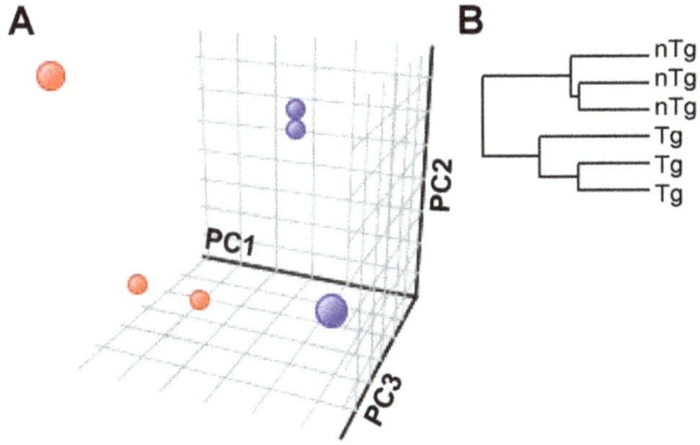

Figure 3. Transcriptional Profiles of *B. theta* Recovered from the Ceca of Monoassociated Rats. (A) 3-dimensional principal components analysis and (B) unsupervised hierarchical clustering of transcriptomes of cecal *B. theta* from 6-week monoassociated rats (PC1 = 36.1%, PC2 = 23.9%, PC3 = 21.7%). Red and blue spheres represent bacterial transcriptomes from *HLA-B27* transgenic (Tg) and non-transgenic (nTg) rats, respectively.

priori defined set of genes shows statistically significant, concordant differences between two biological states.

Virtually all of the significantly affected *B. theta* pathways (FDR q<0.20) were enriched with genes that were downregulated in *B. theta* from Tg rats with colitis compared to *B. theta* from healthy nTg rats (Tables 1 and 2). GO molecular functions involved in translation and ATP production, including "Structural Constituent of Ribosome" and "Hydrogen Ion Transporting ATPase Activity," were significantly enriched with genes that are downregulated in cecal bacteria from Tg rats (Table 1, Figure 4B–C). Similar to the results of the GSEA analysis of GO molecular functions, GSEA analysis of KEGG canonical pathways revealed that "Ribosome" and "Oxidative Phosphorylation" were highly enriched with genes that are downregulated in cecal *B. theta* from Tg rats (Table 2, Figure 4D–E). In addition, "Pyrimidine Metabolism," "Purine Metabolism", "Peptidoglycan Biosynthesis", and "Metabolic Pathways" were significantly enriched with *B. theta* genes that are downregulated in Tg rats with inflammation (Table 2, Figure 4F). These results indicate that colitis is predominantly associated with downregulation of genes in *B. theta* pathways important for energy production, metabolism, and growth.

Luminal *B. theta* viability is preserved during colitis despite down regulation of cell division genes

We next wanted to confirm the results of the pathways analysis by measuring molecular markers of bacterial cell division and quantifying luminal bacterial concentrations. To indirectly test whether cell division was decreased in luminal bacterial from Tg rats with colitis, we measured expression of *fts* genes, which are critical for bacterial septum formation and cell division [29]. We detected significantly fewer transcripts of *ftsK*, *ftsQ*, and *ftsX* in cecal bacteria from Tg compared to nTg rats (Figure 5A). Based on the pathways analysis and qPCR results of *fts* genes, we hypothesized that luminal bacterial numbers would also be decreased in Tg compared to nTg rats. However, while we detected numerically fewer viable bacteria per gram of cecal contents in Tg vs. nTg rats, the difference was not statistically significant (Figure 5B). Moreover, there was no difference in bacterial density in the distal colon of Tg rats compared to nTg rats. Thus, downregulation of genes in metabolic pathways associated with bacterial cell growth and division in cecal *B. theta* from Tg rats did not correlate with a statistically significant decreased density of viable luminal bacteria. These data suggest that in the inflamed intestine, *B. theta* may compensate for downregulated pathways important in bacterial cell growth and division by upregulating other pathways that promote bacterial persistence and maintain viability.

Luminal *B. theta* from rats with colitis upregulate genes with receptor activity

In the pathways analysis we detected only one feature, GO molecular function "Receptor Activity," that was significantly enriched (FDR q<0.2) with genes that are upregulated in *B. theta* from Tg rats with colitis (Table 3, Figure 4A). No KEGG canonical pathways were significantly enriched with genes that are upregulated in cecal *B. theta* from Tg rats (Table 4). Interestingly, 98% of the *B. theta* genes assigned to the GO category "Receptor Activity" encode TonB-dependent receptors probably involved in binding nutrients including iron-siderophore complexes, vitamin B12, and glycans [30,31]. When we examined the list of genes that were most highly upregulated in *B. theta* from Tg rats with colitis, we found that 3 out of the top 5 upregulated *B. theta* genes (BT2259, BT2260, and BT4357) encode TonB-dependent receptors (Table S1). Therefore, we speculate that *B. theta* in rats with colitis may upregulate TonB-dependent receptors to improve nutrient acquisition and viability.

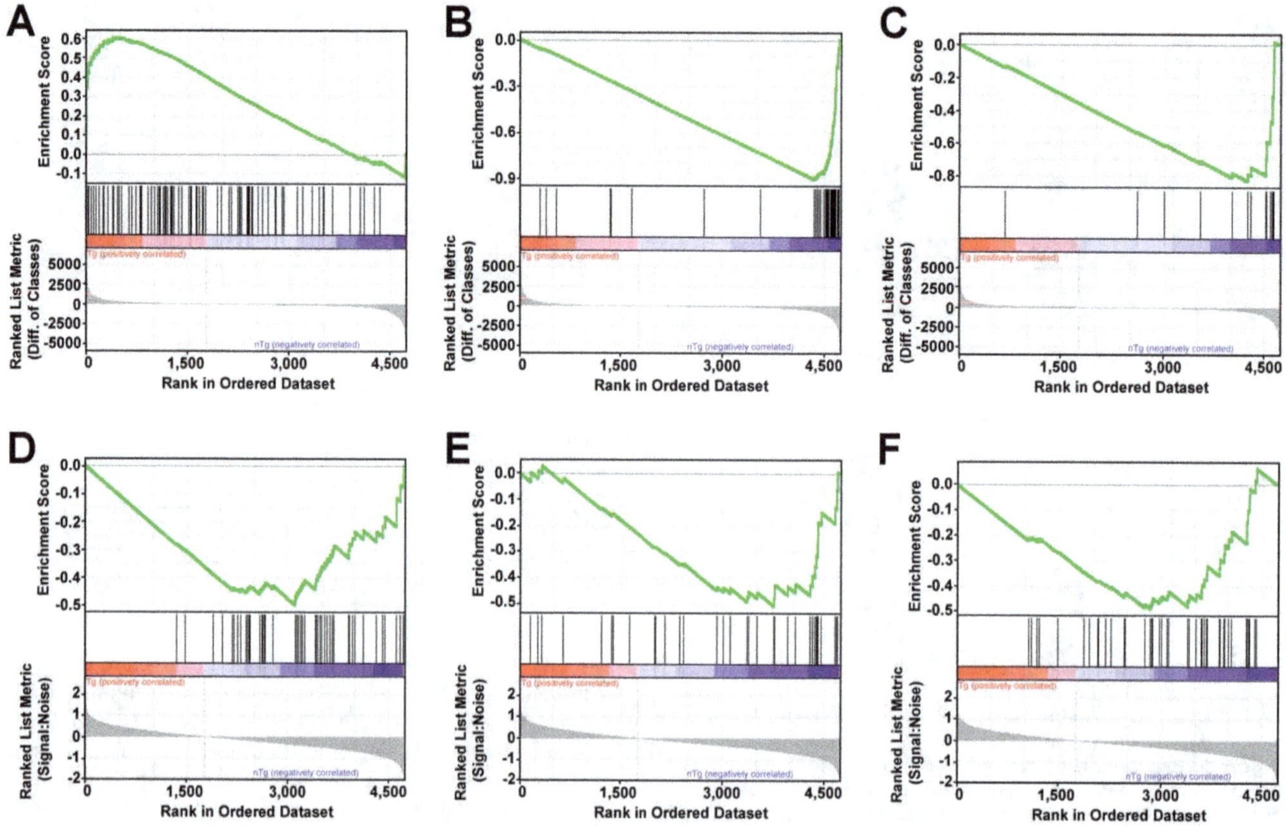

Figure 4. GSEA Enrichment Plots of GO Molecular Functions and KEGG Canonical Pathways With the Largest Normalized Enrichment Scores. (A) Receptor Activity (GO0004872), (B) Structural Constituent of Ribosome (GO0003735), (C) Hydrogen Ion Transporting ATPase Activity (GO0046961), (D) Ribosome, (E) Oxidative Phosphorylation, (F) Pyrimidine Metabolism. Top portions of the plots show the running enrichment score for the gene set as the analysis "walks down" the ranked list. Middle portions of the plots shows where members, indicated by vertical black lines, of the gene set appear in the ranked list of genes. Bottom portions of the plots show the value of the ranking metric as one progresses down the list of ranked genes.

Transgenic rats develop adaptive immune responses to a *B. theta* TonB-dependent receptor

Because we found that expression of TonB-dependent receptors is increased in *B. theta* from rats with colitis, we searched the literature for an association between TonB-dependent receptors and human IBD. Intriguingly, others have previously reported that pediatric IBD patients have increased serum antibody titers against a TonB-dependent receptor from human commensal *Bacteroides caccae* named OmpW. Using sequence alignment, we determined that OmpW shares 27% overall amino acid similarity

Table 1. GO Molecular Functions that are Enriched with Genes Downregulated in *B. theta* from Monoassociated HLA-B27 Tg Rats.

GO Molecular Function	Number of Genes in Pathway	Normalized Enrichment Score	FDR q value
Structural Constituent of Ribosome (GO0003735)	46	−2.01	<0.001
Hydrogen Ion Transporting ATPase Activity (GO0046961)	13	−1.55	0.094
Hydrogen Ion Transporting ATP Synthase Activity (GO0046933)	13	−1.52	0.110
Cation Binding (GO0043169)	54	−1.50	0.101
Protein Binding (GO0005515)	15	−1.50	0.085
Binding (GO0005488)	40	−1.48	0.094
Hydrolase Activity, Acting on Acid Anhydrides, Catalyzing Transmembrane Movement of Substances (GO0016820)	10	−1.44	0.145
Electron Carrier Activity (GO0009055)	36	−1.44	0.130
Cation Transporter Activity (GO0008324)	11	−1.39	0.189
RNA Binding (GO0003723)	38	−1.35	0.257

Table 2. KEGG Canonical Pathways that are Enriched with Genes Downregulated in *B. theta* from Monoassociated HLA-B27 Tg Rats.

KEGG Pathway	Number of Genes in Pathway	Normalized Enrichment Score	FDR q value
Ribosome	51	−1.77	0.048
Oxidative Phosphorylation	35	−1.66	0.098
Pyrimidine Metabolism	42	−1.63	0.081
Purine Metabolism	49	−1.51	0.197
Peptidoglycan Biosynthesis	16	−1.49	0.184
Fructose and Mannose Metabolism	27	−1.44	0.221
Metabolic Pathways	478	−1.44	0.191
Pyruvate Metabolism	25	−1.42	0.195
Aminoacyl-tRNA Biosynthesis	21	−1.41	0.189
Pentose Phosphate Pathway	22	−1.35	0.245

to one of the most highly upregulated TonB-dependent receptors in *B. theta* from Tg rats, BT4357 (Figure 6A) [32,33]. Moreover, amino acid residues 300 to 350 in BT4357 are 58% similar to residues in the corresponding epitope-containing portion of *B. caccae* OmpW [32] (Figure 6A). To determine whether BT4357 is antigenic in Tg rats with colitis, we performed Western Blots using individual sera from *B. theta* monoassociated Tg and nTg rats to detect recombinant protein expressed from a cloned segment of BT4357 (amino acid residues 160–741). We detected BT4357-reactive IgG antibodies in sera from three of four *B. theta* monoassociated Tg rats, but none of five nTg rats (Figure 6B, lower panel). The elevated background signal in Tg samples may be due to increased levels of total serum IgG in these rats. Based on these data, we propose that chronic colitis causes luminal *B. theta* to upregulate the TonB-dependent receptor BT4357, which is antigenic in Tg, but not nTg rats. Whether BT4357 plays a direct role in the pathogenesis of IBD in this animal model remains to be established.

Discussion

B. theta has been implicated in the pathogenesis of human IBD and a model of murine colitis. Here, we show that *B. theta* colonization is also sufficient to induce colitis in *HLA-B27* Tg rats. Furthermore, we demonstrate that chronic intestinal inflammation is associated with transcriptional changes in luminal *B. theta* that suggest decreased bacterial metabolism, growth, and division, but increased nutrient acquisition with the net effect of preserved bacterial viability. We also provide evidence that chronic colitis induces *B. theta* to upregulate expression of a gene that stimulates adaptive immune responses in genetically susceptible animals. Together, these findings indicate that commensal *B. theta* may adapt to intestinal inflammation by shifting cellular resources that would otherwise support cell division to processes that promote microbial persistence, and at the same time activate host immune responses.

The notion that bacteria respond to environmental stimuli by enhancing survival at the expense of growth has been documented elsewhere. For example, a commensal murine isolate of *E. coli* upregulates stress response genes in the IL-10-/- mouse model of colitis that decrease luminal bacterial densities *in vivo*, but have no effect on growth or persistence *in vitro* [28]. Additionally, a survey of many *E. coli* isolates has shown that high levels of σ^s, a transcription factor that controls expression of stress-response genes, correlates with increased resistance to environmental stress, but decreased ability to metabolize low concentrations of nutrients

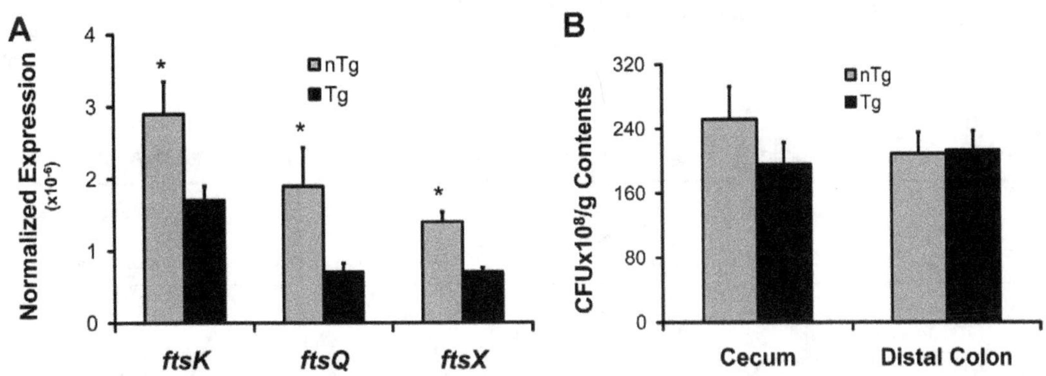

Figure 5. Expression of Cell-Division Genes and Bacterial Density in Cecal Contents from *B. theta* Monoassociated Rats. (A) Normalized expression of *fts* cell-division genes relative to bacterial 16S rRNA in *B. theta* from ceca of 6-week monoassociated rats. (B) Colony forming units (CFU)/g cecal contents from 6-week monoassociated non-transgenic (nTg) and *HLA-B27* transgenic (Tg) rats (mean+SD, n = 4–5 rats/group, *p<0.05).

Table 3. GO Molecular Functions that are Enriched with Genes Upregulated in *B. theta* from Monoassociated HLA-B27 Tg Rats.

GO Molecular Function	Number of Genes in Pathway	Normalized Enrichment Score	FDR q value
Receptor Activity (GO0004872)	93	1.70	0.148
Transporter Activity (GO0005215)	169	1.45	0.742
Sigma Factor Activity (GO0016987)	37	1.29	1.000
Transferase Activity, Transferring Nitrogenous Groups (GO0016769)	10	1.28	0.875
Metallopeptidase Activity (GO0008237)	16	1.27	0.713
Transcription Factor Activity (GO0003700)	140	1.26	0.625
Two-component Sensor Activity (GO0000155)	64	1.12	0.946
Calcium Ion Binding (GO0005509)	26	1.10	0.889
Sequence-Specific DNA Binding (GO0043565)	87	1.06	0.891
Protein Histidine Kinase Activity (GO0004673)	57	1.03	0.896

[34]. Thus, the functional outcome of bacterial responses to environmental conditions can lead to growth or persistence depending on the nature of the stimulus and the genetic composition of the bacteria.

Whether the transcriptional changes noted in *B. theta* monoassociated Tg rats are representative of Bacteroides gene expression in human IBD remains to be determined. The animal model used in our studies has several limitations. While *Bacteroides spp.* are a dominant member of the commensal human gut microbiota, *B. theta* represents a relatively small component of the *Bacteroides* and changes in its transcriptome may not be representative of transcriptional changes that occur in other *Bacteroides spp.* Inflammation in *HLA-B27* Tg rats colonized with commensal bacteria is similar to that observed in human Crohn's disease because it is characterized by a Th-1 predominant immune response and affects both the upper and lower digestive tract and extraintestinal organs [19,20]. However, unlike human Crohn's disease, Tg rats do not typically develop mucosal ulceration. It is also important to note that *B. theta* transcriptional changes in monoassociated rats used in our studies may not reflect those observed in a more natural complex microbiota where other members of the microbial community would likely influence *B. theta* gene regulation. Furthermore, our gene expression studies did not distinguish between luminal and mucosal-associated bacteria, which may be more relevant in host-commensal interactions due to proximity. However, we have previously shown that metagenomic functional profiles of mucosal associated bacteria are similarly diverse as those reported in feces [35].

Interestingly, most of the differentially expressed *B. theta* genes were downregulated in bacteria from Tg rats. Concordantly, more pathways were significantly enriched with genes that were downregulated in bacteria from Tg rats compared to pathways enriched with genes that were upregulated in bacteria from Tg rats. However, the transcriptional changes did not significantly affect luminal bacterial density and it is unknown whether deletion of differentially expressed genes in *B. theta* would affect bacterial viability in animals with colitis. While we have assumed that decreased expression of genes in metabolic and growth-related pathways should result in fewer viable luminal bacteria, it is possible that downregulation of these genes in bacteria does not affect growth. Consistent with this, differentially expressed genes in *B. theta* from the Tg rats did not overlap with genes in *B. theta* from wild-type mice, that when mutated, conferred a competitive growth advantage or disadvantage [36].

Compared to the number of downregulated genes, fewer bacterial genes were upregulated in Tg rats. For instance, *B. theta* upregulate expression of bacterial enzymes that metabolize products of the host innate immune response, including reactive oxygen and nitrogen species that are increased in intestinal tissue from patients with IBD and animals with experimental colitis [37,38]. We found that bacteria from Tg rats with colitis increase expression of genes encoding nitrite reductase (BT1414–1417), an enzyme that detoxifies nitric oxides produced by activated host innate immune cells [39], compared to healthy controls. Expression of this same set of genes was increased in *B. theta* from monoassociated Rag1-/- mice that have increased levels of intestinal inducible nitric oxide synthase [17].

Table 4. KEGG Canonical Pathways that are Enriched with Genes Upregulated in *B. theta* from Monoassociated HLA-B27 Tg Rats.

KEGG Pathway	Number of Genes in Pathway	Normalized Enrichment Score	FDR q value
Nitrogen Metabolism	21	1.29	0.774
Two-component System	15	1.16	0.698
Sphingolipid Metabolism	15	0.87	1.000
Starch and Sucrose Metabolism	28	0.87	1.000
Other Glycan Degradation	24	0.79	0.964
Glycine, Serine, and Threonine Metabolism	20	0.72	0.890

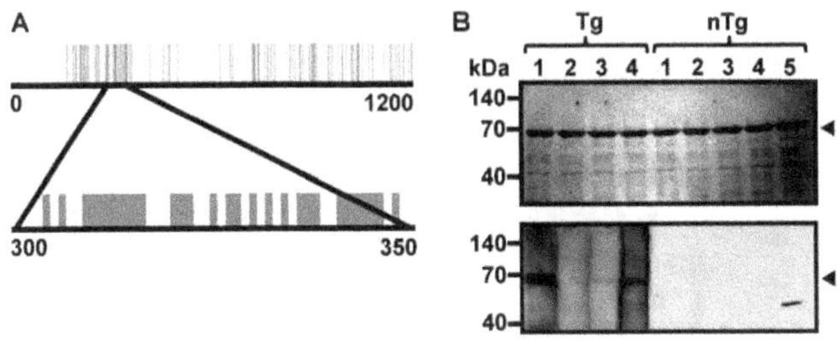

Figure 6. Serologic Responses to Recombinant BT4357 SusC Homolog in *B. theta* Monoassociated Rats. (A) Amino acid sequence alignment of BT4357 and *B. caccae* OmpW using Clustal W2, including a magnified view from residues 300–350. Vertical lines represent identical residues. (B) Ponceau S stained Western Blot membrane demonstrating equivalent amounts of purified recombinant BT4357 fragment in each lane (top panel). Western Blot of strips of the membrane shown in the top panel using sera from individual *B. theta* monoassociated transgenic (Tg) and non-transgenic (nTg) rats and an anti-rat IgG secondary antibody (bottom panel). Predicted size of BT4357 fragment is indicated by the arrowheads.

Many of the other highly upregulated genes encode proteins important for starch utilization by *B. theta*, including several *susC* and *susD* homologues. Similarly, GO molecular function analysis revealed an enrichment in transcripts of genes with receptor activity in bacteria from Tg rats. *B. theta* have evolved mechanisms to utilize carbohydrates from a variety of sources—including dietary and host glycans [27,40]. Genes involved in host mucin-O-glycan metabolism (BT1042–1053, BT4355–4359, and BT0317–0319), which were previously shown to enhance fitness of *B. theta in vivo* and participate in the production of the polysaccharide capsule, are upregulated in bacteria from Tg rats [31,41]. This suggests that colitis is associated either with an altered carbohydrate landscape on the intestinal epithelium or decreased concentrations of dietary glycans in the cecum.

Interestingly, the *B. theta susC* homolog (BT4357) that was most highly upregulated in Tg rats is very similar to *Bacteroides caccae* OmpW, which induces adaptive immune responses in pediatric IBD patients more frequently than in healthy controls [32,33]. Both BT4357 and OmpW are TonB-dependent receptors and belong to a family of receptors that facilitate nutrient acquisition and uptake. In our studies, we found that BT4357 is also antigenic in Tg, but not nTg monoassociated rats suggesting the possibility of a conserved epitope in TonB-dependent receptors across *Bacteroides* species. However, it should be noted that we measured anti-BT4357 IgG in the rat sera, whereas the anti-OmpW antibodies detected in IBD patients were of the IgA isotype. Furthermore, it is possible that the elevated serologic immune responses to BT4357 in Tg rats are due to increased gut permeability during colitis and are not proportional to the expression level of BT4357 in luminal bacteria. While several other bacterial proteins including OmpC, I2 and flagellin have been previously shown to induce elevated antibody responses in IBD patients compared to controls, this is the first report of inflammation-associated upregulation of a bacterial antigen in colitis [42,43]. We speculate that environmental factors in the lumen of the inflamed colon (e.g. altered nutrient availability) cause *B. theta* to induce expression of this TonB-dependent receptor, which is a dominant antigen that may contribute to chronic inflammation. Gnotobiotic studies using BT4357-deficient *B. theta* in Tg rats are needed to test whether immune responses to BT4357 are a cause or effect of colitis. Furthermore, testing sera from IBD patients for anti-BT4357 antibodies could expand the relevance of our findings to human IBD.

In summary, we have observed that the human commensal *B. theta* induces chronic, immune-mediated colitis in HLA-B27 Tg rats, which is associated with significant changes in luminal bacterial transcription that affect metabolic, growth, and nutrient binding pathways. In addition, intestinal inflammation induces *B. theta* to upregulate expression of a nutrient receptor that stimulates adaptive immune responses specifically in rats that are genetically susceptible to colitis. These studies add to a growing body of evidence demonstrating that commensal intestinal microbes actively participate in chronic intestinal inflammation by inducing and reacting to host inflammation. Exploring mechanisms of how host inflammatory factors affect gut commensals and the impact of inflammation-induced microbial transcriptional changes on disease pathogenesis may reveal novel pathways that could be potential therapeutic targets to treat human IBD.

Supporting Information

Figure S1 Real-Time RT-PCR Verification of Microarray Results for Selected *B. theta* Genes. Selected differentially expressed *B. theta* genes from cecal bacteria from 6 week-monoassociated non-transgenic (nTg) and *HLA-B27* transgenic (Tg) rats were quantified using real-time RT-PCR. Results are normalized to bacterial 16S expression (Mean+SD, n = 4–5 rats/group, $*p<0.05$).

Table S1 Upregulated *B. theta* genes in cecal bacteria from Tg vs. nTg Rats.

Table S2 Downregulated *B. theta* genes in cecal bacteria from Tg vs. nTg Rats.

Table S3 Sequences of oligonucleotides used in PCR reactions.

Acknowledgments

We thank Dr. Jeffrey I. Gordon for the kind gift of the custom *B. theta* microarrays. We acknowledge the Gnotobiotic and Histology Cores at the UNC Center for Gastrointestinal Biology and Disease and the University of Chicago Host-Microbe Core of the Digestive Disease Research Core Center.

Author Contributions

Conceived and designed the experiments: JJH YH DAP TF EBC RBS. Performed the experiments: JJH YH DAP LG TF. Analyzed the data: JJH YH DAP LG TF EBC RBS. Contributed reagents/materials/analysis tools: JJH DAP EBC RBS. Wrote the paper: JJH YH.

References

1. Fujiya M, Musch MW, Nakagawa Y, Hu S, Alverdy J, et al. (2007) The Bacillus subtilis quorum-sensing molecule CSF contributes to intestinal homeostasis via OCTN2, a host cell membrane transporter. Cell Host Microbe 1: 299–308.
2. Chow J, Mazmanian SK (2010) A pathobiont of the microbiota balances host colonization and intestinal inflammation. Cell Host Microbe 7: 265–276.
3. Hugot JP, Chamaillard M, Zouali H, Lesage S, Cezard JP, et al. (2001) Association of NOD2 leucine-rich repeat variants with susceptibility to Crohn's disease. Nature 411: 599–603.

4. Ogura Y, Bonen DK, Inohara N, Nicolae DL, Chen FF, et al. (2001) A frameshift mutation in NOD2 associated with susceptibility to Crohn's disease. Nature 411: 603–606.
5. Janowitz HD, Croen EC, Sachar DB (1998) The role of the fecal stream in Crohn's disease: an historical and analytic review. Inflamm Bowel Dis 4: 29–39.
6. Hansen J, Gulati A, Sartor RB (2010) The role of mucosal immunity and host genetics in defining intestinal commensal bacteria. Curr Opin Gastroenterol 26: 564–571.
7. Kotlowski R, Bernstein CN, Sepehri S, Krause DO (2007) High prevalence of Escherichia coli belonging to the B2+D phylogenetic group in inflammatory bowel disease. Gut 56: 669–675.
8. Darfeuille-Michaud A, Boudeau J, Bulois P, Neut C, Glasser AL, et al. (2004) High prevalence of adherent-invasive Escherichia coli associated with ileal mucosa in Crohn's disease. Gastroenterology 127: 412–421.
9. Sokol H, Pigneur B, Watterlot L, Lakhdari O, Bermudez-Humaran LG, et al. (2008) Faecalibacterium prausnitzii is an anti-inflammatory commensal bacterium identified by gut microbiota analysis of Crohn disease patients. Proc Natl Acad Sci U S A 105: 16731–16736.
10. Frank DN, St Amand AL, Feldman RA, Boedeker EC, Harpaz N, et al. (2007) Molecular-phylogenetic characterization of microbial community imbalances in human inflammatory bowel diseases. Proc Natl Acad Sci U S A 104: 13780–13785.
11. Takaishi H, Matsuki T, Nakazawa A, Takada T, Kado S, et al. (2008) Imbalance in intestinal microflora constitution could be involved in the pathogenesis of inflammatory bowel disease. Int J Med Microbiol 298: 463–472.
12. Gophna U, Sommerfeld K, Gophna S, Doolittle WF, Veldhuyzen van Zanten SJ (2006) Differences between tissue-associated intestinal microfloras of patients with Crohn's disease and ulcerative colitis. J Clin Microbiol 44: 4136–4141.
13. Bibiloni R, Mangold M, Madsen KL, Fedorak RN, Tannock GW (2006) The bacteriology of biopsies differs between newly diagnosed, untreated, Crohn's disease and ulcerative colitis patients. J Med Microbiol 55: 1141–1149.
14. Andoh A, Tsujikawa T, Sasaki M, Mitsuyama K, Suzuki Y, et al. (2009) Faecal microbiota profile of Crohn's disease determined by terminal restriction fragment length polymorphism analysis. Aliment Pharmacol Ther 29: 75–82.
15. Edwards LA, Lucas M, Edwards EA, Torrente F, Heuschkel RB, et al. (2011) Aberrant response to commensal Bacteroides thetaiotaomicron in Crohn's disease: an ex vivo human organ culture study. Inflamm Bowel Dis 17: 1201–1208.
16. Hansen JJ, Sartor RB (2007) Insights provided by animal models into the pathogenesis and treatment of IBD. In: Bernstein C, editor. The Inflammatory Bowel Disease Yearbook. London: Remedica. pp. 19–55.
17. Peterson DA, McNulty NP, Guruge JL, Gordon JI (2007) IgA response to symbiotic bacteria as a mediator of gut homeostasis. Cell Host Microbe 2: 328–339.
18. Bloom SM, Bijanki VN, Nava GM, Sun L, Malvin NP, et al. (2011) Commensal Bacteroides species induce colitis in host-genotype-specific fashion in a mouse model of inflammatory bowel disease. Cell Host Microbe 9: 390–403.
19. Hammer RE, Maika SD, Richardson JA, Tang JP, Taurog JD (1990) Spontaneous inflammatory disease in transgenic rats expressing HLA-B27 and human beta 2 m: an animal model of HLA-B27-associated human disorders. Cell 63: 1099–1112.
20. Rath HC, Herfarth HH, Ikeda JS, Grenther WB, Hamm TE, et al. (1996) Normal luminal bacteria, especially Bacteroides species, mediate chronic colitis, gastritis, and arthritis in HLA-B27/human beta2 microglobulin transgenic rats. J Clin Invest 98: 945–953.
21. Rath HC, Wilson KH, Sartor RB (1999) Differential induction of colitis and gastritis in HLA-B27 transgenic rats selectively colonized with Bacteroides vulgatus or Escherichia coli. Infect Immun 67: 2969–2974.
22. Kim SC, Tonkonogy SL, Albright CA, Tsang J, Balish EJ, et al. (2005) Variable phenotypes of enterocolitis in interleukin 10-deficient mice monoassociated with two different commensal bacteria. Gastroenterology 128: 891–906.
23. Li C, Hung Wong W (2001) Model-based analysis of oligonucleotide arrays: model validation, design issues and standard error application. Genome Biol 2: RESEARCH0032.
24. Tusher VG, Tibshirani R, Chu G (2001) Significance analysis of microarrays applied to the ionizing radiation response. Proc Natl Acad Sci U S A 98: 5116–5121.
25. Xu J, Bjursell MK, Himrod J, Deng S, Carmichael LK, et al. (2003) A genomic view of the human-Bacteroides thetaiotaomicron symbiosis. Science 299: 2074–2076.
26. Subramanian A, Tamayo P, Mootha VK, Mukherjee S, Ebert BL, et al. (2005) Gene set enrichment analysis: a knowledge-based approach for interpreting genome-wide expression profiles. Proc Natl Acad Sci U S A 102: 15545–15550.
27. Sonnenburg JL, Xu J, Leip DD, Chen CH, Westover BP, et al. (2005) Glycan foraging in vivo by an intestine-adapted bacterial symbiont. Science 307: 1955–1959.
28. Patwa LG, Fan TJ, Tchaptchet S, Liu Y, Lussier YA, et al. (2011) Chronic intestinal inflammation induces stress-response genes in commensal Escherichia coli. Gastroenterology 141: 1842–1851 e1841–1810.
29. Weiss DS (2004) Bacterial cell division and the septal ring. Mol Microbiol 54: 588–597.
30. Koebnik R (2005) TonB-dependent trans-envelope signalling: the exception or the rule? Trends Microbiol 13: 343–347.
31. Martens EC, Chiang HC, Gordon JI (2008) Mucosal glycan foraging enhances fitness and transmission of a saccharolytic human gut bacterial symbiont. Cell Host Microbe 4: 447–457.
32. Wei B, Dalwadi H, Gordon LK, Landers C, Bruckner D, et al. (2001) Molecular cloning of a Bacteroides caccae TonB-linked outer membrane protein identified by an inflammatory bowel disease marker antibody. Infect Immun 69: 6044–6054.
33. Ashorn S, Honkanen T, Kolho KL, Ashorn M, Valineva T, et al. (2009) Fecal calprotectin levels and serological responses to microbial antigens among children and adolescents with inflammatory bowel disease. Inflamm Bowel Dis 15: 199–205.
34. King T, Ishihama A, Kori A, Ferenci T (2004) A regulatory trade-off as a source of strain variation in the species Escherichia coli. J Bacteriol 186: 5614–5620.
35. Wang Y, Antonopoulos DA, Zhu X, Harrell L, Hanan I, et al. (2010) Laser capture microdissection and metagenomic analysis of intact mucosa-associated microbial communities of human colon. Appl Microbiol Biotechnol 88: 1333–1342.
36. Goodman AL, McNulty NP, Zhao Y, Leip D, Mitra RD, et al. (2009) Identifying genetic determinants needed to establish a human gut symbiont in its habitat. Cell Host Microbe 6: 279–289.
37. Carroll IM, Andrus JM, Bruno-Barcena JM, Klaenhammer TR, Hassan HM, et al. (2007) Anti-inflammatory properties of Lactobacillus gasseri expressing manganese superoxide dismutase using the interleukin 10-deficient mouse model of colitis. Am J Physiol Gastrointest Liver Physiol 293: G729–738.
38. Keshavarzian A, Banan A, Farhadi A, Komanduri S, Mutlu E, et al. (2003) Increases in free radicals and cytoskeletal protein oxidation and nitration in the colon of patients with inflammatory bowel disease. Gut 52: 720–728.
39. Vine CE, Cole JA (2011) Unresolved sources, sinks, and pathways for the recovery of enteric bacteria from nitrosative stress. FEMS Microbiol Lett.
40. Hooper LV, Xu J, Falk PG, Midtvedt T, Gordon JI (1999) A molecular sensor that allows a gut commensal to control its nutrient foundation in a competitive ecosystem. Proc Natl Acad Sci U S A 96: 9833–9838.
41. Martens EC, Koropatkin NM, Smith TJ, Gordon JI (2009) Complex glycan catabolism by the human gut microbiota: the Bacteroidetes Sus-like paradigm. J Biol Chem 284: 24673–24677.
42. Landers CJ, Cohavy O, Misra R, Yang H, Lin YC, et al. (2002) Selected loss of tolerance evidenced by Crohn's disease-associated immune responses to auto- and microbial antigens. Gastroenterology 123: 689–699.
43. Lodes MJ, Cong Y, Elson CO, Mohamath R, Landers CJ, et al. (2004) Bacterial flagellin is a dominant antigen in Crohn disease. J Clin Invest 113: 1296–1306.

16

CCL25/CCR9 Interactions Regulate Large Intestinal Inflammation in a Murine Model of Acute Colitis

Marc-Andre Wurbel[1]*, Maria G. McIntire[2], Peter Dwyer[1], Edda Fiebiger[1]*

1 Division of Gastroenterology and Nutrition, Children's Hospital Boston, and Department of Pediatrics, Harvard Medical School, Boston, Massachusetts, United States of America, **2** Department of Pathology, Harvard Medical School, Brigham and Women's Hospital, Boston, Massachusetts, United States of America

Abstract

Background & Aims: CCL25/CCR9 is a non-promiscuous chemokine/receptor pair and a key regulator of leukocyte migration to the small intestine. We investigated here whether CCL25/CCR9 interactions also play a role in the regulation of inflammatory responses in the large intestine.

Methods: Acute inflammation and recovery in wild-type (WT) and CCR9$^{-/-}$ mice was studied in a model of dextran sulfate sodium (DSS)-induced colitis. Distribution studies and phenotypic characterization of dendritic cell subsets and macrophage were performed by flow cytometry. Inflammatory bowel disease (IBD) scores were assessed and expression of inflammatory cytokines was studied at the mRNA and the protein level.

Results: CCL25 and CCR9 are both expressed in the large intestine and are upregulated during DSS colitis. CCR9$^{-/-}$ mice are more susceptible to DSS colitis than WT littermate controls as shown by higher mortality, increased IBD score and delayed recovery. During recovery, the CCR9$^{-/-}$ colonic mucosa is characterized by the accumulation of activated macrophages and elevated levels of Th1/Th17 inflammatory cytokines. Activated plasmacytoid dendritic cells (DCs) accumulate in mesenteric lymph nodes (MLNs) of CCR9$^{-/-}$ animals, altering the local ratio of DC subsets. Upon re-stimulation, T cells isolated from these MLNs secrete significantly higher levels of TNFα, IFNγ, IL2, IL-6 and IL-17A while down modulating IL-10 production.

Conclusions: Our results demonstrate that CCL25/CCR9 interactions regulate inflammatory immune responses in the large intestinal mucosa by balancing different subsets of dendritic cells. These findings have important implications for the use of CCR9-inhibitors in therapy of human IBD as they indicate a potential risk for patients with large intestinal inflammation.

Editor: Guillaume Dalmasso, Emory Unviersity, United States

Funding: This work was supported by a Crohn's & Colitis Foundation of America Career Development Award (to MAW), by a Pilot Project Grant from the Harvard Digestive Diseases Center P30 DK034854 (to MAW), by a Research Scholar Award from the American Gastroenterological Association (to EF) and by grant R01AI075037 from the National Institutes of Health (to EF). The funders had no role in study design, data collection and analysis, decision to publish, or preparation of the manuscript.

Competing Interests: The authors have declared that no competing interests exist.

* E-mail: marc-andre.wurbel@childrens.harvard.edu (M-AW); edda.fiebiger@childrens.harvard.edu (EF)

Introduction

Crohn's disease and ulcerative colitis represent two clinical subtypes of inflammatory bowel disease (IBD). Infiltration of inflammatory leukocytes into the gastrointestinal mucosa critically regulates development as well as progression of both types of IBD. Tissue- and cell type-specific leukocyte trafficking is orchestrated by chemokines and their receptors. Interaction of CCL25 with CCR9 identifies one of the few non-promiscuous chemokine/receptor pairs involved in gut-specific migration of leukocytes. CCL25 is strongly expressed by the small intestinal epithelium [1,2,3] and regulates trafficking of gut-specific memory/effector T cells via upregulation of the integrin homing receptor $\alpha4\beta7$ and CCR9 [4,5,6,7]. The chemokine itself is dispensable for the development of CCR9^{high} intestinal memory-phenotype T cells. CCX282-B (Traficet-EN, ChemoCentryx) is a small molecule that can antagonize CCR9 function and has already shown promising results in a phase II clinical trial of moderate to severe Crohn's Disease patients as it successfully delays disease progression [8]. As CCL25/CCR9 interactions are currently considered dispensable for the regulation of inflammation in the large intestine, the therapeutic effect of the CCR9-antagonist has not been studied in ulcerative colitis.

Several different murine models have been described to study the pathophysiology of ulcerative colitis [9]. Administration of Dextran Sulfate Sodium (DSS) in drinking water induces a reversible form of colitis in mice [10]. This model is characterized by acute tissue inflammation in the colon and mimics the pathology of human ulcerative colitis. Since immuno-compromised mice such as Recombinase-Activating Gene (RAG) deficient mice or severe combined immune deficiency (SCID) mice lacking the T and B cell compartment remain susceptible in this disease model [11], a central role for monocytes/macrophages (MΦ) and dendritic cells (DCs) was proposed for the pathogenesis of DSS colitis and likewise for human ulcerative colitis. Consequently, inflammatory MΦ were described as antigen-presenting cells (APCs) that activate T cells and induce T cell proliferation in DSS colitis [12,13].

MΦ and intestinal DCs are located in the intestinal lamina propria (LP), Peyer's patches (PPs) and mesenteric lymph nodes (MLN) and are the first APCs to sense and respond to exogenous antigens or tissue injury [14]. Several subpopulations of DCs and MΦ have been described in the intestinal microenvironment [15,16,17]. Their respective functions for the induction of protective immunity versus immune tolerance in the gut remain poorly understood [14]. Recent studies have shown that depletion of DCs during DSS-induced colitis leads to ameliorated or exacerbated symptoms depending on the time point of intervention [18,19,20]. These observations imply that concerted trafficking of different DC subsets is critical for onset and recovery of colitis. CCR9 is a candidate chemokine receptor for the regulation of this type of DC trafficking, because it has been demonstrated that CD11c-positive splenic DCs as well as peritoneal MΦ migrate towards a CCL25 chemotactic gradient [1]. However the role of CCL25/CCR9 interactions during the regulation of large intestinal inflammation has not been studied so far.

Here we describe a so far unanticipated role of CCL25 and CCR9 in the regulation of large intestinal inflammation. We show that CCR9$^{-/-}$ animals display exacerbated colitis. In the absence of physiological CCL25/CCR9 interactions, we detect an imbalance of DC subpopulations and the accumulation of inflammatory MΦ in the lamina propria of the colon and in gut-associated lymphoid tissue.

Materials and Methods

Mice

The generation of CCR9$^{-/-}$ and CCL25$^{-/-}$ mice has been described previously [7,21]. All strains of mice, including C57Bl/6 control mice were bred in the animal facility at Children's Hospital Boston, born and held in the same room under specific pathogen-free conditions. To avoid variations of commensal bacteria in our experiments, littermate controls were used. All animal experiments were approved under animal protocol number 09-03-1326 *by Children's Hospital Boston Institutional Animal Care and Use Committee. Children's Hospital Boston's assurance number is A3303-01. Children's* Hospital Boston is accredited by AAALAC International. All efforts were made to minimize suffering of animals.

Dextran Sulfate Sodium- (DSS) mediated colitis

Sex- and age-matched mice received 2% DSS (36–50 kDa, MP Biomedicals, LCC, Solon, OH) in the drinking water for 7 days followed by 10-day water administration. The animal weight was recorded daily. For flow cytometry, histology and mRNA analysis, mice were euthanized at indicated time points, with day 0 (d0) corresponding to the initiation of DSS treatment. All efforts were made to minimize suffering of animals.

Preparation of cell suspensions

Spleens (SPL) and mesenteric lymph nodes (MLN) were harvested in HBSS with Ca^{2+} and Mg^{2+} supplemented with 2% fetal calf serum (FCS) and 10mM HEPES. SPL and MLN suspensions were obtained by collagenase VIII digestion (Sigma-Aldrich, St. Louis, MO) for 30 min at 37°C. Lamina Propria Lymphocyte (LPL) suspensions were obtained as previously described [7]. Large intestines were flushed and opened longitudinally. To remove intra-epithelial lymphocytes and epithelial cells, intestinal pieces were incubated in HBSS without Ca^{2+}/Mg^{2+} supplemented with 10mM EDTA, 10mM HEPES, 0.5% FCS and 1.5 mM DTET, for 2×20 min at 37°C. Intestinal pieces were digested in HBSS with Ca^{2+}/Mg^{2+}, 20% FCS, 100 U/ml collagenase VIII and 5 μg/ml DNase (Sigma-Aldrich) for 60–90 min at 37°C. LPL were purified over a 40%–100% Percoll gradient (GE Healthcare Bio-Sciences Corp, Piscataway, NJ).

Flow Cytometry Analysis

Cell suspensions from SPL, MLN and large intestinal LP were analyzed by flow cytometry. Cells were stained with FITC-, PE-, PerCP-Cy5.5, PE-Cy7-, APC- or AF-647, APC-Cy7- or APC-eF780-labeled mAbs for MHC II, CD11c, CD11b, Ly6C, PDCA-1, CD103, CD8α, B220, CD19 (BD Biosciences, Franklin Lakes, NJ), CCR9 (eBioscience, San Diego, CA), DX5 and CD3ε (Biolegend, San Diego, CA). Blocking of FcγR-binding was performed using mouse and rat serum (Jackson Immunoresearch, West Grove, PA). Cells were analyzed on a FACS Canto II (BD Biosciences, Franklin Lakes, NJ). Data were collected using FACS Diva software (BD Biosciences) and analyzed with FlowJo software (TreeStar, Ashland, OR).

Histology and IBD scoring

Intestinal samples of the distal colon were harvested, fixed in 10% formalin and embedded in paraffin for H&E staining. Histological IBD scoring was performed blindly by a pathologist as follows: IBD scores corresponding to 0 = normal, 1 = mild, 2 = moderate, 3 = severe were attributed to activity grade, changes of crypt architecture, basal lymphoplasmacytosis, expansion of lamina propria and epithelial hyperplasia. Scores were graphed in a total range of 0–15.

mRNA quantification

Total RNA was extracted with TRIzol™ (Invitrogen, Carlsbad, CA) according to the manufacturer's guidelines. Quantification of total RNA was performed with a Nanodrop™ spectrophotometer (Thermo Scientific). For real-time RT-PCR, cDNA was synthesized with iScript™ Select cDNA Synthesis kit (Biorad, Hercules, CA). Amplification was performed with the iQ5 quantitative PCR System (Biorad) and iQ™ SYBR® Green Supermix (Biorad) on 50ng RNA. CCR9 and CCL25 mRNAs were quantified using β-actin mRNA for normalization. Primer sequences: CCL25 Forward: 5′-ccaaggtgcctttgaagact-3′, CCL25 Reverse: 5′-tcctccagctggtggttact-3′, CCR9 Forward: 5′-ccaggaaatctctggtctgc-3′, CCR9 Reverse: 5′-ctgtggaagcagtggagtca, β-actin Forward: 5′-gctgtattcccctccatcgt -3′, β-actin Reverse: 5′-gccatgttcaatggggtact -5′. For nCounter™ analysis (Nanostring, Seattle, WA), code sets were generated by the GeneSelector algorithm [22]. 250 ng of colonic RNA were hybridized for 16 h, loaded onto the nCounter™ prep-station and quantified with the nCounter™ Digital Analyzer. nCounter data were normalized in two steps according to the manufacturer. We controlled for variations in the efficiency of processing with controls from the manufacturer. Data were normalized to Tomm7, Shfml, Hprtl, Hsp90abl and actb as housekeeping genes.

Cell culture and cytokine measurement

RPMI 1640 medium (GIBCO) supplemented with 10% FCS, 2 mmol/L L-glutamine, 100 U/ml penicillin-streptomycin, and 50 μmol/L 2-mercaptoethanol (Invitrogen) was used for all cultures. 10^6 cells from WT and CCR9$^{-/-}$ MLN harvested at d17 of DSS colitis were activated with immobilized anti-CD3 mAb (145-2C11; 0.5 μg/ml) and soluble anti-CD28 mAb (BD Biosciences). Supernatants were harvested at 72 h for cytokine measurement by BD Cytometric Bead Array (CBA) using a mouse Th1/Th2/Th17 kit according to the manufacturer's guidelines (BD Biosciences). Samples were analyzed on a FACS

Canto II flow cytometer using FACS Diva Software (BD Biosciences) with FCAP Array Software (BD Biosciences).

Enrichment of pDCs

pDCs were enriched by positive selection with PDCA-1 conjugated magnetic beads (Miltenyi Biotec, Auburn, CA) according to manufacturer. Purity was determined by flow cytometry using mAbs anti-MHC II, CD11c, PDCA-1 and B220 and Ly6C. Enrichment led to 90% purity.

Statistical Analysis

Weight loss, Colon length, IBD Scoring and cellular distributions were compared using either Student t-test or ANOVA test. Differences with $p<0.05$ were considered significant. Statistical analysis was performed using Prism (Graph Pad Software, La Jolla, CA). Kaplan-Meier survival curves to DSS-mediated colitis were created using Prism (Graph Pad Software).

Results

CCR9 and CCL25 are expressed in the mucosa of the large intestine

In line with the literature [1,2,3], high levels of CCR9 and CCL25 transcripts were detected in Peyer's Patches (PPs) and in the small intestine (SI). We found low-level expression of CCR9 and CCL25 in the large intestine (LI) of healthy wild-type (WT) mice. Intestinal tissue from CCR9$^{-/-}$ and CCL25$^{-/-}$ animals was used as a specificity control (Figure 1*A*).

We next analyzed whether large intestinal inflammation affects expression levels of CCL25. Acute experimental colitis was induced by addition of DSS in the drinking water for seven days followed by a ten-day recovery period (Figure 1*B*). CCL25 mRNA levels did not change significantly until day 10 (d10). At d13 and at d17, CCL25 transcripts were significantly upregulated (6.9+/−4.8 and 21.5+/−11.2 fold induction, Figure 1*C*). Our data show that CCL25 expression increases during DSS colitis, suggesting a

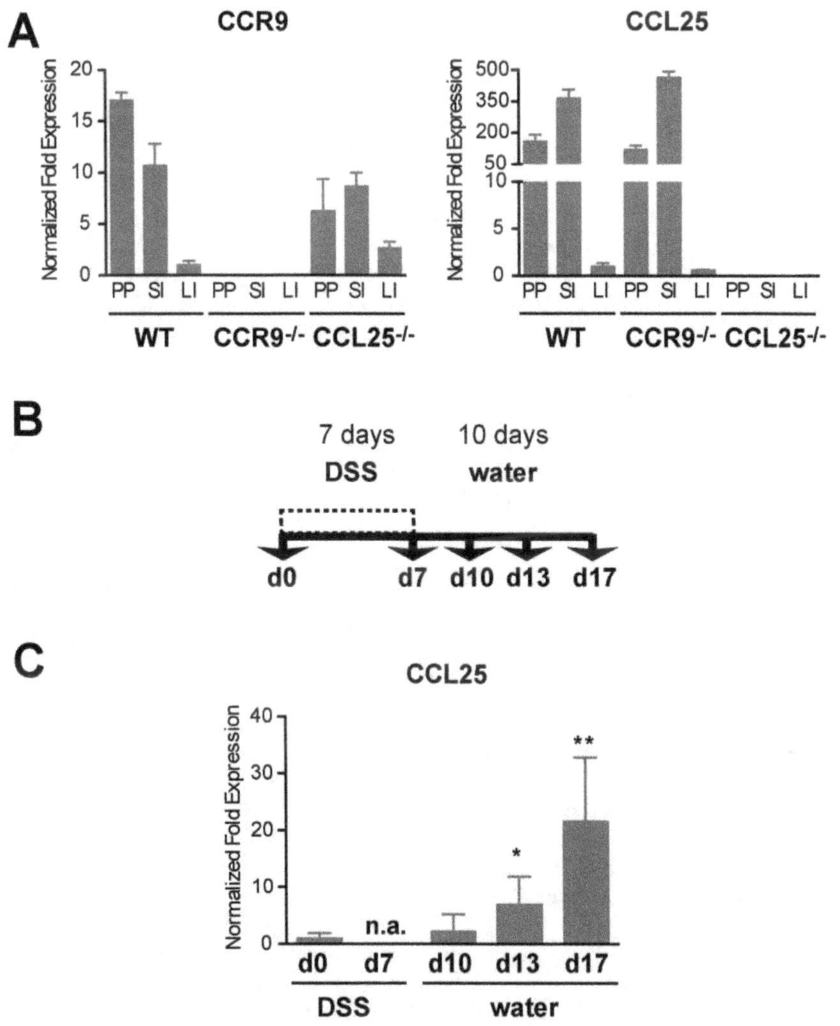

Figure 1. Expression of CCR9 and CCL25 in the large intestine. (**A**) Quantification of CCR9 and CCL25 mRNA levels from intestinal tissues of WT, CCR9$^{-/-}$ and CCL25$^{-/-}$ mice. Y-axis shows expression levels normalized to β-actin mRNA (mean +/− SD, n = 3). PP: Peyer's Patches, SI: Small intestine, LI: Large intestine. Data represent the mean +/− SD of 3 independent experiments, performed in triplicate (**B**) Acute DSS-mediated colitis. Induction phase: 2% DSS in drinking water for 7 days. Recovery: 10 days water. Mice were analyzed at days 0 (d0), d7, d10, d13 and d17. (**C**) CCL25 mRNA expression increases during the recovery phase of DSS-mediated colitis, (mean +/− SD; d0, n = 3; d10, n = 3; d13, n = 5; d17, n = 5; where n corresponds to a single experiments of 3 to 5 pooled intestinal samples).

regulatory role of CCL25/CCR9 interactions during large intestinal inflammation.

CCR9$^{-/-}$ mice show increased susceptibility to acute DSS colitis

DSS colitis is dependent on the duration and dose of DSS administration as well as the genetic background of the animals [10,23,24]. We next compared the susceptibility of CCR9$^{-/-}$ and WT mice to 3% DSS, as commonly used in C57Bl/6 mice. Surprisingly, administration of this DSS concentration induced a mortality of 100% in CCR9$^{-/-}$ animals during the recovery phase (data not shown). We thus decreased the DSS concentration to 2% resulting in a reduction of mortality to 30.65% (Figure 2*A*). Both strains were susceptible to DSS colitis as evidenced by body weight loss (Figure 2*B*). Maximal weight loss occurred in WT mice by d10 and in CCR9$^{-/-}$ mice by d12. CCR9$^{-/-}$ mice lost significantly more weight than WT animals. In contrast to WT mice, CCR9$^{-/-}$ animals were unable to regain their initial body weight during the water administration phase (Figure 2*B*). Like CCR9$^{-/-}$ animals, CCL25$^{-/-}$ mice were more susceptible to DSS colitis (Figure S1). Since similar results were obtained with the CCL25$^{-/-}$ strain, these data show that the exacerbated colitis is a consequence of impaired CCL25/CCR9 interaction.

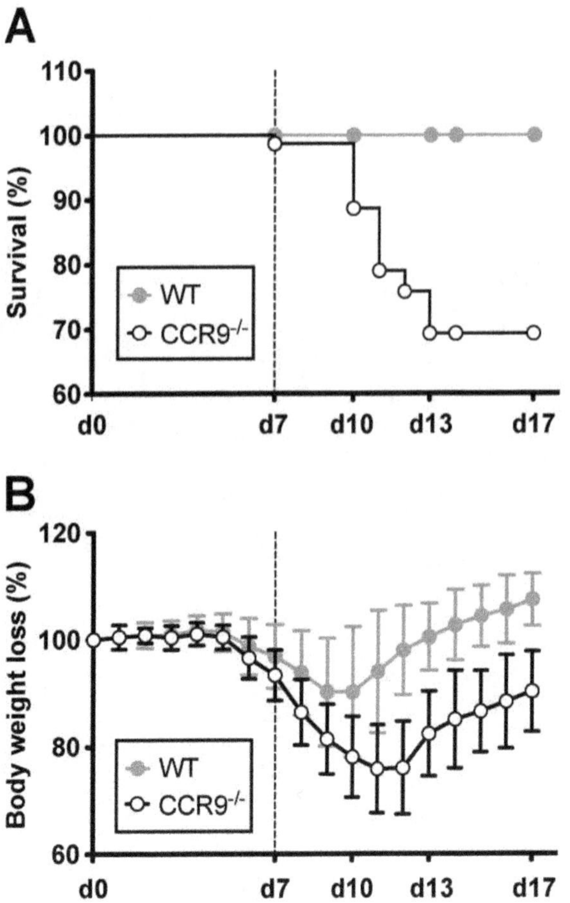

Figure 2. CCR9$^{-/-}$ mice show increased mortality and delayed recovery during DSS-mediated colitis. (**A**) 30.65% mortality was observed in CCR9$^{-/-}$ mice (open circles, n = 78). WT mice are shown in gray circles (n = 66). Data are representative of 17 pooled experiments. (**B**) CCR9$^{-/-}$ mice showed a more pronounced body weight loss than WT. Body weight was monitored daily and is expressed as percent of weight at d0 (data represent the mean +/− SD of 17 pooled experiments of 3–5 mice per group). Open circles show CCR9$^{-/-}$ mice, gray circles WT.

Exacerbated IBD symptoms in CCR9$^{-/-}$ animals

We next analyzed how the increased susceptibility to DSS colitis affects IBD symptoms in CCR9$^{-/-}$ animals. According to the weight loss data in WT animals, IBD scoring of H&E sections of the distal colon peaked at d10 and reversed during water administration by d13. In contrast, CCR9$^{-/-}$ mice showed persistent intestinal inflammation until d17 (Figure 3*A* and Table S1). Intestinal inflammation in CCR9$^{-/-}$ mice was characterized by an increase of cellular activity with granulocytic infiltration, expansion of the lamina propria and more pronounced basal lymphoplasmacytosis (Figure 3*B*). Epithelial hyperplasia, frequent crypt abscesses and mucosal ulceration also persisted until d17 (Figure 3*B*). As opposed to WT animals, CCR9$^{-/-}$ mice still showed shortening of the colon at the end of the DSS cycle (Figure 3*C* and Table S2). CCL25 transcripts levels were not upregulated in CCR9$^{-/-}$ large intestinal mucosa (Figure S2), probably due to the altered ratio of infiltrating cells to resident cells when compared to WT mucosa at the same time point (Figure S2). In summary, these experiments describe exacerbated IBD symptoms in the absence of CCR9 expression.

The gut-associated lymphoid tissue and the intestinal mucosa of CCR9$^{-/-}$ mice show multiple signs of exacerbated inflammation after DSS colitis

As recruitment and activation of intestinal MΦ has been described in human ulcerative colitis and murine DSS colitis [10,17], we analyzed the numbers and phenotype of MΦ in gut-associated lymphoid tissue and intestinal mucosa. The cellularity of lymphoid organs during DSS colitis was similar in WT and CCR9$^{-/-}$ animals (Figure S3). At d17, however, a 3-fold increase of MΦ was detected in MLNs of CCR9$^{-/-}$ animals compared to WT mice. MΦ in both strains expressed the surface markers F4/80 and Ly6C, suggesting an inflammatory phenotype [15] (Figure 4*A*). CCR9$^{-/-}$ MΦ expressed higher levels of MHC II than WT cells, indicating that these MΦ are more activated [25].

We next compared mRNA expression patterns of the large intestinal tissue of WT and CCR9$^{-/-}$ animals at steady state and at d17 using nCounter^{TM} mRNA analysis. This digital methodology allows for a direct analysis of mRNA copy numbers without amplification steps [22]. In line with our flow cytometry analysis, the increase in inflammatory MΦ at d17 was reflected by increased expression of CD64 and Arginase1 (Figure 4*B*). As a reflection of recent tissue inflammation, mRNA levels of TNFα, IL-1β and IL-6 were increased at d17 (Figure 4*C*). CCR9$^{-/-}$ animals consistently showed increased levels of all transcripts when compared to WT (Figures 4*B* and 4*C*). Exacerbated IBD in CCR9$^{-/-}$ mice further correlated with upregulation of IFNγ, IL-17A and IL-17F. No induction of IL-4 mRNA was observed (Figure 4*C*).

We next studied cytokine production of T cells isolated from MLNs at d17 after stimulation with anti-CD3ε/CD28 mAbs (Figure 4*D* and 4*E*). T cells from CCR9$^{-/-}$ animals produced higher levels of TNFα, IFNγ, IL-2, IL-6 and IL-17A than WT cells. Production of IL-4 and IL-10 was significantly down-regulated in CCR9$^{-/-}$ mice. In summary, this set of data describes an exacerbated inflammatory immune response of the Th1/Th17 immunophenotype with higher numbers of tissue macrophages in the large intestinal mucosa and gut-associated lymphoid tissues of CCR9$^{-/-}$ mice.

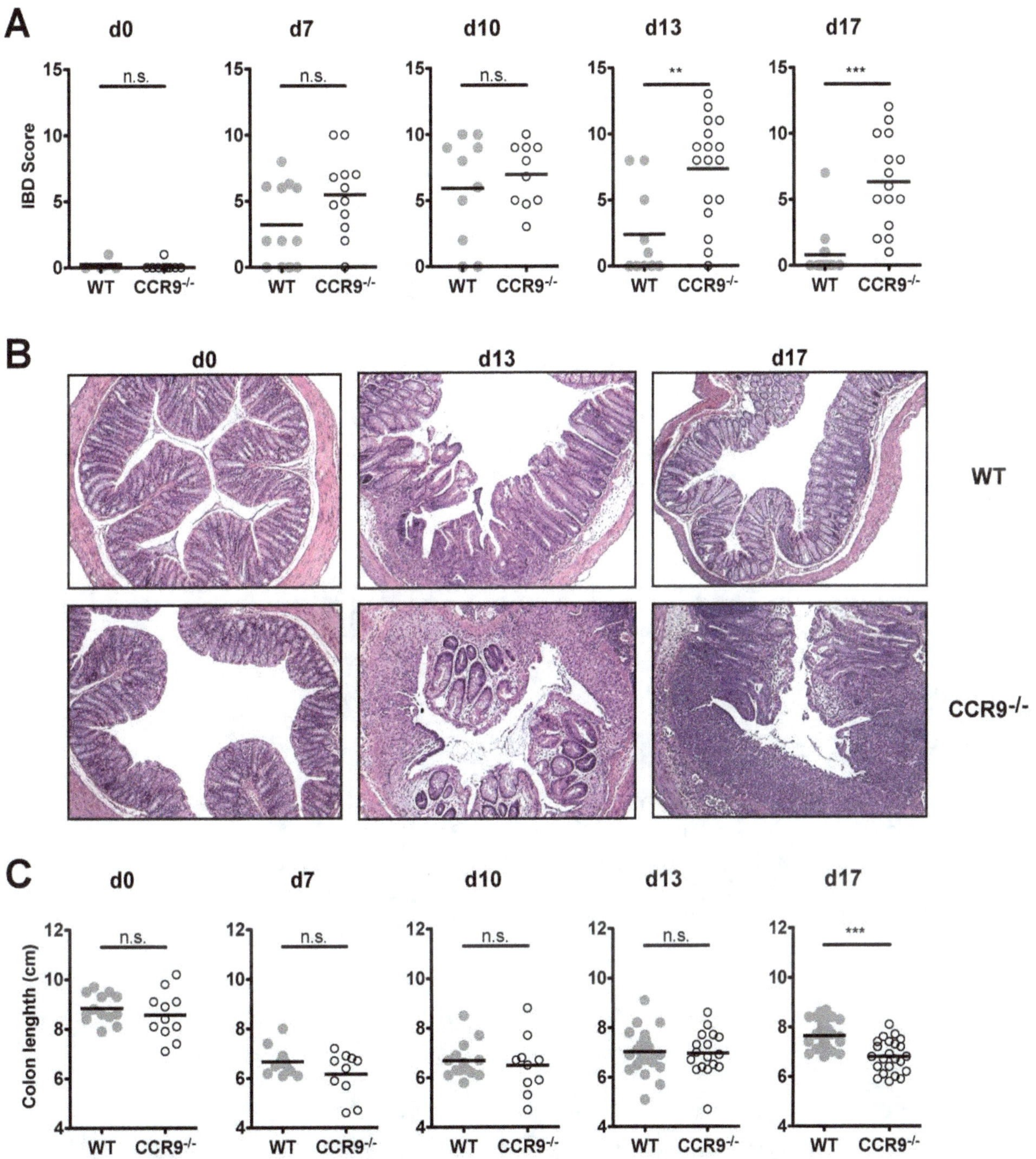

Figure 3. Exacerbation of DSS-mediated colitis in CCR9$^{-/-}$ mice. (**A**) Higher IBD scores during the recovery phase in CCR9$^{-/-}$ animals. WT mice are depicted in gray circles (n = 51), CCR9$^{-/-}$ mice in open circles (n = 63). (**B**) Representative H&E sections from colons of WT and CCR9$^{-/-}$ mice (d0, d13 and d17; 10×-magnification). CCR9$^{-/-}$ intestinal mucosa displays exacerbated IBD symptoms. (**C**) Significant colon shortening in CCR9$^{-/-}$ mice (open circles) at d17. Colon length was measured from d0 to d17. ***P<0.005, n.s. not significant.

Exacerbated DSS colitis correlates with the accumulation of activated plasmacytoid DCs in MLNs

DCs are gatekeepers for the induction of adaptive immune responses and different DC subpopulations are also considered key regulators of inflammatory immune responses [14]. In particular, expression of CCR9 on plasmacytoid DCs (pDCs) defines a tolerogenic subpopulation [26]. We therefore compared the distribution of DC subsets in CCR9$^{-/-}$ and WT animals at steady state and during DSS colitis.

We first confirmed that a subset of pDCs from MLNs and spleen of WT animals expresses high levels of CCR9 [26,27] (Figure 5*A* and data not shown). Then, we analyzed distribution of DC subpopulations in CCR9$^{-/-}$ and WT animals by assessing the ratio between pDCs and conventional DCs (cDCs). According to the literature [15], cDCs were gated based on expression of high levels of CD11c and MHC II pDCs were defined as MHC II^{low}, CD11c^{low} and PDCA-1^{+} cells [28]. The relative distribution of

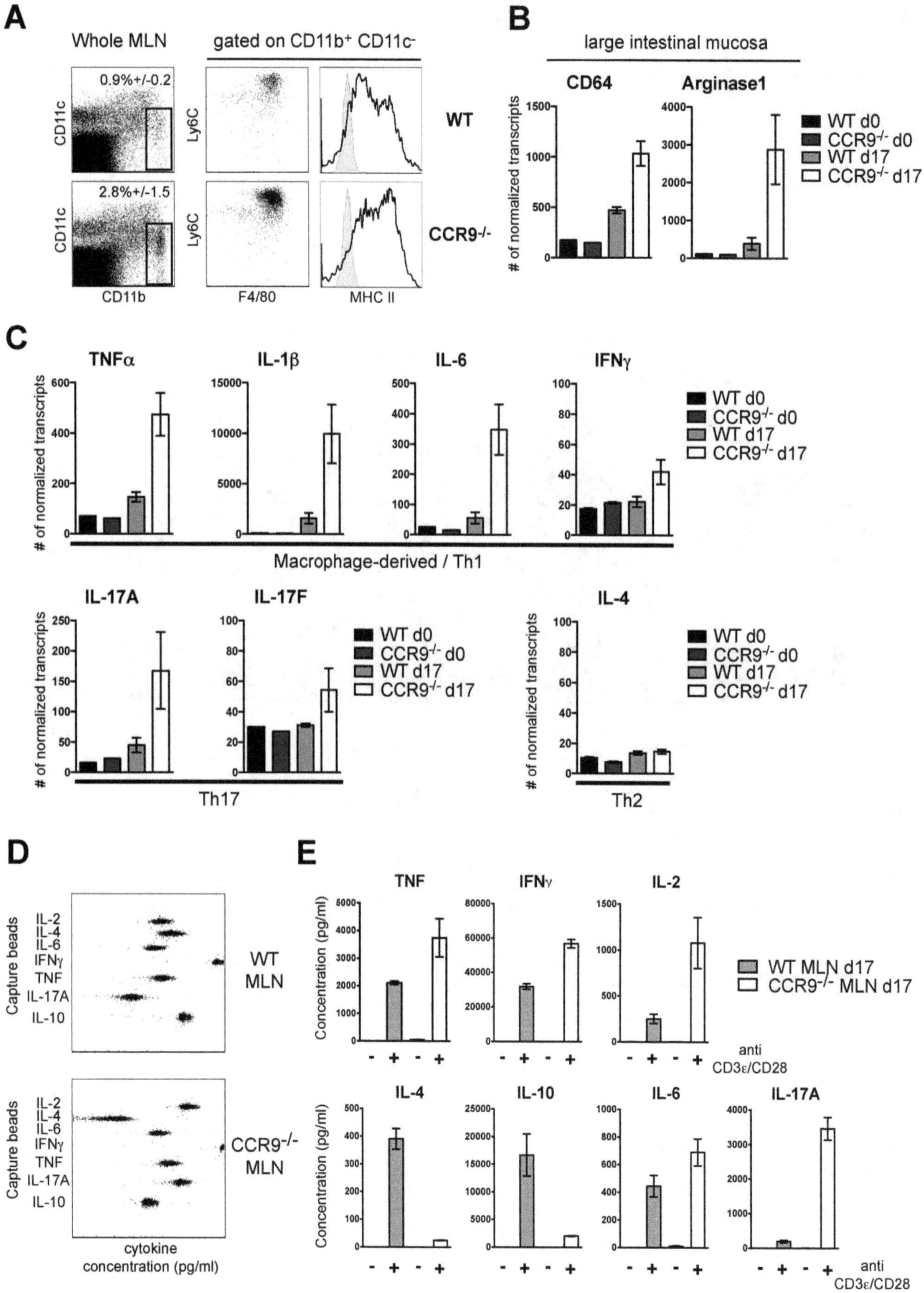
A
Whole MLN
gated on CD11b+ CD11c-
0.9%+/-0.2
2.8%+/-1.5
CD11c
Ly6C
CD11b
F4/80
MHC II
WT
CCR9-/-
B
large intestinal mucosa
CD64
Arginase1
# of normalized transcripts
WT d0
CCR9-/- d0
WT d17
CCR9-/- d17
C
TNFα
IL-1β
IL-6
IFNγ
Macrophage-derived / Th1
IL-17A
IL-17F
IL-4
Th17
Th2
D
Capture beads
IL-2
IL-4
IL-6
IFNγ
TNF
IL-17A
IL-10
WT MLN
CCR9-/- MLN
cytokine concentration (pg/ml)
E
TNF
IFNγ
IL-2
IL-4
IL-10
IL-6
IL-17A
Concentration (pg/ml)
WT MLN d17
CCR9-/- MLN d17
anti CD3ε/CD28

Figure 4. The gastrointestinal tract of CCR9$^{-/-}$ animals shows multiple signs of exacerbated tissue inflammation. (**A**) Accumulation of inflammatory macrophages. Flow cytometry analysis of MLNs of WT and CCR9$^{-/-}$ animals. Frequencies of inflammatory macrophages were determined in MLN suspensions with anti-CD11c, CD11b, F4/80, Ly6C and MHC-II (in black) overlaid on isotype control mAbs (in gray). Data represent the mean (+/− SD) of 3 independent experiments of 3–5 pooled mice per genotype. (**B and C**) mRNA profiling of large intestinal tissues. Total RNA was prepared from the colon of WT and CCR9$^{-/-}$ mice at d0 and d17 and was analyzed with the nCounter™ system (mean +/− SD of 3–5 animals per group of 2 independent experiments). (**B**) Macrophage accumulation is reflected by increased mRNA levels of CD64 and Arginase1. (**C**) Comparison of tissue immunophenotype of the large intestinal mucosa before and after DSS-mediated colitis in WT and CCR9$^{-/-}$ animals. (**D and E**) T cell re-stimulation assay for cytokine production. (**D**) Representative cytometry bead array assay for Th1/Th2/Th17 cytokines. (**E**) Production of TNFα, IFNγ, IL-2, IL-6 and IL-17A is upregulated while production of IL-10 and IL-4 is down-regulated in T cells from CCR9$^{-/-}$ animals. Quantification of cytokine production from WT (gray bars) and CCR9$^{-/-}$ cells (open bars). Data represent one experiment out of 3 independent experiments, performed in triplicate (mean +/− SD) of 3 pooled WT MLN and 3 pooled CCR9$^{-/-}$ MLN cell suspensions reactivated in vitro with anti-CD3ε/anti-CD28 mAbs for 72 h.

cDCs subsets based on expression of CD8α, CD11b and CD103 did not differ in lymphoid organs or large intestinal tissues at steady state between the two strains (data not shown). In line with the literature, our results showed an increase in the pDC/cDC ratio in SPL and MLN due to an accumulation of pDCs in CCR9$^{-/-}$ mice (Figure 5*B*). The pDC/cDC ratio in the colon of both strains was comparable.

We next analyzed the effects of DSS colitis on the distribution of pDCs in MLNs and observed a biphasic pattern. At d10, a drop in pDC numbers was detected in WT and CCR9$^{-/-}$ mice. Then, we observed an accumulation of pDCs, which was significantly more pronounced in CCR9$^{-/-}$ when compared to WT animals (2-fold at d13, 4-fold at d17, Figure 5*C*). The enhanced accumulation of pDCs observed in CCR9$^{-/-}$ animals significantly shifted the pDC/cDC ratio in MLNs at d13 and d17. The relative distribution of cDCs and their subsets during DSS colitis was comparable in both strains (Figure S4 and S5). The pDC/cDC ratio in the colon (Figure 5E) and in the SPL (Figure S6) was not affected.

Since the severity of colitis symptoms in mice is partly dependent on the DSS dose [10,23], we hypothesized that a higher dose of DSS might induce a comparable accumulation of pDCs in MLNs of WT animals. Administration of 4% DSS indeed induced accumulation of pDCs when compared to 2% DSS (Figure 5*C* and 5*D*). We detected a pDC subset that expresses CCR9. The majority of accumulating pDCs, however, were lacking CCR9 expression (Figure 5*D*), implying that these pDCs have an inflammatory rather than a tolerizing immune phenotype [26].

We compared maturation/activation levels of the accumulating pDCs by comparing MHC II, CD80 and CD86 expression levels. Low expression levels of CD11b on WT and CCR9$^{-/-}$ pDCs (Figure 6*A*, left) confirmed that these cells were different from the activated macrophages described in Figure 4. By gating on the CD11b^{low} PDCA-1^{+} population, we confirmed that the pDCs were MHC II^{+} (Figure 6*A*, right) and CD11c^{low} and Ly6C^{high} (data not shown). Comparative analysis of expression levels of MHC II, CD80 and CD86 showed that these surface markers were upregulated in pDCs from CCR9$^{-/-}$ animals (Figure 6*B*). Despite the different activation level, pDCs isolated from MLNs of WT and CCR9$^{-/-}$ animals at d17 showed the same plasmacytoid morphology (Figure 6*C*). In summary, these data show that activated pDCs accumulate in the gut-associated lymphoid tissue of CCR9$^{-/-}$ animals.

Discussion

The results presented in this study identify a novel role of CCL25/CCR9 interactions in the pathogenesis of a well-established acute colitis model mediated by oral administration of DSS. In our study, DSS specifically targets the large intestine, but not the small intestine, and we show that CCL25 expression is upregulated after acute large intestinal inflammation. When studying CCR9$^{-/-}$ mice with the DSS model, we found that the large intestinal mucosa displays characteristics of enhanced tissue inflammation resulting in exacerbated IBD symptoms and a delay in recovery from tissue injury. Thus, our findings are of high relevance for clinical care of human IBD as they point to potential detrimental effects of CCR9-blocking therapy for patients suffering from inflammation in the large intestine, as commonly observed in ulcerative colitis. This suggests that blocking CCL25/CCR9 interactions in ulcerative colitis patients may lead to an inefficiency in resolving intestinal inflammation or, at worst case, even exacerbated IBD symptoms. An oral CCR9 antagonist (CCX282-B) is currently used in a Phase II clinical trial for the treatment of Crohn's disease and has shown efficacy in the treatment of patients with moderate to severe small bowel Crohn's disease [8]. This compound has shown potent inhibition of CCL25-mediated chemotaxis of CCR9-expressing cells [29]. However, contradicting results have emerged in the role of CCL25/CCR9 interactions in the experimental small intestinal inflammation of the TNF$^{\Delta are}$ mouse model that mimics human Crohn's Disease. Walters et al. showed that the orally bioavailable CCR9 antagonist CCX282-B can ameliorate, in one single experiment, the severity of small intestinal chronic inflammation of TNF$^{\Delta are}$ mice [29]. Apostolaki et al. demonstrated that the development of intestinal inflammation in the TNF$^{\Delta are}$ mouse model is critically dependent on β7 integrin-mediated T-lymphocyte recruitment, while the function of the CCL25/CCR9 axis in T-cell specific mucosal recruitment appears dispensable in this model [30]. The fact that Walters et al. did not provide the CCR9 antagonist orally but subcutaneously may explain such discrepancy. Oral administration of CCR9 antagonists should thus be evaluated in animal models of large intestinal inflammation.

In the SAMP1/Yit chronic ileitis mouse model that shares similarities with the TNF$^{\Delta are}$ mouse model, Matsuzaki et al. showed that antibodies against the α4β7-integrin ligand MAdCAM-1 significantly inhibited adhesion of T lymphocytes to microvessels of the terminal ileum of SAMP1/Yit mice, and led to a strong chronic ileitis suppressive effect [31]. Although antibody blockade of CCL25/CCR9 interactions ameliorated early, but not late, SAMP1/Yit chronic murine ileitis [32], it would be very interesting to test whether the CCR9 antagonist CCX282-B and/or CCR9-deficiency in the SAMP1/Yit ileitis model can ameliorate small intestinal chronic inflammation as well. The fact that these studies were focused on small intestinal but not large intestinal inflammation, made CCL25 and CCR9 attractive candidates for the treatment of Crohn's disease but not ulcerative colitis. However, prior to this study, no work has been presented on CCL25/CCR9 interactions in an experimental acute colitis mouse model mediated by DSS exposure.

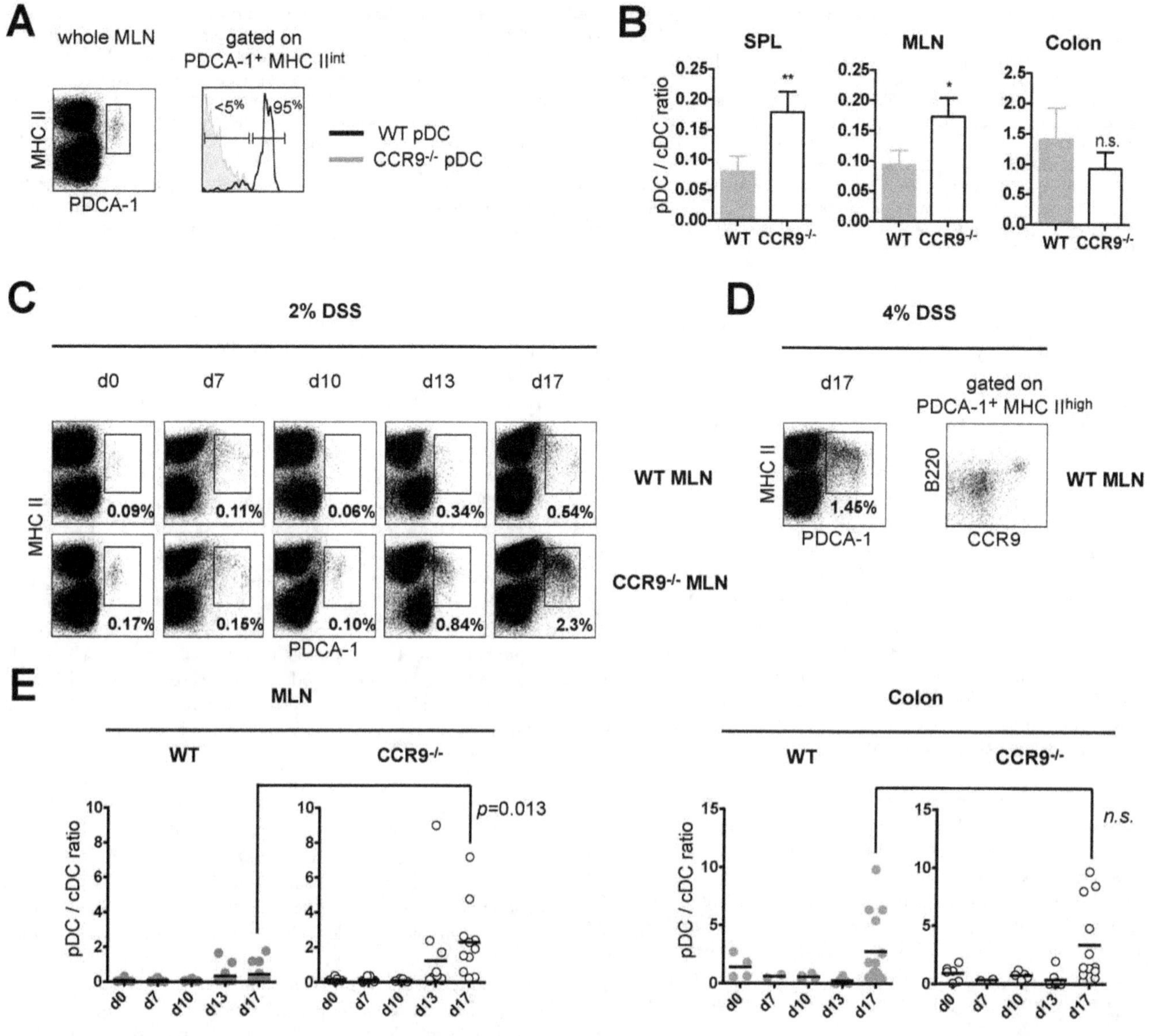

Figure 5. CCR9$^{-/-}$ mice show altered ratios of dendritic cell subpopulations at steady state and during DSS-mediated colitis. (**A**) WT MLNs contain CCR9^{+} and CCR9^{-} pDCs gated as MHC II^{int} and PDCA-1^{high} (left dot plot). CCR9 expression in WT pDCs (black line, right histogram) is overlaid on CCR9$^{-/-}$ pDCs (in gray, right histogram) (**B**) Steady state distribution of pDCs and cDCs is altered in SPL and MLN of CCR9$^{-/-}$ mice. No significant difference between strains is observed in the colon. cDCs were defined as CD11c^{high} and MHC II^{high} cells by flow cytometry. Ratio of subpopulations is expressed on the y-axis as pDC/cDC cells. Data represent the mean +/− SD of 4 independent experiments of 3–5 pooled mice per group. (**C**) Accumulation of pDCs in MLNs of CCR9$^{-/-}$ animals. Percentages of pDCs in WT and CCR9$^{-/-}$ MLN are depicted in bold from d0 to d17 of DSS colitis. (**D**) Accumulation of pDCs correlates with the level of tissue damage. Increase of DSS concentration to 4% augments the number of CCR9$^{low/-}$ B220^{+} PDCA-1^{+} MHC II$^{int/high}$ cells in MLNs of WT animals. (**E**) DSS-mediated tissue inflammation alters pDC/cDC ratios in MLN of CCR9$^{-/-}$ animals. Data points correspond to individual experiments corresponding to 17 DSS colitis experiments harvested at different time point using 3–5 pooled mice per genotype.

Our data on the gastrointestinal expression pattern of CCL25 support the findings of Stenstad et al. showing expression of this chemokine in the colon [33]. To date, only low expression levels at steady state were described. We show here that inflammation increases CCL25 expression in the large intestinal mucosa. It has been described that the small intestinal mucosa reacts to injection of the inflammatory cytokine TNFα with rapid upregulation of CCL25 [34]. Our data suggest that the colonic mucosa reacts similarly to inflammation, presumably to attract CCR9-positive leukocytes to participate in the mucosal immune response.

The most compelling argument for a physiologic role of CCL25/CCR9 interactions during an inflammatory response in the colon is derived from the increased susceptibility to colitis and the high mortality rate observed in CCR9$^{-/-}$ animals. Increased IBD scores, more pronounced weight loss, a delay in recovery from acute inflammation and the inability to regain initial body weight during the experimental time period support the critical role for CCL25/CCR9 dependent trafficking events during the acute and recovery phase of DSS colitis. The altered microenvironment of the large intestine appears to favor CCL25/CCR9-independent migration of pro-inflammatory leukocytes in

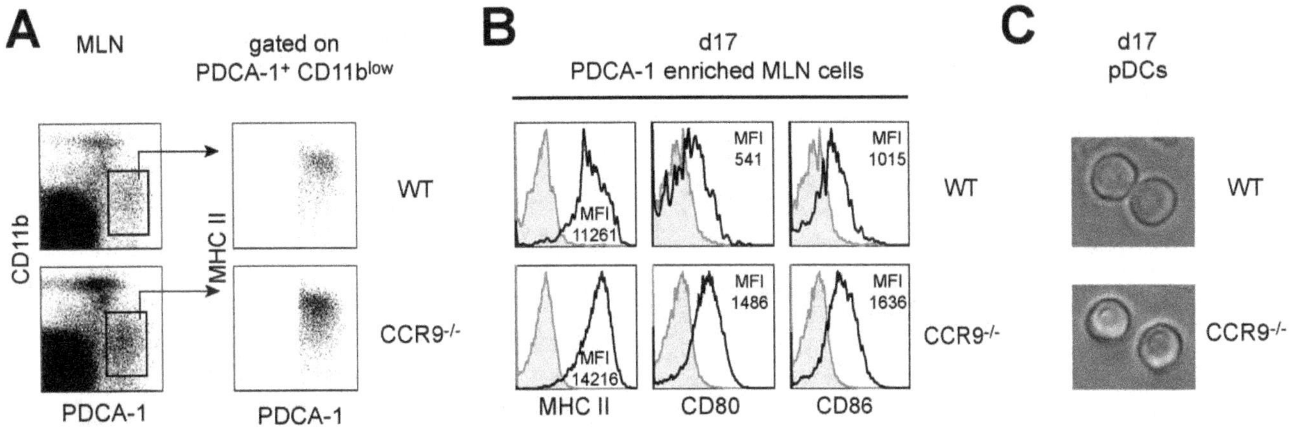

Figure 6. pDCs from CCR9$^{-/-}$ MLNs are more activated than WT pDCs. (**A**) pDCs of WT and CCR9$^{-/-}$ mice express low levels of CD11b in contrast to inflammatory macrophages. pDCs were defined as CD11b^{low} MHC II$^{int/high}$ PDCA-1^{+}. (**B**) CCR9$^{-/-}$ pDCs show signs of phenotypic maturation. Maturation levels were assessed by comparing expression levels of MHC II and costimulatory molecules CD80 and CD86. (**C**) Morphology of pDCs isolated from WT and CCR9$^{-/-}$ animals.

CCR9$^{-/-}$ animals. This situation is highly relevant for our understanding of the therapeutic effects of CCR9-antagonists as this type of medication could result in a comparable scenario in human IBD patients.

To date, targeting of chemokine receptors such as CCR2, CCR5, CCR6, CXCR3, CXCR4 and CX3CR1 by gene disruption or antagonistic peptides has been found to protect animals from DSS colitis [35,36,37,38,39]. The mechanism commonly proposed is that interference with chemokine receptor function is beneficial, because these receptors are potentially pro-inflammatory. In contrast, we show that CCR9$^{-/-}$ and CCL25$^{-/-}$ animals respond with exacerbated IBD symptoms. To our knowledge, this is the first report to show that interference with a chemokine/receptor pair aggravates IBD symptoms. As a mechanism, we propose that CCL25/CCR9 interactions are critical components of an anti-inflammatory tissue response in the colon.

The interpretation of our results as a consequence of an impaired anti-inflammatory response in CCR9$^{-/-}$ animal is supported by our data in two ways: the pronounced accumulation of activated inflammatory macrophages and the increased expression of the pro-inflammatory cytokines IL-1β, IL-6, and TNF-α in the large intestinal mucosa. Expression of the latter cytokines is not only described for animal models of colitis [40,41] but also for human IBD [42,43], underlining the relevance of the murine model for human disease. Unlike other models of murine colitis [44], our model shows that the absence of CCR9 does not change the immune profile of the inflammatory response. Only higher levels of Th1- and Th17-type inflammatory cytokines, but no Th2-type immune responses, were detected. Additionally, high levels of IL-17A and IL-17F were detected as part of the aggravated immunophenotype of CCR9$^{-/-}$ mice both at the mRNA level and the protein level. As IL-17 is considerably increased in chronic IBD patients [45], it is conceivable that the CCL25/CCR9 interactions are playing a physiological role during the development of the chronic disease symptoms as well. Melgar *et al.* showed that a single cycle of high-dose DSS can induce chronic inflammation over time in wild type C57Bl/6 mice [24]. Along this line, we have preliminary evidence that a single cycle of low-dose DSS is sufficient in CCR9$^{-/-}$ C57Bl/6 animals to induce chronic IBD (data not shown). Further investigation will determine whether CCL25/CCR9 interactions play a role in DSS chronic colitis.

The delayed recovery from acute colitis is further characterized by an accumulation of pDCs and a change of the pDC/cDC ratio in the gut-associated lymphoid tissue in CCR9$^{-/-}$ mice. pDCs have been described as immune suppressive APCs [46] that can induce systemic tolerance to T cell-mediated delayed-type hypersensitivity after oral sensitization [47]. pDCs are also discussed as regulators of DSS colitis [48]. However, Hadeiba et al. described a significant difference in the ability of pDCs subsets to promote tolerance [26]. In fact, CCR9 expression delineates a tolerogenic pDC subset while CCR9-negative pDCs were unable to prevent T cell activation/proliferation. Our results also suggest the concerted action of two functionally distinct pDCs subsets: a CCR9-positive tolerogenic pDC subset that regulates the inflammatory response during and after DSS colitis and a CCR9-negative predominantly inflammatory pDC subset. When regulatory pDCs lose CCR9 expression due to genetic manipulation, they also lose their ability to migrate in response to CCL25 upregulation in the colon and become trapped in the MLN. Alternatively, CCR9 expression by itself could influence the tolerogenic potential of these pDCs. One might even argue that the subset of CCR9-positive regulatory pDCs is underrated in WT animals, as these cells are likely to escape detection by flow cytometry once they have reached large intestinal LP. These cells likely down-regulate their surface chemokine receptors in response to CCL25. The CCR9-negative pDCs appear inflammatory in our model as demonstrated by the correlation of exacerbated IBD symptoms with the expansion of this pDC subset. In CCR9$^{-/-}$ mice, the altered microenvironment might also favor CCL25/CCR9-independent tissue homing of inflammatory pDCs. Additionally, the impaired balance of DCs subpopulations may contribute to the enhanced activation of the immune system and the failure to recover from tissue injury in the absence of physiological CCL25/CCR9 interactions. It now will be important to study if the impaired ratio of inflammatory and regulatory pDCs, the expanded macrophage population or both cell types regulate the exacerbated IBD symptoms in CCR9$^{-/-}$ animals. The question whether this phenotype is actually exacerbated IBD or rather an impaired ability to recover from acute large intestinal inflammation also requires further analysis.

Prevention of the CD45RB^{high} CD4+ T cell transfer colitis model in immuno-compromised animals can be achieved by cotransferring Regulatory T cells (Tregs) [49]. Given the fact that CCR9-expressing pDCs are inducers of T regulatory cell functions, further examination of Tregs distribution and function would determine whether Tregs play a role in DSS colitis recovery and whether or not it is CCL25/CCR9 dependent.

In summary, our study shows that impairment of CCL25/CCR9-interaction has profound negative effects on the regulation of the local inflammatory immune response. While a phase II clinical study with a CCR9-inhibitor suggests a therapeutic benefit for Crohn's disease patients [8], our results strongly suggest that this form of therapeutic intervention could have detrimental effects when offered to patients that suffer from ulcerative large intestinal-specific inflammation.

Supporting Information

Figure S1 CCL25$^{-/-}$ mice show increased susceptibility to DSS colitis comparable to CCR9$^{-/-}$ animals. (**A**) A mortality rate of 38% was observed in CCL25$^{-/-}$ (blue circles) mice exposed to DSS for 7 days and 10 days of water when compared to control CCL25$^{-/-}$ mice exposed to water only (black circles). Data represent survival of 5 mice per group in 5 independent experiments; P value = 0.0166 (Log-rank Test). (**B**) Delayed recovery in CCL25$^{-/-}$ mice is evidenced by significant weight loss and inability to recover to initial body weight. Body weight was monitored daily and is expressed as percent of body weight measured at d0. Data are displayed as the mean +/− SD of the mean of 5 independent experiments, each with 5 mice per group. Blue circles show CCL25$^{-/-}$ mice exposed to DSS colitis, black circles CCL25 control mice.

Figure S2 CCL25 mRNA expression increases during the recovery phase of DSS-mediated colitis in WT intestinal mucosa but not CCR9$^{-/-}$ large intestinal mucosa. Y-axis shows expression CCL25 levels normalized to β-actin mRNA. Data represent the mean +/− SD; d10, n = 3; d13, n = 5; d17, n = 5; where n corresponds to the number of experiments of 3 to 5 pooled large intestinal samples.

Figure S3 Cellularity in SPL and MLN of WT and CCR9$^{-/-}$ animals during DSS colitis is comparable. Collagenase digestion of SPL and MLN was performed at indicated time points. Cell suspensions were counted with a Casy® automatic cell counter. Each data point represents a single mouse, WT mice are depicted in gray circles and CCR9$^{-/-}$ mice are depicted in open circles. Horizontal black bars represent the mean of SPL and MLN cell numbers from d0 to d17. SPL: spleen, MLN: mesenteric lymph nodes.

Figure S4 Distribution of pDCs and cDCs in WT and CCR9$^{-/-}$ mice during DSS colitis. Cell suspensions were prepared from WT and CCR9$^{-/-}$ SPL, MLN and colonic mucosa and were analyzed by flow cytometry. Frequencies of pDCs (PDCA-1^{+} MHC II$^{int/high}$) and cDCs (CD11c^{high} MHC II^{high}) were determined and are graphed as percentages of total leukocytes. Each data point represents a single animal. WT mice are depicted as gray circles and CCR9$^{-/-}$ mice as open circles. Horizontal black bars represent the mean of pDCs and cDCs frequencies determined by flow cytometry from d0 to d17.

Figure S5 Flow cytometry analysis of cDCs subsets in WT and CCR9$^{-/-}$ animals at d17 of DSS colitis. Cell suspensions from SPL, MLN and colonic mucosa were analyzed by flow cytometry. Frequencies of cDCs subsets (CD11c^{high} MHC II^{high}) were determined and subsets were further analyzed based on expression of CD11b and CD103. Percentages of cDCs subsets are expressed as percentage of total cDCs and numbers are shown in red in each graph. Dot plots are representative of 5 independent experiments. We did not observe any statistically significant differences in the frequencies of all cDC subsets analyzed.

Figure S6 Ratio of DC subsets in the spleen of CCR9$^{-/-}$ animals compares to WT spleens during DSS colitis. Quantification of pDC/cDC ratios at d0, d7, d10, d13 and d17 in WT (gray circles, left graph) and CCR9$^{-/-}$ mice (open circles, right graph) by flow cytometry using a lineage negative staining to remove any CD3^{+}, CD19^{+} and CD11b^{high} cells. Each data point corresponds to one experiment using 3–5 pooled animals. Horizontal black bars represent the mean of pDC/cDC ratios from d0 to d17.

Table S1 IBD scoring. Values represent the mean ± SEM of IBD scores depicted in Figure 3a.

Table S2 Colon Length. Values represent the mean ± SEM of colon length depicted in Figure 3c.

Acknowledgments

We thank Dr. Barbara Platzer for helpful critical suggestions and Michael Pardo for critically reading the manuscript.

Author Contributions

Conceived and designed the experiments: MAW MGM PD EF. Performed the experiments: MAW MGM PD. Analyzed the data: MAW MGM. Contributed reagents/materials/analysis tools: MAW MGM PD EF. Wrote the paper: MAW EF MGM. Supported MAW in performing data acquisition and maintenance of the animal colony: PD.

References

1. Vicari AP, Figueroa DJ, Hedrick JA, Foster JS, Singh KP, et al. (1997) TECK: a novel CC chemokine specifically expressed by thymic dendritic cells and potentially involved in T cell development. Immunity 7: 291–301.
2. Papadakis KA, Prehn J, Nelson V, Cheng L, Binder SW, et al. (2000) The role of thymus-expressed chemokine and its receptor CCR9 on lymphocytes in the regional specialization of the mucosal immune system. J Immunol 165: 5069–5076.
3. Wurbel MA, Philippe JM, Nguyen C, Victorero G, Freeman T, et al. (2000) The chemokine TECK is expressed by thymic and intestinal epithelial cells and attracts double- and single-positive thymocytes expressing the TECK receptor CCR9. Eur J Immunol 30: 262–271.
4. Johansson-Lindbom B, Svensson M, Wurbel MA, Malissen B, Marquez G, et al. (2003) Selective generation of gut tropic T cells in gut-associated lymphoid tissue (GALT): requirement for GALT dendritic cells and adjuvant. J Exp Med 198: 963–969.
5. Mora JR, Bono MR, Manjunath N, Weninger W, Cavanagh LL, et al. (2003) Selective imprinting of gut-homing T cells by Peyer's patch dendritic cells. Nature 424: 88–93.
6. Stenstad H, Ericsson A, Johansson-Lindbom B, Svensson M, Marsal J, et al. (2006) Gut-associated lymphoid tissue-primed CD4+ T cells display CCR9-dependent and -independent homing to the small intestine. Blood 107: 3447–3454.

7. Wurbel MA, Malissen M, Guy-Grand D, Malissen B, Campbell JJ (2007) Impaired Accumulation of Antigen-Specific CD8 Lymphocytes in Chemokine CCL25-Deficient Intestinal Epithelium and Lamina Propria. J Immunol 178: 7598–7606.
8. Keshav S, Johnson D, Bekker P, Schall TJ (2009) PROTECT-1 Study Demonstrated Efficacy of the Intestine-Specific Chemokine Receptor Antagonist CCX282-B (Traficet-EN) in Treatment of Patients with Moderate to Severe Crohn's Disease. Gastroenterology 136: A-65.
9. Blumberg RS, Saubermann LJ, Strober W (1999) Animal models of mucosal inflammation and their relation to human inflammatory bowel disease. Curr Opin Immunol 11: 648–656.
10. Okayasu I, Hatakeyama S, Yamada M, Ohkusa T, Inagaki Y, et al. (1990) A novel method in the induction of reliable experimental acute and chronic ulcerative colitis in mice. Gastroenterology 98: 694–702.
11. Dieleman LA, Ridwan BU, Tennyson GS, Beagley KW, Bucy RP, et al. (1994) Dextran sulfate sodium-induced colitis occurs in severe combined immunodeficient mice. Gastroenterology 107: 1643–1652.
12. Shintani N, Nakajima T, Sugiura M, Murakami K, Nakamura N, et al. (1997) Proliferative effect of dextran sulfate sodium (DSS)-pulsed macrophages on T cells from mice with DSS-induced colitis and inhibition of effect by IgG. Scand J Immunol 46: 581–586.
13. Shintani N, Nakajima T, Okamoto T, Kondo T, Nakamura N, et al. (1998) Involvement of CD4+ T cells in the development of dextran sulfate sodium-induced experimental colitis and suppressive effect of IgG on their action. Gen Pharmacol 31: 477–481.
14. Kelsall B (2008) Recent progress in understanding the phenotype and function of intestinal dendritic cells and macrophages. Mucosal Immunol 1: 460–469.
15. Geissmann F, Manz MG, Jung S, Sieweke MH, Merad M, et al. (2010) Development of monocytes, macrophages, and dendritic cells. Science 327: 656–661.
16. Coombes JL, Powrie F (2008) Dendritic cells in intestinal immune regulation. Nat Rev Immunol 8: 435–446.
17. Weber B, Saurer L, Mueller C (2009) Intestinal macrophages: differentiation and involvement in intestinal immunopathologies. Semin Immunopathol 31: 171–184.
18. Abe K, Nguyen KP, Fine SD, Mo JH, Shen C, et al. (2007) Conventional dendritic cells regulate the outcome of colonic inflammation independently of T cells. Proc Natl Acad Sci U S A 104: 17022–17027.
19. Berndt BE, Zhang M, Chen GH, Huffnagle GB, Kao JY (2007) The role of dendritic cells in the development of acute dextran sulfate sodium colitis. J Immunol 179: 6255–6262.
20. Qualls JE, Tuna H, Kaplan AM, Cohen DA (2009) Suppression of experimental colitis in mice by CD11c+ dendritic cells. Inflamm Bowel Dis 15: 236–247.
21. Wurbel MA, Malissen M, Guy-Grand D, Meffre E, Nussenzweig MC, et al. (2001) Mice lacking the CCR9 CC-chemokine receptor show a mild impairment of early T- and B-cell development and a reduction in T-cell receptor gammadelta(+) gut intraepithelial lymphocytes. Blood 98: 2626–2632.
22. Geiss GK, Bumgarner RE, Birditt B, Dahl T, Dowidar N, et al. (2008) Direct multiplexed measurement of gene expression with color-coded probe pairs. Nat Biotechnol 26: 317–325.
23. Egger B, Bajaj-Elliott M, MacDonald TT, Inglin R, Eysselein VE, et al. (2000) Characterisation of acute murine dextran sodium sulphate colitis: cytokine profile and dose dependency. Digestion 62: 240–248.
24. Melgar S, Karlsson A, Michaelsson E (2005) Acute colitis induced by dextran sulfate sodium progresses to chronicity in C57BL/6 but not in BALB/c mice: correlation between symptoms and inflammation. Am J Physiol Gastrointest Liver Physiol 288: G1328–1338.
25. Mosser DM, Edwards JP (2008) Exploring the full spectrum of macrophage activation. Nat Rev Immunol 8: 958–969.
26. Hadeiba H, Sato T, Habtezion A, Oderup C, Pan J, et al. (2008) CCR9 expression defines tolerogenic plasmacytoid dendritic cells able to suppress acute graft-versus-host disease. Nat Immunol 9: 1253–1260.
27. Wendland M, Czeloth N, Mach N, Malissen B, Kremmer E, et al. (2007) CCR9 is a homing receptor for plasmacytoid dendritic cells to the small intestine. Proc Natl Acad Sci U S A 104: 6347–6352.
28. Blasius AL, Giurisato E, Cella M, Schreiber RD, Shaw AS, et al. (2006) Bone marrow stromal cell antigen 2 is a specific marker of type I IFN-producing cells in the naive mouse, but a promiscuous cell surface antigen following IFN stimulation. J Immunol 177: 3260–3265.
29. Walters MJ, Wang Y, Lai N, Baumgart T, Zhao BN, et al. (2010) Characterization of CCX282-B, an orally bioavailable antagonist of the CCR9 chemokine receptor, for treatment of inflammatory bowel disease. J Pharmacol Exp Ther 335: 61–69.
30. Apostolaki M, Manoloukos M, Roulis M, Wurbel MA, Muller W, et al. (2008) Role of beta7 integrin and the chemokine/chemokine receptor pair CCL25/CCR9 in modeled TNF-dependent Crohn's disease. Gastroenterology 134: 2025–2035.
31. Matsuzaki K, Tsuzuki Y, Matsunaga H, Inoue T, Miyazaki J, et al. (2005) In vivo demonstration of T lymphocyte migration and amelioration of ileitis in intestinal mucosa of SAMP1/Yit mice by the inhibition of MAdCAM-1. Clin Exp Immunol 140: 22–31.
32. Rivera-Nieves J, Ho J, Bamias G, Ivashkina N, Ley K, et al. (2006) Antibody Blockade of CCL25/CCR9 Ameliorates Early but not Late Chronic Murine Ileitis. Gastroenterology 131: 1518–1529.
33. Stenstad H, Svensson M, Cucak H, Kotarsky K, Agace WW (2007) Differential homing mechanisms regulate regionalized effector CD8{alpha}beta+ T cell accumulation within the small intestine. Proc Natl Acad Sci U S A 104: 10122–10127.
34. Hosoe N, Miura S, Watanabe C, Tsuzuki Y, Hokari R, et al. (2004) Demonstration of functional role of TECK/CCL25 in T lymphocyte-endothelium interaction in inflamed and uninflamed intestinal mucosa. Am J Physiol Gastrointest Liver Physiol 286: G458–466.
35. Andres PG, Beck PL, Mizoguchi E, Mizoguchi A, Bhan AK, et al. (2000) Mice with a selective deletion of the CC chemokine receptors 5 or 2 are protected from dextran sodium sulfate-mediated colitis: lack of CC chemokine receptor 5 expression results in a NK1.1+ lymphocyte-associated Th2-type immune response in the intestine. J Immunol 164: 6303–6312.
36. Varona R, Cadenas V, Flores J, Martinez AC, Marquez G (2003) CCR6 has a non-redundant role in the development of inflammatory bowel disease. Eur J Immunol 33: 2937–2946.
37. Tokuyama H, Ueha S, Kurachi M, Matsushima K, Moriyasu F, et al. (2005) The simultaneous blockade of chemokine receptors CCR2, CCR5 and CXCR3 by a non-peptide chemokine receptor antagonist protects mice from dextran sodium sulfate-mediated colitis. Int Immunol 17: 1023–1034.
38. Mikami S, Nakase H, Yamamoto S, Takeda Y, Yoshino T, et al. (2008) Blockade of CXCL12/CXCR4 axis ameliorates murine experimental colitis. J Pharmacol Exp Ther 327: 383–392.
39. Kostadinova FI, Baba T, Ishida Y, Kondo T, Popivanova BK, et al. (2010) Crucial involvement of the CX3CR1-CX3CL1 axis in dextran sulfate sodium-mediated acute colitis in mice. J Leukoc Biol.
40. Garside P (1999) Cytokines in experimental colitis. Clin Exp Immunol 118: 337–339.
41. Jurjus AR, Khoury NN, Reimund JM (2004) Animal models of inflammatory bowel disease. J Pharmacol Toxicol Methods 50: 81–92.
42. Rogler G, Andus T (1998) Cytokines in inflammatory bowel disease. World J Surg 22: 382–389.
43. Autschbach F, Giese T, Gassler N, Sido B, Heuschen G, et al. (2002) Cytokine/chemokine messenger-RNA expression profiles in ulcerative colitis and Crohn's disease. Virchows Arch 441: 500–513.
44. Nguyen DD, Maillard MH, Cotta-de-Almeida V, Mizoguchi E, Klein C, et al. (2007) Lymphocyte-dependent and Th2 cytokine-associated colitis in mice deficient in Wiskott-Aldrich syndrome protein. Gastroenterology 133: 1188–1197.
45. Kaser A, Blumberg RS (2008) Adaptive immunity in inflammatory bowel disease: state of the art. Curr Opin Gastroenterol 24: 455–461.
46. Villadangos JA, Young L (2008) Antigen-presentation properties of plasmacytoid dendritic cells. Immunity 29: 352–361.
47. Goubier A, Dubois B, Gheit H, Joubert G, Villard-Truc F, et al. (2008) Plasmacytoid dendritic cells mediate oral tolerance. Immunity 29: 464–475.
48. Sainathan SK, Hanna EM, Gong Q, Bishnupuri KS, Luo Q, et al. (2008) Granulocyte macrophage colony-stimulating factor ameliorates DSS-induced experimental colitis. Inflamm Bowel Dis 14: 88–99.
49. Uhlig HH, Coombes J, Mottet C, Izcue A, Thompson C, et al. (2006) Characterization of Foxp3+CD4+CD25+ and IL-10-secreting CD4+CD25+ T cells during cure of colitis. J Immunol 177: 5852–5860.

17

Effects of Dietary Glutamine on the Homeostasis of CD4+ T Cells in Mice with Dextran Sulfate Sodium-Induced Acute Colitis

Yuan-Chin Hsiung[1], Jun-Jen Liu[2], Yu-Chen Hou[3], Chiu-Li Yeh[4], Sung-Ling Yeh[1]*

1 School of Nutrition and Health Sciences, Taipei Medical University, Taipei, Taiwan, **2** School of Medical Laboratory Science and Biotechnology, Taipei Medical University, Taipei, Taiwan, **3** Department of Surgery, National Taiwan University Hospital, Taipei, Taiwan, **4** Department of Food and Nutrition, Chinese Culture University, Taipei, Taiwan

Abstract

This study investigated the effects of dietary glutamine (Gln) on T-helper (Th) and T regulatory (Treg) cell homeostasis and colonic inflammatory mediator expression in mice with dextran sulfate sodium (DSS)-induced colitis. Mice were randomly assigned to 4 groups with 2 normal control (C and G) and 2 DSS-treated groups (DC and DG). The C and DC groups were fed a common semipurified diet, while the G and DG groups received an identical diet except that part of the casein was replaced by Gln, which provided 25% of the total amino acid nitrogen. Mice were fed the diets for 10 days. On day 6, mice in the normal control groups were given distilled water, while those in the DSS groups were given distilled water containing 1.5% DSS for 5 d. At the end of the experiment, the mice were sacrificed for further examination. Results showed that DC group had higher plasma haptoglobin, colonic weight, immunoglobulin G, inflammatory cytokine and nuclear factor (NF)-κB protein levels. Gln administration lowered inflammatory mediators and NF-κB/IκBα ratio in colitis. Compared with the DC group, the percentages of interleukin-17F and interferon-γ in blood and transcription factors, T-bet and RAR-related orphan receptor-γt, gene expressions in mesenteric lymph nodes were lower, whereas blood Foxp3 was higher in the DG group. Also, DG group had lower colon injury score. These results suggest that Gln administration suppressed Th1/Th17 and Th-associated cytokine expressions and upregulated the expression of Tregs, which may modulate the balance of Th/Treg and reduce inflammatory reactions in DSS-induced colitis.

Editor: Simon Patrick Hogan, Cincinnati Children's Hospital Medical Center, University of Cincinnati College of Medicine, United States of America

Funding: This study was supported by the National Science Council grant NSC100-2320-B-038-007-MY3, Taipei, Taiwan. The funders had no role in study design, data collection and analysis, decision to publish, or preparation of the manuscript.

Competing Interests: No conflicts of interest, financial or otherwise, are declared by the authors.

* E-mail: sangling@tmu.edu.tw

Introduction

Inflammatory bowel disease (IBD), which includes Crohn's disease (CD) and ulcerative colitis (UC), refers to chronic inflammatory disorders that may affect the entire gastrointestinal tract [1]. The precise etiology of IBD remains unidentified [2]. A recent study indicated that genetic factors, epithelial barrier functions, gut microbiota, and the host immune system are involved in the development and course of IBD [3].

CD4$^+$ helper T (Th) cells play major roles in both the induction and persistence of IBD by producing proinflammatory cytokines. Th cells are traditionally divided into Th1 and Th2 subsets, characterized by distinct cytokines and effector functions. Interferon (IFN)-γ is produced by Th1 lymphocytes, and interleukin (IL)-4 is a Th2 cytokine. Classically, CD is considered a Th1-mediated disease, whereas UC exerts a Th2-like response [4–6]. A recent study suggested that the Th17-cell-driven immune response, which produces excess IL-17A, IL-17F, and IL-22, plays a critical role in the pathogenesis of both CD and UC [7]. An additional Th cell subset which produces IL-22 was identified and designated Th22. Th22 may also participate in the immune response of IBD, but the exact role remains ambiguous [8,9]. Regulatory T (Treg) cells are a distinct T cell subset with opposing actions to Th17. Treg cells are implicated in suppressing an excessive T cell response [10]. The intestinal mucosa is normally maintained in an equilibrium state in which the protective immunity and tolerance to self-antigens and commensal bacteria are balanced. This tolerance is maintained by Treg cells in the gut by inhibiting the proliferation and effector functions of other T cells [11]. Recent studies indicated that IBD is associated with a decrease in Treg cells and increase in Th17 cells in peripheral blood [12,13].

Glutamine (Gln) is the most abundant free amino acid in the plasma and tissue pool. It serves as an important fuel source for rapidly dividing cells, especially lymphocytes and enterocytes. Although it is a non-essential amino acid, many studies showed that Gln has immunomodulatory properties and is considered conditionally essential for patients with catabolic conditions [14–17]. Shiomi et al. [18] reported that Gln levels of serum and colon tissues were significantly lower in the acute phase of colonic inflammation, and Gln supplementation attenuated the degree of microscopic injury induced by dextran sulfate sodium (DSS). Previous studies showed that Gln therapy improves outcomes of in vitro and in vivo experimental colitis models, and is able to attenuate proinflammatory mediator expressions in experimental colitis [19,20]. A recent study performed by our laboratory found that pretreatment with alanyl-Gln injection suppresses Th cell-associated cytokine expression and reduces inflammatory responses in mice with acute DSS-induced colitis [21]. However, studies concerning the effect of dietary Gln on the balance of Th/Treg cells and colonic tissue damage in IBD are rare. Therefore, this study investigated the effects of dietary Gln supplementation on Th/Treg cell homeostasis, colonic cell apoptosis and inflammatory mediator expression in mice with DSS-induced acute colitis.

Materials and Methods

Animal preparations

Male C57BL/6 mice at 8~12 weeks old and weighing 22~25 g at the beginning of the experiment were used in this study. All mice were housed in cages in a temperature- and humidity-controlled room and were allowed free access to a standard chow diet for 1 wk before the study. Care of laboratory animals was in full compliance with the *Guide for the Care and Use of Laboratory Animals* (National Research Council, 1996), and protocols were approved by the institutional Animal Care and Use Committee of Taipei Medical University.

Experimental procedures

Thirty-two mice were assigned to 4 groups with 2 normal control (C and G) and 2 DSS-treated groups (DC and DG). The C and DC groups were fed a common semipurified diet, while the G and DG groups received an identical diet except that part of the casein was replaced by Gln, which provided 25% of total amino acid nitrogen. The 2 diets were isocaloric and isonitrogenous (Table 1). The amount of GLN used is known to have an immunomodulatory effect on catabolic conditions [22]. The mice were not paired fed because the food intakes between the 2 control groups and 2 DSS-treated groups were comparable. The diets were fed for 10 days. On day 6, mice in the normal control groups were given distilled water, and those in the DSS groups were given distilled water containing 1.5% (wt/vol) DSS (MW 40 kDa; MP Biomedicals, Solon, OH) for 5 d. During the experimental period, the body weight (BW) was recorded daily. At the end of the experiment (day 11), mice were anesthetized with an intraperitoneal Zoletil (20 mg/kg) injection and sacrificed by cardiac puncture. Whole blood was centrifuged at 3000×*g* for 10 min at 4°C to obtain plasma. The mesenteric lymph nodes (MLNs) were removed and processed for RNA isolation. The colon was cut close to the ileocecal valve, and the length and weight were measured. The luminal content of the colon was collected by flushing each specimen with 2 ml of ice-cold phosphate-buffered saline (PBS). Colon lavage fluid (CLF) was centrifuged at 2000×*g* for 10 min at 4°C, and supernatants were collected and kept at −80°C until being processed for further analyses. Sections (1 cm) of the distal colon were cut out and fixed with buffered 4% paraformaldehyde for a histopathological examination.

Measurements of haptoglobin in plasma

Plasma samples were used to determine the concentration of haptoglobin by an enzyme-linked immunosorbent assay (ELISA) kit (ICL, Newberg, OR). Procedures followed the manufacturer's instructions.

Distribution of T lymphocyte subpopulations in blood

To determine the phenotypes of helper T lymphocytes in the blood, 100-μl aliquots of whole blood were incubated with Pacific blue-conjugated anti-mouse CD4 (BD Biosciences, San Jose, CA). Another 100 μl of whole blood was incubated with Pacific blue-conjugated anti-mouse CD4 and APC-conjugated anti-mouse CD25 (eBioscience, San Diego, CA) for 30 min to analyze the Treg cell percentage. After lysing red blood cells, the remaining leukocytes were fixed and permeated for intracellular cytokine staining. The following antibodies (Abs) were used for intracellular

Table 1. Composition of the experimental diets (g/kg).

Component	Control diet	Glutamine diet
Soybean oil	100	100
Casein	200	150
Glutamine	0	41.7
Salt mixture†	35	35
Vitamin mixture‡	10	10
Methyl cellulose	31	31
Choline bitartrate	2.5	2.5
Methionine	3	3
Corn starch	626.8	618.5

†The salt mixture contained the following (mg/g): calcium phosphate dibasic, 500; sodium chloride, 74; potassium sulfate, 52; potassium citrate monohydrate, 20; magnesium oxide, 24; manganese carbonate, 3.5; ferric citrate, 6; zinc carbonate, 1.6; curpric carbonate, 0.3; potassium iodate, 0.01; sodium selenite, 0.01; and chromium potassium sulfate, 0.55.
‡The vitamin mixture contained the following (mg/g): thiamin hydrochloride, 0.6; riboflavin, 0.6; pyridoxine hydrochloride, 0.7; nicotinic acid, 3; calcium pantothenate, 1.6; D-biotin, 0.05; cyanocobalamin, 0.001; retinyl palmitate, 1.6; DL-α-tocopherol acetate, 20; cholecalciferol, 0.25; and menaquinone, 0.005.

Table 2. Sequences of oligonucleotide primers used in the PCR amplification.

Gene	Primer sequences (5′ to 3′)
T-bet	F: TGTTCCCAGCCGTTTCTACC
	R:GCTCGGAACTCCGCTTCATA
GATA-3	F: TGACGGAAGAGGTGG ACGTA
	R:GGATACCTCTGCACCGTAGC
RORγt	F: TGCAAGACTCATCGACAAGG
	R: AGGGGATTCAACATCAGTGC
AhR	F: AGGATCGGGGTACCAGTTCA
	R:CTCCAGCGACTGTGTTTTGC
Foxp3	F: AGCGAGTGTCCCTGCTCTCCC
	R: CTTCTGTCTGGAGTGGCTGGGTGT
Muc2	F: ATGCCCACCTCCTCAAAGAC
	R: GTAGTTTCCGTTGGAACAGTGAA
Tff3	F: TTGCTGGGTCCTCTGGGATAG
	R: TACACTGCTCCGATGTGACAG
Hsp72	F: GCTGGCTAGGAGACAGATATGTGGC
	R: AAAGCCCACGTGCAATACACAAAGT
Bcl-xL	F: GGCACTGTGCGTGGAAAGCGTA
	R: CCGCCGTTCTCCTGGATCCA
18 s	F: CGCGGTTCTATTTTGTTGGT
	R: AGTCGGCATCGTTTATGGTC

T-bet, T-box expressed in T cells; ROR-γt, RAR-related orphan receptor gamma t; AhR, aryl hydrocarbon receptor; Foxp3, forhead box p 3.

Table 3. Histological score of colitis.

Feature	Score	Description
Loss of epithelium	0	None
	1	0%~25% loss of epithelium
	2	26%~50% loss of epithelium
	3	>50% loss of epithelium
Length of crypts	0	None to length of crypts 85% normal thickness
	1	Length of crypts 85%~70% normal thickness
	2	Length of crypts 70%~50% normal thickness
	3	Length of crypts <50% normal thickness
Infiltration of leukocytes	0	None
	1	Mild
	2	Moderate
	3	Severe

cytokine staining: Alexa Fluor® 488-conjugated anti-mouse IL-4 (eBioscience), Alexa Fluor® 647-conjugated anti-mouse IFN-γ (Biolegend, San Diego, CA), fluorescein isothiocyanate (FITC)-conjugated anti-mouse IL-17A (eBioscience), phycoerythrin (PE)-conjugated anti-mouse IL-17F (eBioscience), and PerCP-eFluor® 710-conjugated anti-mouse IL-22 (eBioscience). For intracellular staining of forhead box p3 (Foxp3), leukocytes were fixed and permeated with Foxp3 staining buffer (eBioscience) and PE-conjugated anti-mouse Foxp3 (Biolegend). Cells were analyzed with a FACS *Canto II* flow cytometer (BD Biosciences). Lymphocytes were gated with characteristic low forward- and side-scatter profiles. Phenotypes of Th cells are presented as percentages of Th-associated cytokine-expressing cells among Th cells ($CD4^+$ lymphocytes). Treg cells are presented as a percentage of $CD4^+CD25^+Foxp3^+$ cells among lymphocytes or a percentage of Foxp3-expressing cells among $CD4^+CD25^+$ cells.

Table 4. Colonic length and weight, and immunoglobulin (Ig) levels in lavage fluid and haptoglobin concentrations in plasma of experimental mice.

	C	G	DC	DG
Colon				
Length (cm)	5.76±0.40	5.53±0.32	4.63±0.69*	4.95±0.49*
Weight (g)	0.23±0.03	0.26±0.04	0.30±0.04*	0.26±0.05
IgA (μg/mg protein)	15.01±0.06	15.02±0.06	17.18±0.54	16.85±0.52
IgG (μg/mg protein)	20.53±2.77	17.00±4.38	105.53±4.17*#	41.23±6.44
MCP-1 (pg/ml)	60.30±1.48	63.62±1.17	102.6±2.70*	74.06±0.68
TNF-α (pg/ml)	43.52±0.71	41.85±0.16	61.70±1.01*#	48.38±1.44
Plasma				
Haptoglobin (μg/ml)	14.43±0.14	15.31±0.42	121.21±8.50*#	40.87±1.8

Data are expressed as the mean ± SEM. Differences among groups were analyzed by ANOVA using Tukey's test.
*Significantly differs from the C group.
#Significantly differs from the DG group ($p<0.05$).

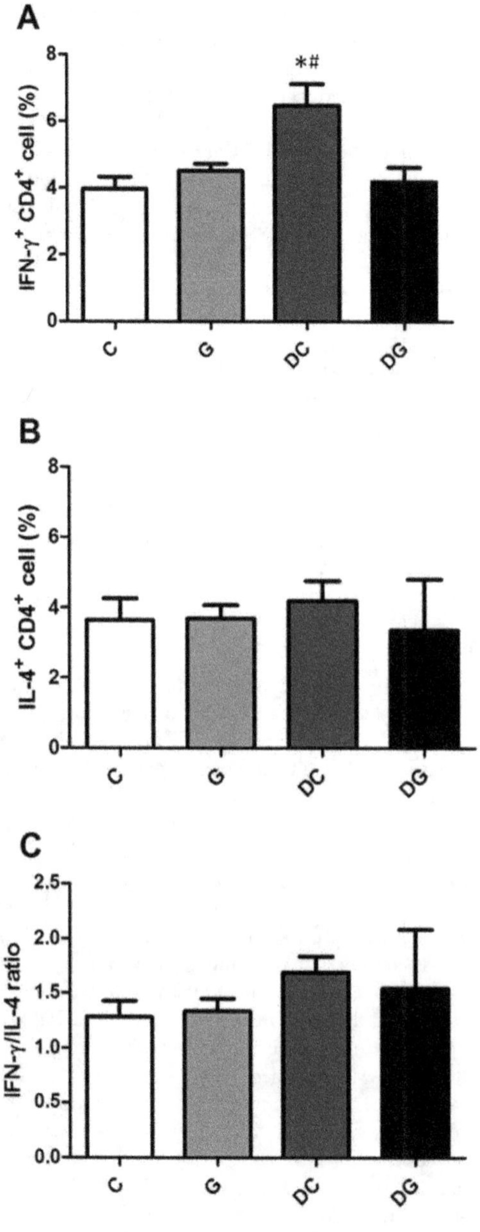

Figure 1. Percentage of Th1/Th2 cell subpopulations in the blood. Lymphocytes were gated according to their size and granularity using light scatter detectors (FSC/SSC). CD4-positive lymphocytes were considered Th cells and were gated to determine the expression of intracellular cytokines. A, B: Percentages of interferon (IFN)-γ- and interleukin (IL)-4-expressing $CD4^+$ lymphocytes. C: IFN-γ/IL-4 ratio. Data are presented as the mean ± SEM. Differences among groups were analyzed by ANOVA using the Tukey's test. *Significantly differs from the C group. #Significantly differs from the DG group ($p<0.05$).

RNA extraction and quantitative real-time reverse-transcription polymerase chain reaction (RT-qPCR)

Total RNA was isolated from MLNs using the Trizol reagent (Invitrogen, Carlsbad, CA). RNA (1 μg) was reverse-transcribed using random hexamer primers with a complementary (c)DNA synthesis kit (Fermentas, Glen Burnie, MD) according to standard

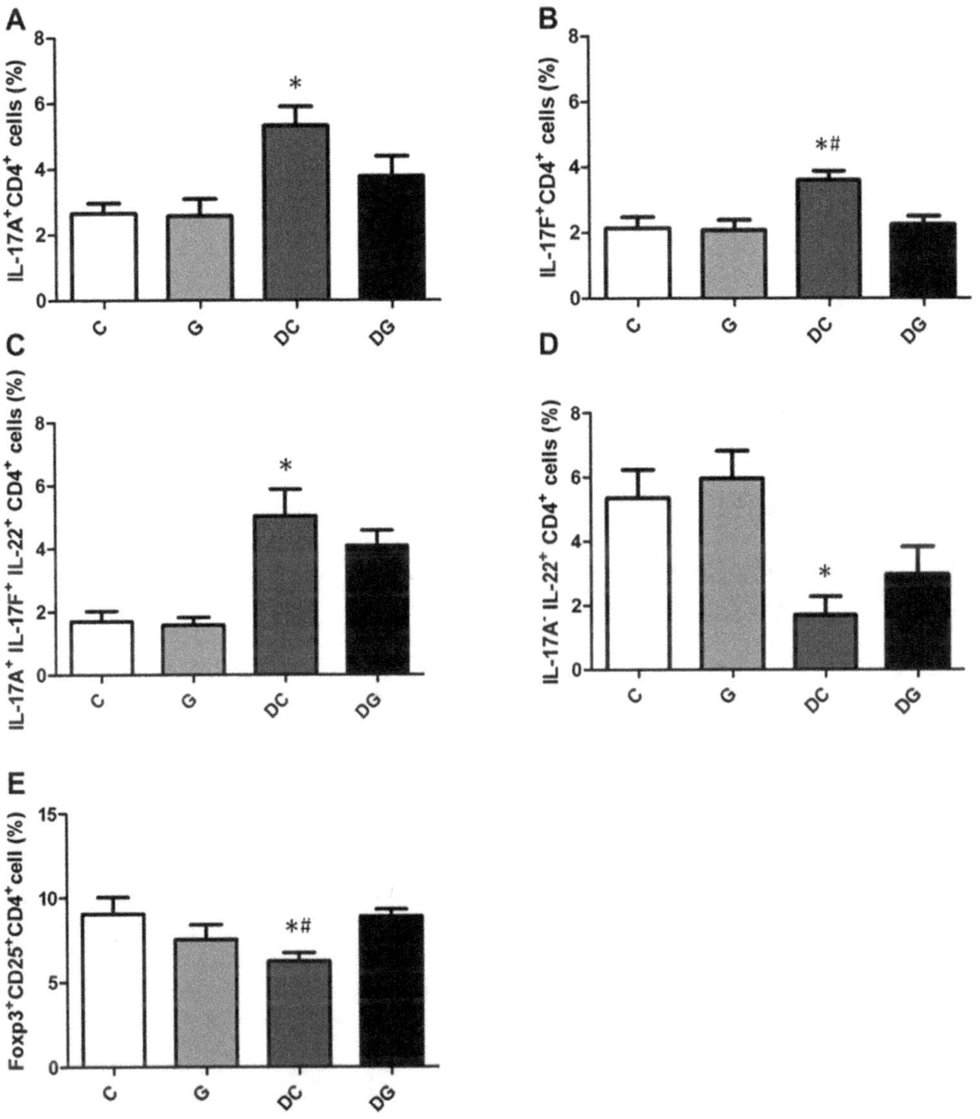

Figure 2. Percentages of Th17/Th22-associated cytokine-producing cell and Treg cell populations in the blood. CD4-positive lymphocytes were gated to analyze intracellular cytokine expressions by flow cytometry. A: Expression of intracellular interleukin (IL)-17A. B: Expression of intracellular IL-17F. C: Triple expression of intracellular IL-17A, IL-17F, and IL-22. D: IL-22$^+$ and IL-17A$^-$Th cells. E: Percentage of Treg cells. Data are presented as the mean ± SEM. Differences among groups were analyzed by an ANOVA using Tukey's test. *Significantly differs from the C group. #Significantly differs from the DG group ($p<0.05$).

protocols. A real-time RT-PCR was carried out in optical 96-well plates on an ABI 7300 Real-Time PCR System (Applied Biosystems, Foster City, CA). Primers used in this study are listed in Table 2. The expression of each gene was assayed in a total volume of 25 µl containing 1× SYBR green master mix reagent (Applied Biosystems), 100 nM of each primer, and 50 ng of cDNA. Amplification was performed according to the thermocycling protocol recommended by the PCR system, with a final dissociation curve (DC) analysis. No-template controls and a melting curve analysis were used to confirm the specificity of the real-time PCR. All samples were analyzed in triplicate, and multiples of change of messenger (m)RNA were calculated by the equation $2^{-\Delta\Delta Ct}$ (ΔCt indicates the difference of threshold cycles between the test gene and 18 s, and $\Delta\Delta$Ct indicates the difference of ΔCt between the colitis and normal control groups).

Immunoglobulin (Ig) and cytokine concentrations in CLF

Ig, macrophage chemoattractant protein (MCP)-1 and tumor necrosis factor (TNF)-α were determined by enzyme-linked immunosorbent assay (ELISA) kits. Antibodies specific for IgA, IgG, MCP-1 and TNF-α (eBioscience) were coated onto wells of microtiter strips provided. Procedures followed the manufacturer's instructions. Levels of Igs and cytokines were determined by detecting an Ab conjugated to horseradish peroxidase.

Immunoblotting

Colon tissues were homogenized in lysis buffer (50 mMTris (pH 7.4), 1% sodium dodecylsulfate (SDS), and 10 mM EDTA) containing a protease inhibitor cocktail (Sigma) to prepare whole-tissue lysates. The homogenates were centrifuged at 15,000× g for 15 min, and the supernatants were used for immunoblotting. Protein concentrations of the supernatant were determined using a

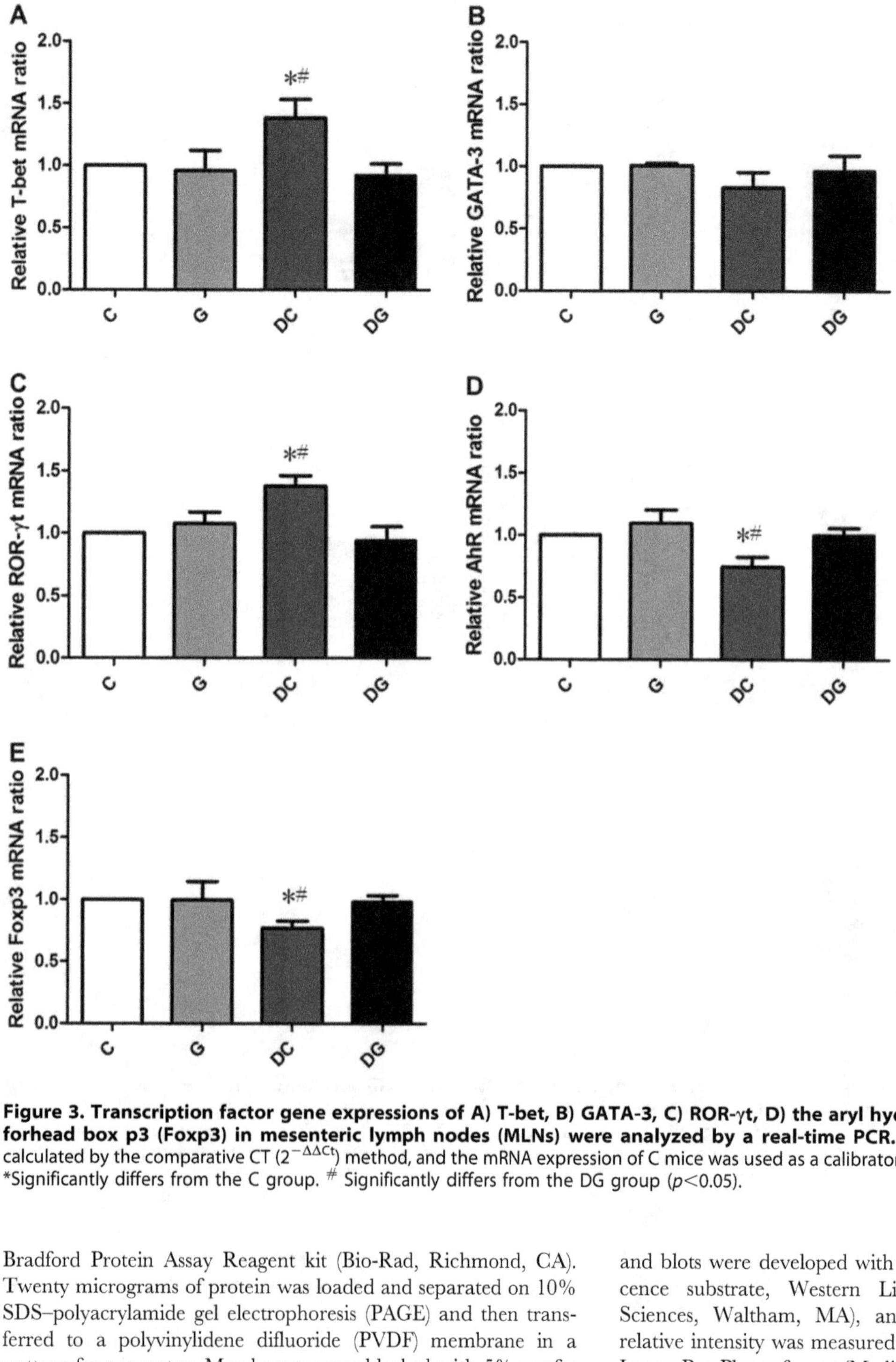

Figure 3. Transcription factor gene expressions of A) T-bet, B) GATA-3, C) ROR-γt, D) the aryl hydrocarbon receptor (AhR), and E) forhead box p3 (Foxp3) in mesenteric lymph nodes (MLNs) were analyzed by a real-time PCR. Quantitation of mRNA changes was calculated by the comparative CT ($2^{-\Delta\Delta Ct}$) method, and the mRNA expression of C mice was used as a calibrator. Data are shown as the mean ± SEM. *Significantly differs from the C group. # Significantly differs from the DG group ($p<0.05$).

Bradford Protein Assay Reagent kit (Bio-Rad, Richmond, CA). Twenty micrograms of protein was loaded and separated on 10% SDS–polyacrylamide gel electrophoresis (PAGE) and then transferred to a polyvinylidene difluoride (PVDF) membrane in a wettransfer apparatus. Membranes were blocked with 5% nonfat milk in Tris-buffered saline (TBS) for 30 min and then incubated with antibodies overnight at 4°C. Polyclonal rabbit antibodies against poly (adenosine diphosphate-ribose) polymerase (PARP) were purchased from Cell Signaling Technology (Danvers, MA). Polyclonal rabbit antibodies against nuclear factor (NF)-κB p65 or IκBα were purchased from Santa Cruz Biotechnology (Santa Cruz, CA). A monoclonal mouse antibody against β-actin was purchased from Sigma. After washing 3 times in TBS-T (TBS containing 0.1% Tween-20), membranes were incubated with horseradish peroxidase (HRP)-conjugated species-specific antibodies for 1 h. Membranes were then washed with TBS-T for 30 min, and blots were developed with the high-sensitivity chemiluminescence substrate, Western Lighting Ultra (PerkinElmer Life Sciences, Waltham, MA), and exposed to X-ray films. The relative intensity was measured to quantify the protein level using Image-Pro Plus software (Media Cybernetics, Bethesda, MD). All blots were normalized against actin to adjust for the amount of protein loaded.

Histopathology

After being embedded in paraffin, specimens of the distal colon were sectioned at 5 μm, mounted on glass slides and stained with hematoxylin and eosin for the histopathology analysis. Digital images at 40× magnification per section were captured with a Zeiss Axiphot light microscope (Carl Zeiss MicroImaging LLC, Thornwood, NY) and a Nikon D1X digital camera (Tokyo, Japan). Five fields per section were examined to determine the

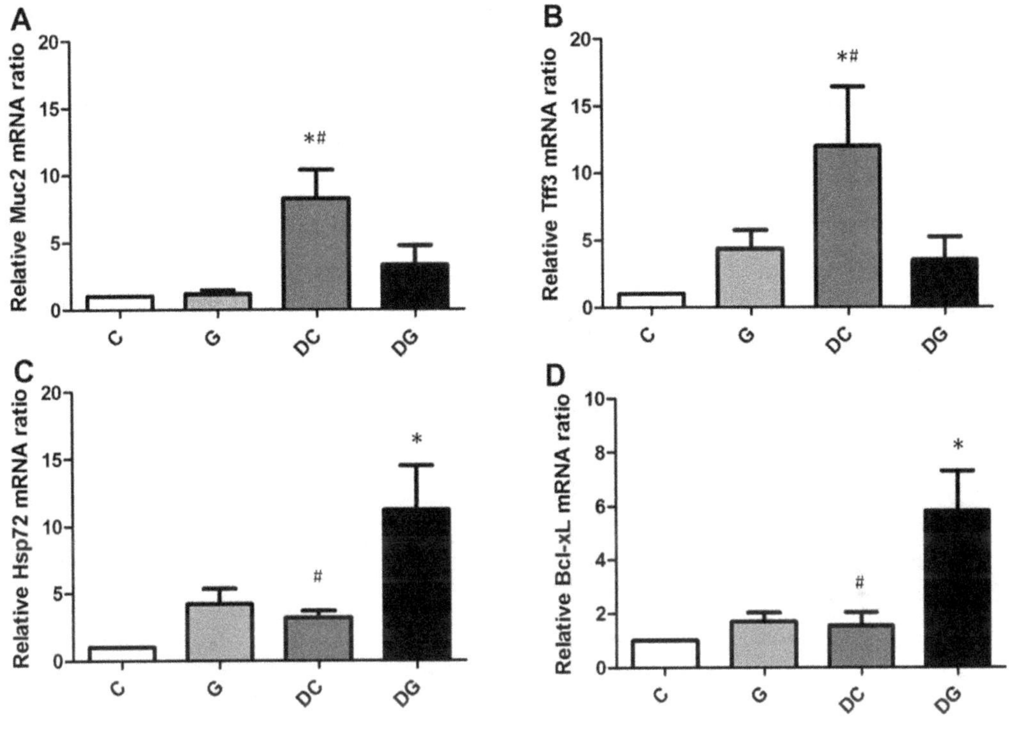

Figure 4. mRNA expressions of mucosal recovery-related and antiapoptotic genes in colon tissues. mRNA levels were analyzed by a real-time PCR. A: Expression of Muc2 mRNA. B: Expression of Tff3 mRNA. C: Expression of Hsp72 mRNA. D: Expression of Bcl-xL mRNA. Quantitation of mRNA changes was calculated by the comparative CT ($2^{-\Delta\Delta Ct}$) method, and mRNA expression of C mice was used as a calibrator. Data are shown as the mean ± SEM. *Significantly differs from the C group. #Significantly differs from the DG group (P<0.05).

morphological lesions and changes in the colon mucosa. The degree of IBD was measured by the modified scoring system of Iba et al. [23]. Inflammatory colitis was scored from 0 to 3 for lesions based on loss of epithelium, length of crypts, and infiltration of leukocytes (Table 3). The total histological score ranged from 0 to 9, which represented the summed scores of loss of epithelium, length of crypts and infiltration of leukocytes, with a higher score indicating more-severe disease.

Statistical analysis

All data are expressed as the mean ± standard error of the mean (SEM). Differences among groups were analyzed by an analysis of variance (ANOVA) using Tukey's test. A two-way ANOVA using the Bonferroni posttest was used to analyze differences among groups. A p value of <0.05 was considered statistically significant.

Results

BW changes of the mice

There were no differences in the initial BWs among the 4 groups. Clinical symptoms of exposure to DSS for 5 d were BW loss and the presence of blood in the feces. The BWs did not differ between the C and G groups during the experimental period (data not shown). Weight loss was observed at day (d)11 in the DC group compared to the C group (20.7±1.7 vs. 24.5±0.6 g, $p<0.05$). Also, the BW of the DC group was less than that of the DG group on d11 (20.7±1.7 vs. 22.9±1.4 g, $p<0.05$).

Colon weight and length, Ig, cytokines and plasma haptoglobin concentrations

There were no differences in colonic weight or length, Ig in lavage fluid, or plasma haptoglobin concentrations between the C and G groups. Mice that received DSS had a significantly shorter colon length, and the DC group had a higher colon weight than the C group. Also, the DC group had significantly higher colonic IgG and plasma haptoglobin levels than those of the control and DG groups. MCP-1 levels were significantly higher in the DC group than the C group. Also, the DC group had higher TNF-α levels than the C and DG group (Table 4).

Percentage of blood T cell subpopulations

There were no differences in percentages of Th cell subpopulations between the C and G group. Percentages of IFN-γ-expressing $CD4^+$ cells were higher in the DC group than in the C and DG groups. No differences in IL-4-expressing $CD4^+$ cells or the IFN-γ/IL-4 ratio were detected among the 4 groups (Figure 1). The DC group had significantly higher percentages of IL-17A, IL-17F, and $IL\text{-}17A^+IL\text{-}17F^+IL\text{-}22^+$-expressing $CD4^+$ cells while lower $IL\text{-}17A^-IL\text{-}22^+$ Th22 cells than those in the C group. Also, $Foxp3^+CD4^+CD25^+$ Treg cells were lower in the DC group than the C and DG groups. The DG group had lower IL-17F-expressing $CD4^+$ cells and higher $Foxp3^+CD4^+CD25^+$ Treg cells than the DC group but showed no differences from the C group (Figure 2).

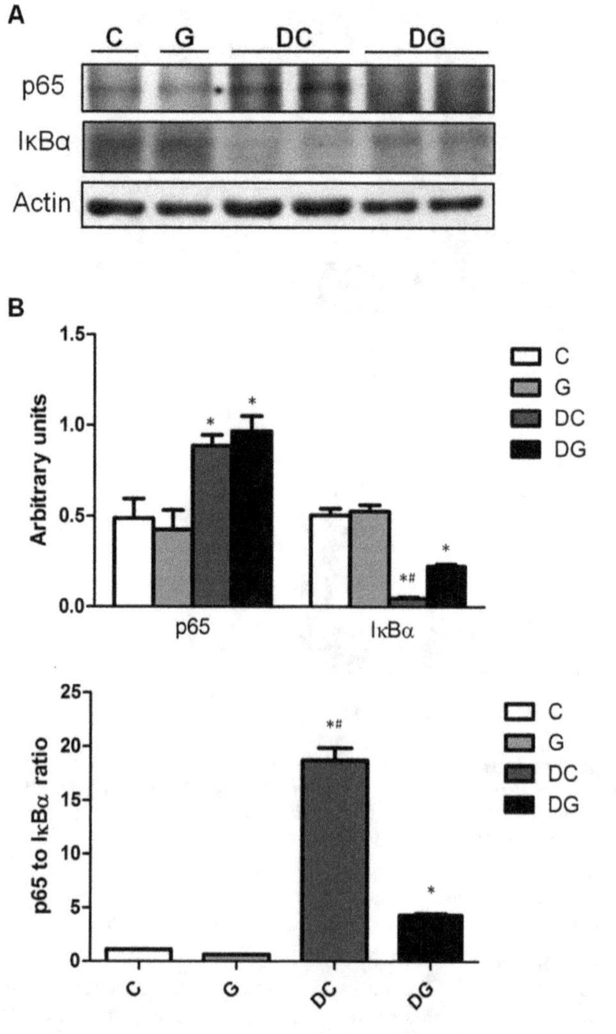

Figure 5. Protein levels of nuclear factor (NF)-κB p65 and inhibitory factor κBα (IκBα) in colon tissues. a Protein expressions of NF-κB p65 and IκBα. Whole-tissue lysates were analyzed by immunoblotting, and b-actin was used as a loading control. b Densitometric analysis of the blot corrected by the protein loading control. c The ratio of NF-κB p65 to IκBα. Results of the densitometric analysis are shown as the mean ± SEM. *Significantly differs from the C group. #Significantly differs from the DG group ($P<0.05$).

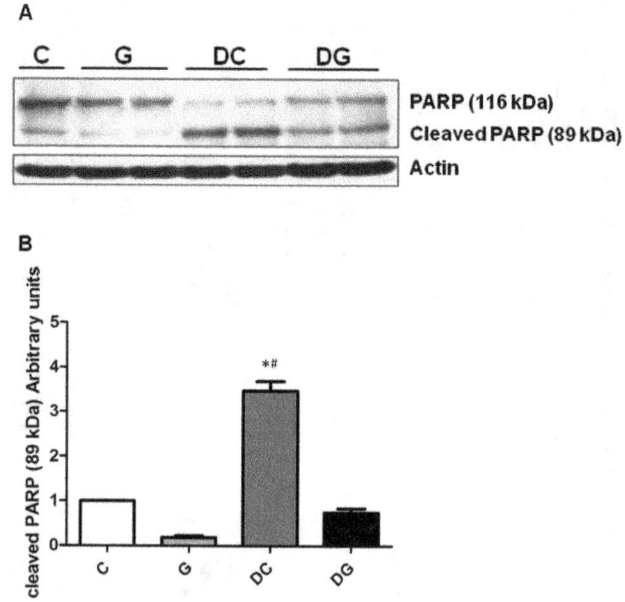

Figure 6. Protein levels of PARP and cleaved PARP in colon tissues. A: protein expressions of PARP and cleaved PARP. Whole-tissue lysates were analyzed by immunoblotting, and β-actin was used as a loading control. B: densitometric analysis of the blot corrected by the protein loading control. Results of the densitometric analysis are shown as the mean ± SEM. *Significantly differs from the C group. #Significantly differs from the DG group ($P<0.05$).

Gene expressions in MLNs and colon tissues

mRNA levels of T-box expressed in T cells (T-bet) and RAR-related orphan receptor gamma t (ROR-γt) were higher whereas the aryl hydrocarbon receptor (AhR) and Foxp3 gene expressions in MLN were lower in the DC group than in the C and DG group (Figure 3). Mucin 2 (Muc2) and trefoil factor 3 (Tff3) mRNA levels in the colon tissues were significantly higher in the DC group than the other 3 groups. The DG group had the highest gene expressions of Hsp72 and antiapoptotic Bcl-xL in colon tissues among the 4 groups (Figure 4).

Protein levels of PARP and NF-κB/IκBα in colon tissues

Compared to the NC group, the DS and DG groups had significantly higher NF-κB p65 whereas lower IκBα expressions. The NF-κB/IκBα ratio was lower in the DG group than the DC group (Figure 5). DC group showed significantly higher protein levels of cleaved PARP than the C and DG group (Figure 6).

Histopathological aspects of the colon

Colon section from the C and G groups showed intact epithelium, a well-defined gland, and no leukocyte infiltration in the mucosa. In contrast, the DC group showed mucosal ulceration, infiltration of leukocytes, crypt distortion, and hyperplastic epithelium, and had a significantly higher colon injury score than the C and DG groups (Figure 7).

Discussion

In this study, dietary Gln was administered for 5 d before colitis was induced, and was sustained through the period of DSS-induced colitis. Because IBD is a disease that flares up with remissions and relapses, this model mimics the preventive oral Gln administration to the acute phase of IBD patients in order to resolve the inflammation of colitis. We did not include an amino acid mixture without Gln group in this study, because previous study had shown that Gln, but not isonitrogenous non-amino acid mixture, promotes T lymphocyte response [24]. A study conducted by our laboratory previously compared intraperitoneal injection of Gln dipeptide and identical amount of amino acid solution in a mouse colitis model. Our results also showed that compared with the mixed amino acid solution group, Gln administration reduced inflammatory mediator production and leukocyte infiltration into tissues [21]. We analyzed the distribution of blood T cell populations including Th1, Th2, Th17, Th22, and Treg cells, because the balance between Th and Treg cells and the cytokine profiles derived from these T cells play major roles in the inflammation of IBD [12,25,26]. T-bet, GATA-3, ROR-γt, AhR, and Foxp3 are transcription factors that respectively participate in the differentiation of Th1, Th2, Th17, Th22, and Treg cells. Since the colon is the main site of injury in IBD, gene expressions of transcription factors in MLNs were also

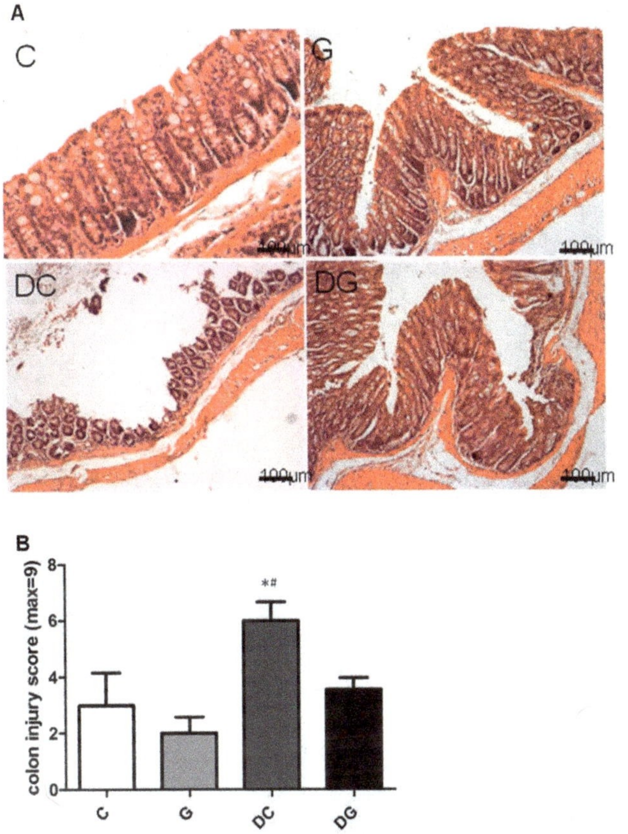

Figure 7. Histopathology of colon tissues. A: Hematoxylin and eosin staining of colon tissues from mice in the C, G, DC, and DG groups. B: Histological scores of colitis. Data are presented as the mean ± SEM., which were determined as described in "Materials and Methods." Differences among groups were analyzed by a one-way ANOVA using Tukey's test. *Significantly differs from the C group. #Significantly differs from the DG group ($p<0.05$).

analyzed to evaluate the polarization of Th subsets and Treg cells. The findings of this study showed that dietary Gln supplementation before and during colitis modulate the homeostasis of Th and Treg cells that may mitigate colonic inflammatory reactions. Besides, the partial elemental component provided by Gln diet may also have favorable effect on treating IBD.

Cytokines are key players in innate and adaptive immune responses in mucosal inflammation. A previous study indicated that different models of IBD produced specific cytokine profiles in the initiation and perpetuation of disease pathogenesis [27]. Those investigators suggested that cytokine profiling can be used as diagnostic and prognostic tools in IBD. Our results showed that percentages of blood IFN-γ, IL-17A, and IL-17F together with the mRNA expressions of T-bet and ROR-γt in MLNs were upregulated in the DC group. This result is consistent with a previous report which also showed that DSS-induced acute colitis was characterized by polarization toward the Th1-Th17 panel [27]. Th22 is a newly identified subset of Th cells. Th22 appears to be regulated by the AhR transcription factor and plays a critical role in mucosal healing through epithelial proliferation and increased mucus production. Activation of the AhR ameliorates the inflammation and disease activity of colitis mice [28–30]. Our results showed that DSS administration reduced the population of blood Th22 cells and mRNA levels of the AhR in MLNs indicating that Th22 expression was suppressed in mice with acute colitis. These findings were consistent with previous studies that Th22 and AhR expressions are downregulated in actively inflamed colitis tissue of IBD patients and experimental colitis models [9,29].

Treg cells express the CD4 and CD25 surface markers. Foxp3 is a key transcription factor of Treg cell development and function, and is the best marker for defining murine Treg cells [10,31]. Treg cells were shown to suppress a number of additional T cell-mediated responses in vitro and in vivo and are effective in the prevention and downregulation of IBD in animal models [32–34]. Results of this study found that percentages of blood Treg cells and mRNA levels of Foxp3 in MLNs significantly decreased in the DC group. Our findings are consistent with previous reports which also found that Treg cells decreased in the blood and inflamed colon tissue of IBD patients [13,35–37].

Haptoglobin is an acute-phase protein, which is used as a marker of systemic inflammation to monitor disease activity in experimental colitis in rodent models [38]. IgA is the main Ig produced by the intestinal mucosa. In this study, IgA levels did not differ among the control and DSS colitis groups. This result is similar with a report by Macpherson et al. [39], who also found no difference in colonic IgA concentrations between IBD patients and controls. In contrast to IgA, IgG is considered a specific index for grading disease activity in patients with IBD [40]. We also found dramatically higher levels in the DSS colitis group. MCP-1 is a chemotactic and activating factor for mononuclear phagocytes. MCP-1 and TNF-α are important mediators involved in the inflammatory and immune responses. NF-κB is a widely expressed inducible transcription factor that is an important regulator of genes involved in inflammatory response. NF-κB DNA binding is inhibited by IκBα. The higher NF-κB/IκBα ratio indicates higher NF-κB activation. The significantly elevated plasma haptoglobin and intraluminal mediators accompanied with higher NF-κB/IκBα ratio indicated that experimental colitis was active.

Previous study demonstrated that DSS results in epithelial damage by inhibiting proliferation and inducing apoptosis [41]. There is a layer of mucus formed by mucins lining the gastrointestinal tract to act as a lubricant and provide protection of mucosal barrier. Muc2 is one of the predominant mucins detected in the colorectum. Trefoils are a group of small peptides that have important roles in epithelial protection and mucosal healing [42]. Trefoil factor family (Tff)3 is one of the Tff peptides found throughout the small and large intestines. Previous studies found that Muc2 and Tff3 genes were up-regulated during colitis induction, and suggested that their mRNA levels could be used as early markers of inflammation [43]. The higher Muc2 and Tff3 mRNA expressions in the DC group may indicate more severe mucosal damage that required to be repaired. Apoptosis is a form of cell death, which is controlled by intracellular proteases of the caspase family. Caspases cleave various cellular substrates including PARP and thereby induce the typical alterations of apoptotic cells [44]. The result of this study showed that the protein levels of cleaved PARP in colon tissue were elevated in the DC group suggested DSS-induced apoptosis is initiated.

In this study, we found that dietary Gln supplementation resulted in several beneficial effects that were not observed in colitis mice without Gln administration. First, the DSS-induced Th1–Th17 response and decreased Th22 and Treg cell expressions were inhibited by Gln administration. These findings were partly similar to a previous study which used an intraperitoneal injection of Gln in mice with DSS-induced colitis [21]. Second, transcription factor gene expressions corresponding to Th and Treg cells in MLNs were consistent with the T cell response in the blood indicating that Gln has a regulatory role in systemic and local T cell polarization in acute colitis. Third, dietary Gln supplementation lowered the plasma haptoglobin and intraluminal inflammatory mediators. The lower NF-κB/IκBα ratio further supports the role of Gln in reducing colitic inflammation. Fourth, Gln prevented the apoptosis of colon cells possibly by reducing caspase activities and enhancing colonic antiapoptotic Bcl-xL gene expression. The higher heat shock protein (Hsp) expression may also play roles in inhibiting apoptosis. Hsp is vital to cellular and tissue protection after stress or injury. Previous study indicated that Gln protected gut mucosa from injury by inducing Hsp72 expression [45,46]. The chaperone property of Hsp72 is related to the cytoprotective effects and the ability to inhibit apoptosis [47,48]. The lower colonic Muc2 and Tff3 mRNA expressions observed in the DSS-Gln group were consistent with the histological findings that damage to the colonic mucosa was less severe in the colitis group with Gln supplementation.

Gln is the primary fuel source for immune cells. Also, it is a precursor for the endogenous antioxidant, glutathione. Previous studies demonstrated that Gln enhanced IL-2 production, promoted T cell proliferation, and decreased T cell apoptosis possibly through certain redox-based mechanisms [49,50]. In addition, IL-2 was found to maintain Foxp3 Treg cells and inhibit the polarization of Th17 cells [51,52]. However, elucidating the mechanisms responsible for the effects of Gln on regulating T cell polarization and the association between CD4+ T cell homeostasis and inflammatory response requires further investigation.

In summary, this study showed for the first time that in a DSS-induced acute colitis model, dietary Gln supplementation suppressed Th1/Th17-associated cytokine expressions while enhancing Th22 and Treg cell expressions. Also, systemic and intraluminal inflammatory proteins and the apoptosis of colonic cells were reduced. These results suggest that Gln treatment modulates the homeostasis between Treg and Th cells, and ameliorates the disease severity of acute DSS-induced colitis.

Author Contributions

Conceived and designed the experiments: Y. Hsiung SLY. Performed the experiments: Y. Hsiung. Analyzed the data: Y. Hsiung JJL Y. Hou CLY. Prepared figures: Y. Hsuing. Wrote the manuscript: SLY. Edited and revised the manuscript: JJL.

References

1. Triantafillidis JK, Nasioulas G, Kosmidis PA (2009) Colorectal cancer and inflammatory bowel disease: epidemiology, risk factors, mechanisms of carcinogenesis and prevention strategies. Anticancer Res 29: 2727–2737.
2. Maloy KJ, Powrie F (2011) Intestinal homeostasis and its breakdown in inflammatory bowel disease. Nature 474: 298–306.
3. Kaser A, Zeissig S, Blumberg RS (2010) Inflammatory bowel disease. Annu Rev Immunol 28: 573–621.
4. Bouma G, Strober W (2003) The immunological and genetic basis of inflammatory bowel disease. Nat Rev Immunol 3: 521–533.
5. Fuss IJ, Neurath M, Boirivant M, Klein JS, de la Motte C, et al. (1996) Disparate CD4+ lamina propria (LP) lymphokine secretion profiles in inflammatory bowel disease. Crohn's disease LP cells manifest increased secretion of IFN-gamma, whereas ulcerative colitis LP cells manifest increased secretion of IL-5. J Immunol 157: 1261–1270.
6. Nielsen OH, Koppen T, Rudiger N, Horn T, Eriksen J, et al. (1996) Involvement of interleukin-4 and -10 in inflammatory bowel disease. Dig Dis Sci 41: 1786–1793.
7. Boirivant M, Cossu A (2012) Inflammatory bowel disease. Oral Dis 18: 1–15.
8. Zhang N, Pan HF, Ye DQ (2011) Th22 in inflammatory and autoimmune disease: prospects for therapeutic intervention. Mol Cell Biochem 353: 41–46.
9. Leung JM, Davenport M, Wolff MJ, Wiens KE, Abidi WM, et al. (2013) IL-22-producing CD4+ cells are depleted in actively inflamed colitis tissue. Mucosal Immunol. doi: 10.1038/mi.2013.31.
10. Sakaguchi S, Yamaguchi T, Nomura T, Ono M (2008) Regulatory T cells and immune tolerance. Cell 133: 775–787.
11. Sakaguchi S, Sakaguchi N, Asano M, Itoh M, Toda M (1995) Immunologic self-tolerance maintained by activated T cells expressing IL-2 receptor alpha-chains (CD25). Breakdown of a single mechanism of self-tolerance causes various autoimmune diseases. J Immunol 155: 1151–1164.
12. Eastaff-Leung N, Mabarrack N, Barbour A, Cummins A, Barry S (2010) Foxp3+ regulatory T cells, Th17 effector cells, and cytokine environment in inflammatory bowel disease. J Clin Immunol 30: 80–89.
13. Maul J, Loddenkemper C, Mundt P, Berg E, Giese T, et al. (2005) Peripheral and intestinal regulatory CD4+ CD25(high) T cells in inflammatory bowel disease. Gastroenterology 128: 1868–1878.
14. Wilmore DW (2001) The effect of glutamine supplementation in patients following elective surgery and accidental injury. J Nutr 131: 2543S–2549S; discussion 2550S–2541S.
15. Lacey JM, Wilmore DW (1990) Is glutamine a conditionally essential amino acid? Nutr Rev 48: 297–309.
16. Kim H (2011) Glutamine as an immunonutrient. Yonsei Med J 52: 892–897.
17. Parry-Billings M, Evans J, Calder PC, Newsholme EA (1990) Does glutamine contribute to immunosuppression after major burns? Lancet 336: 523–525.
18. Shiomi Y, Nishiumi S, Ooi M, Hatano N, Shinohara M, et al. (2011) GCMS-based metabolomic study in mice with colitis induced by dextran sulfate sodium. Inflamm Bowel Dis 17: 2261–2274.
19. Kretzmann NA, Fillmann H, Mauriz JL, Marroni CA, Marroni N, et al. (2008) Effects of glutamine on proinflammatory gene expression and activation of nuclear factor kappa B and signal transducers and activators of transcription in TNBS-induced colitis. Inflamm Bowel Dis 14: 1504–1513.
20. Xue H, Sufit AJ, Wischmeyer PE (2011) Glutamine therapy improves outcome of in vitro and in vivo experimental colitis models. JPEN J Parenter Enteral Nutr 35: 188–197.
21. Chu CC, Hou YC, Pai MH, Chao CJ, Yeh SL (2012) Pretreatment with alanyl-glutamine suppresses T-helper-cell-associated cytokine expression and reduces inflammatory responses in mice with acute DSS-induced colitis. J Nutr Biochem 23: 1092–1099.
22. Yeh CL, Hsu CS, Yeh SL, Lin MT, Chen WJ (2006) Dietary glutamine supplementation reduces cellular adhesion molecule expression and tissue myeloperoxidase activity in mice with gut-derived sepsis. Nutrition 22: 408–413.
23. Iba Y, Sugimoto Y, Kamei C, Masukawa T (2003) Possible role of mucosal mast cells in the recovery process of colitis induced by dextran sulfate sodium in rats. Int Immunopharmacol 3: 485–491.
24. Kew S, Wells SM, Yaqoob P, Wallace FA, Miles EA, et al. (1999) Dieatry glutamine enhances murine T lymphocyte responsiveness. J Nutr 129: 1524–1531.
25. Baumgart DC, Carding SR (2007) Inflammatory bowel disease: cause and immunobiology. Lancet 369: 1627–1640.
26. Boden EK, Snapper SB (2008) Regulatory T cells in inflammatory bowel disease. Curr Opin Gastroenterol 24: 733–741.
27. Alex P, Zachos NC, Nguyen T, Gonzales L, Chen TE, et al. (2009) Distinct cytokine patterns identified from multiplex profiles of murine DSS and TNBS-induced colitis. Inflamm Bowel Dis 15: 341–352.
28. Benson JM, Shepherd DM (2011) Aryl hydrocarbon receptor activation by TCDD reduces inflammation associated with Crohn's disease. Toxicol Sci 120: 68–78.
29. Monteleone I, Rizzo A, Sarra M, Sica G, Sileri P, et al. (2011) Aryl hydrocarbon receptor-induced signals up-regulate IL-22 production and inhibit inflammation in the gastrointestinal tract. Gastroenterology 141: 237–248, 248 e231.
30. Singh NP, Singh UP, Singh B, Price RL, Nagarkatti M, et al. (2011) Activation of aryl hydrocarbon receptor (AhR) leads to reciprocal epigenetic regulation of FoxP3 and IL-17 expression and amelioration of experimental colitis. PLoS One 6: e23522.
31. Vignali DA, Collison LW, Workman CJ (2008) How regulatory T cells work. Nat Rev Immunol 8: 523–532.
32. Maloy KJ, Powrie F (2001) Regulatory T cells in the control of immune pathology. Nat Immunol 2: 816–822.
33. Shevach EM (2002) CD4+ CD25+ suppressor T cells: more questions than answers. Nat Rev Immunol 2: 389–400.
34. Sakaguchi S, Sakaguchi N, Shimizu J, Yamazaki S, Sakihama T, et al. (2001) Immunologic tolerance maintained by CD25+ CD4+ regulatory T cells: their common role in controlling autoimmunity, tumor immunity, and transplantation tolerance. Immunol Rev 182: 18–32.
35. Takahashi M, Nakamura K, Honda K, Kitamura Y, Mizutani T, et al. (2006) An inverse correlation of human peripheral blood regulatory T cell frequency with the disease activity of ulcerative colitis. Dig Dis Sci 51: 677–686.
36. Saruta M, Yu QT, Fleshner PR, Mantel PY, Schmidt-Weber CB, et al. (2007) Characterization of FOXP3+CD4+ regulatory T cells in Crohn's disease. Clin Immunol 125: 281–290.
37. Yu QT, Saruta M, Avanesyan A, Fleshner PR, Banham AH, et al. (2007) Expression and functional characterization of FOXP3+ CD4+ regulatory T cells in ulcerative colitis. Inflamm Bowel Dis 13: 191–199.
38. Melgar S, Karlsson A, Michaelsson E (2005) Acute colitis induced by dextran sulfate sodium progresses to chronicity in C57BL/6 but not in BALB/c mice: correlation between symptoms and inflammation. Am J Physiol Gastrointest Liver Physiol 288: G1328–1338.

39. Macpherson A, Khoo UY, Forgacs I, Philpott-Howard J, Bjarnason I (1996) Mucosal antibodies in inflammatory bowel disease are directed against intestinal bacteria. Gut 38: 365–375.
40. Choudari CP, O'Mahony S, Brydon G, Mwantembe O, Ferguson A (1993) Gut lavage fluid protein concentrations: objective measures of disease activity in inflammatory bowel disease. Gastroenterology 104: 1064–1071.
41. Renes IB, Verburg M, Van Nispen DJ, Taminiau JA, Buller HA, et al. (2002) Epithelial proliferation, cell death, and gene expression in experimental colitis: alterations in carbonic anhydrase I, mucin MUC2, and trefoil factor 3 expression. Int J Colorectal Dis 17: 317–326.
42. Kindon H, Pothoulakis C, Thim L, Lynch-Devaney K, Podolsky DK (1995) Trefoil peptide protection of intestinal epithelial barrier function: cooperative interaction with mucin glycoprotein. Gastroenterology 109: 516–523.
43. Hoebler C, Gaudier E, De Coppet P, Rival M, Cherbut C (2006) MUC genes are differently expressed during onset and maintenance of inflammation in dextran sodium sulfate-treated mice. Dig Dis Sci 51: 381–389.
44. Fischer U, Janicke RU, Schulze-Osthoff K (2003) Many cuts to ruin: a comprehensive update of caspase substrates. Cell Death Differ 10: 76–100.
45. Cuzzocrea S, Ianaro A, Wayman NS, Mazzon E, Pisano B, et al. (2003) The cyclopentenone prostaglandin 15-deoxy-delta(12,14)- PGJ2 attenuates the development of colon injury caused by dinitrobenzene sulphonic acid in the rat. Br J Pharmacol 138: 678–688.
46. Wischmeyer PE, Musch MW, Madonna MB, Thisted R, Chang EB (1997) Glutamine protects intestinal epithelial cells: role of inducible HSP70. Am J Physiol 272: G879–884.
47. Lanneau D, Brunet M, Frisan E, Solary E, Fontenay M, et al. (2008) Heat shock proteins: essential proteins for apoptosis regulation. J Cell Mol Med 12: 743–761.
48. Sreedhar AS, Csermely P (2004) Heat shock proteins in the regulation of apoptosis: new strategies in tumor therapy: a comprehensive review. Pharmacol Ther 101: 227–257.
49. Chang WK, Yang KD, Chuang H, Jan JT, Shaio MF (2002) Glutamine protects activated human T cells from apoptosis by up-regulating glutathione and Bcl-2 levels. Clin Immunol 104: 151–160.
50. Chang WK, Yang KD, Shaio MF (1999) Lymphocyte proliferation modulated by glutamine: involved in the endogenous redox reaction. Clin Exp Immunol 117: 482–488.
51. Chen Q, Kim YC, Laurence A, Punkosdy GA, Shevach EM (2011) IL-2 controls the stability of Foxp3 expression in TGF-beta-induced Foxp3+ T cells in vivo. J Immunol 186: 6329–6337.
52. Laurence A, Tato CM, Davidson TS, Kanno Y, Chen Z, et al. (2007) Interleukin-2 signaling via STAT5 constrains T helper 17 cell generation. Immunity 26: 371–381.

18

Tristetraprolin Mediates Anti-Inflammatory Effect of Carbon Monoxide against DSS-Induced Colitis

Yeonsoo Joe[1], Md. Jamal Uddin[1], Min Zheng[1,2], Hyo Jeong Kim[1], Yingqing Chen[1], Nal Ae Yoon[1], Gyeong Jae Cho[3], Jeong Woo Park[1]*, Hun Taeg Chung[1]*

1 Department of Biological Sciences, University of Ulsan, Ulsan, Korea, **2** Department of Thoracic and Cardiovascular Surgery, Affiliated Hospital of Yanbian University, Yanji, China, **3** Department of Anatomy, School of Medicine and Institute of Health Sciences, Gyeongsang National University, Jinju, Korea

Abstract

Endogenous carbon monoxide (CO) exerts anti-inflammatory effects. Tristetraprolin (TTP) is known to destabilize pro-inflammatory transcripts. Here we found that exogenous CO enhanced the decay of *TNF-α* mRNA and suppressed TNF-α expression in LPS-activated macrophages from wild-type (WT) mice. However, *TTP* deficiency abrogated the effects of exogenous CO. While CO treatment prior to DSS administration in WT mice significantly reduced inflammatory cytokine levels and colitis, it failed to reduce the pro-inflammatory cytokine levels and colitis in TTP knockout (KO) mice. Our results demonstrate that TTP is a key factor mediating the anti-inflammatory action of CO in DSS-induced colitis.

Editor: Benoit Foligne, Institut Pasteur de Lille, France

Funding: This study was supported by the Bio & Medical Technology Development Program of the National Research Foundation (NRF) funded by the Korean government (MEST) (2012M3A9C3048687). The funders had no role in study design, data collection and analysis, decision to publish, or preparation of the manuscript.

Competing Interests: The authors have declared that no competing interests exist.

* E-mail: chung@ulsan.ac.kr (HTC); jwpark@ulsan.ac.kr (JWP)

Introduction

Endogenous CO is one of the three products of heme degradation created by heme oxygenase-1 (HO-1), the other two being Fe^{2+} and biliverdin [1]. These byproducts have recently been shown to have strong cytoprotective effects. This is thought to result from their anti-inflammatory, anti-apoptotic, and anti-oxidant actions [2]. Interestingly, recent studies have shown that the exogenous application of CO or CO-releasing molecules (CO-RMs) can also confer protective effects in models of inflammatory stress or tissue injury [3]. In intestinal inflammation, exogenous CO reduces the severity of disease activity [4,5]. Recently, CO-RMs have been used in biological systems to deliver CO in a controlled manner, while keeping carbon monoxy hemoglobin levels stable [6]. CO-RM-derived CO has been shown to inhibit various inflammatory states [7]. In particular, CO-RM ameliorates DSS-induced colitis by inhibition of neutrophil infiltration and TNF-α production [8]. Hence, CO might be a novel and important molecule in the treatment of intestinal inflammation.

Inflammatory bowel diseases (IBD) are inflammatory disorders related to a dysfunction in the innate responses to bacterial products. Multiple genetic defects have been linked to immune dysfunction [9], but the precise pathogenesis of IBD remains unclear. Various models of experimental IBD have been developed to investigate the pathogenesis. The administration of dextran sulfate sodium (DSS) induces a reversible form of colitis in mice [10]. This model is characterized by acute tissue inflammation in the colon and mimics the pathology of human ulcerative colitis. In this colitis model, expression of pro-inflammatory cytokines is upregulated [11]. Since immuno-compromised mice lacking the T and B cell compartments remain susceptible in this model [12], macrophages and dendritic cells (DCs) are proposed to play a central role in the pathogenesis of DSS-induced colitis. Macrophages and intestinal DCs are the first antigen presenting cells (APCs) to sense and respond to exogenous antigens or tissue injury [13] and to activate T cells and induce T cell proliferation in DSS-induced colitis [14].

The inflammatory response has been reported to be modulated by post-transcriptional control [15]. The post-transcriptional control of inflammatory transcripts is strongly dependent on AU-rich element (ARE)-mediated mechanisms [16]. The destabilizing function of AREs is believed to be regulated by ARE-binding proteins [17]. Tristetraprolin (TTP) is an ARE-binding protein that promotes degradation of a number of inflammatory mediators [18–20]. TTP-knockout mice develop severe inflammatory arthritis, autoimmune dysfunction, and myeloid hyperplasia, demonstrating the importance of TTP in limiting the inflammatory response [21].

Here we describe a so far unanticipated role of TTP in the anti-inflammatory function of CO in DSS-induced colitis. We found that TTP deficiency exacerbates disease severity and blocks the anti-inflammatory activity of CO in DSS-induced colitis. We provide evidence that CO induces the expression of TTP, and in turn, TTP plays an important role in the CO-induced anti-inflammatory effect through destabilization of *TNF-α* transcripts.

Methods

Cells

Peripheral macrophages were isolated from wild-type (WT) and TTP knockout (KO) mice according to previously described methods [22]. Peritoneal macrophages and murine monocyte macrophage cells (RAW264.7) were cultured in DMEM supplemented with 10% FBS. Cells were exposed for 4 h to LPS (1 μg/ml, L-2654, Sigma, USA) in the presence or absence of tricarbonyldichlororuthenium (II) dimer (CORM-2; Sigma, USA) (5, 10, 20, and 50 μM), and TTP and TNF-α levels were determined at the end of the incubation. Inactive CORM-2 (iCORM-2) was used as a negative control [23] to assess whether the effects observed were due to the CO liberated by the CORM-2 or were caused by other components of the molecules.

Mice and Ethics Statement

TTP knockout (KO) mice were kindly provided by Dr. Perry J Blackshear (Laboratory of Signal Transduction, National Institute of Environmental Health Sciences, USA). Mice were bred in the animal facility at the University of Ulsan and were born and housed in the same room under specific pathogen-free conditions. In all experiments, sex- and age-matched littermates were used as controls. All mice were handled in accordance with the guidelines of the Institutional Animal Care and Use Committee (IACUC) of the Immunomodulation Research Center (IRC), University of Ulsan. All animal procedures were approved by IACUC of IRC (Permit Number: UOU-2012-005). All surgery was performed under sodium pentobarbital anesthesia, and all efforts were made to minimize suffering.

Dextran Sulfate Sodium (DSS)-mediated Colitis

Acute colitis was induced with 2% (w/v) dextran sulfate sodium (DSS) (36–50 kDa, MP Biomedicals) dissolved in drinking water for 7 days followed by normal drinking water until the end of the experiment. The DSS solutions were made fresh every day.

CO Inhalation Treatment

After treatment with DSS for 7 days, mice were exposed to CO at a concentration of 250 ppm in an exposure chamber (LB Science, Daejeon, Korea) at room temperature for 3 h a day for 5 days. A CO analyzer (Tongoy Control Technology, Beijing, China) was used to continuously measure the CO levels in the cage in order to maintain the CO concentration at 250 ppm. The animals were divided into three groups: a sham group, a DSS-induced colitis group, and a DSS-induced colitis group treated with CO inhalation.

Evaluation of Colitis Severity

The clinical activity score was determined daily by scoring changes in animal weight, occult blood positivity, gross bleeding, and stool consistency. We used five grades of weight loss (0, no loss or weight gain; 1, 1–5% loss; 2, 5–10% loss; 3, 10–20% loss; 4, > 20% loss), three grades of stool consistency (0, normal; 2, loose; and 4, diarrhea), and three grades of occult blood (0, negative; 2, occult blood-positive; and 4, gross bleeding). These scores were added to generate a clinical activity score ranging from 0 to 12.

After determining the clinical activity score, mice were sacrificed, the entire colon was removed from the cecum to the anus, and the colon length was measured as an indirect marker of inflammation. The distal colon was fixed in 10% buffered formalin for histological analysis. Sections 5 μm thick were prepared and stained with hematoxylin and eosin (H&E).

Determination of TNF-α Levels

The concentration of TNF-α in the supernatant of cultured cells or mucosal homogenates was analyzed using DuoSet ELISA Development Systems (R&D Systems, Minneapolis, MN, USA).

Plasmids, Transfections and Luciferase Assay

The genomic sequence of the mouse *TTP* gene (GenBank accession number NT_187034) was used to engineer PCR cloning primers: 5′-GAGCTCTTCTATCTTTCTGTAACCCAC-3′, 5′-CTCGAGTGGCAGAGAGATCCATGGTGG-3′. Underlined letters are restriction enzyme sites. A 1309-base pair (bp) genomic fragment containing the 5′-flanking region of the *TTP* gene was isolated by PCR amplification from mouse genomic DNA. Construct pGL3/mTTP p-1309 contains the -1309 bp promoter region of the mouse TTP gene up to nucleotide +48 base pair (*i.e.*, downstream from the mouse TTP mRNA cap site) inserted into the *Sac*I and *Xho*I sites of the pGL3 basic vector (Promega). A pRL-SV40 *Renilla* luciferase construct was purchased from Promega (E2231).

RAW264.7 cells were transfected with luciferase reporter constructs using the Neon^{TM} transfection system (Invitrogen). Lysates of the transfected cells were mixed with luciferase assay reagent (Promega), and the chemiluminescent signal was measured in a Wallac Victor 1420 Multilabel Counter (EG&G Wallac, Turku, Finland). Firefly luciferase of pGL3/mTTP p-1309 was normalized to *Renilla* luciferase of pRL-SV40 in each sample.

Actinomycin D-based RNA Kinetic Analysis

Peritoneal macrophages were exposed to 10 μM CORM-2 (Sigma) and 1 μg/ml LPS (Sigma) for 20 min. After incubation for 24 h, cells were incubated with 5 μg/ml actinomycin D (Sigma) to stop transcription, and cells were collected at 0, 15, 30, 45, and 60 min after addition of actinomycin D and analyzed for *TNF-α* mRNA by quantitative RT-PCR.

Quantitative Real-time PCR and Semi-qRT-PCR

Total RNAs were extracted from cells and colon of WT and TTP KO mice using the RNeasy Mini Kit (Qiagen). For RNA kinetic analysis, 3 μg of DNase I-treated total RNA was reverse transcribed using oligo-dT and Superscript II reverse transcriptase (Invitrogen) according to the manufacturer's instructions. qRT-PCR was performed by monitoring the increase in fluorescence in real-time of the SYBR Green dye (QIAGEN, Hilden, Germany) using StepOnePlus^{TM} Real-time PCR systems (Applied Biosystems). Semi-qRT-PCR was performed using Taq polymerase (Solgent, Daejeon, Korea) and PCR primer pairs:

GAPDH, 5′-ATGACAACTTTGGCATTGTG-3′ and 5′-CATACTTGGCAGGTTTCTCC-3′; 18S rRNA, 5′-CAGTGAAACTGCGAATGGCT-3′ and 5′-TGCCTTCCTTGGATGTGGTA-3′; KC (CXCL1), 5′-TTGTGCGAAAAGAAGTGCAG-3′ and 5′-TACAAACACAGCCTCCCACA-3′; IL-6, 5′-ACAAGTCGGAGGCTTAATTACACAT-3′ and 5′-TTGCCATTGCACAACTCTTTTC-3′; TNF-α, 5′-AGGCTGCCCCGACTACGT-3′ and 5′-GACTTTCTCCTGGTATGAGATAGCAAA-3′; MIP-2 (CXCL2), 5′-CACTCTCAAGGGCGGTCAAA-3′ and 5′-TACGATCCAGGCTTCCCGGGT-3′.

Myeloperoxidase (MPO) Assay

The MPO enzyme activity in colonic tissues was analyzed using Mouse Myeloperoxidase DuoSet (R&D Systems, Minneapolis, MN).

Statistical Analysis

For statistical comparisons, p-values were determined using Student's t test.

Results

CO Induces *TTP* mRNA in Macrophages

CO has been reported to suppress the production of inflammatory cytokines [7]. However, the molecular basis by which CO mediates such anti-inflammatory functions is unknown. TTP enhances degradation of various inflammatory cytokines [18–20]. This prompted us to evaluate the functional link between CO and TTP in macrophages, with the hypothesis that CO increases the expression of TTP, which in turn mediates the anti-inflammatory activity of CO by enhancing the degradation of mRNAs of inflammatory cytokine genes. To test this hypothesis, we initially determined the effect of CORM-2 on the expression level of TTP in macrophages. CORM-2 treatment significantly increased TTP transcripts in a dose-dependent manner (Fig. 1A). This effect appeared to be strictly dependent on the CO released by CORM-2, since iCORM-2, which does not liberate CO, did not have any effect on TTP level (Fig. 1A).

The experiments above indicate that CORM-2 is able to induce *TTP* transcription. We next tested whether CORM-2 was able to transactivate the *TTP* promoter in a reporter assay. RAW264.7 cells were transiently transfected with pGL3/mTTP p-1309 construct containing the $-1261 \sim +48$ promoter region of the mouse TTP gene followed by treatment with CORM-2. CORM-2 treatment significantly stimulated the *TTP* promoter at 4 h after the treatment in a dose-dependent manner (Fig. 1B). These data indicate that CORM-2 enhances the *TTP* promoter and thus increases TTP transcript level.

TTP Deficiency Abrogates the Anti-inflammatory Effect of CORM-2 in Macrophages

Our next goal was to determine whether TTP deficiency affects the anti-inflammatory effect of CORM-2 in macrophages. To test this, we treated peritoneal macrophages from wild-type and TTP KO mice with LPS in the presence or absence of CORM-2 and analyzed TNF-α expression by ELISA and RT-PCR. LPS treatment caused a significant increase in TNF-α in macrophages from both wild-type and TTP KO mice (Figs. 2A and 2B). However, although CORM-2 significantly inhibited the production of TNF-α induced by LPS in macrophages from wild-type mice, deficiency of TTP blocked the inhibitory effect of CORM-2 on LPS-induced production of TNF-α (Figs. 2A and 2B). These results suggest that TTP deficiency suppresses the anti-inflammatory effect of CORM-2 in macrophages.

We next determined whether CORM-2 could decrease the stability of *TNF-α* mRNA induced by LPS in macrophages. In macrophages from wild-type mice, CORM-2 treatment significantly decreased the stability of *TNF-α* mRNA (Fig. 2C), indicating that the inhibitory effect of CORM-2 on the TNF-α production in macrophages results from enhancing the decay of *TNF-α* mRNA. To determine whether TTP deficiency affects the CORM-2-induced destabilization of *TNF-α* in macrophages, macrophages from TTP KO mice were treated with LPS in the presence or absence of CORM-2. In contrast to the macrophages from wild-type mice, CORM-2 treatment did not decrease the half-life of *TNF-α* mRNA in macrophages from TTP KO mice (Fig. 2C), suggesting that TTP deficiency blocks the CORM-2-induced destabilization of *TNF-α* mRNA.

TTP Knockout Increases Susceptibility of Mice to DSS-induced Colitis

Administration of DSS increases the levels of pro-inflammatory cytokines [11]. Thus, it is possible to predict that TTP deficiency exacerbate DSS-induced colitis. To test this hypothesis, we assessed the effect of TTP knockout on intestinal inflammation in a DSS-induced colitis model. During the course of DSS treatment, TTP KO mice displayed a higher clinical score determined at day 12 after treatment (Fig. 3A). Colon shortening, a macroscopic parameter of colitis severity, was more pronounced in DSS-treated TTP KO mice than in DSS-treated WT mice (colon length, 3.50±0.13 cm vs. 4.07±0.13 cm; Figs. 3B and 3C). No significant difference was observed in the colon length between untreated WT and TTP KO mice. In addition, histological study showed that DSS treatment resulted in greater loss of epithelial crypts and massive infiltration of inflammatory cells into the mucosa in TTP KO mice than in WT mice (Fig. 3D). The activity of myeloperoxidase (MPO), a marker for neutrophil infiltration, in the colon of DSS-treated TTP KO mice was also increased compared with that in DSS-treated WT mice (Fig. 3E). Next, we determined the effects of TTP deficiency on the DSS-induced production of inflammatory cytokines. It has been reported that DSS can develop colitis in the absence of TNF-α [24]. Thus, we analyzed the levels of pro-inflammatory cytokines including IL-6, CXCL1, and CXCL2 as well as TNF-α. As shown in Fig. 3F, TTP

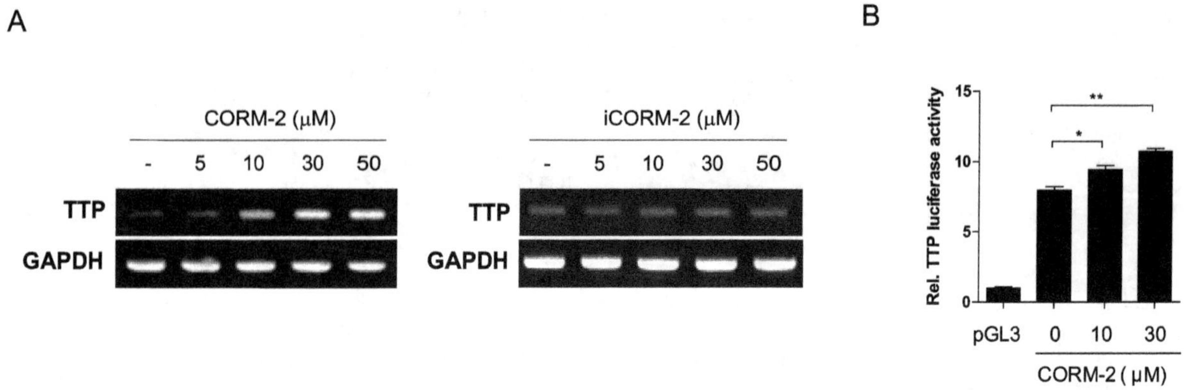

Figure 1. CORM-2 induces TTP promoter activity and *TTP* mRNA in macrophages. A. RAW264.7 cells were incubated with different concentration of CORM-2 or iCORM-2 for 4 h. *TTP* mRNA expression was determined by semi-quantitative RT-PCR. B. RAW264.7 cells were transfected with pGL3/mTTP P-1309 containing the mouse *TTP* promoter. After 24 h, cells were treated with different concentrations of CORM-2 for 4 h, and luciferase activity was determined. The level of firefly luciferase activity was normalized using *Renilla* luciferase activity. The relative luciferase activity is presented as a fold increase over untreated cells. Values are mean ± SD (n = 3). *, $p<0.05$; **, $p<0.01$.

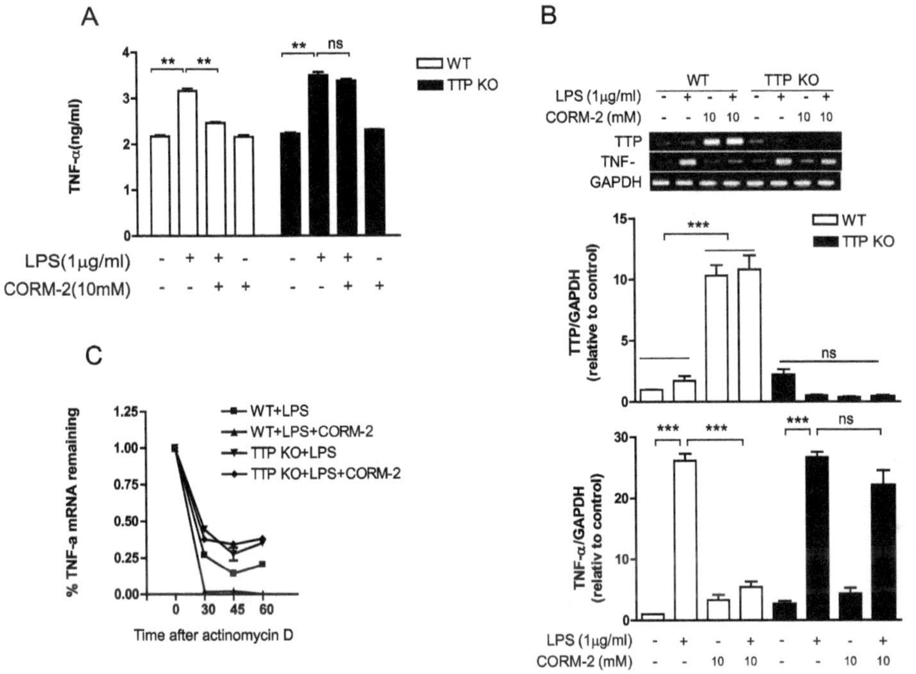

Figure 2. TTP deficiency blocks the anti-inflammatory function of CORM-2 in macrophages. Peritoneal macrophages were harvested from WT and TTP KO mice. Cells were treated with 1 μg/ml LPS in the presence of 10 μM CORM-2 for 4 h. A. TNF-α in the supernatant of cells was determined by ELISA. Data shown are mean ± SD (n = 3). **, $p<0.01$. B. The expression levels of *TTP* and *TNF-α* mRNA were determined by semi-quantitative RT-PCR. C. Expression of *TNF* mRNA in macrophages was determined by quantitative real-time PCR at indicated times after the addition of 5 μg/ml actinomycin D. Values are mean ± SD (n = 3). ***, $p<0.001$. The band densities in the agarose gel were quantified by PhosphorImager, normalized to the internal control GAPDH and expressed as percentage (%) of the value of untreated control cells. Data shown are mean ± SD (n = 3). ***, p<0.005. ns, not significant.

KO mice showed a marked increase in DSS-induced production of TNF-α, IL-6, CXCL1, and CXCL2 in colon tissues. Overall, these results demonstrate that TTP deficiency aggravates inflammation in a mouse model of colitis.

TTP is Required for the CO-mediated Protection Against DSS-induced Colitis

Based on our findings that CORM-2 increases TTP levels, and in turn, TTP mediates the anti-inflammatory effect of CORM-2 in macrophages and TTP deficiency exacerbates DSS-induced colitis, we hypothesized that exogenous CO and CO-RM may protect mice from DSS-induced colitis through a TTP–dependent mechanism. To assess whether TTP is required for the anti-inflammatory effects of exogenous CO in DSS-induced colitis, we administered 2% DSS to wild-type mice and TTP KO mice with or without exposure to exogenous CO. CO inhalation treatment significantly decreased the levels of inflammatory cytokines (TNF-α and IL-6) and chemokines (CXCL1 and CXCL2) induced by DSS in wild-type mice (Fig. 3F). However, in TTP KO mice, the inhibitory effect of CO on the production of inflammatory cytokines and chemokines was blocked (Fig. 3F). In addition, CO decreased the susceptibility of wild-type mice to DSS-induced colitis as determined by clinical score (Fig. 3A), colon length (Figs. 3B and 3C), and neutrophil infiltration (Figs. 3D and 3E). However, in TTP KO mice, CO treatment did not change the severity of DSS-induced colitis in TTP KO mice (Figs. 3A–F). Collectively, our data suggest that TTP is required for the anti-inflammatory effect of CO in the DSS-induced colitis model.

Discussion

The administration of CO or CO-RMs can inhibit the production of inflammatory cytokines and protect animals against inflammatory diseases [3]. However, the basic mechanisms underlying the anti-inflammatory function of CO are not clear. In this study, we provide evidence that CO exerts its inhibitory effects through induction of TTP expression in macrophages; CORM-2 increases the *TTP* promoter activity and the expression of TTP, decreases the stability of *TNF-α* mRNA induced by LPS in a TTP-dependent manner, and CO decreases the levels of *TNF-α*, *IL-6*, *CXCL1*, and *CXCL2* induced by LPS, while TTP deficiency blocks the anti-inflammatory effect of CO. These results indicate that TTP induced by CO-RM mediates the anti-inflammatory function of CO-RM in macrophages. Here we did not analyze the mechanisms for the CO-RM-induced expression of TTP. It has been reported that CO activates STAT3 [25] and STAT3 binds to TTP promoter region and induces TTP expression in macrophages [26]. Thus, it is possible to predict that the CO/STAT3 pathway enhances the *TTP* promoter activity and increases *TTP* expression. Further studies are required to elucidate the mechanisms involved in the induction of *TTP* by CO-RM.

The expression of inflammatory cytokines is associated with the development of intestinal inflammation in both animal models of colitis [27] and human IBD [28]. In the DSS-induced colitis model, expression of pro-inflammatory cytokines and chemokines is upregulated [11]. The mRNAs of these inflammatory cytokines contain AREs within their 3′UTR, and their expression can be down-regulated by TTP [18–20]. Thus, mice lacking the *TTP* gene may lose their ability to down-regulate the production of

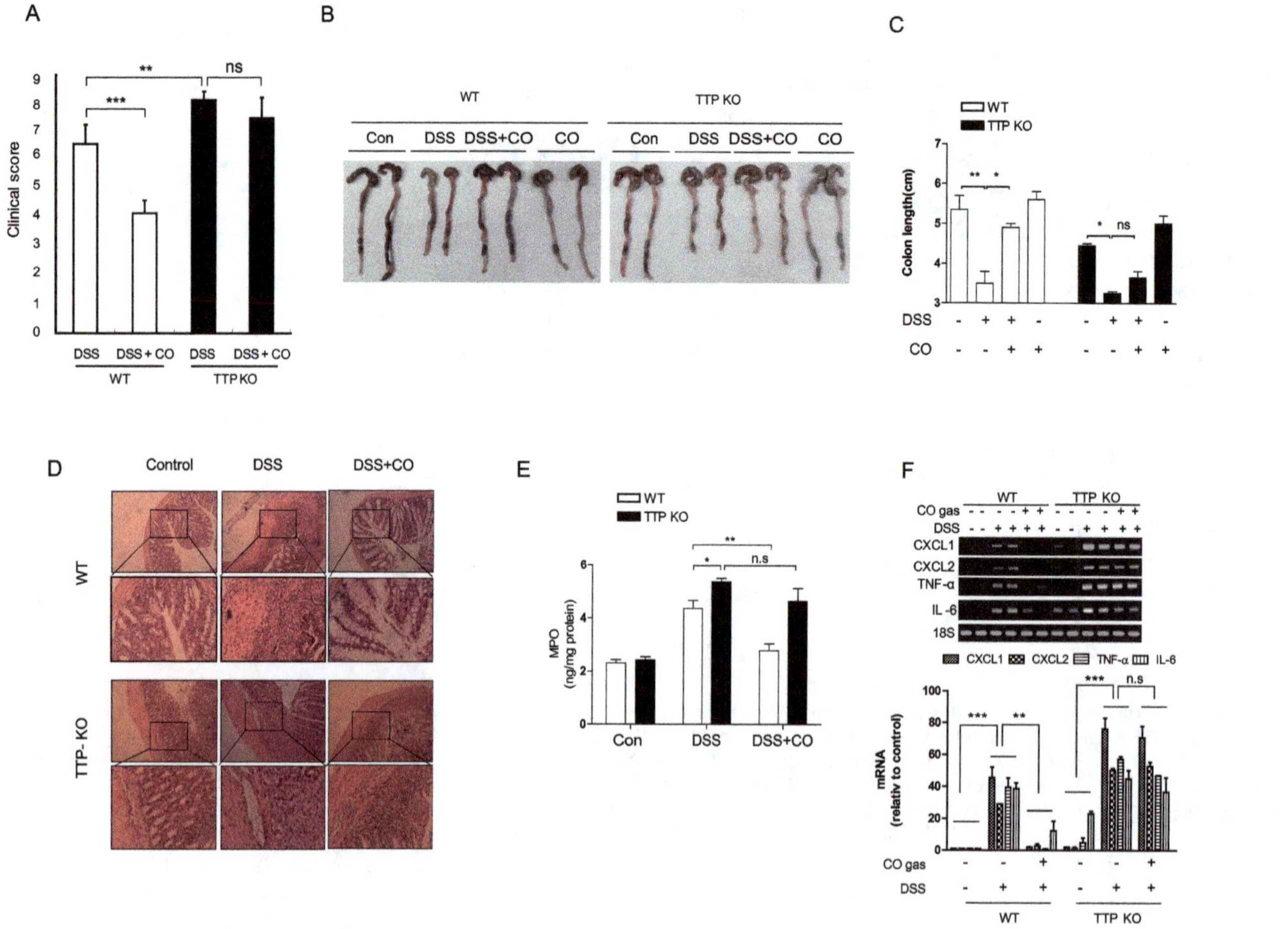

Figure 3. TTP deficiency blocks the anti-inflammatory function of CO in DSS-induced colitis. After treatment with 2% (w/v) DSS for 7 days, WT and TTP KO mice were exposed to CO at a concentration of 250 ppm for 5 days and analyzed for colitis. A. Clinical scores were assessed as described in Materials and Methods. Data are mean ± SD for 5 mice (**, $p<0.01$; ***, $p<0.005$). ns, not significant. B and C. Colon length. B. Representative images of 5 tests conducted in each group. C. Data are mean ± SD for 5 mice (*, $p<0.05$; **, $p<0.01$). D. Representative H&E sections of each group from colons of WT and TTP KO mice. E. Neutrophil infiltration into the colon, quantified by measuring MPO activity. Data are mean ± SD for 5 mice (*, $p<0.05$; **, $p<0.01$). F. Colonic cytokine/chemokine mRNA levels, analyzed by semi-quantitative RT-PCR. Data represent 1 of 3 independent experiments with similar results. The band densities in the agarose gel were quantified by PhosphorImager, normalized to the internal control GAPDH and expressed as percentage (%) of the value of untreated control cells. Data shown are mean ± SD (n = 3). **, $p<0.01$; ***, $p<0.005$. ns, not significant.

inflammatory cytokines in response to tissue damage in the colon, resulting in exacerbated colitis. Consistently, we found that the TTP KO mice treated with DSS displayed increased susceptibility to colitis, decreased colon length, and increased neutrophil infiltration and expression of pro-inflammatory cytokines such as *TNF-α*, *IL-6*, *CXCL1*, and *CXCL2* in the large intestinal mucosa. Considering the facts that these inflammatory cytokines are described for both animal models of colitis [27] and human IBD [28], it is possible to predict that decreased level and/or activity of TTP in ulcerative colitis patients may lead to a defect in resolution of intestinal inflammation and exacerbated IBD symptoms.

It has been reported that CO-RM can protect against DSS-induced colitis [8]. The exacerbated colitis in TTP KO mice led us to test whether CO-RM can ameliorate DSS-induced colitis in TTP KO mice as well. Consistent with a previous report [8], we observed that, in wild-type mice, CO ameliorated DSS-induced colitis by inhibition of neutrophil infiltration and inflammatory cytokine production. However, under conditions of CO exposure, TTP deficiency prevented the anti-inflammatory effect of CO in DSS-induced colitis. Previously it has been reported that HO-1 mediates the inhibitory effect of CO on chronic colitis [4]. Our data indicate that TTP is a key regulator of intestinal inflammatory diseases and CO-mediated anti-inflammatory function. Previously, it has been reported that TTP-knockout mice develop severe inflammatory arthritis, demonstrating the importance of TTP in limiting the inflammatory response [21].

In conclusion, our study with an intestinal inflammation models shows that CO-mediated protection operates in part by inducing TTP, which leads to the down-regulation of inflammatory cytokines and chemokines. TTP deficiency exacerbates DSS-induced colitis and abrogates the protective effect of CO against DSS-induced colitis. Taken together, these data demonstrate for the first time a dependence on TTP in the CO-induced protection against DSS-induced colitis. The finding that TTP plays important roles in protection against DSS-induced colitis makes CO-TTP pathway an attractive candidate for the treatment of ulcerative colitis.

Author Contributions

Conceived and designed the experiments: JWP HTC. Performed the experiments: YJ MJU MZ HJK YC NAY GJC. Analyzed the data: YJ GJC JWP HTC. Contributed reagents/materials/analysis tools: GJC. Wrote the paper: JWP.

References

1. Maines MD (1997) The heme oxygenase system: a regulator of second messenger gases. Annu Rev Pharmacol Toxicol 37: 517–554.
2. Morse D, Choi AM (2005) Heme oxygenase-1: from bench to bedside. Am J Respir Crit Care Med 172: 660–670.
3. Motterlini R, Otterbein LE (2010) The therapeutic potential of carbon monoxide. Nat Rev Drug Discov 9: 728–743.
4. Hegazi RA, Rao KN, Mayle A, Sepulveda AR, Otterbein LE, et al. (2005) Carbon monoxide ameliorates chronic murine colitis through a heme oxygenase 1-dependent pathway. J Exp Med 202: 1703–1713.
5. Naito Y, Uchiyama K, Takagi T, Yoshikawa T (2012) Therapeutic potential of carbon monoxide (CO) for intestinal inflammation. Curr Med Chem 19: 70–76.
6. Motterlini R, Clark JE, Foresti R, Sarathchandra P, Mann BE, et al. (2002) Carbon monoxide-releasing molecules: characterization of biochemical and vascular activities. Circ Res 90: E17–24.
7. Cepinskas G, Katada K, Bihari A, Potter RF (2008) Carbon monoxide liberated from carbon monoxide-releasing molecule CORM-2 attenuates inflammation in the liver of septic mice. Am J Physiol Gastrointest Liver Physiol 294: G184–191.
8. Takagi T, Naito Y, Uchiyama K, Suzuki T, Hirata I, et al. (2011) Carbon monoxide liberated from carbon monoxide-releasing molecule exerts an anti-inflammatory effect on dextran sulfate sodium-induced colitis in mice. Dig Dis Sci 56: 1663–1671.
9. Xavier RJ, Podolsky DK (2007) Unravelling the pathogenesis of inflammatory bowel disease. Nature 448: 427–434.
10. Okayasu I, Hatakeyama S, Yamada M, Ohkusa T, Inagaki Y, et al. (1990) A novel method in the induction of reliable experimental acute and chronic ulcerative colitis in mice. Gastroenterology 98: 694–702.
11. Yan Y, Kolachala V, Dalmasso G, Nguyen H, Laroui H, et al. (2009) Temporal and spatial analysis of clinical and molecular parameters in dextran sodium sulfate induced colitis. PLoS One 4: e6073.
12. Dieleman LA, Ridwan BU, Tennyson GS, Beagley KW, Bucy RP, et al. (1994) Dextran sulfate sodium-induced colitis occurs in severe combined immunodeficient mice. Gastroenterology 107: 1643–1652.
13. Kelsall B (2008) Recent progress in understanding the phenotype and function of intestinal dendritic cells and macrophages. Mucosal Immunol 1: 460–469.
14. Shintani N, Nakajima T, Sugiura M, Murakami K, Nakamura N, et al. (1997) Proliferative effect of dextran sulfate sodium (DSS)-pulsed macrophages on T cells from mice with DSS-induced colitis and inhibition of effect by IgG. Scand J Immunol 46: 581–586.
15. Stoecklin G, Anderson P (2006) Posttranscriptional mechanisms regulating the inflammatory response. Adv Immunol 89: 1–37.
16. Khabar KS (2005) The AU-rich transcriptome: more than interferons and cytokines, and its role in disease. J Interferon Cytokine Res 25: 1–10.
17. Shyu AB, Wilkinson MF (2000) The double lives of shuttling mRNA binding proteins. Cell 102: 135–138.
18. Carballo E, Lai WS, Blackshear PJ (1998) Feedback inhibition of macrophage tumor necrosis factor-alpha production by tristetraprolin. Science 281: 1001–1005.
19. Kratochvill F, Machacek C, Vogl C, Ebner F, Sedlyarov V, et al. (2011) Tristetraprolin-driven regulatory circuit controls quality and timing of mRNA decay in inflammation. Mol Syst Biol 7: 560.
20. Molle C, Zhang T, Ysebrant de Lendonck L, Gueydan C, Andrianne M, et al. (2013) Tristetraprolin regulation of interleukin 23 mRNA stability prevents a spontaneous inflammatory disease. J Exp Med 210: 1675–1684.
21. Taylor GA, Carballo E, Lee DM, Lai WS, Thompson MJ, et al. (1996) A pathogenetic role for TNF alpha in the syndrome of cachexia, arthritis, and autoimmunity resulting from tristetraprolin (TTP) deficiency. Immunity 4: 445–454.
22. Kumagai K, Itoh K, Hinuma S, Tada M (1979) Pretreatment of plastic Petri dishes with fetal calf serum. A simple method for macrophage isolation. J Immunol Methods 29: 17–25.
23. Sawle P, Foresti R, Mann BE, Johnson TR, Green CJ, et al. (2005) Carbon monoxide-releasing molecules (CO-RMs) attenuate the inflammatory response elicited by lipopolysaccharide in RAW264.7 murine macrophages. Br J Pharmacol 145: 800–810.
24. Naito Y, Takagi T, Handa O, Ishikawa T, Nakagawa S, et al. (2003) Enhanced intestinal inflammation induced by dextran sulfate sodium in tumor necrosis factor-alpha deficient mice. J Gastroenterol Hepatol 18: 560–569.
25. Zhang X, Shan P, Alam J, Fu XY, Lee PJ (2005) Carbon monoxide differentially modulates STAT1 and STAT3 and inhibits apoptosis via a phosphatidylinositol 3-kinase/Akt and p38 kinase-dependent STAT3 pathway during anoxia-reoxygenation injury. J Biol Chem 280: 8714–8721.
26. Joe Y, Kim HJ, Kim S, Chung J, Ko MS, et al. (2011) Tristetraprolin mediates anti-inflammatory effects of nicotine in lipopolysaccharide-stimulated macrophages. J Biol Chem 286: 24735–24742.
27. Garside P (1999) Cytokines in experimental colitis. Clin Exp Immunol 118: 337–339.
28. Autschbach F, Giese T, Gassler N, Sido B, Heuschen G, et al. (2002) Cytokine/chemokine messenger-RNA expression profiles in ulcerative colitis and Crohn's disease. Virchows Arch 441: 500–513.

19

Interferon-γ Induces Expression of MHC Class II on Intestinal Epithelial Cells and Protects Mice from Colitis

Christoph Thelemann[1], Remzi Onur Eren[1], Manuel Coutaz[1], Jennifer Brasseit[2], Hanifa Bouzourene[3], Muriel Rosa[1], Anais Duval[1], Christine Lavanchy[1], Vanessa Mack[1], Christoph Mueller[2], Walter Reith[4], Hans Acha-Orbea[1]*

1 Department of Biochemistry, University of Lausanne, Epalinges, Switzerland, **2** Institute of Pathology, University of Bern, Bern, Switzerland, **3** Unilabs Pathologie Suisse Romande, Epalinges, Switzerland, **4** Department of Pathology and Immunology, University of Geneva, Geneva, Switzerland

Abstract

Immune responses against intestinal microbiota contribute to the pathogenesis of inflammatory bowel diseases (IBD) and involve $CD4^+$ T cells, which are activated by major histocompatibility complex class II (MHCII) molecules on antigen-presenting cells (APCs). However, it is largely unexplored how inflammation-induced MHCII expression by intestinal epithelial cells (IEC) affects $CD4^+$ T cell-mediated immunity or tolerance induction *in vivo.* Here, we investigated how epithelial MHCII expression is induced and how a deficiency in inducible epithelial MHCII expression alters susceptibility to colitis and the outcome of colon-specific immune responses. Colitis was induced in mice that lacked inducible expression of MHCII molecules on all nonhematopoietic cells, or specifically on IECs, by continuous infection with *Helicobacter hepaticus* and administration of interleukin (IL)-10 receptor-blocking antibodies (anti-IL10R mAb). To assess the role of interferon (IFN)-γ in inducing epithelial MHCII expression, the T cell adoptive transfer model of colitis was used. Abrogation of MHCII expression by nonhematopoietic cells or IECs induces colitis associated with increased colonic frequencies of innate immune cells and expression of proinflammatory cytokines. $CD4^+$ T-helper type (Th)1 cells - but not group 3 innate lymphoid cells (ILCs) or Th17 cells - are elevated, resulting in an unfavourably altered ratio between $CD4^+$ T cells and forkhead box P3 $(FoxP3)^+$ regulatory T (Treg) cells. IFN-γ produced mainly by $CD4^+$ T cells is required to upregulate MHCII expression by IECs. These results suggest that, in addition to its proinflammatory roles, IFN-γ exerts a critical anti-inflammatory function in the intestine which protects against colitis by inducing MHCII expression on IECs. This may explain the failure of anti-IFN-γ treatment to induce remission in IBD patients, despite the association of elevated IFN-γ and IBD.

Editor: Muriel Moser, Université Libre de Bruxelles, Belgium

Funding: The project was funded by a Swiss National Science Fellowship to HAO No 310030_132492, Website: http://www.snf.ch/E/Pages/default.aspx. The funders had no role in study design, data collection and analysis, decision to publish, or preparation of the manuscript.

Competing Interests: The authors have declared that no competing interests exist.

* E-mail: hans.acha-orbea@unil.ch

Introduction

IBDs are chronic and recurring inflammatory disorders affecting the human gastrointestinal tract. There are two major clinical forms of IBD, Crohn's disease and ulcerative colitis. Progression of Crohn's disease is mainly driven by $CD4^+$ Th1 and Th17 cells, and IFN-γ is a signature cytokine of the disease [1,2].

MHCII-mediated antigen presentation is fundamental for driving $CD4^+$ T cell orchestrated immune responses. MHCII is primarily expressed on professional APCs, which induce both effector T cell activation and $FoxP3^+$ Treg cell-mediated tolerance [3]. However, under inflammatory conditions, MHCII is typically also induced on nonhematopoietic cells [4]. IECs are able to process and present gut luminal antigens as they express the MHCII antigen-presentation machinery and antigens in the context of MHCII molecules [5,6,7,8,9,10]. However, as it remains debated whether IECs are able to provide sufficient costimulation for immunogenic T cell activation [11,12,13], it is controversial whether their function as nonprofessional APCs promotes $CD4^+$ T cell-dependent tolerance or boosts immune responses *in situ.* Previous observations obtained mainly from *in vitro* or *ex vivo* studies might not reflect the more complex situation *in vivo* [14,15,16].

Cell-type-specific expression of the MHCII antigen-presentation machinery is directed by the class II transactivator (CIITA). CIITA expression is tightly regulated by the differential usage of three independent promoters, pI, pIII and pIV [4]. pI is active in myeloid cells. pIII activity is mainly restricted to lymphoid cells. Importantly for this study, pIV−/− mice display a selective abrogation of inducible MHCII expression in nonhematopoietic cells, including IECs. These mice lack positive selection of $CD4^+$ T cells due to the absence of MHCII on cortical thymic epithelial cells (cTECs) [17]. However, $CD4^+$ T cell development is restored by introducing a CIITA transgene (Tg) driven by the keratin-14 (K14) promoter: The resulting pIV−/− K14 CIITA Tg mice harbour normal repertoires of $CD4^+$ T cells and display normal levels of MHCII on professional APCs, which depend on pI and pIII, but lack inducible MHCII expression on nonhematopoietic cells [4,17,18].

To investigate the *in vivo* role of nonhematopoietic MHCII expression on the outcome of gut-specific immune responses and pathology, we administered interleukin (IL)-10 receptor-blocking antibodies (anti-IL10R mAb) to pIV−/− K14 CIITA Tg and control mice infected chronically with *H. hepaticus*. In comparison to the control mice, the absence of epithelial MHCII expression led to colitis characterised by enhanced colonic infiltration of innate effector cells and elevated expression of proinflammatory chemokines and cytokines. This resulted in increased infiltration of inflammatory $CD4^+$ Th1 cells and an increased ratio between $CD4^+$ T cells and $FoxP3^+$ Treg cells. A deficiency in IFN-γ, or its neutralization, resulted in the absence or reduced levels of epithelial MHCII expression, respectively, suggesting that mainly T cell-derived IFN-γ is required to induce epithelial MHCII expression. These findings reveal a critical role of IFN-γ-induced epithelial MHCII expression in contributing to intestinal homeostasis by exerting an anti-inflammatory effect *in vivo*, which is consistent with the failure to attenuate IBD with anti-IFN-γ treatment.

Materials and Methods

Animals

Mice were on a C57BL/6 background and were used between 6–10 weeks of age. pIV−/− K14 CIITA Tg mice were described previously [18]. C57BL/6 mice were obtained from Harlan Laboratories. Heterozygous control mice were obtained by crossing pIV−/− K14 CIITA Tg with WT C57BL/6 mice. $pIV^{fl/fl}$ vil-Cre Tg mice and $pIV^{fl/fl}$ littermates were generated by crossing Vil-Cre-ER^{T2} mice [19] and $pIV^{fl/fl}$ mice [17]. Rag1−/− IFN-γ−/− mice were obtained by crossing Rag1−/− mice [20] and IFN-γ−/− mice [21]. Mice were housed in specific-pathogen-free (SPF) facilities at the Universities of Lausanne or Bern. All experiments were approved by the institutional, Swiss federal and cantonal veterinary authorities (Permit number 1521.3), and all efforts were made to minimise suffering.

Anti-IL-10R mAb-induced Colitis Model

Experimental mice were obtained from *H. hepaticus* infected parents. Prior and during *in vivo* experiments, the intestinal flora of mice was synchronized by repeatedly exchanging feces among experimental groups. Comparable *H. hepaticus* loads in individual mice were confirmed by qPCR (details in Methods S1). Mice were treated i.p. with 0.5 mg per injection of mAb 1B1.3a (anti–IL-10R), or isotype control mAb Y13-259 (anti-p21 Ras Epitope within amino acids 62–76), in PBS on days 0, 4, 7, 11, 14, 18, 21, and 25. For *in vivo* IFN-γ neutralization, mice were treated i.p. with 400 mg per injection of mAb XMG1.2 (anti-IFN-γ), or isotype control mAb Y13-259, in PBS on days 11, 14, 18, 21, 25, and 28. Weight of mice was followed daily during treatment until day 28. Mice were sacrificed for analysis 1 wk after the last anti-IL-10R mAb injection.

$CD4^+$ T-cell Transfer Colitis Model

Colitis was induced by adoptive transfer of 2×10^5 $CD4^+$ $CD25^-$ $CD45RB^{hi}$ FACS-sorted T cells from WT or IFN-γ−/− mice into Rag1−/− or Rag1−/− IFN-γ−/− mice. Animals were sacrificed at days 21–26 post $CD4^+$ T cell transfer at the onset of severe clinical signs of colitis (diarrhoea, severe weight loss).

Colon Histopathological Analysis

Intestinal tissues of the mid-colon were immediately frozen in Tissue-Tek O.C.T. compound (Sakura). 4–5 µm cross-sections were stained with hematoxylin and eosin, and inflammation was assessed blinded by a clinical pathologist on a scale of 0–15 according to the following criteria: Presence of lymphocyte infiltration in the mucosa (0–1 score), submucosa (0–1 score) and/or muscularis propia (0–1 score), cryptitis (0–3 score), ulceration (0–3 score), crypt erosion/destruction (0–3 score). The degree of inflammation was graded semi-quantitatively from 0 to 3 as follows: 0, no evidence of inflammation; 1, mild inflammation; 2, moderate inflammation; 3, severe inflammation. Microscopic images were acquired using a DFC295 camera connected to a DMIL LED light microscope via the FireCam Software (Leica Microsystems).

Detection of Fecal Serum Albumin

Fresh feces were collected, lyophilized, and suspended in PBS. Fecal albumin levels were determined using the "Mouse albumin ELISA kit" (Bethyl Laboratories).

Cell Preparations and Purifications

Single cell suspensions from colonic epithelial and lamina propria tissue fractions were obtained using a modification of an established protocol [22]. Briefly, longitudinally-cut colon samples were washed in PBS, further cut into small pieces, and incubated twice in Hank's balanced-salt solution (HBSS) containing 5 mM EDTA and 2 mM DTT in a shaking incubator (37°C, 220 rpm) for 30 minutes to isolate cells from the intestinal epithelium. To derive lamina propria mononuclear cells, the tissue was further incubated in HBSS containing 0.1 U/mL collagenase D and 50 U/mL DNase I (both Roche) in a shaking incubator (37°C, 220 rpm) for 2–3 cycles of 30–40 minutes. After each incubation cycle, the collected fraction was sequentially filtered through a 70 µm and 40 µm cell strainer (BD Biosciences). For eventual further enrichment of lymphocytes via gradient centrifugation, derived cell fractions were resuspended in 40% Percoll (v/v) (GE Healthcare), layered on top of 80% Percoll (v/v) and centrifuged for 20 min at 1000×g at RT. Lymphocytes were recovered at the 40%/80% Percoll interphase. Single cell suspensions from lymphoid organs were obtained by mashing the organs through a 40 µm cell strainer.

Flow Cytometry

Single cell suspensions were incubated with anti-FcγRII/III (2.4G2). The following antibodies (clones) were used for surface staining: anti-CD3ε (145-2C11), anti-CD4 (RM4-5), anti-CD8 (53-6.7), anti-CD11b (M1/70), anti-CD11c (N418), anti-CD25 (PC61.5), anti-CD40 (1C10), anti-CD44 (IM7), anti-CD45.2 (104), anti-CD62L (MEL-14), anti-CD90.2 (53-2.1), anti-Ly-6C (HK1.4), anti-Sca-1 (D7), anti-EpCAM (G8.8) (all from eBioscience), anti-CD80 (16-10A1), anti-CD86 (GL-1), anti-MHCII (M5/114.15.2), anti-Ly-6G (1A8) (all from Biolegend). Dead cells were excluded by eF506 viability staining. For transcription factor staining, cells were fixed and permeabilized using the transcription factor staining kit and were stained with anti-FoxP3 (FJK-16s) (both eBioscience). Samples were measured on an LSR II flow cytometer (BD Biosciences), and analysed via the FlowJo software (Tree Star).

qPCR

Small colonic explants were shock frozen in liquid nitrogen before homogenisation using the Tissue Lyser II. RNA was isolated by the RNeasy mini kit (both Qiagen). cDNA was generated with the Superscript II reverse transcriptase kit (Life Technologies) and random nonamer primers. cDNA concentrations were adjusted and qPCR reactions were performed using the SYBR Green Master Mix (Roche) on a LightCycler 480 machine (Roche). The following primer sequences were used (from 5′ to 3′):

ccl3 forward CCAAGTCTTCTCAGCGCCAT, reverse TCCGGCTGTAGGAGAAGCAG; *ccl4* forward TCTTGCTCGTGGCTGCCT, reverse GGGAGGGTCAGAGCCCA; *ccl5* forward CCTCACCATCATCCTCACTGC, reverse TCTTCTCTGGGTTGGCACACA; *ifn-g* forward GGATGCATTCATGAGTATTG, reverse CTTTTCCGCTTCCTGAGG; *il-1b* forward CAACCAACAAGTGATATTCTCCATG, reverse GTGCCGTCTTTCATTACACAG; *il-6* forward GAGGATACCCTCCCAACAGACC, reverse AAGTGCATCATCGTTGTTCATACA; *Il-23p19* forward AGCGGGACATATGAATCTACTAAGAGA, reverse GTCCTAGTAGGGAGGTGTGAAGTTG; *t-bet* forward CAACAACCCCTTTGCCAAAG, and reverse TCCCCCAAGCAGTTGACAGT; *ror-γt* forward CCGCTGAGAGGGCTTCAC, and reverse TGCAGGAGTAGGCCACATTACA; *tbp* forward CCTTCACCAATGACTCCTATGAC, reverse CAAGTTTACAGCCAAGATTCAC; *b-actin* forward GCACAGCTTCTTTGCAGCTCCTTCG, reverse TTTGCACATGCCGGAGCCGTTG. Gene expression for each individual sample was normalised to the housekeeping genes TBP and β-actin via the qBASE PLUS software (Biogazelle).

Detection of Secreted Cytokines in Colon Explants

Longitudinally-cut specimens of the mid-colon were rinsed with PBS and cultured for 6 h in IMDM +10% FCS $+5\times10^{-5}$ M 2-ME at 37°C, 5% CO_2. Debris was removed by centrifugation. IFN-γ (BD Biosciences) and IL-17A (eBioscience) were measured by ELISA. All other molecules were detected using the Mouse cytokine 20-Plex (Life Technologies) on a Luminex xMAP analyser (Merck Millipore). Concentrations were normalized to the weight of the colon explants.

Statistical Analysis

Differences in weight gain between groups of mice were assessed by a repeated two-way analysis of variance (ANOVA), followed by a Bonferroni post-hoc test. For all other experiments, differences between groups were determined by the student's unpaired t test or, when the normality test failed, by the Mann-Whitney Rank Sum test. *P* values are indicated when considered statistically significant (*$P<0.05$, **$P<0.01$, and ***$P<0.001$).

Results

Characterisation of T cells in pIV−/− K14 CIITA Tg Mice

It was previously shown that pIV−/− K14 CIITA Tg mice are deficient in nonhematopoietic MHCII expression but harbour normal thymic and peripheral CD4$^+$ T cell populations displaying WT T cell receptor Vβ-chain repertoires [18]. Frequencies of CD4$^+$ T cells, including FoxP3$^+$ Treg cells, in colon-draining mesenteric and caudal lymph nodes, the colonic intestinal epithelium (cIE) and lamina propria (cLP) were found to be comparable between pIV−/− K14 CIITA Tg, heterozygous and WT mice (Figure S1). We also observed a normal distribution of CD4$^+$ effector, memory, naïve and FoxP3$^+$ T cell subsets in the thymus, spleen and peripheral lymph nodes (Figure S2). Finally, we examined CD4$^+$ T cell-dependent B cell responses *in vivo* in pIV−/− K14 CIITA Tg mice upon immunisation with 4-Hydroxy-3-nitrophenylacetyl-hapten-23-conjugated chicken γ-globulin (NP_{23}-CGG) or ovalbumin. Systemic antigen-specific antibody responses in pIV−/− K14 CIITA Tg mice were comparable to WT mice (Figure S3). In line, affinity maturation, assessed by detection of NP_4-specific total serum IgG in NP_{23}-CGG immunised mice, was similar to WT mice (Figure S3A). These results confirm that the phenotypes and functions of CD4$^+$ T cells, including FoxP3$^+$ Treg cells, in the colon and in primary and secondary lymphoid organs of pIV−/− K14 CIITA Tg mice are comparable to those of WT mice.

Anti-IL-10R mAb Treatment during Chronic *H. hepaticus* Infection in the Absence of Inducible Nonhematopoietic MHCII Expression Leads to Colitis

To assess susceptibility to bacterial-driven intestinal inflammation, experimental mice chronically infected since birth with *H. hepaticus* were treated with anti-IL-10R mAb. Prior and during the treatment period, we synchronized the microbiome by repeatedly exchanging feces among mice, based on the recent observation that co-housed mice adopt each others' microbial configuration in the fecal content [23,24]. In addition, the low to undetectable colonic MHCII expression in the steady state (shown below) should not influence the flora. Notably, *H. hepaticus* loads were comparable in all experimental mice before and after anti-IL10R mAb treatment (Figure S4). It is important to mention that this experimental system is different from the previously published colitis model based on induction of chronic colitis by acute *H. hepaticus* infection [25]. In contrast, in our setting, chronically infected WT mice should not develop colitis.

To evaluate whether the absence of inducible nonhematopoietic MHCII expression (shown below) alters susceptibility to bacterial-driven colitis, pIV−/− K14 CIITA Tg mice and heterozygous controls chronically infected since birth with *H. hepaticus* were treated with anti-IL-10R mAb. In contrast to MHCII-competent controls, pIV−/− K14 CIITA Tg mice gained significantly less weight (Figure 1A), displayed significantly elevated fecal serum albumin levels reflecting augmented protein-losing enteropathy (Figure 1B), and developed a mild but prominent diarrhoea that was not observed in heterozygous control mice (not shown). Histopathological examinations of colon sections revealed an exacerbated inflammation in pIV−/− K14 CIITA Tg mice (Figures 1C–D). pIV−/− K14 CIITA Tg mice exhibited a diffuse colonic mononuclear cell infiltration, whereas heterozygous controls displayed only focal infiltration (not shown).

We next used a conditional knockout system to determine whether the observed pathology is due to the lack of inducible MHCII expression on IECs. Mice in which pIV is flanked by loxP sites (pIV$^{fl/fl}$) were crossed with mice harbouring a transgene in which expression of tamoxifen-inducible Cre-recombinase is controlled by an IEC-specific villin promoter (vil-Cre Tg). In pIV$^{fl/fl}$ vil-Cre Tg mice, tamoxifen induces pIV excision exclusively in IECs. Upon the administration of tamoxifen and anti-IL-10R mAb pIV$^{fl/fl}$ vil-Cre Tg mice displayed increased colitis susceptibility (Figures S5A–C), indicating that the absence of inducible MHCII expression specifically on IECs significantly exacerbates chronic *H. hepaticus*-mediated colitis. However, we noted that tamoxifen altered the homeostatic composition of gut lymphocytes (not shown) and affected colitis in control mice. This is consistent with the fact that tamoxifen substantially affects the murine gastrointestinal tract [26,27]. Due to the adverse effects of tamoxifen we focussed on the constitutively pIV-depleted mice for further experiments.

Colitic pIV−/− K14 CIITA Tg Mice Display Increased Innate Effector Cell Infiltration and Elevated Expression of Proinflammatory Chemokines and Cytokines

We next sought to identify the major cellular and molecular players mediating exacerbated inflammation and tissue damage in colitic pIV−/− K14 CIITA Tg mice. Infiltration of Ly6G$^+$

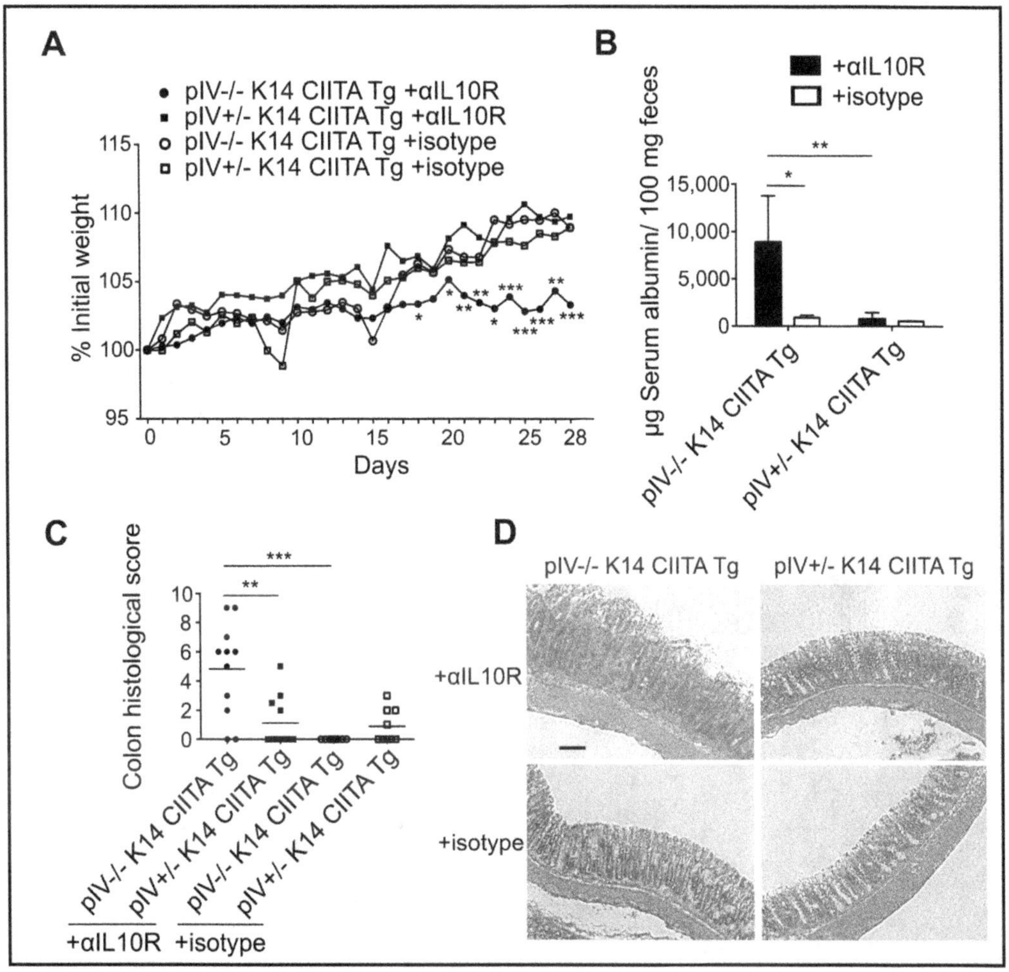

Figure 1. Chronic *H. hepaticus* infection plus anti-IL10R mAb treatment induces colitis in pIV−/− K14 CIITA Tg mice. (A) Development of body weight during anti-IL-10R mAb or isotype treatment of *H. hepaticus*-infected pIV−/− K14 CIITA Tg mice or pIV+/− K14 CIITA Tg controls (n = 9–11 per group). (B) Serum albumin concentrations in feces collected on days 26–30 (n = 6–8 per group). Data are shown as mean and s.d. and represent two pooled experiments. (C–D) Colon histopathological analysis on day 32; (C) colitis scores, data displayed as mean, and (D) representative photomicrographs of colon sections, stained with hematoxylin and eosin. Bar, 100 μm. Data represent three pooled experiments (n = 9–11 per group). αIL10R, anti-interleukin-10 receptor monoclonal antibodies;

neutrophils was increased in the colons of colitic pIV−/− K14 CIITA Tg mice, which was significant in the cIE but not the cLP (Figure 2A). CD11b$^+$ Ly6C$^+$ inflammatory monocytes were significantly elevated in both the cIE and cLP (Figure 2B). These innate effector cell subsets are also augmented in IBD patients [2]. We also noted a mild increase in CD11c$^+$ DCs in the inflamed colons (Figure S6). mRNA quantification revealed a significant elevation of mRNAs encoding the proinflammatory chemokines CCL3, CCL4 and CCL5 in the colons of colitic pIV−/− K14 CIITA Tg mice (Figure 2C). These chemokines recruit innate effector cells and T cells to sites of inflammation [28]. Moreover, mRNAs encoding the inflammatory cytokines IL-1β and IL-6 were significantly increased (Figure 2C). We also found enhanced colonic secretion of proinflammatory IL-1β, tumour necrosis factor (TNF)-α and IL-12p40, as well as CXCL9 and vascular endothelial growth factor (VEGF) in colitic pIV−/− K14 CIITA Tg mice (Figure 2D). Increased expression of IL-1β, TNF-α, IL-6 and IL-12p40 was previously observed in IBD patients [1,2]. CXCL9 secreted by innate effector cells was shown to promote T cell activation and recruitment [29]. VEGF is known to increase vascular permeability and inflammatory leukocyte extravasation in IBD and experimental colitis [30]. In summary, the cellular and molecular mediators of intestinal inflammation in colitic pIV−/− K14 CIITA Tg mice display similarities to those in IBD, underlining the physiological relevance of the applied colitis model.

Exacerbated Colitis in pIV−/− K14 CIITA Tg Mice Correlates with the Inability of IECs to Upregulate MHCII Expression

We next examined whether exacerbated colitis in pIV−/− K14 CIITA Tg mice correlates with the loss of inducible MHCII expression by IECs. IECs in anti-IL-10R-treated heterozygous control mice upregulated MHCII expression, while this was not observed in colitic pIV−/− K14 CIITA Tg mice or healthy isotype-treated controls (Figure 3). The same was true in the inducible IEC-specific MHCII knock-out system (Figure S5D). Confocal microscopy revealed that IECs from anti-IL-10R-treated heterozygous mice expressed MHCII molecules on the basolateral and apical surface (Figure S7). Since the provision of costimulation by APCs is a prerequisite for immunogenic T cell activation, we

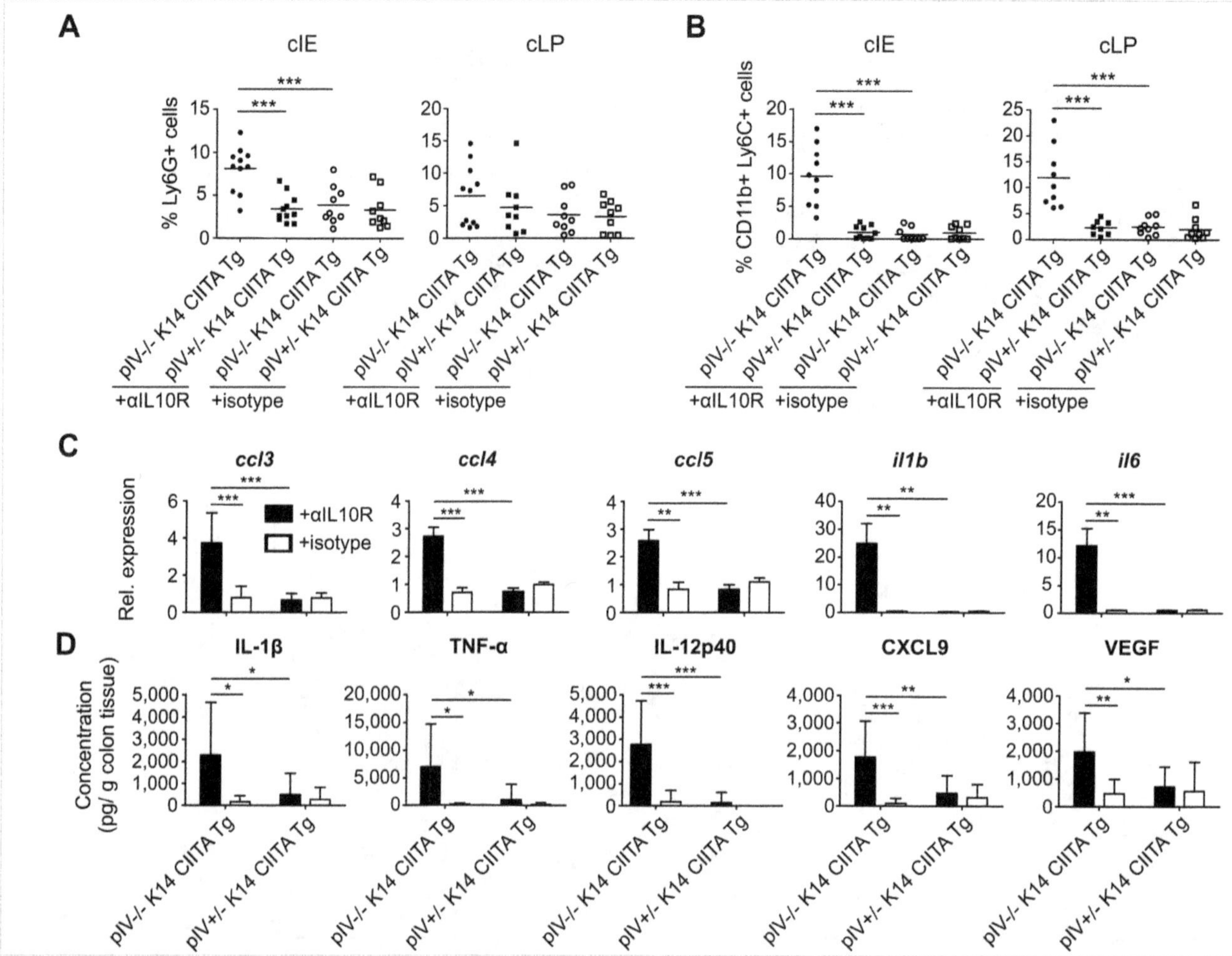

Figure 2. Innate effector cells and proinflammatory cytokines are elevated in colitic pIV−/− K14 CIITA Tg mice. (A–B) Frequency of Ly6G$^+$ neutrophil granulocytes (A) and CD11b$^+$ Ly6C$^+$ inflammatory monocytes (B) isolated from the colonic intestinal epithelium (cIE, left panel) and the colonic lamina propria (cLP, right panel) of *H. hepaticus*-infected pIV−/− K14 CIITA Tg mice or pIV+/− K14 CIITA Tg controls. (C) *ccl3, ccl4, ccl5, il1b* and *il6* mRNA expression levels in colon explants. (D) IL-1β, TNF-α, IL-12p40, CXCL9 and VEGF secretion upon *ex vivo* organ culture of colon explants. All data represent three pooled experiments ($n = 9$–11 per group). αIL10R, anti-interleukin-10 receptor monoclonal antibodies; IL, interleukin; TNF, tumor necrosis factor; VEGF, vascular endothelial growth factor;

examined whether IECs express costimulatory molecules in healthy and/or colitic mice. We did not detect induction of the classical costimulatory molecules CD40, CD80 and CD86 (Figure S8). Collectively, these results confirm that exacerbated colitis in pIV−/− K14 CIITA Tg mice correlates with the inability of IECs to express MHCII.

Colitic pIV−/− K14 CIITA Tg Mice Display Elevated Frequencies of Colonic CD4$^+$ Th1 Cells and an Increased CD4$^+$ T cell: FoxP3$^+$ Treg Cell Ratio

We next investigated the impact of deficient epithelial MHCII expression on intestinal T cells during colitis. We observed an increase in colonic CD4$^+$ but not CD8$^+$ T cells in colitic pIV−/− K14 CIITA Tg mice, which was significant in the cIE but not the cLP (Figures 4A–B). Colitic heterozygous mice only displayed a mild elevation of CD4$^+$ T cells. Similarly, CD4$^+$ T cells were significantly elevated in colitic pIV$^{fl/fl}$ vil-Cre Tg mice, which lack MHCII expression specifically on IECs (Figure S5E). Examination of T cell polarization revealed significantly augmented expression of mRNAs encoding the Th1 signature factors T-bet and IFN-γ, as well as IFN-γ secretion, in inflamed colons of pIV−/− K14 CIITA Tg mice (Figures 4C–D).

Natural cytotoxicity-triggering receptor (NCR$^-$) group 3 innate lymphoid cells (ILC) cells were recently identified as important cellular mediators of *H. hepaticus*-driven innate colitis [31,32]. However, we did neither detect a specific increase in these cells (Figure S6B) nor in the expression of *ror-γt*, *il23p19* or IL-17A, which are diagnostic for group 3 ILCs and Th17 responses (Figure S9). Thus, although we do not exclude a contribution of these cells to the inflammatory process, they are unlikely to play a dominant role in the increased pathology observed in our system.

Interestingly, we observed that colonic CD4$^+$ T cells from colitic pIV−/− K14 CIITA Tg mice displayed a mildly reduced expression of the co-inhibitory marker programmed cell death (PD)-1 when compared to heterozygous mice (not shown). We also found a significantly increased CD4$^+$ T cell: FoxP3$^+$ Treg cell ratio in the cIE of colitic pIV−/− K14 CIITA Tg mice compared to identically treated heterozygous control mice (Figure 4E). The majority of FoxP3$^+$ cells lacked neuropillin (Nrp)-1 expression in both anti-IL-10R-treated groups (not shown), suggesting that the

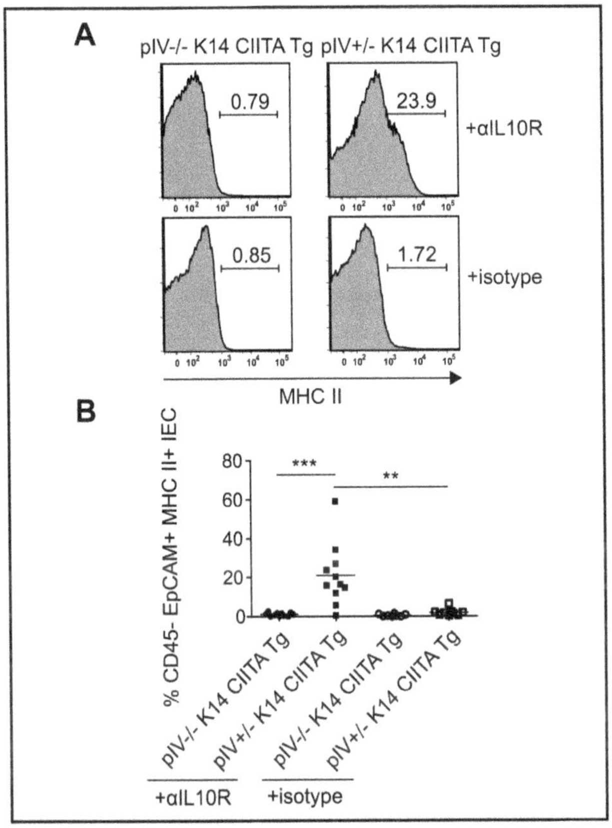

Figure 3. Colitic pIV−/− K14 CIITA Tg mice lack inducible MHCII expression by colonic IECs. (A–B) Frequency of $CD45.2^{-}$ $EpCAM^{+}$ $MHCII^{+}$ IECs isolated from anti-IL-10R mAb or isotype treated, *H. hepaticus*-infected pIV−/− K14 CIITA Tg mice or pIV+/− K14 CIITA Tg controls. Representative histograms (A) and summarized data as mean (B) from three pooled experiments ($n = 8$–11 per group). αIL10R, anti-interleukin-10 receptor monoclonal antibodies; IEC, intestinal epithelial cell;

majority of colonic Treg cells were generated peripherally [33]. Taken together, these results indicate that MHCII expression by IECs attenuates bacterial-driven colitis by preventing exacerbated effector Th1 cell accumulation and the establishment of an unfavourably altered ratio between conventional $CD4^{+}$ T cells and $FoxP3^{+}$ Treg cells.

Epithelial MHCII Expression is Induced by IFN-γ Mainly Derived from $CD4^{+}$ T cells

To examine whether IFN-γ is responsible for inducing epithelial MHCII expression we made use of the adoptive transfer colitis model in which lymphocyte-deficient mice develop colitis upon transfer of $CD4^{+}$ $CD45RB^{hi}$ T cells [34]. Transfer of WT $CD4^{+}$ T cells into Rag1−/− IFN-γ−/− mice resulted in prominent upregulation of epithelial MHCII expression, which was markedly reduced when IFN-γ−/− $CD4^{+}$ T cells were transferred into IFN-γ-competent Rag1−/− mice (Figure 5A). Notably, IECs did not upregulate MHCII expression when both donor and recipient mice lacked IFN-γ (Figure 5A). Importantly, all experimental groups developed severe colitis as assessed by histopathology (Brasseit *et al.*, manuscript in preparation). These results indicate that IFN-γ is the major cytokine driving MHCII expression on IECs during adoptive transfer colitis, and that $CD4^{+}$ T cells represent the major source of IFN-γ in this process.

To evaluate whether IFN-γ-induced epithelial MHCII expression protects against colitis we administered neutralizing anti-IFN-γ mAb to pIV+/− K14 CIITA Tg mice 11 days after initial anti-IL-10R treatment to avoid interference with T cell polarization. Neutralization of IFN-γ in anti-IL-10R-treated pIV+/− K14 CIITA Tg mice reduced MHCII expression by IECs as compared to isotype-treated mice (Figure 5B). Importantly, this resulted in elevated frequencies of $CD4^{+}$ T cells in the cIE of anti-IFN-γ mAb-treated mice, comparable to pIV−/− K14 CIITA Tg mice (Figure 5C). In addition, preliminary data indicates that the $CD4^{+}$ T cell: $FoxP3^{+}$ Treg cell ratio is mildly elevated in anti-IFN-γ-administered pIV+/− K14 CIITA Tg mice compared to isotype-treated mice (not shown). Collectively, these findings suggest that IFN-γ-mediated MHCII expression by IECs plays an anti-inflammatory role by reducing the accumulation of colitogenic $CD4^{+}$ T cells during chronic bacterial-driven colitis.

Discussion

We report here that the abrogation of inducible MHCII expression on IECs during chronic *H. hepaticus* infection and anti-IL-10R mAb treatment leads to overt colitis associated with an augmented accumulation of $CD4^{+}$ Th1 cells and an increased $CD4^{+}$ T cell:$FoxP3^{+}$ Treg cell ratio. In contrast, heterozygous control mice do not develop intestinal pathology as assessed by clinical parameters, despite the fact that they display increased MHCII expression by IECs and exhibit mildly elevated levels of infiltrating $CD4^{+}$ T cells. Finally, we show that epithelial MHCII expression is induced by IFN-γ produced mainly by $CD4^{+}$ T cells.

We also examined whether NCR^{-} group 3 ILCs - which were recently described to have a major role in murine innate colitis [31,32] - or Th17 cells might be responsible for promoting intestinal inflammation in the absence of nonhematopoietic MHCII. However, we observed comparable group 3 ILC frequencies in all anti-IL-10R mAb-administered animal groups, and no increase in associated factors ROR-γt, IL-23 and IL-17A. Thus, albeit group 3 ILCs and Th17 cells may play an important role in colitis, we exclude a decisive role in determining disease severity in our model.

Induction of MHCII on IECs correlated with a protection against colitis in heterozygous mice, indicating that the low-levels of IFN-γ observed in heterozygous mice were sufficient to maintain intestinal homeostasis via the upregulation of MHCII expression during chronic *H. hepaticus* infection and anti-IL-10R treatment. IECs are well known to fulfil diverse functions crucial for intestinal homeostasis, including the capacity to modulate intestinal immune responses [3]. Here we expand these previous findings by reporting an MHCII-dependent anti-inflammatory role of IECs that confers protection against colitis induced by chronic *H. hepaticus* colonization.

Previous studies examining potential antigen-presentation functions of IECs and their consequences for intestinal inflammation generated conflicting results and relied almost exclusively on *in vitro* or *ex vivo* assays [14,15,16]. One recent *in vivo* study using a mouse model in which MHCII is expressed solely on IECs indicated that antigen presentation by bone marrow-derived APCs is indispensable for triggering severe bacterial-driven intestinal pathology [35].

Immunogenic T cell activation requires TCR-MHCII-dependent signals, the presence of polarizing cytokines and the provision of costimulation. Whether IECs can express classical costimulatory molecules remains a matter of debate [11,12,13]. In our model we did not observe expression of the classical costimulatory molecules CD40, CD80 or CD86 on $MHCII^{+}$ IECs. Antigen-presentation in

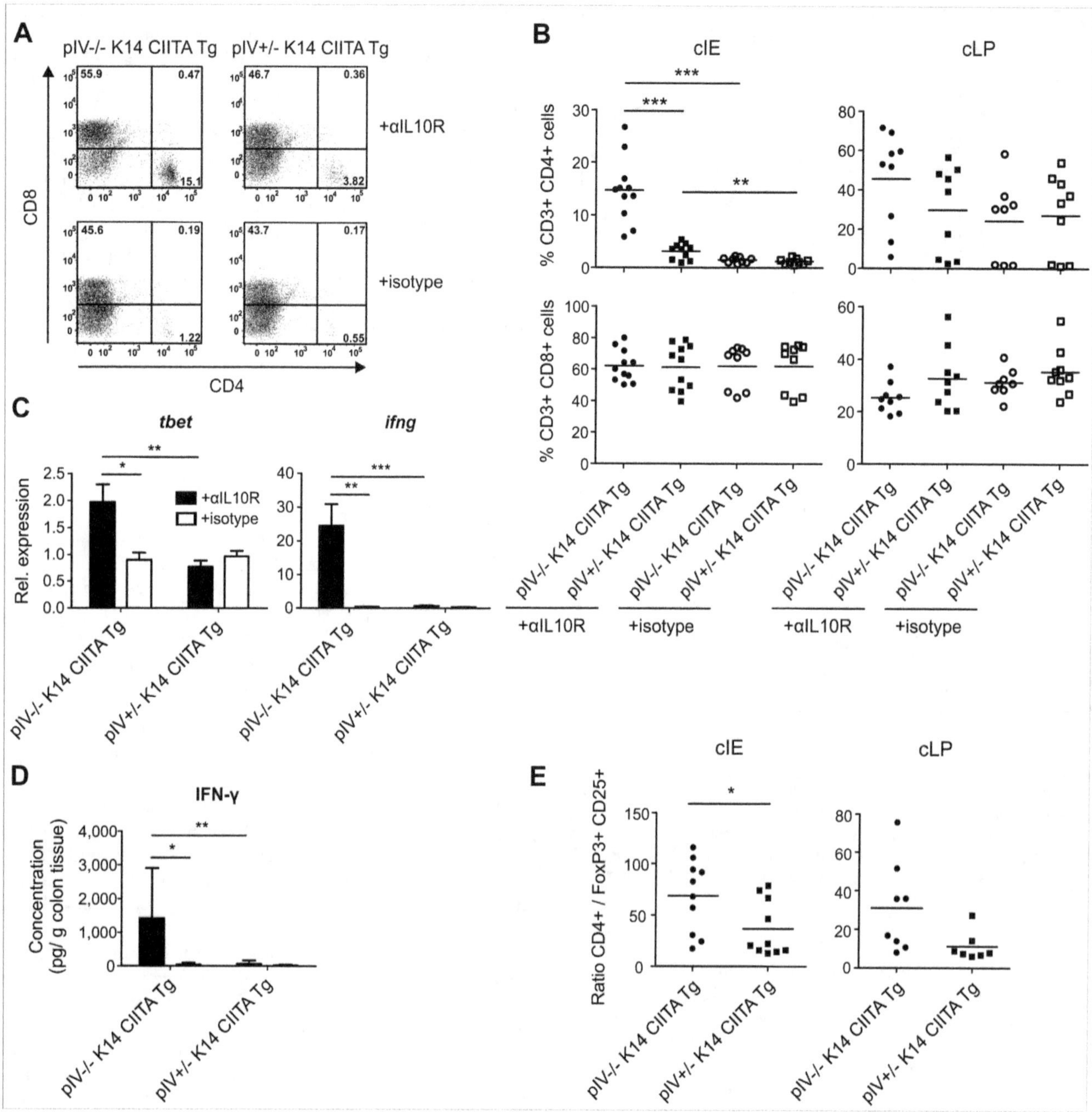

Figure 4. Colitic pIV−/− K14 CIITA Tg mice display elevated Th1 cells, IFN-γ, and CD4⁺ T cell: FoxP3⁺ Treg cell ratios. (A–B) Frequency of $CD3^+$ $CD4^+$ and $CD8^+$ T cells isolated from anti-IL-10R mAb or isotype treated, *H. hepaticus*-infected pIV−/− K14 CIITA Tg mice or pIV+/− K14 CIITA Tg controls. Representative histograms from the colonic intestinal epithelium (cIE) (A) and summarized data (B) from cIE (left) and the colonic lamina propria (cLP) (right) as mean. (C) *ifng* and *tbet* mRNA expression levels in colon explants. (D) IFN-γ secretion upon *ex vivo* organ culture of colon explants as means and s.d. (A–D) Data represent three pooled experiments ($n = 9–11$ per group). (E) Ratio of absolute numbers of $CD4^+$ T cells:absolute numbers of $CD25^+$ $FoxP3^+$ Treg cells from cIE (left) and cLP (right) as mean from two pooled experiments ($n = 7–10$ per group). αIL10R, anti-interleukin-10 receptor monoclonal antibodies; FoxP3, forkhead box P3; IFN, interferon;

the absence of costimulatory molecules has been proposed to limit $CD4^+$ T cell responses [36], which is consistent with the finding that IECs are not *bona fide* professional APCs capable of promoting severe colitis *in vivo* [35]. However, non-classical costimulatory molecules, such as IcosL, PD-L1 or LFA3 have been proposed to be used by IECs to interact with $CD4^+$ T cells [12,37].

The anti-inflammatory cytokine IL-10 is critical for maintaining local tissue homeostasis in the presence of intestinal *H. hepaticus* infection. First indications for this came from early observations in IL-10-deficient mice that developed spontaneous colitis under conventional housing conditions which was significantly less severe (or even absent) when mice were held under SPF conditions [38]. Deliberate infection of SPF-housed IL-10−/− mice with *H. hepaticus* significantly exacerbated the development of colitis [39], and susceptibility to colitis induction is re-established in WT mice, treated with anti-IL-10R mAb following *H. hepaticus* infection [25].

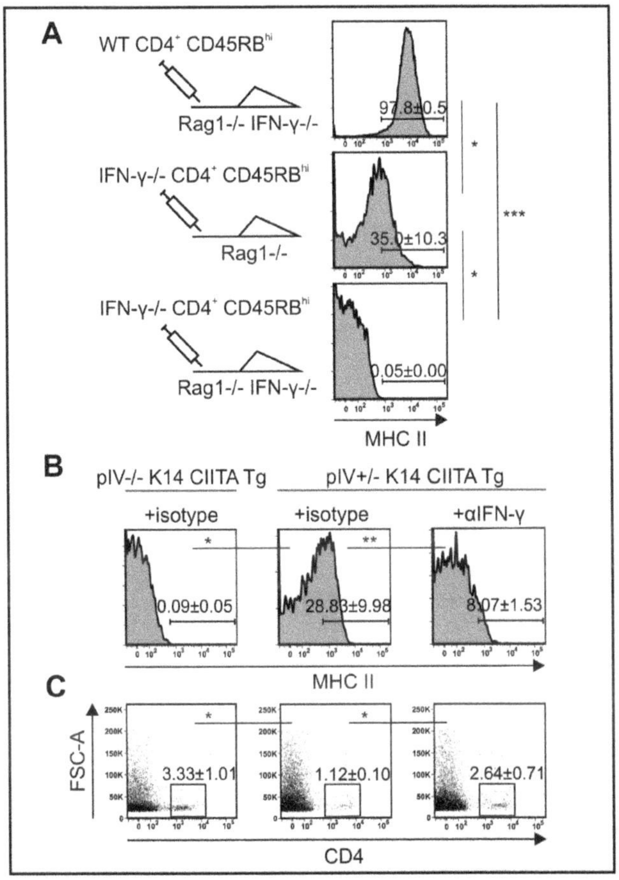

Figure 5. IFN-γ induces MHCII expression on IECs. (A) Frequency of CD45.2⁻ EpCAM⁺ MHCII⁺ intestinal epithelial cells (IEC) isolated from Rag1−/− or Rag1−/− IFN-γ−/− mice that were adoptively transferred with CD4⁺ CD45RB^hi T cells from WT or IFN-γ−/− mice shown as means and SEM in representative histograms ($n = 3$ mice per group). (B–C) Frequency of CD45.2⁻ EpCAM⁺ MHCII⁺ IECs (B) and CD4⁺ T cells from the colonic intestinal epithelium (C) isolated from *H. hepaticus*-infected, anti-IL-10R mAb-administered pIV−/− K14 CIITA Tg, pIV+/− K14 CIITA Tg or pIV+/− K14 CIITA Tg that were treated with neutralizing anti-IFN-γ mAb. Shown are representative FACS plots, means and SEM from two pooled experiments ($n = 4$–7 mice per group). αIFN-y, anti-interferon-γ monoclonal antibodies; FSC, forward scatter; IFN, interferon; Rag, recombination activating gene; WT, wild type;

Furthermore, *H. hepaticus* was shown to induce colitis in lymphocyte-deficient 129/SvEv Rag2−/− mice [32,40,41]. However, adoptive transfer of Treg cells inhibits the development of gut inflammation in this colitis model [41,42,43], which depends on the ability of transferred cells to express IL-10 [43,44]. Similarly, IL-10 is important to prevent colitis in humans, as certain variants of early-onset IBD observed in infants and small children appear to be a monogenic diseases caused by deleting mutations in IL-10 or its receptor (reviewed in [45]).

In contrast, the complex role of IFN-γ during *H. hepaticus*-induced colitis is incompletely understood. Injection of IFN-γ-neutralizing mAb into *H. hepaticus*-infected IL-10−/− mice suggested that IFN-γ is required for disease onset but not for the chronicity of colitis [39,46]. Similarly, *H. hepaticus*-infected IFN-γ−/− mice treated with anti-IL-10R mAb developed less intestinal inflammation than WT mice [25], suggesting a contribution of IFN-γ to colitis development. In contrast, the severity of *H. hepaticus*-induced colitis in mice lacking both IL-10 and IFN-γ was comparable to mice lacking IL-10 alone [46], indicating that IFN-γ does not favour colitis development. Recently, it was reported that during the course of *H. hepaticus*-mediated colitis, induced Th17 cells switch phenotype to become IFN-γ⁺ ex-Th17 cells [47]. These results imply A) the potential existence of alternative pathways affecting colitis development following acute *H. hepaticus* infection, e.g. via the increase of inflammatory Th17 cells in the absence of IFN-γ, and B) that IFN-γ may have both pro- and anti-inflammatory effects on the outcome of *H. hepaticus*-mediated colitis [25]. Our results expand these previous observations by demonstrating that IFN-γ-mediated upregulation of MHCII molecules on IECs plays an anti-inflammatory role that reduces infiltrating CD4⁺ effector T cell frequencies and avoids the establishment of a pathologically altered CD4⁺ T cell:FoxP3⁺ Treg cell ratio in the colon. Of note, IFN-γ was reported to feature anti-inflammatory properties in the context of oral tolerance [48].

Our findings may help to explain why anti-IFN-γ treatments have consistently failed to induce remission in patients with active IBD despite the association of enhanced IFN-γ expression with IBD [49]. Moreover, this study paves the way for further work on the MHCII-dependent tolerogenic function of IECs as a potential therapeutic target in patients suffering from inflammatory disorders of the intestine.

Supporting Information

Figure S1 Intestinal FoxP3⁺ Treg cell frequencies in healthy pIV−/− K14 CIITA Tg mice. (A–D) Healthy pIV−/− K14 CIITA Tg, pIV+/− K14 CIITA Tg and C57BL/6 WT mice were subjected to flow cytometry. (A) Mesenteric lymph node (mLN), (B) caudal lymph node (cLN), (C) colonic intestinal epithelium (cIE) and (D) colonic lamina propria (cLP) cells were gated on CD45.2⁺ CD4⁺ cells, and from there on FoxP3⁺ cells. Data shown represents mean and s.d. ($n = 3$ per group). FoxP3, forkhead box P3; WT, wild type;

Figure S2 Lymphoid organ T cell frequencies in healthy pIV−/− K14 CIITA Tg mice. (A–C) Thymus (THY), spleen (SPL) and pooled peripheral lymph nodes (LN) of healthy pIV−/− K14 CIITA Tg, pIV+/− K14 CIITA Tg and C57/BL6 wild type (WT) mice were subjected to flow cytometry. Dead cells were excluded and CD3⁺ cells were gated on (A) CD4 and CD8. (B) CD4⁺ CD8⁻ T cells were gated on CD44 and CD62L to identify effector (T_{eff}, CD44⁺ CD62L⁻), memory (T_{mem}, CD44⁺ CD62L⁺) and naïve T (T_{naive}, CD44⁻ CD62L⁺) cells. (C) CD4⁺ T cells were gated on CD25 and FoxP3. Data shown represents mean and s.d. ($n = 3$ per group) from one experiment out of at least two experiments.

Figure S3 Similar specific total IgG responses upon exogenous antigen immunisation in pIV−/− K14 CIITA Tg mice. (A–B) pIV−/− K14 CIITA Tg, pIV+/− K14 CIITA Tg and B6 WT mice were immunised with 4-Hydroxy-3-nitrophenylacetyl hapten-conjugated chicken gamma globulin (NP_{23}-CGG) or ovalbumin. Serum was analysed for the presence of antigen-specific total IgG against either (A) NP_4 and (B) ovalbumin. Data represent mean and s.d. ($n = 7$–8 per group) from two pooled experiments. IgG, immunoglobulin G;

Figure S4 *H. hepaticus* colonization levels before and after anti-IL-10R treatment. Fresh fecal specimens from pIV−/− K14 CIITA Tg and pIV+/− K14 CIITA Tg mice were collected on days −4 to −2 before anti-IL-10R administration, and on days 26–28 of the experiment. Total fecal DNA was isolated and *H. hepaticus* DNA was quantified by qPCR and normalized to the dry weight of the fecal pellet. Each symbol represents a single animal. αIL10R, anti-interleukin-10 receptor monoclonal antibodies;

Figure S5 *H. hepaticus* infection plus anti-IL10R mAb treatment induces exacerbated colitis in pIV$^{fl/fl}$ vil-Cre Tg mice. (A) Development of body weight during anti-IL-10R mAb or isotype treatment of *H. hepaticus*-infected, tamoxifen-administered pIV$^{fl/fl}$ vil-Cre Tg mice or pIV$^{fl/fl}$ controls. Data are shown as mean. (B) Serum albumin concentrations in feces collected on days 26–30. Data are shown as mean and s.d. (C) Colitis scores upon organ collection on day 32. Data displayed as mean. (D) Frequency of CD45.2^{-} EpCAM^{+} MHCII^{+} IECs. Representative histograms (left) and summarized data (right) as mean. (E) Frequency of CD3^{+} CD4^{+} and CD8^{+} T cells in the cIE. Representative histograms (left) and summarized data (right) as mean. All data represent $n = 3–5$ per group. αIL10R, anti-interleukin-10 receptor monoclonal antibodies;

Figure S6 Levels of colonic DC and group 3 ILCs in colitic pIV−/− K14 CIITA Tg. (A) Frequency of Ly6C^{-} CD11c^{+} conventional DCs in the cIE and cLP and (B) CD45.2^{+} Lin^{-} (CD11b, Gr-1, B220) CD3ε^{-} Thy1^{high} Sca-1^{+} group 3 ILCs in the cLP isolated from anti-IL-10R mAb or isotype treated, *H. hepaticus*-infected pIV−/− K14 CIITA Tg mice or pIV+/− K14 CIITA Tg controls. (A) Representative histograms (left) display the cIE and data (right) represent mean ($n = 9–11$ per group) from three pooled experiments. (B) dot plots showed represent $n = 3–4$ per group. αIL10R, anti-interleukin-10 receptor monoclonal antibodies;

Figure S7 Colonic IECs from anti-IL-10R-treated pIV+/− K14 CIITA Tg mice express MHCII molecules apically and basolaterally. (A and B) *H. hepaticus*-infected pIV−/− K14 CIITA Tg or pIV+/− K14 CIITA Tg control mice were treated with anti-IL-10R mAb or isotype control mAb. Mid-colon sections were stained with DAPI (blue) to label nuclei and anti-MHCII mAb (red). (A) Representative pIV−/− K14 CIITA Tg mouse and (B) representative pIV+/− K14 CIITA Tg mouse. Right upper panel depicts a region with MHCII^{-} IECs; Right lower panel depicts a region with MHCII^{+} IECs. Bar, 20 μm.
(TIF)

Figure S8 Colitic mice do not induce the expression of CD40, CD80 and CD86 on colonic IECs. (A–C) CD45.2^{-} EpCAM^{+} IECs isolated from anti-IL-10R mAb or isotype treated, *H. hepaticus*-infected pIV−/− K14 CIITA Tg mice or pIV+/− K14 CIITA Tg controls were analysed for the expression of classical costimulatory molecules by flow cytometry. (A) Frequency of CD40, (B) CD80 or (C) CD86. Histograms represent $n = 3–5$ per group. αIL10R, anti-interleukin-10 receptor monoclonal antibodies;

Figure S9 Expression levels of Th17- and group 3 ILC-associated factors. (A–B) *H. hepaticus*-infected pIV−/− K14 CIITA Tg or pIV+/− K14 CIITA Tg control mice were treated with anti-IL-10R mAb or isotype control mAb. (A) *ror-γt* and *il23p19* mRNA expression levels in colon explants. Data represent $n = 9–11$ per group from three pooled experiments. (B) IL-17A secretion upon *ex vivo* organ culture of colon explants. Data represent $n = 6$ per group from two pooled experiments. Data displayed as mean and s.d. αIL10R, anti-interleukin-10 receptor monoclonal antibodies;

Methods S1 Additional methods applied to generate supporting figures.

Acknowledgments

We thank Amy Beebe (Merck Research Labs) for providing the anti-IL-10R mAb; Beat Imhof for providing the hybridoma Y13-259; Sylvie Robine for providing vil-Cre Tg mice; Benjamin Weber and Nina Dickgreber for providing technical protocols; Catherine Ronet for providing qPCR primer sequences; Jean-Christophe Stehle and Janine Horlbeck for preparation and staining of histological samples; Danny Labes and Anne Wilson for advice in flow cytometry.

Author Contributions

Conceived and designed the experiments: HAO WR CM CT JB. Performed the experiments: CT ROE MC JB MR AD CL VM. Analyzed the data: CT ROE MC JB HB. Contributed reagents/materials/analysis tools: WR. Wrote the paper: CT WR CM HAO.

References

1. Strober W, Fuss IJ (2011) Proinflammatory cytokines in the pathogenesis of inflammatory bowel diseases. Gastroenterology 140: 1756–1767.
2. Brown SJ, Mayer L (2007) The immune response in inflammatory bowel disease. Am J Gastroenterol 102: 2058–2069.
3. Maloy KJ, Powrie F (2011) Intestinal homeostasis and its breakdown in inflammatory bowel disease. Nature 474: 298–306.
4. Reith W, LeibundGut-Landmann S, Waldburger JM (2005) Regulation of MHC class II gene expression by the class II transactivator. Nat Rev Immunol 5: 793–806.
5. Kaiserlian D, Vidal K, Revillard JP (1989) Murine enterocytes can present soluble antigen to specific class II-restricted CD4+ T cells. Eur J Immunol 19: 1513–1516.
6. Buning J, Hundorfean G, Schmitz M, Zimmer KP, Strobel S, et al. (2006) Antigen targeting to MHC class II-enriched late endosomes in colonic epithelial cells: trafficking of luminal antigens studied in vivo in Crohn's colitis patients. FASEB J 20: 359–361.
7. Bland PW, Warren LG (1986) Antigen presentation by epithelial cells of the rat small intestine. I. Kinetics, antigen specificity and blocking by anti-Ia antisera. Immunology 58: 1–7.
8. Mayer L, Shlien R (1987) Evidence for function of Ia molecules on gut epithelial cells in man. J Exp Med 166: 1471–1483.
9. Hershberg RM, Framson PE, Cho DH, Lee LY, Kovats S, et al. (1997) Intestinal epithelial cells use two distinct pathways for HLA class II antigen processing. J Clin Invest 100: 204–215.
10. Hershberg RM, Cho DH, Youakim A, Bradley MB, Lee JS, et al. (1998) Highly polarized HLA class II antigen processing and presentation by human intestinal epithelial cells. J Clin Invest 102: 792–803.
11. Sanderson IR, Ouellette AJ, Carter EA, Walker WA, Harmatz PR (1993) Differential regulation of B7 mRNA in enterocytes and lymphoid cells. Immunology 79: 434–438.
12. Framson PE, Cho DH, Lee LY, Hershberg RM (1999) Polarized expression and function of the costimulatory molecule CD58 on human intestinal epithelial cells. Gastroenterology 116: 1054–1062.
13. Nakazawa A, Watanabe M, Kanai T, Yajima T, Yamazaki M, et al. (1999) Functional expression of costimulatory molecule CD86 on epithelial cells in the inflamed colonic mucosa. Gastroenterology 117: 536–545.
14. Dotan I, Allez M, Nakazawa A, Brimnes J, Schulder-Katz M, et al. (2007) Intestinal epithelial cells from inflammatory bowel disease patients preferentially stimulate CD4+ T cells to proliferate and secrete interferon-gamma. Am J Physiol Gastrointest Liver Physiol 292: G1630–1640.
15. Westendorf AM, Fleissner D, Groebe L, Jung S, Gruber AD, et al. (2009) CD4+Foxp3+ regulatory T cell expansion induced by antigen-driven interaction with intestinal epithelial cells independent of local dendritic cells. Gut 58: 211–219.
16. Cruickshank SM, McVay LD, Baumgart DC, Felsburg PJ, Carding SR (2004) Colonic epithelial cell mediated suppression of CD4 T cell activation. Gut 53: 678–684.

17. Waldburger JM, Suter T, Fontana A, Acha-Orbea H, Reith W (2001) Selective abrogation of major histocompatibility complex class II expression on extrahematopoietic cells in mice lacking promoter IV of the class II transactivator gene. J Exp Med 194: 393–406.
18. Irla M, Hugues S, Gill J, Nitta T, Hikosaka Y, et al. (2008) Autoantigen-specific interactions with CD4+ thymocytes control mature medullary thymic epithelial cell cellularity. Immunity 29: 451–463.
19. el Marjou F, Janssen KP, Chang BH, Li M, Hindie V, et al. (2004) Tissue-specific and inducible Cre-mediated recombination in the gut epithelium. Genesis 39: 186–193.
20. Mombaerts P, Iacomini J, Johnson RS, Herrup K, Tonegawa S, et al. (1992) RAG-1-deficient mice have no mature B and T lymphocytes. Cell 68: 869–877.
21. Dalton DK, Pitts-Meek S, Keshav S, Figari IS, Bradley A, et al. (1993) Multiple defects of immune cell function in mice with disrupted interferon-gamma genes. Science 259: 1739–1742.
22. Weigmann B, Tubbe I, Seidel D, Nicolaev A, Becker C, et al. (2007) Isolation and subsequent analysis of murine lamina propria mononuclear cells from colonic tissue. Nat Protoc 2: 2307–2311.
23. Henao-Mejia J, Elinav E, Jin C, Hao L, Mehal WZ, et al. (2012) Inflammasome-mediated dysbiosis regulates progression of NAFLD and obesity. Nature 482: 179–185.
24. Elinav E, Strowig T, Kau AL, Henao-Mejia J, Thaiss CA, et al. (2011) NLRP6 inflammasome regulates colonic microbial ecology and risk for colitis. Cell 145: 745–757.
25. Kullberg MC, Jankovic D, Feng CG, Hue S, Gorelick PL, et al. (2006) IL-23 plays a key role in Helicobacter hepaticus-induced T cell-dependent colitis. J Exp Med 203: 2485–2494.
26. Verdu EF, Deng Y, Bercik P, Collins SM (2002) Modulatory effects of estrogen in two murine models of experimental colitis. Am J Physiol Gastrointest Liver Physiol 283: G27–36.
27. Huh WJ, Khurana SS, Geahlen JH, Kohli K, Waller RA, et al. (2012) Tamoxifen induces rapid, reversible atrophy, and metaplasia in mouse stomach. Gastroenterology 142: 21–24 e27.
28. Zimmerman NP, Vongsa RA, Wendt MK, Dwinell MB (2008) Chemokines and chemokine receptors in mucosal homeostasis at the intestinal epithelial barrier in inflammatory bowel disease. Inflamm Bowel Dis 14: 1000–1011.
29. Farber JM (1990) A macrophage mRNA selectively induced by gamma-interferon encodes a member of the platelet factor 4 family of cytokines. Proc Natl Acad Sci U S A 87: 5238–5242.
30. Krishnan K, Arnone B, Buchman A (2011) Intestinal growth factors: potential use in the treatment of inflammatory bowel disease and their role in mucosal healing. Inflamm Bowel Dis 17: 410–422.
31. Spits H, Artis D, Colonna M, Diefenbach A, Di Santo JP, et al. (2013) Innate lymphoid cells - a proposal for uniform nomenclature. Nat Rev Immunol 13: 145–149.
32. Buonocore S, Ahern PP, Uhlig HH, Ivanov, II, Littman DR, et al. (2010) Innate lymphoid cells drive interleukin-23-dependent innate intestinal pathology. Nature 464: 1371–1375.
33. Yadav M, Louvet C, Davini D, Gardner JM, Martinez-Llordella M, et al. (2012) Neuropilin-1 distinguishes natural and inducible regulatory T cells among regulatory T cell subsets in vivo. J Exp Med 209: 1713–1722, S1711–1719.
34. Morrissey PJ, Charrier K, Braddy S, Liggitt D, Watson JD (1993) CD4+ T cells that express high levels of CD45RB induce wasting disease when transferred into congenic severe combined immunodeficient mice. Disease development is prevented by cotransfer of purified CD4+ T cells. J Exp Med 178: 237–244.
35. Maggio-Price L, Seamons A, Bielefeldt-Ohmann H, Zeng W, Brabb T, et al. (2012) Lineage targeted MHC-II transgenic mice demonstrate the role of dendritic cells in bacterial-driven colitis. Inflamm Bowel Dis.
36. Schwartz RH (2003) T cell anergy. Annu Rev Immunol 21: 305–334.
37. Nakazawa A, Dotan I, Brimnes J, Allez M, Shao L, et al. (2004) The expression and function of costimulatory molecules B7H and B7-H1 on colonic epithelial cells. Gastroenterology 126: 1347–1357.
38. Kuhn R, Lohler J, Rennick D, Rajewsky K, Muller W (1993) Interleukin-10-deficient mice develop chronic enterocolitis. Cell 75: 263–274.
39. Kullberg MC, Ward JM, Gorelick PL, Caspar P, Hieny S, et al. (1998) Helicobacter hepaticus triggers colitis in specific-pathogen-free interleukin-10 (IL-10)-deficient mice through an IL-12- and gamma interferon-dependent mechanism. Infect Immun 66: 5157–5166.
40. Ward JM, Anver MR, Haines DC, Melhorn JM, Gorelick P, et al. (1996) Inflammatory large bowel disease in immunodeficient mice naturally infected with Helicobacter hepaticus. Lab Anim Sci 46: 15–20.
41. Erdman SE, Poutahidis T, Tomczak M, Rogers AB, Cormier K, et al. (2003) CD4+ CD25+ regulatory T lymphocytes inhibit microbially induced colon cancer in Rag2-deficient mice. Am J Pathol 162: 691–702.
42. Kullberg MC, Jankovic D, Gorelick PL, Caspar P, Letterio JJ, et al. (2002) Bacteria-triggered CD4(+) T regulatory cells suppress Helicobacter hepaticus-induced colitis. J Exp Med 196: 505–515.
43. Maloy KJ, Salaun L, Cahill R, Dougan G, Saunders NJ, et al. (2003) CD4+CD25+ T(R) cells suppress innate immune pathology through cytokine-dependent mechanisms. J Exp Med 197: 111–119.
44. Erdman SE, Rao VP, Poutahidis T, Ihrig MM, Ge Z, et al. (2003) CD4(+)CD25(+) regulatory lymphocytes require interleukin 10 to interrupt colon carcinogenesis in mice. Cancer Res 63: 6042–6050.
45. Glocker EO, Kotlarz D, Klein C, Shah N, Grimbacher B (2011) IL-10 and IL-10 receptor defects in humans. Ann N Y Acad Sci 1246: 102–107.
46. Kullberg MC, Rothfuchs AG, Jankovic D, Caspar P, Wynn TA, et al. (2001) Helicobacter hepaticus-induced colitis in interleukin-10-deficient mice: cytokine requirements for the induction and maintenance of intestinal inflammation. Infect Immun 69: 4232–4241.
47. Morrison PJ, Bending D, Fouser LA, Wright JF, Stockinger B, et al. (2013) Th17-cell plasticity in Helicobacter hepaticus-induced intestinal inflammation. Mucosal Immunol.
48. Lee HO, Miller SD, Hurst SD, Tan LJ, Cooper CJ, et al. (2000) Interferon gamma induction during oral tolerance reduces T-cell migration to sites of inflammation. Gastroenterology 119: 129–138.
49. Cottone M, Orlando A, Renna S (2010) Investigational agents for Crohn's disease. Expert Opin Investig Drugs 19: 1147–1159.

20

Colonic miRNA Expression/Secretion, Regulated by Intestinal Epithelial PepT1, Plays an Important Role in Cell-to-Cell Communication during Colitis

Saravanan Ayyadurai[1]*, Moiz A. Charania[1], Bo Xiao[1], Emilie Viennois[1,2], Yuchen Zhang[1], Didier Merlin[1,2]

1 Department of Biology and Chemistry, Center for Diagnostics and Therapeutics, Georgia State University, Atlanta, Georgia, United States of America, **2** Veterans Affairs Medical Center, Decatur, Georgia, United States of America

Abstract

PepT1 is a member of the proton-oligopeptide cotransporter family SLC15, which mediates the transport of di/tripeptides from intestinal lumen into epithelial cells. MicroRNAs (miRNAs), a small noncoding RNAs (21–23 nucleotides), post-transcriptionally regulate gene expression by binding to the 3′-untranslated regions (UTRs) of their target mRNAs. Although the role of most miRNAs remains elusive, they have been implicated in vital cellular functions such as intestinal epithelial cells differentiation, proliferation, and apoptosis. In the present study, we investigated the effect of intestinal epithelial PepT1 expression on microRNA (miRNA) expression/secretion in the colons of control mice and in mice with experimentally induced colonic inflammation (colitis). The colonic miRNA expression was deregulated in both colitis and control mice but the deregulation of miRNA expression/secretion was specific to colonic tissue and did not affect other tissues such as spleen and liver. Intestinal epithelial PepT1-dependent deregulation of colonic miRNA expression not only affects epithelial cells but also other cell types, such as intestinal macrophages. Importantly, we found the miRNA 23b which was known to be involved in inflammatory bowel disease was secreted and transported between cells to impose a gene-silencing effect on recipient intestinal macrophages. Based on our data, we may conclude that the expression of a specific protein, PepT1, in the intestine affects local miRNA expression/secretion in the colon on a tissue specific manner and may play an important role during the induction and progression of colitis. Colonic miRNA expression/secretion, regulated by intestinal epithelial PepT1, could play a crucial role in cell-to-cell communication during colitis.

Editor: Josep Bassaganya-Riera, Virginia Tech, United States of America

Funding: This work was supported by the department of veteran's affairs (Didier Merlin). The funders had no role in study design, data collection and analysis, decision to publish, or preparation of the manuscript.

Competing Interests: The authors have declared that no competing interests exist.

* E-mail: sayyadurai@gsu.edu

Introduction

PepT1 is a di/tripeptide transporter [1–3] highly expressed in epithelial cells of the small intestine, and poorly expressed in the colon [4,5]. However, colonic PepT1 expression is enhanced under conditions of chronic inflammation such as Inflammatory Bowel Disease (IBD) [4,6,7]. Recently, a polymorphism of the hPepT1 gene has been shown to be associated with IBD susceptibility, indicating a direct involvement of this transporter in IBD [8]. Also, it has been shown that PepT1 expressed in immune cells played an important role in promoting the immune response during experimentally induced colitis compared to the knock-out mice [9]. Recent study showed that IL-16 induces intestinal inflammation by up regulating PepT1 expression in puffer fish intestine and it subsequently transported the bacterial peptide fMLP which triggers the intestinal inflammation [7].

To specifically examine the role played by hPepT1 in intestinal epithelial cells (IECs) (including colonocytes) during intestinal inflammation, we generated a transgenic mouse model, in which hPepT1 was specifically expressed in IECs under the control of a villin promoter (villin-hPepT1 mice). Western blotting confirmed expression of hPepT1 in the colonocytes of transgenic mice (TG) but not those of wild-type (WT) mice [10]. The mice appeared healthy and exhibited normal body weight, breeding behavior, and general appearance. The morphology of the gastrointestinal tract as judged by histological examination appeared normal [10]. Immunohistochemical analysis verified hPepT1 membrane staining of colonocytes in villin-hPepT1 Tg mice, but not in WT mice [10]. In addition, apical membrane vesicles prepared from colonocytes of villin-hPepT1 mice, expressed significantly higher levels of functional hPepT1 compared to WT mice [10]. Together, the results clearly showed that villin-hPepT1 mice express hPepT1 in the colonic mucosa, which has also been observed in IBD patients [4,6] and therefore represents an appropriate model in which the pathogenic role of hPepT1 in IBD may be explored.

To assess the effect of hPepT1 expression in colonocytes during inflammation, colitis was induced using dextran sulfate sodium (DSS) and TNBS [10–14]. Such treatment induced a more drastic weight loss in villin-hPepT1 mice with a higher clinical score compared to WT mice [10]. The severity of DSS-induced colitis in villin-hPepT1 mice was accompanied by a rise in inflammation, as noted by colonoscopy, with massive mucosal erythema and bleeding. DSS treatment increased the extent of histological damage in villin-hPepT1 mice as shown by almost complete crypt disruption and inflammatory infiltration throughout the mucosa

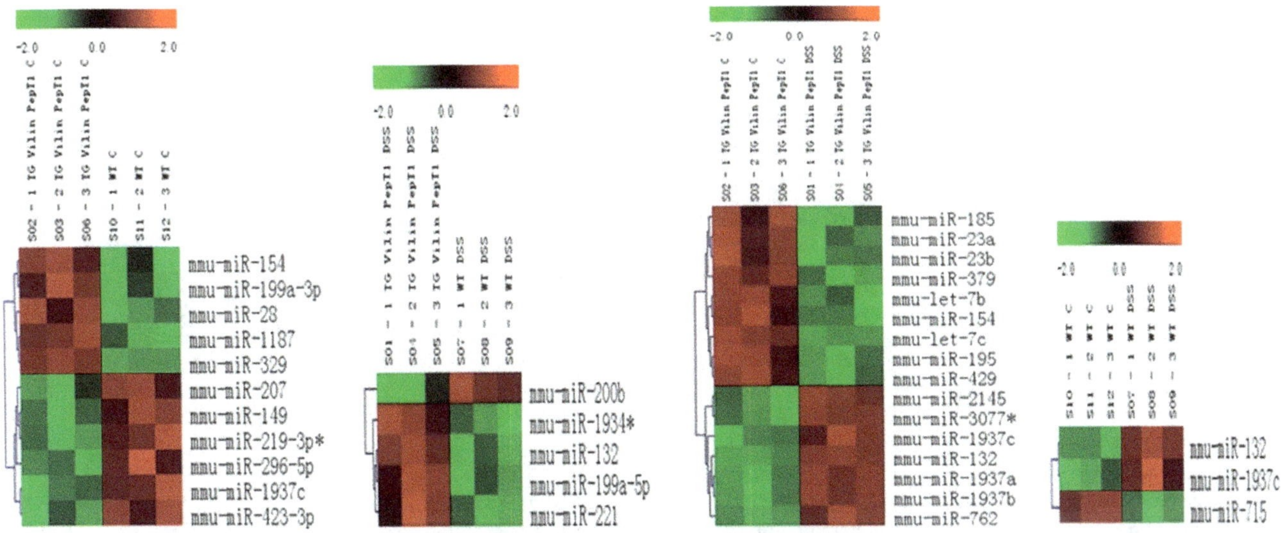

FVB WT H_2O vs Villin-hPepT1 H_2O | **FVB WT DSS vs Villin-hPepT1 DSS** | **Villin-hPepT1 DSS vs Villin-PepT1 H_2O** | **FVB WT DSS vs FVB WT H_2O**

Figure 1. Clustering graph of miRNAs. microRNA microarray results demonstrated that villin-hPepT1 and FVB WT mice treated with and without DSS expressed different miRNA profiles. miRNAs expressed with a p value of <0.01 and signal >500.

and submucosa, consistent with the marked increase noted in colonic MPO activity compared to that of WT mice. Importantly, villin-hPepT1 animals also exhibited a marked increase in DSS-induced colonic levels of the pro-inflammatory cytokines such as IL-1β, IL-6, TNF-α and IFN-γ, compared to WT animals [10]. Our studies demonstrated that IEC-specific hPepT1 expression exacerbated the susceptibility of mice to DSS-induced colitis and reduced intestinal recovery and healing after induction of inflammation.

microRNA (miRNA), described in *Caenorhabditis elegans* in 1993 [15,16] are 18 to 22 nucleotides in length [17] and negatively regulate target mRNAs by binding to their 3′- untranslated region (UTR) [18–20]. Each miRNA can target hundreds of mRNAs within a given cell type [21] and a single mRNA is the target of multiple miRNAs [22,23]. Thus, miRNAs contribute to the regulation of over 30% of protein-coding genes [24]. MiRNAs have been shown to play important roles in various biological processes including immunity, cell proliferation and development [25–27] and intestinal epithelial cell differentiation [28,29]. Many studies have examined global miRNA expression in health and disease conditions [17,30–35]. Tissue specific miRNAs from mouse have already been investigated [36]. Recently, we have shown the tissue specific expression of CD98 on miRNA expression in the same tissue [37]. In the present study, we investigated the effect of intestinal epithelial PepT1 expression on miRNA expression in the colon of control mice and in mice experiencing inflammation.

Materials and Methods

Generation of hPepT1 transgenic mice

Homozygous villin-hPepT1 mice were previously generated [10] and FVB WT mice were used as controls. All animal procedures were approved by the Animal Care Committee of Emory University and Georgia State University and were conducted in accordance to the *Guide for the Care of Use of Laboratory Animals* from the US Public Health Service.

Induction of colitis

Six week old villin-hPepT1 and FVB WT male mice were used for this study. Colitis was induced by the addition of 3% (w/v) dextran sodium sulfate (DSS; molecular weight 36,000–50,000 Da; MP Biomedicals, LLC, OH) to the drinking water [9]. Physical characteristics such as body weight and pro and anti-inflammatory cytokine profile were matched with previously reported [10]. The mice were humanly euthanized, and colon, spleen and liver tissue were processed further by extracting total RNA for microarray analysis and immunohistochemistry after 7 days of DSS treatment.

RNA extraction and miRNA expression analysis by miRNA Microarray

Total RNA containing miRNA was extracted from the liver, spleen and colon of mice by RNeasy Plus Mini kit (Qiagen, Valencia, CA) according to the manufacturer's instruction given in Qiagen supplementary protocol for purification of miRNA from animal tissue. The yield and quality of RNA was verified. A size fractionation step with YM-100 Microcon filter was done which isolates nucleotides of ~200 bp or less (LC Sciences, Houston, TX). MicroRNA microarrays were performed by using the µParaflo® microfluidic chip technology (LC Sciences). Probes for the arrays were developed using version 16 of the miRBase sequence database updated with 1145 miRNAs (http://www.lcsciences.com/applications/transcriptomics/mirna-profiling/mirna/). Data analysis for the arrays was performed using *t*-test, ANOVA and/or clustering analysis. We compared transcripts of FVB WT H_2O vs villin-hPepT1 H_2O, FVB WT H_2O vs villin-hPepT1 treated with DSS, FVB WT H_2O vs FVB WT DSS-treated and villin-hPepT1 H_2O vs villin-hPepT1 DSS-treated (Fig. 1).

Real-time RT-PCR analysis

cDNA was generated from the total RNAs isolated above using the NCode™ miRNA first-strand cDNA synthesis kit (Invitrogen, Carlsbad, CA) or Maxima first strand cDNA synthesis kit (Thermo

Scientific, Glen-Burnie, MD) as previously described [38]. Levels of mature miRNAs expression were quantified by qRT-PCR using Maxima® SYBR Green/ROX qPCR Master Mix (Thermo Scientific, Pittsburgh, PA). The universal reverse primer provided in the NCode™ miRNA first-strand cDNA synthesis kit and the specific microRNA forward primers were used. Small RNA 234 or cel-mir-39 was used as housekeeping gene. Fold-induction was calculated using the Ct method as follows: $\Delta\Delta Ct = (Ct_{Target} - Ct_{housekeeping})_{group\ 1} - (Ct_{Target} - Ct_{housekeeping})_{group\ 2}$, and the final data were derived from $2^{-\Delta\Delta CT}$. All primers used for qRT-PCR are described in Table S5.

miRNA target prediction

To determine the potential target genes of detected miRNAs, three different miRNA target prediction algorithms were used: PicTar (http://pictar.mdc-berlin.de) [39], MicroCosm (http://www.ebi.ac.uk/enright-srv/microcosm/htdocs/targets/v5/) [40] and TargetScan (http://www.targetscan.org/) [41]. The Matchminer program (http://discover.nci.nih.gov/matchmi ner/index.jsp) [42] was then used to determine genes that were identified by at least two algorithms.

DAVID gene functional annotation tool

DAVID (the Database for Annotation, Visualization and Integrated Discovery) is a bioinformatics resource developed by the Laboratory of Immunopathogenesis and Bioinformatics [43]. All tools in the DAVID Bioinformatics Resources aim to provide functional interpretation of large lists of genes derived from genomic studies, such as microarray and proteomics studies. DAVID can be found at http://david.niaid.nih.gov or http://david.abcc.ncifcrf.gov. The DAVID Functional Annotation Tool mainly provides typical batch annotation and gene-GO term enrichment analysis to highlight the most relevant GO terms associated with a given gene list. The *p*-values associated with each annotation term inside each cluster are used to rank their biological significance. Thus, the top ranked annotation groups most likely have consistently lower p-values for their annotation members.

The miRNAs predicted common protein targets from the Matchminer program were later analyzed. The functional annotation of each protein was analyzed through clusters formed by DAVID. Each cluster that scored an enrichment score of >1.0 were taken for analysis and the *p*-value of each annotation cluster verified.

Western blot analysis

Approximately 1.0 cm piece of colon were homogenized in radioimmunoprecipitation assay buffer (RIPA) (150 mM NaCl, 0.5% sodium deoxycholate, 50 mM Tris-HCl, pH 8, 0.1% SDS, 0.1% Nonidet P-40) supplemented with protease inhibitors (Roche Diagnostics, Indianapolis, IN) on ice. The homogenates were centrifuged at 12,000 rpm for 10 min at 4°C. Total cell lysates were resolved on 10% polyacrylamide gels (Bio-Rad, Hercules, CA) and transferred to nitrocellulose membranes (Bio-Rad). Membranes were then probed with Marcksl-1 (Proteintech, 10002-2-AP, Chicago, IL) and beta-tubulin (Sigma- Aldrich, T8328, St Louis, MO). After washes, membranes were incubated with appropriate horseradish peroxidase-conjugated secondary antibody (GE Healthcare Biosciences, Pittsburgh, PA), and blots were detected using the Enhanced Chemiluminescence Detection kit (GE Healthcare Biosciences).

Immunohistochemistry

Paraffin-embedded tissue sections (5-µm) were deparaffinized in xylene and rehydrated in an ethanol gradient. Epitope retrieval was done by treating with 10 mM sodium citrate buffer (pH 6.0) and 10 mM citric acid (4:1 ratio) at 120°C for 10 min in a pressure cooker. Sections were blocked with 5% goat serum and then incubated with Marcksl-1 (1:100 dilution) overnight at 4°C. After washing with phosphate buffered saline (PBS), sections were incubated with Alexa-Fluor 568 phalloidin (Invitrogen, 1:5000) and horseradish peroxidase-conjugated secondary antibody for 45 minutes at room temperature in the dark. Sections were mounted in mounting medium with 4′, 6-diamidino-2-phenylindole (DAPI) (Vector Laboratories, Burlingame, CA) and cover slipped. Images were acquired using an Olympus microscope equipped with an Hamamatsu Digital Camera ORCA-03G.

Secreted miRNA in colon culture

DSS treated villin-hpepT1 and FVB WT along with H_2O control mouse colons were cut and washed three times in sterile PBS and cultured in RPMI media without serum at 37°C for 24 hrs. The supernatant was collected and centrifuged to sediment the tissue particles. Cel-miR-39 was used as an invariant control for the conditioned medium RNA extraction and qRT-PCR analysis as described earlier [44,45]. 10 µL of 0.1 nM cel-miR-39 was added to each 1 mL aliquot of supernatant and vortexed for 30s. miRNAs extraction was performed using the Norgen Biotek Exosome RNA extraction kit (Norgen Biotek, Ontario, Canada) according to the manufacturer's instructions and the RNA yield was verified. miRNA profiles from the conditioned medium or blank medium were assessed by qRT-PCR and further confirmed by Signosis miRNA expression plate assay according to the manufacturer's protocol (Signosis Inc, Sunnyvale, CA) and chemiluminescence was measured in a Biotek synergy 2.0 microplate reader (Biotek, Winooski, VT).

miRNA uptake experiment in macrophages

Although many miRNA's up or down regulated in our study, it has been reported that miRNA 23a and miRNA 23b have a potential roles in ulcerative colitis and Crohn's disease in patients [46]. Therefore, we chose miRNA 23b for further study. MiRNA 23b uptake by macrophages was assessed using Cy3 labeled dsRNA 23b (5′-Cy3 labeled antisense strand) (Integrated DNA Technologies, Coralville, IA). 3×10^4 macrophage (RAW-264.7) cells were grown in 6 chamber BD falcon culture slides (BD Bioscience, Bedford, MA) at 37°C with 5% CO_2 for 24 h. The Cy3 labeled miRNA 23b at 50 nM concentration was added into the culture medium and incubated at 37°C with 5% CO_2 for 24 h. Cells were washed with PBS and stained with Alexa Fluor 488 phalloidin (Invitrogen) and vectashield mounting medium with DAPI (Vector Laboratories, Burlingame, CA) and the slides were examined under microscope for miRNA 23b uptake by macrophages.

Targeting Marcksl-1 3′UTR by miRNA 23b in macrophages

To examine whether miRNA-23b directly targets the 3′UTR of Marcksl-1 mRNA, Marcksl-1 3′UTR was cloned downstream in pEZX vector with neomycin/kanamycin selection with a luciferase reporter gene (Luc-Marcksl-1 3′UTR) (Genecopoeia, Rockville, MD). Precursor miRNA-23b cloned in CMV promoter with ampicillin selection (Genecopoeia, Rockville, MD). The constructs were transfected in XL gold ultracompetent cells (Agilent Technologies, Santa Clara, CA) and selected with appropriate antibiotic selection media. The plasmid extraction was done using

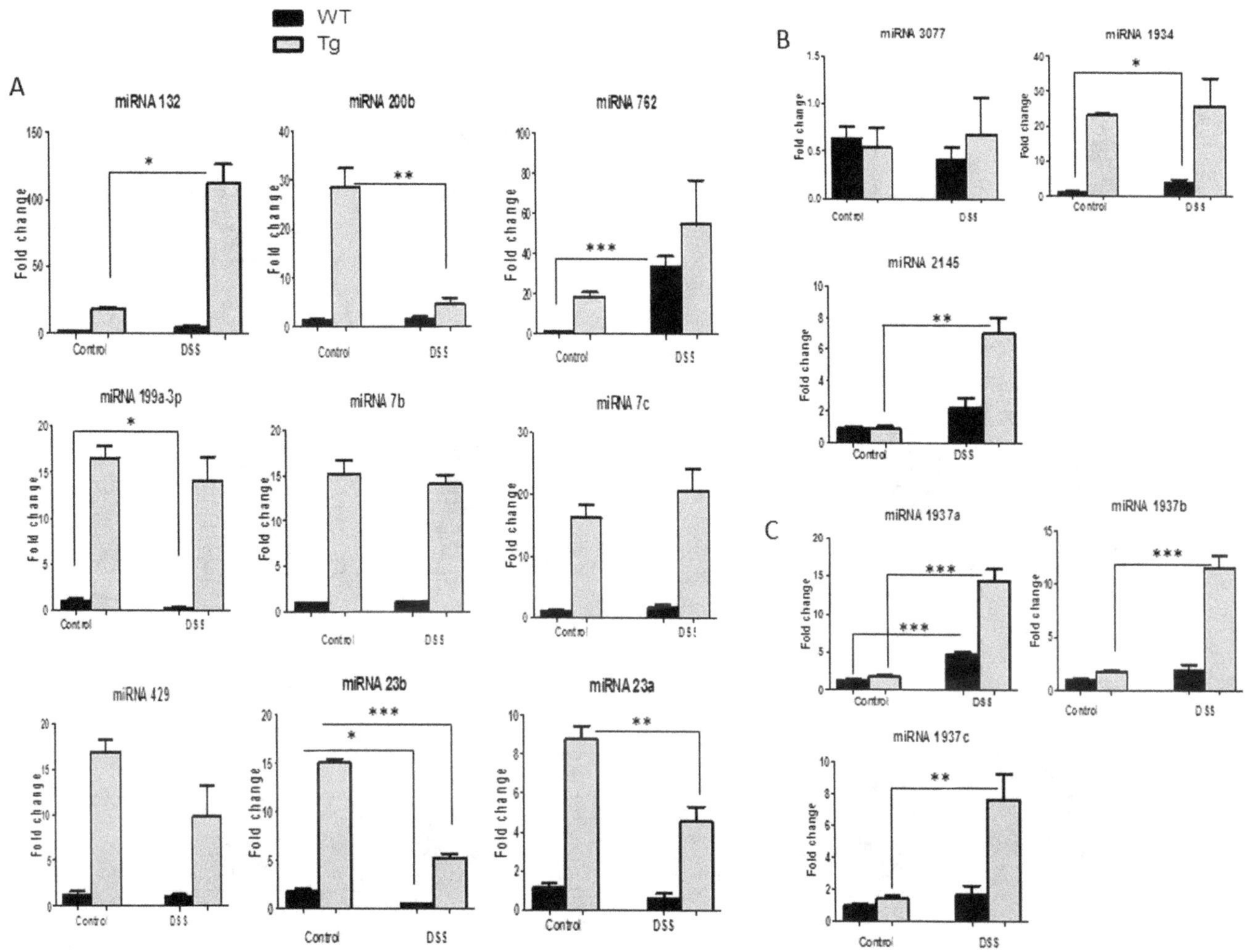

Figure 2. Colonic miRNA expression levels are modulated in villin-hPepT1 and FVB WT mice with and without DSS. miRNAs expressed with the a p-value of <0.01 and signal >500 in microRNA microarray were analyzed by qRT-PCR (Fig. 2A). miRNA 3077, miRNA 1934, miRNA 2145 were not associated with any target mRNAs so these three miRNAs were excluded from further analysis (Fig. 2B) and the mature mmu-miR-1937a, mmu-miR-1937b, and mmu-miR-1937c are fragments of tRNA (www.mirbase.org) so we eliminated these from further analyses (Fig. 2C). Difference in miRNA expression noted as * $p<0.05$, ** $p<0.001$ and *** $p<0.0001$. Values represent means ± SEM of n = 6/group.

Qiagen Medi-plasmid extraction kit (Qiagen, Valencia, CA). The plasmid concentration and the constructs position were verified using restriction enzymes. RAW-264.7 cells were grown in 6 well plate (3.3×10^5) and Luc-Marcksl-1 3′UTR construct was co-transfected with miRNA-23b precursor. As controls, Luc-Marcksl-1 3′UTR and miRNA-23b precursor constructs alone transfected in RAW 264.7 cells using Lipofectamine 2000 (Life Technologies, Grand Island, NY) in Opti-MEM reduced serum medium (GIBCO, Life Technologies, Grand Island, NY). Only RAW 264.7 cells used as negative control. After 4 h of transfection, serum-free DMEM medium was added (cellgro, Manassas, VA). Transfected cells were incubated at 37°C for 24 h with 5% CO_2. After incubation, the cells were washed with sterile PBS and luciferase assay was carried out according to the manufactures protocol (Genecopoeia, Rockville, MD). The targeting of miRNAs Marcksl-1 3′UTR was then assessed by measuring luciferase activity in these cells.

Statistical analysis

Values were expressed as means ± standard error of mean (SEM). Statistical analysis was performed using unpaired two-tailed t-test by GraphPad Prism 5 software. $p<0.05$ were considered statistically significant.

Results

Differential effects of colonic PepT1 expression on colonic miRNA synthesis

The expression of colonic miRNA transcripts was compared between WT and villin-hPepT1 mice either treated with DSS, or not, at the significance levels of $p<0.01$, $p<0.05$, and $p<0.1$ (Table S1). Although large numbers of miRNAs were differentially expressed, many yielded low signal strengths (<500). These miRNAs and those for which the differential p-values greater than 0.01, were excluded from analysis (Fig. 1). Of the 15 miRNAs that met our stringent criteria, 3 were discarded: the mature miRNAs, mmu-miR-1937a, mmu-miR-1937b, and mmu-miR-1937c are in fact fragments of tRNA (www.mirbase.org) (Fig. 2C). The remaining 12 miRNAs with differential p-values<0.01 and of signal strengths >500 were further analyzed by qRT-PCR to determine fold changes (Fig. 2A and Fig. 2B). The data were compared with the differential expression levels detected upon

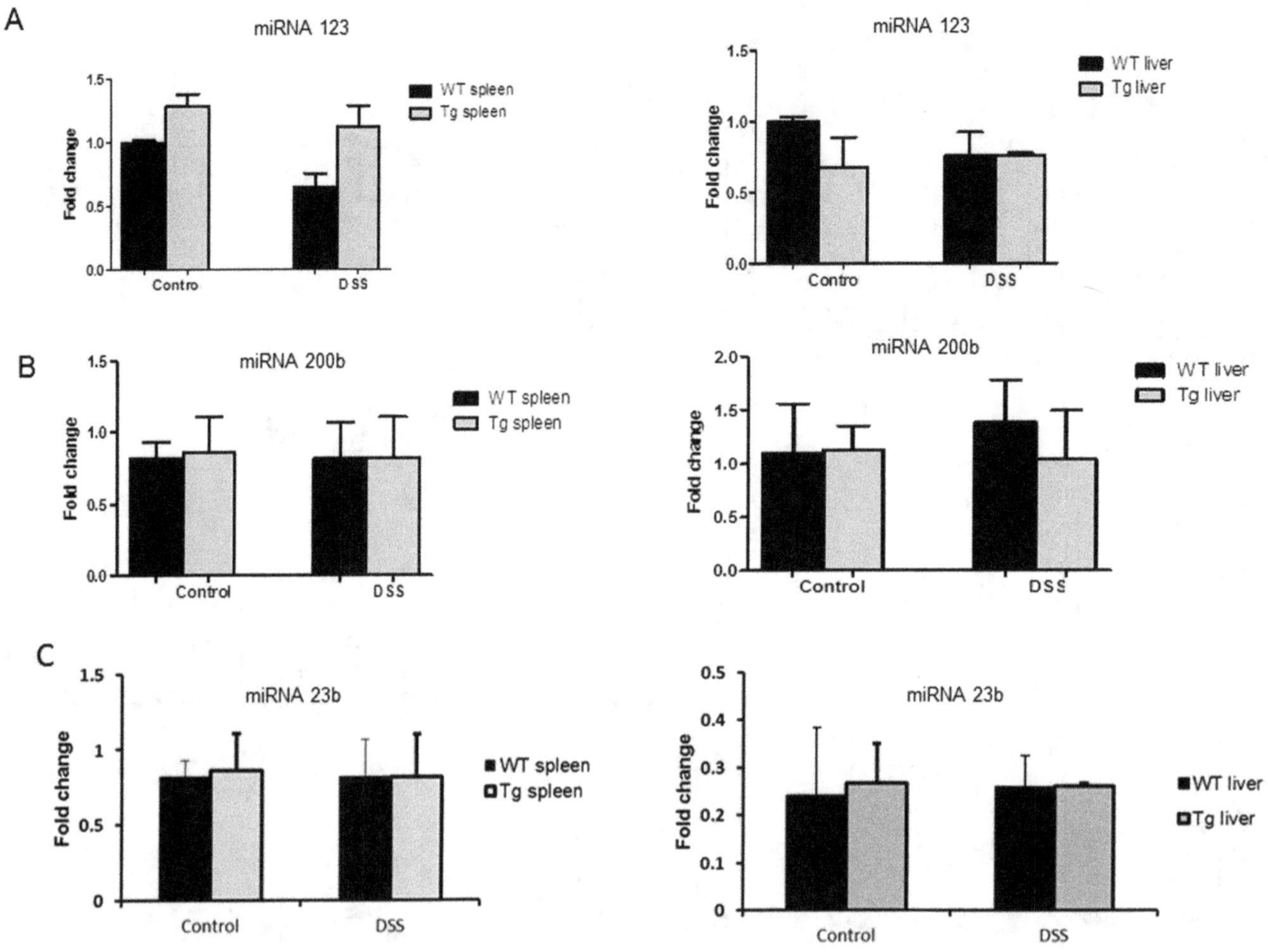

Figure 3. hPepT1 regulates miRNA 132, miRNA 200b and miRNA 23b expression in colon- specific manner. Upon exposure to DSS or normal drinking water, intestinal epithelial PepT1 overexpression did not affect the expression level of miRNA 132 (Fig. 3A), miRNA 200b (Fig. 3B) and miRNA 23b (Fig. 3C) in liver or spleen. Values represent means ± SEM of n = 6/group.

microarray analysis (Table S1). Out of 12 microRNAs, 10 were differentially expressed, with statistical significance, when non-treated WT and villin-hPepT1 mice were compared (the Student's *t*-test values were 0.001–0.04 with p-values<0.01; the fold changes yielded upon qRT-PCR analysis were comparable).

Intestinal epithelial PepT1 expression upregulates basal colonic miRNA expression

First, we investigated the effect of intestinal epithelial PepT1 expression on colonic (epithelial and non-epithelial cells) miRNA expression in untreated mice. The expression levels of the 12 relevant miRNAs, as calculated by qRT-PCR, were in agreement with the miRNA microarray data (Fig. 2A and 2B). A total of 10 colonic miRNAs (miRNA 132, 200b, 762, 199a-3p, 7b, 7c, 429, 23b, 23a, and 1934) were upregulated in villin-hPepT1 mice compared to WT animals. In contrast, miRNAs 3077 and 2145 were expressed at similar levels in both mouse strains (Fig. 2B). Importantly, we found that intestinal epithelial PepT1 overexpression did not affect the expression level of any of these 12 miRNAs in other tissues, including the liver and spleen. We herein represented miRNA 132 (Fig. 3A), miRNA 200b (Fig. 3B) and miRNA 23b (Fig. 3C) in liver and spleen respectively. Thus, overexpression of intestinal epithelial PepT1 specifically upregulated 10 colonic miRNAs. Next, we identified the mRNAs targeted by these miRNAs using Pictar, MicroCosm and Targetscan algorithms. Matchminer program was then employed to identify target genes detected by at least two of the former algorithms. miRNA 3077, miRNA 1934 and miRNA 2145 were not found to target any mRNA and these three miRNAs were excluded from further analysis (Fig. 2B). The remaining nine miRNAs potentially regulated the expression of 704 genes (Table S2).

DAVID functional annotation clustering of villin-hPepT1 and WT at the basal level identified a total of 30 clusters of 453 genes; 161 genes were not part of any of these clusters. The most enriched functional groups (score >1.0) included eleven clusters of genes that were potentially downregulated. These genes are involved in transcription regulation, protein biosynthesis, cell division, endocytosis and calcium binding domains (Table 1) and (Table S3).

Intestinal epithelial PepT1 expression deregulates colonic miRNA expression under induced colitis

To investigate the effect of intestinal epithelial PepT1 expression on colonic miRNA expression after induction of colitis, villin-hPepT1 and WT mice were treated with DSS (given in drinking

Table 1. DAVID functional annotation clustering of villin-hPepT1 and FVB WT at the basal level.

Annotation cluster	Enrichment score	Enriched functional group gene annotation/function	Total gene count
1	4.77	Transcription and Transcription regulation	144
		Nucleus	128
		DNA - binding	54
2	3.31	Isopeptide bond	18
		Ubl conjugation	27
		Cross-links: glycyl lysine isopeptide (Lys-Gly) (interchain with G-Cter in SUMO)	10
3	2.17	Nucleotide-binding	64
		atp-binding	51
		Transferase	53
		Kinase	28
		Domain: protein kinase	22
		Binding site: ATP	24
		Nucleotide phosphate-binding region: ATP	35
		Serine/threonine-protein kinase	17
		Active site: protein acceptor	24
4	2.05	Golgi apparatus	28
		Topological domain: Lumenal	20
		glycosyltransferase	11
		Signal-anchor	17
5	2	Domain:W2	5
		Initiation factor	4
		Protein biosynthesis	5
6	1.83	Repeat: LDL-receptor class B1–20	71
		Repeat: LDL-receptor class A1–8	27
		Domain: EGF-like1–8	45
		Domain: EGF-like 2;calcium binding	3
		Endocytosis	6
		Short sequence modif: Endocytosis signal	3
7	1.56	Nucleotide binding	6
		P-Loop	6
		GTP binding	4
8	1.37	Calcium and calcium binding region 1–2	41
		Domain: EF-hand 1–3	24
9	1.35	Cell division	13
		Cell cycle	19
		Mitosis	8
10	1.12	Short sequence motif: DEAD box	4
		Short sequence motif: Q box	4
		Domain: Helicase C-terminal	6
		Domain: Helicase ATP binding	6
		Helicase	6
11	1.1	Domain: WW 1–3	9

The common proteins were clustered into 30 groups, but based on enrichment score >1.0. 11 groups were considered to be the potential targets with a total of 1100 genes.

water) for 7 days and the levels of the nine colonic miRNAs described above were measured. As shown in Fig. 2A, DSS did not significantly affect the expression levels of colonic miRNAs 762,199a-3p, 429, 7b, or 7c in Tg mice, nor those of miRNAs 132, 200b, 7b, 7c, 429, or 23a in WT mice, compared to the levels seen in untreated WT or Tg mice. In contrast, colonic miRNA 762 was up-regulated and colonic miRNA 199a-3p and miRNA 23b significantly down-regulated after DSS treatment in WT mice

Table 2. miRNAs differentially expressed after DSS treatment in colon.

Upregulated miRNAs		Downregulated miRNAs	
Name	Fold change	Name	Fold change
mmu-miR-132	7.81	mmu-miR-200b	−6.05
mmu let-7c	1.27	mmu-miR-429	−1.71
		mmu-miR-23b	−2.85
		mmu-miR-23a	−1.92

miRNA microarray with the fold change (up-regulated and/or down-regulated) listed in the table.

(Fig. 2A). Interestingly, colonic miRNAs 200b, 23b, and 23a were down-regulated, and 132 up-regulated in villin-hPepT1 mice after DSS-treatment (Fig. 2A). However, the expression levels of all nine miRNAs were significantly higher in DSS-treated villin-hPepT1 compared to DSS treated WT mice (Fig. 2A). The miRNA fold changes observed in microarray and verified by qRT-PCR are listed in Table 2.

Upon DSS exposure, intestinal epithelial PepT1 overexpression did not affect the level of miRNA expression in other tissues such as liver or spleen (Fig. 3A, 3B and 3C). These results suggest that the mRNAs targeted by the nine colonic miRNAs could be differentially expressed in mice over expressing intestinal epithelial PepT1 compared to animals in which intestinal epithelial PepT1 is not expressed or expressed at low basal levels.

DAVID functional annotation clustering of villin-hPepT1 and FVB WT upon DSS treatment identified a total of 15 clusters of 196 genes; 83 genes were not part of any of these clusters (Table S4). The most enriched functional groups identified 4 clusters of genes involved in transcription, ion channel and transport, transcription, calcium binding and DNA binding (Table 3).

Deregulation of colonic miRNAs occurs not only in epithelial cells but also in immune cells such as macrophages

The miRNA expression analysis was performed with the whole colon RNA, therefore the observed differences in colonic miRNA expression likely reflect changes in both epithelial and non-epithelial (*i.e.*, immune) cells. For this purpose, we looked at the mRNA and protein expression of a non-epithelial protein macrophage myristoylated alanine-rich C kinase substrate (Marcksl-1), a potential target gene of miRNA 23a and 23b (Table S2). We chose miRNA 23b for our study as it was previously shown to be involved in chronically active Crohn's disease [47], and active ulcerative colitis [46]. In addition, Marcksl-1 is specifically expressed in macrophages [48] and has been associated with gastrointestinal and inflammatory disease [49], apoptosis and immune response [50,51]. As shown in Fig. 4A and 4B, qRT-PCR and western blot analysis of Marcksl-1 mRNA and protein levels upon DSS treatment were up-regulated in WT mice compared to villin-hPepT1 and were in agreement with colonic miRNA 23b expression levels after DSS treatment (Fig. 2A). The anti-Marcksl-1 immunofluorescence from the colon tissue of WT and villin-hPepT1 mice with and without DSS treatment also showed the WT DSS-treated mice had higher protein accumulation compared to DSS-treated villin-hPepT1 mice (Fig. 4C).

Intestinal epithelial PepT1 expression up-regulates the secretion of colonic miRNA 23b

An analysis of miRNA 23b secretion was performed in colon cultures from villin-hPepT1 and FVB WT mice with or without DSS treatment. Secreted miRNA 23b in the colon culture medium was assessed using a miRNA plate assay method and qRT-PCR. The levels of secreted miRNA 23b were higher in colonic tissues from villin-hPepT1 control mice compared to colonic tissues from FVB WT mice (Fig. 5A and 5B). Notably, DSS treatment significantly reduced the levels of secreted miRNA 23b in the colon culture medium coming from both WT and villin-hPepT1 control mice (Fig. 5A and 5B). These results showed that

Table 3. DAVID functional annotation clustering of villin-hPepT1 and FVB WT treated with DSS.

Annotation cluster	Enrichment score	Enriched functional group gene annotation/function	Total gene count
1	2.96	Transcription and Transcription regulation	68
		Nucleus	59
		Activator	14
		DNA – binding	26
2	1.92	Isopeptide bond	9
		Ubl conjugation	13
		Cross-links: glycyl lysine isopeptide (Lys-Gly) (interchain with G-Cter in SUMO)	5
3	1.79	Calcium and calcium-binding region 1 and 2	26
		Domin:EF-hand 1, 2 and 3	17
4	1.12	Potassium and Potassium transport	10
		Potassium channel	4
		Voltage-gated channel	5
		Ion transport	9
		Ionic channel	5

The common proteins obtained from the matchminer software were clustered in to 15 groups but based on enrichment score >1.0, a total of 4 groups were considered to be the potential targets with a total of 270 genes.

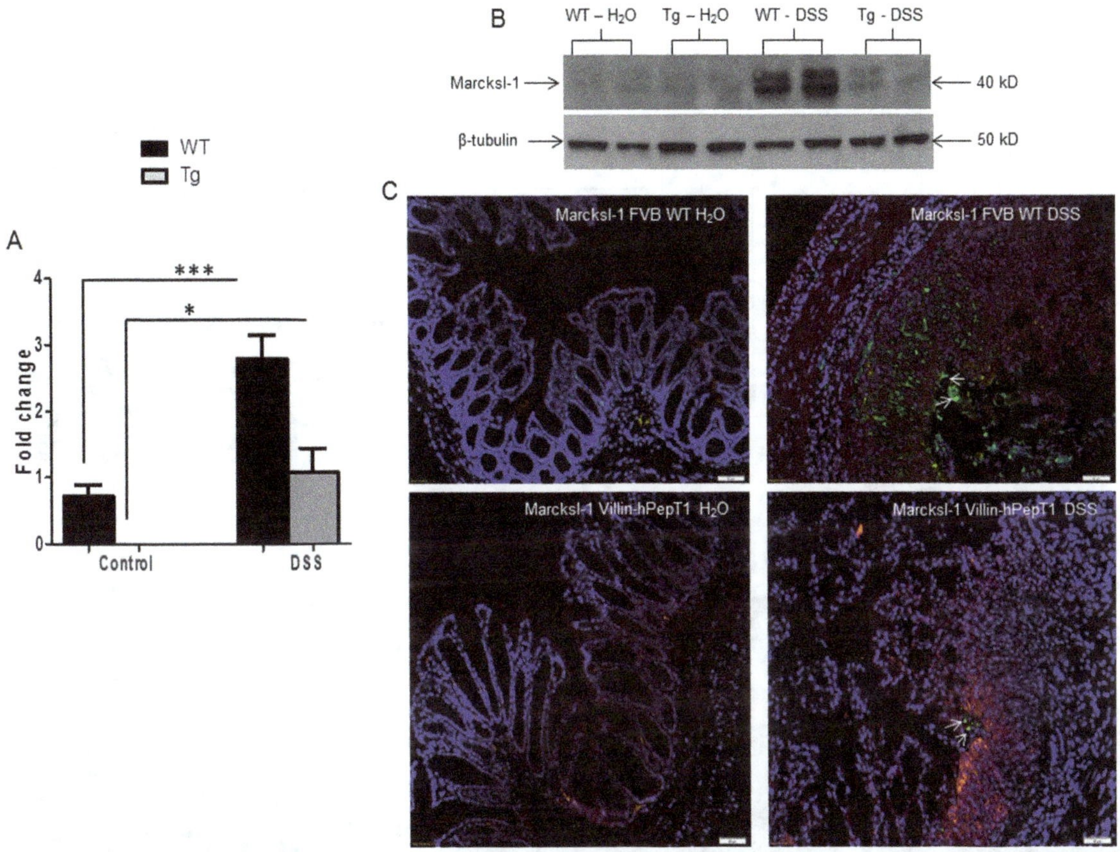

Figure 4. Marcksl-1 is regulated by colonic miRNA 23b in DSS-treated FVB WT mice. Marcksl-1 mRNA fold level was quantified by qRT-PCR (Fig. 4A). Western blot demonstrated protein expression was observed at high level in WT DSS-treated mice and at low level Marcksl-1 and/or not at all in villin-hPepT1 DSS-treated mice compared to their respective control groups. Beta tubulin, 50 kDa was used as a loading control (Fig. 4B). Immunofluorescence staining of Marcksl-1 protein expression (green) in FVB WT DSS mice compared to villin-hPepT1 DSS treated mice (Fig. 4C). Marcksl-1 (FITC - green), nuclear staining (DAPI - blue) and F-actin staining (TRITC - red) and separate pictures were taken at 40× for each filter and merged. Values represent means ± SEM of n = 6/group. $^{*}p<0.05$ and $^{***}p<0.0001$. Scale bar = 50 μm.

an increase in intestinal epithelial PepT1 expression enhanced the secretion of miRNA 23b from colonic tissue. Interestingly, up-regulated levels of colonic miRNA 23b secretion induced by intestinal epithelial hPepT1 expression remained higher in colonic tissue expressing hPepT1 compared with colonic tissue with no or low PepT1 expression (Fig. 5A and 5B).

Colonic miRNA 23b is actively up-taken by colonic macrophages

Next, we investigated the possible uptake of secreted colonic miRNA 23b by colonic macrophages. To examine this possibility, we labeled the 5′-end of dsmiRNA 23b with Cy3 and assessed its uptake behavior into macrophages. As shown in Figure 5C, Cy3-labeled miRNA 23b was effectively taken up by macrophages incubated in the presence of 50 nM Cy3-labeled miRNA 23b for 24 hours at 37°C and pH 7.2. In addition, miRNA 23b uptake by macrophages was inhibited at 4°C (Fig. 5D), indicating that it is an active energy-dependent process. We also observed that miRNA 23b uptake by macrophages occurs at pH 7.0, 7.2 or 7.8 (Fig. 5E), but not at pH 6.0 or 6.5 (Fig. 5F). This latter observation is consistent with an endocytosis-mediated uptake mechanism. Taken together, our results demonstrated that secreted colonic miRNA 23b may be actively taken up by macrophages via an endocytosis/phagocytosis-mediated mechanism.

MiRNA 23b directly targets the Marcksl-1 3′UTR in macrophages

To examine whether miRNA 23b directly targets the 3′UTR of Marcksl-1 mRNA, Marcksl-1 3′UTR was cloned into a luciferase reporter gene (Luc-Marcksl-1 3′UTR), and this construct was transfected into RAW 264.7 cells in the presence of miRNA 23b precursor or alone. The targeting of miRNAs to Marcksl-1 3′UTR was then assessed by measuring luciferase activity in these cells. As shown in Fig. 6, miRNA 23b co-transfected with Luc-Marcksl-1 3′UTR significantly reduced luciferase activity in macrophage cells after 24 h of transfection. In contrast, Luc-Marcksl-1 3′UTR luciferase activity remained unchanged. The reduction of luciferase activity indicated that miRNA 23b targeted Marcksl-1 in its 3′UTR.

Discussion

It has been recently reported that specific human colonic miRNAs are differentially expressed in IBD [30–32]. However, the mechanism underlying this deregulation has not been studied. To examine the effects of colonic PepT1 expression on colonic miRNA expression in untreated mice and in mice with DSS-induced colitis, we used a Tg mouse strain specifically overexpressing hPepT1, (villin-hPepT1) in colonic epithelial cells (IECs) driven by the villin promoter [10]. Our results show that

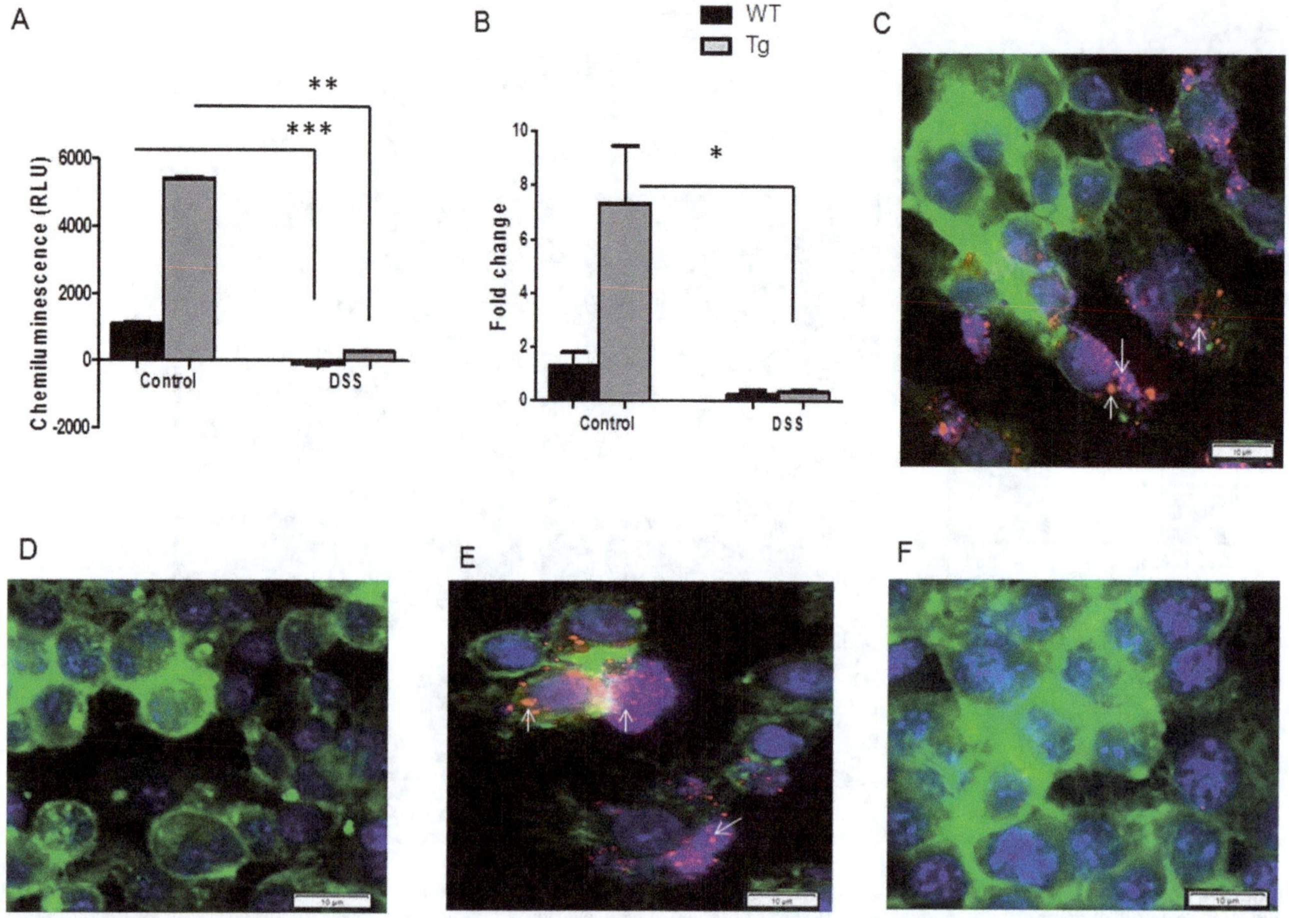

Figure 5. Secretory miRNA in colon culture medium. miRNA 23b in conditioned medium was measured by miRNA plate assay chemiluminescence method (Fig. 5A) and qRT-PCR (Fig. 5B). Cy3 labelled miRNA 23b uptake by macrophage (Fig. 5C). miRNA 23b uptake at 4°C (Fig. 5D), miRNA 23b uptake at pH 7.0 (Fig. 5E) and pH 6.5 (Fig. 5F). F-actin (FITC - green), nuclear staining (DAPI - blue) and Cy3 labelled miRNA 23b (TRITC -filter setting used) are stained and separate pictures were taken at 60× for each filter and merged respectively. Values represent means ± SEM of n = 6/group. *$p<0.05$, **$p<0.001$ and ***$p<0.0001$. Scale bar = 10 μm.

overexpression of PepT1 in IECs alters the profile of miRNA expression in colonic cells, including both epithelial and non-epithelial cells such as intestinal macrophages. In contrast, the expression of miRNAs in non-colonic tissues was not affected in villin-hPepT1 mice. This latter observation demonstrates that the expression of intestinal epithelial PepT1 specifically deregulates the expression of colonic miRNAs. Our results demonstrate that expression of a specific protein involved in IBD (PepT1) may

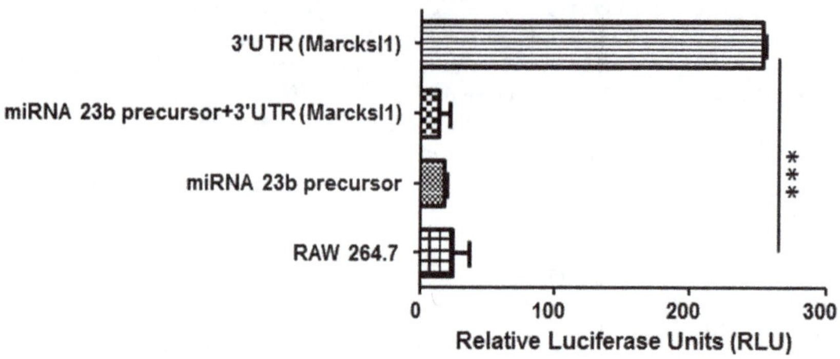

Figure 6. MiR-23b directly targets the Marcksl-1 3′UTR in macrophages. Marcksl-1 3′UTR was cloned into a luciferase reporter gene (Luc-Marcksl-1 3′UTR), and transfected into RAW 264.7 cells in the presence or absence of miRNA 23b precursor. The targeting of miRNAs to Marcksl-1 3′UTR was then assessed by measuring luciferase activity in these cells. The miRNA 23b co-transfected with Luc-Marcksl-1 3′UTR significantly reduced luciferase activity in macrophage cells after 24 h of transfection. In contrast, Luc-Marcksl-1 3′UTR had an increase of luciferase activity. Values represent means ± SEM of n = 3 and ***$p<0.0001$.

deregulate colonic miRNAs under conditions of both active (DSS) and non-active (without DSS) inflammation. Interestingly, these changes were initiated by intestinal epithelial PepT1 expression. These data predict that in a disease state such as intestinal inflammation, IECs over-expressing PepT1 can communicate directly with IECs and/or indirectly through cell/cell interactions; hence, epithelial PepT1 affects miRNA expression in other cells that are in contact with IECs. For example, recent studies have shown that extracellular vesicles contain functional mRNA, miRNA, and DNA molecules that can be taken up by target (acceptor) cells, indicating that these vesicles are a main mechanism for cell-to-cell communication [52–56]. It has recently been demonstrated by Kosaka *et al.* and other groups, that a tumor-suppressive miRNA is secreted and transported between cells to impose a gene-silencing effect on recipient cells [44,45,57]. miRNAs have been found in extracellular space such as plasma, urine, saliva and constitute a form of cell-cell communication [58–61]. Although we do not understand the cellular machinery responsible for the secretion of miRNAs, it is known that they are packaged into exosomes, microvesicles and apoptotic bodies by a broad range of cell types [62–64]. Intriguingly, most extracellular miRNAs are found outside of any lipid-containing vesicle. They are rather associated with RNA-binding proteins (*e.g.*, Argonaute 1 and 2), which may help protect them from the abundant nucleases found in the extracellular space [65]. It has been previously shown by others that under laboratory conditions colon tissues can be cultured and shown to maintain viability [66–68]. Here, we demonstrated that colonic tissue secretes miRNA 23b and this secretion is regulated by the expression of intestinal epithelial hPepT1. Interestingly, we have demonstrated that miRNA 23b is actively taken up by macrophages, presumably through endocytosis. In addition, we have demonstrated that miRNA 23b directly targets the Marcksl-1 3′UTR in macrophages. Our results suggest that IECs may secrete miRNAs that are taken up by other cell types such as macrophages, resulting in regulation of recipient cell target genes such as Marcksl-1.

It has been previously shown that miRNA 23a and miRNA 23b are involved in active ulcerative colitis [46] and chronically active Crohn's disease [32]. These results are consistent with the observed colonic expression of miRNA 23a and 23b in WT and villin-hPepT1 mice with or without DSS treatment (Fig. 2A). Macrophage expression of Marcksl-1, one of the predicted target genes of miRNA 23a and 23b (Table S2), has been suggested to protect the intestine against inflammation [49]. Interestingly, we have observed that, although Marcksl-1 is specifically expressed in macrophages [48], its mRNA and protein expression profile are altered during disease conditions in hPepT1 Tg mouse model. We have indeed demonstrated that Marcksl-1 expression is increased to a lesser extent in intestinal macrophages during DSS-induced colitis in villin-hPepT1 mice than in WT mice. This observation may suggest that Marcksl-1 expression in intestinal macrophages is repressed by the more prominent elevation of miRNA 23b in inflamed villin-hPepT1 mice compared with inflamed WT mice. In addition, the low expression of Marcksl-1 in intestinal macrophages in villin-hPepT1 mice under colitis conditions may explain the greater degree of intestinal inflammation in these mice that over-express PepT1 in IECs.

Herein, we have shown that miRNA 23b expression levels were higher in the colonic tissues (but not other tissues) of villin-hPepT1 mice compared to WT mice, regardless of DSS treatment. Thus, overexpression of intestinal epithelial PepT1 specifically up-regulated colonic miRNA 23b in villin-hPepT1 mice. MiRNA-23b expression was lower in DSS-treated villin-hPepT1 mice compared to untreated villin-hPepT1 mice. However, miRNA 23b expression was higher in DSS-treated villin-hPepT1 mice compared to DSS-treated WT mice. The latter observation suggests that the level of miRNA 23b expression in DSS-treated villin-hPepT1 mice (but not that in DSS-treated WT mice) could be sufficient to target and repress Marcksl-1 expression, which is lower in DSS-treated villin-hPepT1 mice than in DSS-treated WT mice (Figure 4B and 4C). However, miRNA-23b over-expression in untreated villin-hPepT1 mice does not appear to affect Marcksl-1 expression, which is extremely low in non-inflamed intestine (Figure 4C). Collectively, these results show that local expression of a specific colonic protein may affect colonic miRNA expression/secretion. In addition, colonic miRNA expression/secretion, regulated by intestinal epithelial PepT1, may play an important role in cell-to-cell communication during colitis. Together, these results suggest that miRNA-23b expression may play a role in regulating Marcksl-1 during intestinal inflammation.

Supporting Information

Table S1 List of miRNAs differentially expressed in microRNA microarray. The transcripts listed in the table having a statistically significant *p*-value of $p<0.1$ and having a signal of >500.

Table S2 The potential mRNA targets for the nine selected miRNA were obtained from 3 different software Pictar, MicroCosm and Targetscan. The common protein list was obtained from matchminer program by determining the genes that were identified by at least two algorithms. A total of 704 genes were potentially regulated by the 9 miRNA revealed from this software. These miRNA were sub-divided into two groups based on their expression levels in either FVB WT or villin-hPepT1 mice upon DSS treatment.

Table S3 DAVID functional annotation clustering of villin-hPepT1 and FVB WT at basal level. The common obtained from the matchminer software proteins were clustered into 30 groups.

Table S4 DAVID functional annotation clustering of villin-hPepT1 and FVB WT mice treated with DSS. The common proteins obtained from the matchminer software were clustered into 15 groups.

Table S5 List of primers used in this study.

Author Contributions

Conceived and designed the experiments: SA DM. Performed the experiments: SA MC BX. Analyzed the data: SA MC EV YZ DM. Contributed reagents/materials/analysis tools: SA DM. Wrote the paper: SA DM.

References

1. Dalmasso G, Nguyen HT, Charrier-Hisamuddin L, Yan Y, Laroui H, et al. (2010) PepT1 mediates transport of the proinflammatory bacterial tripeptide L-Ala-{gamma}-D-Glu-meso-DAP in intestinal epithelial cells. Am J Physiol Gastrointest Liver Physiol 299: G687–696.

2. Buyse M, Tsocas A, Walker F, Merlin D, Bado A (2002) PepT1-mediated fMLP transport induces intestinal inflammation in vivo. Am J Physiol Cell Physiol 283: C1795–1800.
3. Buyse M, Charrier L, Sitaraman S, Gewirtz A, Merlin D (2003) Interferon-gamma increases hPepT1-mediated uptake of di-tripeptides including the bacterial tripeptide fMLP in polarized intestinal epithelia. Am J Pathol 163: 1969–1977.
4. Merlin D, Si-Tahar M, Sitaraman SV, Eastburn K, Williams I, et al. (2001) Colonic epithelial hPepT1 expression occurs in inflammatory bowel disease: transport of bacterial peptides influences expression of MHC class 1 molecules. Gastroenterology 120: 1666–1679.
5. Ziegler TR, Fernandez-Estivariz C, Gu LH, Bazargan N, Umeakunne K, et al. (2002) Distribution of the H+/peptide transporter PepT1 in human intestine: up-regulated expression in the colonic mucosa of patients with short-bowel syndrome. Am J Clin Nutr 75: 922–930.
6. Wojtal KA, Eloranta JJ, Hruz P, Gutmann H, Drewe J, et al. (2009) Changes in mRNA expression levels of solute carrier transporters in inflammatory bowel disease patients. Drug metabolism and disposition: the biological fate of chemicals 37: 1871–1877.
7. Wang P LY, Wen Y, Yu DY, Ge L, Dong WR, et al. (2013) IL-16 Induces Intestinal Inflammation via PepT1 Upregulation in a Pufferfish Model: New Insights into the Molecular Mechanism of Inflammatory Bowel Disease. journal of immunology. pp. 1413–1427.
8. Zucchelli M, Torkvist L, Bresso F, Halfvarson J, Hellquist A, et al. (2009) PepT1 oligopeptide transporter (SLC15A1) gene polymorphism in inflammatory bowel disease. Inflamm Bowel Dis 15: 1562–1569.
9. Ayyadurai S, Charania MA, Xiao B, Viennois E, Merlin D (2013) PepT1 expressed in immune cells has an important role in promoting the immune response during experimentally induced colitis. Lab Invest 93: 888–899.
10. Dalmasso G, Nguyen HT, Ingersoll SA, Ayyadurai S, Laroui H, et al. (2011) The PepT1-NOD2 signaling pathway aggravates induced colitis in mice. Gastroenterology 141: 1334–1345.
11. Yan Y, Kolachala V, Dalmasso G, Nguyen H, Laroui H, et al. (2009) Temporal and spatial analysis of clinical and molecular parameters in dextran sodium sulfate induced colitis. PLoS One 4: e6073.
12. Dalmasso G, Charrier-Hisamuddin L, Nguyen HT, Yan Y, Sitaraman S, et al. (2008) PepT1-mediated tripeptide KPV uptake reduces intestinal inflammation. Gastroenterology 134: 166–178.
13. Laroui H, Dalmasso G, Nguyen HT, Yan Y, Sitaraman SV, et al. (2010) Drug-loaded nanoparticles targeted to the colon with polysaccharide hydrogel reduce colitis in a mouse model. Gastroenterology 138: 843–853 e841–842.
14. Laroui H, Ingersoll SA, Liu HC, Baker MT, Ayyadurai S, et al. (2012) Dextran sodium sulfate (DSS) induces colitis in mice by forming nano-lipocomplexes with medium-chain-length fatty acids in the colon. PLoS One 7: e32084.
15. Lee RC, Feinbaum RL, Ambros V (1993) The C. elegans heterochronic gene lin-4 encodes small RNAs with antisense complementarity to lin-14. Cell 75: 843–854.
16. Wightman B, Ha I, Ruvkun G (1993) Posttranscriptional regulation of the heterochronic gene lin-14 by lin-4 mediates temporal pattern formation in C. elegans. Cell 75: 855–862.
17. Wu WK, Law PT, Lee CW, Cho CH, Fan D, et al. (2011) MicroRNA in colorectal cancer: from benchtop to bedside. Carcinogenesis 32: 247–253.
18. Ambros V (2001) microRNAs: tiny regulators with great potential. Cell 107: 823–826.
19. Bartel DP (2004) MicroRNAs: genomics, biogenesis, mechanism, and function. Cell 116: 281–297.
20. Davis BN, Hata A (2009) Regulation of MicroRNA Biogenesis: A miRiad of mechanisms. Cell communication and signaling : CCS 7: 18.
21. Lim LP, Lau NC, Garrett-Engele P, Grimson A, Schelter JM, et al. (2005) Microarray analysis shows that some microRNAs downregulate large numbers of target mRNAs. Nature 433: 769–773.
22. Baek D, Villen J, Shin C, Camargo FD, Gygi SP, et al. (2008) The impact of microRNAs on protein output. Nature 455: 64–71.
23. Lewis BP, Shih IH, Jones-Rhoades MW, Bartel DP, Burge CB (2003) Prediction of mammalian microRNA targets. Cell 115: 787–798.
24. Lewis BP, Burge CB, Bartel DP (2005) Conserved seed pairing, often flanked by adenosines, indicates that thousands of human genes are microRNA targets. Cell 120: 15–20.
25. Taganov KD, Boldin MP, Baltimore D (2007) MicroRNAs and immunity: tiny players in a big field. Immunity 26: 133–137.
26. Stefani G, Slack FJ (2008) Small non-coding RNAs in animal development. Nature reviews Molecular cell biology 9: 219–230.
27. Bueno MJ, Perez de Castro I, Malumbres M (2008) Control of cell proliferation pathways by microRNAs. Cell Cycle 7: 3143–3148.
28. Dalmasso G, Nguyen HT, Yan Y, Laroui H, Srinivasan S, et al. (2010) MicroRNAs determine human intestinal epithelial cell fate. Differentiation 80: 147–154.
29. McKenna LB, Schug J, Vourekas A, McKenna JB, Bramswig NC, et al. (2010) MicroRNAs control intestinal epithelial differentiation, architecture, and barrier function. Gastroenterology 139: 1654–1664, 1664 e1651.
30. Dalal SR, Kwon JH (2010) The Role of MicroRNA in Inflammatory Bowel Disease. Gastroenterology & hepatology 6: 714–722.
31. Pekow JR, Kwon JH (2012) MicroRNAs in inflammatory bowel disease. Inflammatory bowel diseases 18: 187–193.
32. Wu F, Zhang S, Dassopoulos T, Harris ML, Bayless TM, et al. (2010) Identification of microRNAs associated with ileal and colonic Crohn's disease. Inflammatory bowel diseases 16: 1729–1738.
33. Bartels CL, Tsongalis GJ (2009) MicroRNAs: novel biomarkers for human cancer. Clinical chemistry 55: 623–631.
34. Bartels CL, Tsongalis GJ (2010) [MicroRNAs: novel biomarkers for human cancer]. Annales de biologie clinique 68: 263–272.
35. Nguyen HT, Dalmasso G, Yan Y, Laroui H, Dahan S, et al. (2010) MicroRNA-7 modulates CD98 expression during intestinal epithelial cell differentiation. J Biol Chem 285: 1479–1489.
36. Lagos-Quintana M, Rauhut R, Yalcin A, Meyer J, Lendeckel W, et al. (2002) Identification of tissue-specific microRNAs from mouse. Current biology : CB 12: 735–739.
37. Charania MA, Ayyadurai S, Ingersoll SA, Xiao B, Viennois E, et al. (2012) Intestinal epithelial CD98 synthesis specifically modulates expression of colonic microRNAs during colitis. Am J Physiol Gastrointest Liver Physiol 302: G1282–1291.
38. Viennois E, Chen F, Laroui H, Baker MT, Merlin D (2013) Dextran sodium sulfate inhibits the activities of both polymerase and reverse transcriptase: lithium chloride purification, a rapid and efficient technique to purify RNA. BMC Res Notes 6: 360.
39. Krek A, Grun D, Poy MN, Wolf R, Rosenberg L, et al. (2005) Combinatorial microRNA target predictions. Nat Genet 37: 495–500.
40. Griffiths-Jones S, Saini HK, van Dongen S, Enright AJ (2008) miRBase: tools for microRNA genomics. Nucleic Acids Res 36: D154–158.
41. Grimson A, Farh KK, Johnston WK, Garrett-Engele P, Lim LP, et al. (2007) MicroRNA targeting specificity in mammals: determinants beyond seed pairing. Mol Cell 27: 91–105.
42. Bussey KJ, Kane D, Sunshine M, Narasimhan S, Nishizuka S, et al. (2003) MatchMiner: a tool for batch navigation among gene and gene product identifiers. Genome biology 4: R27.
43. Huang da W, Sherman BT, Lempicki RA (2009) Systematic and integrative analysis of large gene lists using DAVID bioinformatics resources. Nature protocols 4: 44–57.
44. Kosaka N, Iguchi H, Yoshioka Y, Hagiwara K, Takeshita F, et al. (2012) Competitive interactions of cancer cells and normal cells via secretory microRNAs. The Journal of biological chemistry 287: 1397–1405.
45. Kosaka N, Iguchi H, Yoshioka Y, Takeshita F, Matsuki Y, et al. (2010) Secretory mechanisms and intercellular transfer of microRNAs in living cells. The Journal of biological chemistry 285: 17442–17452.
46. Wu F, Zikusoka M, Trindade A, Dassopoulos T, Harris ML, et al. (2008) MicroRNAs are differentially expressed in ulcerative colitis and alter expression of macrophage inflammatory peptide-2 alpha. Gastroenterology 135: 1624–1635 e1624.
47. Wu F, Zhang S, Dassopoulos T, Harris ML, Bayless TM, et al. (2010) Identification of microRNAs associated with ileal and colonic Crohn's disease. Inflamm Bowel Dis 16: 1729–1738.
48. Li J, Aderem A (1992) MacMARCKS, a novel member of the MARCKS family of protein kinase C substrates. Cell 70: 791–801.
49. Fang K, Bruce M, Pattillo CB, Zhang S, Stone R 2nd, et al. (2011) Temporal genomewide expression profiling of DSS colitis reveals novel inflammatory and angiogenesis genes similar to ulcerative colitis. Physiological genomics 43: 43–56.
50. Saban R, D'Andrea MR, Andrade-Gordon P, Derian CK, Dozmorov I, et al. (2007) Regulatory network of inflammation downstream of proteinase-activated receptors. BMC physiology 7: 3.
51. Wang J, Jarrett J, Huang CC, Satcher RL Jr, Levenson AS (2007) Identification of estrogen-responsive genes involved in breast cancer metastases to the bone. Clinical & experimental metastasis 24: 411–422.
52. Valadi H, Ekstrom K, Bossios A, Sjostrand M, Lee JJ, et al. (2007) Exosome-mediated transfer of mRNAs and microRNAs is a novel mechanism of genetic exchange between cells. Nat Cell Biol 9: 654–659.
53. Mittelbrunn M, Gutierrez-Vazquez C, Villarroya-Beltri C, Gonzalez S, Sanchez-Cabo F, et al. (2011) Unidirectional transfer of microRNA-loaded exosomes from T cells to antigen-presenting cells. Nat Commun 2: 282.
54. Montecalvo A, Larregina AT, Shufesky WJ, Stolz DB, Sullivan ML, et al. (2012) Mechanism of transfer of functional microRNAs between mouse dendritic cells via exosomes. Blood 119: 756–766.
55. Baj-Krzyworzeka M, Szatanek R, Weglarczyk K, Baran J, Urbanowicz B, et al. (2006) Tumour-derived microvesicles carry several surface determinants and mRNA of tumour cells and transfer some of these determinants to monocytes. Cancer Immunol Immunother 55: 808–818.
56. Ehnfors J, Kost-Alimova M, Persson NL, Bergsmedh A, Castro J, et al. (2009) Horizontal transfer of tumor DNA to endothelial cells in vivo. Cell Death Differ 16: 749–757.
57. Furuta K, Lichtenberger R, Helariutta Y (2012) The role of mobile small RNA species during root growth and development. Current opinion in cell biology 24: 211–216.
58. Jin XF, Wu N, Wang L, Li J (2013) Circulating microRNAs: a novel class of potential biomarkers for diagnosing and prognosing central nervous system diseases. Cell Mol Neurobiol 33: 601–613.
59. Lasser C (2013) Identification and analysis of circulating exosomal microRNA in human body fluids. Methods Mol Biol 1024: 109–128.

60. Luo X, Stock C, Burwinkel B, Brenner H (2013) Identification and evaluation of plasma MicroRNAs for early detection of colorectal cancer. PLoS One 8: e62880.
61. Moldovan L, Batte K, Wang Y, Wisler J, Piper M (2013) Analyzing the circulating microRNAs in exosomes/extracellular vesicles from serum or plasma by qRT-PCR. Methods Mol Biol 1024: 129–145.
62. Hannafon BN, Ding WQ (2013) Intercellular Communication by Exosome-Derived microRNAs in Cancer. Int J Mol Sci 14: 14240–14269.
63. Chen X, Liang H, Zhang J, Zen K, Zhang CY (2012) Secreted microRNAs: a new form of intercellular communication. Trends Cell Biol 22: 125–132.
64. Muralidharan-Chari V, Clancy JW, Sedgwick A, D'Souza-Schorey C (2010) Microvesicles: mediators of extracellular communication during cancer progression. J Cell Sci 123: 1603–1611.
65. Chatterjee S, Fasler M, Bussing I, Grosshans H (2011) Target-mediated protection of endogenous microRNAs in C. elegans. Dev Cell 20: 388–396.
66. Dame MK, Bhagavathula N, Mankey C, DaSilva M, Paruchuri T, et al. (2010) Human colon tissue in organ culture: preservation of normal and neoplastic characteristics. In Vitro Cell Dev Biol Anim 46: 114–122.
67. Nguyen HT, Dalmasso G, Powell KR, Yan Y, Bhatt S, et al. (2009) Pathogenic bacteria induce colonic PepT1 expression: an implication in host defense response. Gastroenterology 137: 1435–1447 e1431-1432.
68. Charania MA, Laroui H, Liu H, Viennois E, Ayyadurai S, et al. (2013) Intestinal epithelial CD98 directly modulates the innate host response to enteric bacterial pathogens. Infect Immun 81: 923–934.

21

Ginsenoside Metabolite Compound K Promotes Recovery of Dextran Sulfate Sodium-Induced Colitis and Inhibits Inflammatory Responses by Suppressing NF-κB Activation

Juan Li[1], Wei Zhong[1], Weiwei Wang[1], Shaoping Hu[1], Jiahui Yuan[1], Bing Zhang[2], Tianhui Hu[1]*, Gang Song[1]*

1 Cancer Research Center, Medical College of Xiamen University, Xiamen, China, **2** Department of Basic Medicine, Medical College of Xiamen University, Xiamen, China

Abstract

Phytogenic compounds with anti-oxidant and anti-inflammatory properties, such as ginsenoside metabolite compound K (CK) or berberine (BBR), are currently discussed as promising complementary agents in the prevention and treatment of cancer and inflammation. The latest study showed that ginsenoside Rb1 and its metabolites could inhibit TNBS-induced colitis injury. However, the functional mechanisms of anti-inflammation effects of ginsenoside, particularly its metabolite CK are still not clear. Here, using dextran sulfate sodium (DSS)-induced colitis in mice, clinical parameters, intestinal integrity, pro-inflammatory cytokines production, and signaling pathways in colonic tissues were determined. In mild and sever colitis mice, CK and BBR (as a positive agent) alleviated colitis histopathology injury, ameliorated myeloperoxidase (MPO) activity, reduced pro-inflammatory cytokines production, such as, IL-6, IL-1β, TNF-α, and increased anti-inflammatory cytokine IL-10 production in both mice colon tissues and blood. Nevertheless, the results revealed that CK and BBR inhibited NF-κB p65 nuclear translocation, downregulated p-IκBα and upregulated IκBα, indicating that CK, as well as BBR, suppressed the activation of the NF-κB pathway in the progression of colitis with immunofluorescence, immunohistochemical and western blotting analysis. Furthermore, CK inhibited pro-inflammatory cytokines production in LPS-activated macrophages *via* down-regulation of NF-κB signaling pathway. Taken together, our results not only reveal that CK promotes the recovery of the progression of colitis and inhibits the inflammatory responses by suppressing NF-κB activation, but also suggest that CK downregulates intestinal inflammation through regulating the activation of macrophages and pro-inflammatory cytokines production.

Editor: Lucienne Chatenoud, Université Paris Descartes, France

Funding: This work was supported by the grants from the National Natural Science Foundation of China (31071187, 81172284, 81272721), the Fundamental Research Funds for the Central Universities (2010121102), Xiamen Municipal Science and Technology Innovation Fund Project (3502Z20114018), and the Program for New Century Excellent Talents in Fujian Province University. The funders had no role in study design, data collection and analysis, decision to publish, or preparation of the manuscript.

Competing Interests: The authors have declared that no competing interests exist.

* E-mail: thu@xmu.edu.cn (TH); gangsongsd@xmu.edu.cn (GS)

Introduction

Inflammatory bowel disease (IBD), which includes ulcerative colitis and Crohn's disease, is associated with chronic, relapsing inflammation of the intestinal tract. Evidence from immunological, microbiological, and genetic studies suggest that IBD results from dysregulation of the mucosal immune system leading to excessive immunological responses to intestinal microflora, or changes in the composition of intestinal microflora and/or deranged epithelial barrier function that elicits pathological responses from the normal mucosal immune system in genetically susceptible hosts [1–5]. Nevertheless, acute intestinal inflammation is usually followed by physiologic healing of the damaged tissue and restoration of the normal structure and function of the intestine [6]. If the innate physiologic healing doesn't work, acute inflammation can develop and character by continues events of injury, which associated with the innate immune system responses [7]. Moreover, in IBD and experimental model of autoimmune colitis in mice, when the innate immune responses are initiated by inflammation lesions, innate immune cells such as macrophage and intestinal epithelium cells will secret several cytokines and chemokines, including IL-6, IL-1β, TNF-α, which trigger the adaptive immune system including T and B cell-mediated responses [6–8]. Strikingly, unrestrained reaction may exaggerate inflammatory response and lead to intestinal damage [9]. Therefore, appropriate regulation of the innate immune reaction is very important to the severity of inflammation, so a clear understanding of the mechanism of the development and progression of IBD and colitis is crucial for researching new effective drugs on its therapy.

Nowadays, lots of Chinese herbal medicines, such as ginsenosides and berberine (BBR), have shown various beneficial therapy effects, including cancers and inflammations [10–17]. Compound K (20-O-beta-D-glucopyranosyl-20(S)-protopanaxadiol (structure shown in Fig. 1A) is the main metabolite of the protopanaxadiol type of ginsenoside produced by intestinal bacteria after oral

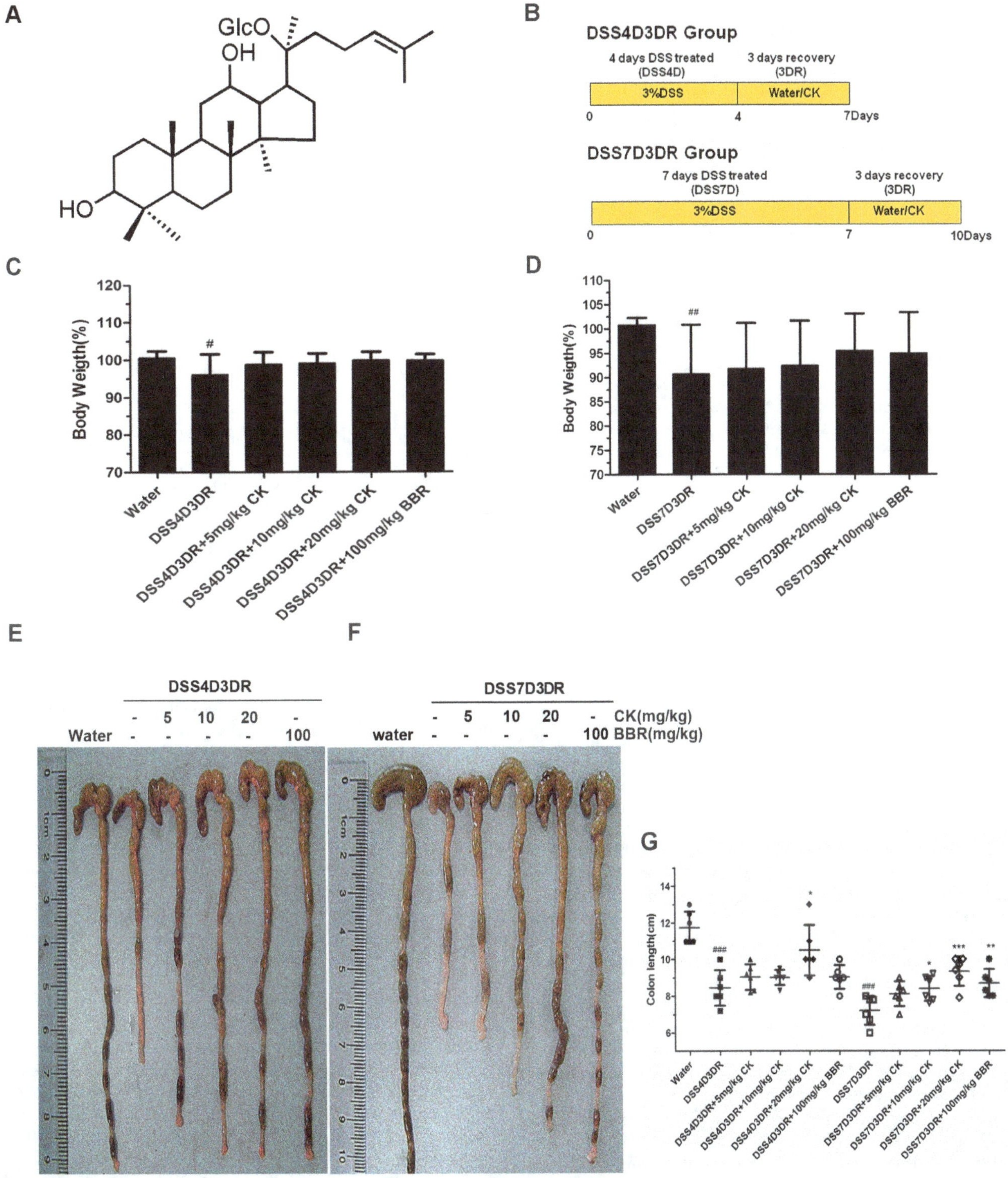

Figure 1. Anti-inflammatory influences of CK in DSS-induced colitis in mice. (A) The chemical structure of CK. The structure was elucidated to be 20-O-(β-D-glucopyranosyl)-20(S)-protopanaxadiol. (B) DSS-induced intestinal injury and inflammation in mice. Mice were administered 3% DSS in drinking water to induce colitis. CK and BBR were intraperitoneal injection for mild colitis group (4-day DSS treatment and 3-day recovery) and severe colitis group (7-day DSS treatment and 3-day recovery). Control mice received water alone. (C) The body weight of mild colitis mice were measured every day and presented as percentage of original body weight. Mild colitis mice: 4-day DSS treatment and 3-day recovery, from day 1 to day 7. (D) The body weight of mice were measured every day and presented as percentage of original body weight. Severe colitis mice: 7-day DSS treatment and 3-day recovery, from day 1 to day 10. (E) The colon morphology of mild colitis group. (F) The colon morphology of severe colitis group. (G) The lengths of colon were measured when mice were euthanized. n = 6. # $p<0.05$ compared with the control group. ## $p<0.01$, ### $p<0.001$ compared with the control group. *p compared with DSS4D3DR or DSS7D3DR group. *$p<0.05$, **$p<0.01$, ***$p<0.001$.

administration of ginseng extracts and is speculated to be the major form of protopanaxadiol saponin absorbed from the intestine [10,11]. Several studies have shown that CK possesses various chemopreventive and chemotherapeutic activities, including attenuation of hepatic lipid accumulation [11], antigenotoxicity and anticlastogenicity [12], reverse of multidrug resistance [13], and antitumor action [14,15]. Our previous work have confirmed the effects of CK on suppression of hepatocellular carcinoma cells survival and its mechanisms of anti-metastatic growth associated with NF-κB p65 nuclear export and the inhibition of MMP2/9 expression [13]. Moreover, CK can also inhibitgrowth of gastric carcinoma and colorectal cancer (CRC) via regulating different pathways [10,14,15]. A latest study indicated that ginsenoside Rb1 and its metabolites inhibited TNBS-induced colitis injury, and reduced pro-inflammatory cytokines production in colon tissues [12]. However, the functional mechanisms of anti-inflammation effects of ginsenoside, especially its metabolites, are still not clear. The purpose of this work was to determine the inhibitory effects of CK on the progression of DSS-induced colitis, and to explore its efficiency mechanism. In this study, 4 days DSS-induced mild colitis mice and 7 days DSS-induced sever colitis mice *in vivo* and RAW 264.7 macrophages *in vitro* were used.

BBR (C20H19NO5) is an isoquinoline alkaloid isolated from coptidis rhizoma and cortex phellodendri [16,17]. Previous studies have reported that BBR have therapeutic effects on DSS-induced colitis, including amelioration of colon injury, decrease of pro-inflammatory cytokines production and inhibition of the NF-κB pathway activation in colon tissues. BBR alsopromoted the peritoneal macrophage apoptosis, and regulated inflammatory responses by decreasing pro-inflammatory cytokines production in colonic macrophages and epithelial cells [1]. Thus, BBR was used as a positive agent for treating colitis mice here.

Our data showed that both in mild colitis groups and sever colitis groups, CK potently alleviated the colon histomorphology injury, promoted the recovery of the colitis and reduced pro-inflammatory cytokines production in a concentration-dependent manner. In addition, immunofluorescence, immunohistochemical and western blotting analysis indicated that CK inhibited colon tissues' NF-κB pathway activation in a concentration-dependent manner. As in the inflammation function cycle, the macrophages stimulated and secreted cytokines and then regulated the innate inflammatory systems [18,19]. According to what we have found, and to verify the functional mechanisms of CK in the intestinal disorder, LPS-stimulated macrophages (RAW 264.7 cells) treated with or without CK or BBR for 10 h, and then cytokines production and signaling pathways were determined *in vitro*. The results demonstrated that CK reduced the pro-inflammatory cytokines levels in LPS-stimulated macrophages by suppressing NF-κB activation in a dose-dependent manner.

Based on the existing data concerning CK, our present study assessed anti-colitis activity of CK with different inflammatory indexes and determined that CK promotes the recovery of colitis in mice associated with regulation of innate immune cells, such as macrophages, by suppressing NF-κB pathway activation. These finding may provide new point on CK treated intestinal inflammatory disorder.

Materials and Methods

Mice and Ethics Statement

Male BALB/C mice, weighing 180–200 g were used between periods of 3–5 weeks. All experimental mice were maintained under SPF conditions and raised under standard conditions (12-hour day-night rhythm) in Xiamen University Laboratory Animal Center. All animal procedures were approved by the Animal Care and Use Committee of Xiamen University (license No: SYXK [Min] 2008-0003, issued on May 6, 2008).

Reagents and Cell Culture

Dextran Sulfate Sodium (molecular weight 36–50 kDa, MP Biomedical, Solon, OH), CK (CK was prepared and identified as in our previous publication (Fig. 1A, >98% pure as determined by HPLC) and BBR (Sigma-Aldrich, St. Louis, MO) were prepared and identified as in our previous publications [1,13]. Antibodies NF-κB (p65) and IκBa were provided by Santa Cruz. p-IκBα purchased from Cell Signaling. The mouse RAW 264.7 macrophage cell line was obtained from the Institute of Biochemistry and Cell Biology, Chinese Academy of Sciences in Shanghai, and was cultured in DMEM medium containing 10% FBS, 1% glutamine, 100,000 IU/l penicillin, and 100 mg/l streptomycin at 37°C with 5% CO_2 and 95% air.

DSS-induced Colitis in Mice and CK Treatment

The curative effects of CK were investigated in the male BALB/C mice. The mice were divided into twelve groups, those are, normal control group and mild DSS-induced colitis groups (DSS four days) and sever colitis groups (DSS seven days) treated with or without CK (5, 10 or 20 mg/kg) or BBR (100 mg/kg). Colitis were induced by the orally administered of 3% (w/v) DSS solution double distilled water every day. The normal control group was treated with double distilled water alone. CK (5, 10 or 20 mg/kg) or BBR (100 mg/kg) was intraperitoneal injection into mice every day after DSS treatment to the day before sacrifice for 3 days. To assess the extent to which colitis was induced, the mice were examined daily for body weight, stool consistency, and blood in the stool.

Analysis of Colon Injury

Paraffin-embedded tissue sections of Swiss-rolled whole colon (rolled from the distal end to the proximal end) were stained with hematoxylin and eosin for light microscopic examination to assess colon injury and inflammation. Samples from the entire colon were examined by a pathologist blinded to treatment conditions. A modified combined scoring system including degree of inflammation (scale of 0–3) and crypt damage (0–4), percentage of area involved by inflammation (0–4) and crypt damage (0–4), and depth of inflammation (0–3) was applied for assessing colitis induced by DSS. The total score is 0 (normal) to 18 (severe colitis).

Blood Samples and Mice Tissues

7 days and 10 days after CK injection, the mice were scarified, a 1 ml sample of orbital blood were collected and the abdomens were opened along the median line, and then was rapidly excised, the colon gently with ice-cold PBS, placed on ice, and opened longitudinally. The colon was incised, and the fecal contents were washed out gently with of PBS. The blood samples were injected into dry test tubes and separated by centrifugation, and the serum was stored at −80°C until use. And then the colon was embed into the dry tubes and stored at −80°C until use.

Immunofluorescence Staining

The colon tissues were fixed in 10% formaldehyde and embedded in paraffin. Tissue sections were permeabilized and blocked in PBS containing 0.3% Triton X-100 (Sigma-Aldrich, Milwaukee, WI) and 10% goat serum, followed by staining with primary antibodies for p65 (1:300) over night at 4°C and an Cy3

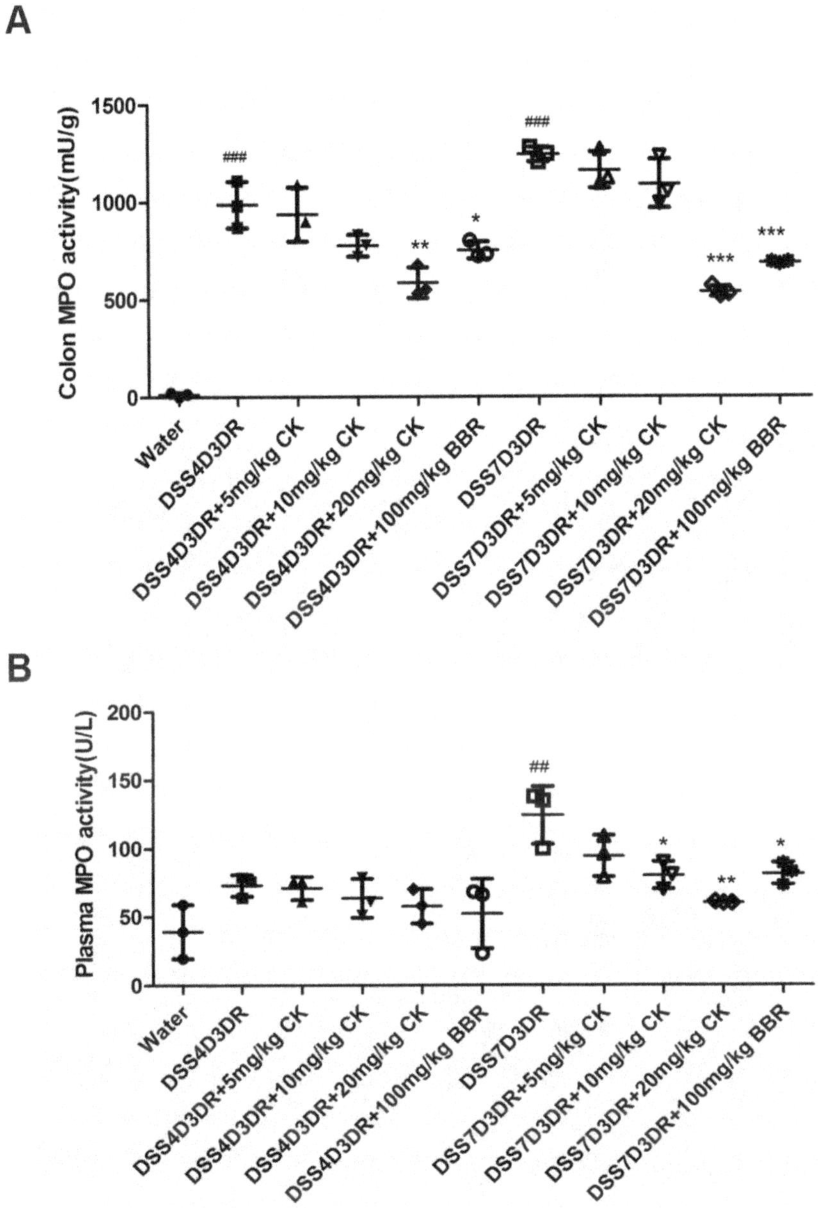

Figure 2. The MPO levels in colon tissues and mice plasma. (A) The levels of MPO in colon tissues. (B) The levels of MPO in mice plasma. ## $p<0.01$, ### $p<0.01$ compared with the control group. *p compared with DSS4D3DR or DSS7D3DR group. n = 3. *$p<0.05$, **$p<0.01$, ***$p<0.001$.

secondary antibody (1:200). p65 proteins were then detected and immunolocalized using Vectashield Mounting Medium containing DAPI. All the sections observed using fluorescence microscopy. Cultured cells immunofluorescence staining was performed as previously described [14]. Image-pro plus software was used to quantify the staining density. Based on the principles of equidistance, we randomly chose five views of distal end of colon in each section using 20X image, quantified the IOD and then averaged IOD of each section. Every group has prepared 10 sections. The averaged IOD of each group was compared by Student's t-test.

Immunohistochemical Staining

The colon tissues sections immunohistochemical staining was performed as previously described [13,14]. As a negative control, the primary antibody was replaced with normal mouse IgG. The method of quantify the staining density is the same as immunofluorescence staining analysis.

Detection of MPO Activity in Colon Tissues and Blood Plasma

This performs of MPO activity as described by the manufacturer (Nanjing Jiancheng Bioengineering Institute, China). Briefly, the colon was weighted, fixed with 19 fold phosphate buffer two, homogenated. The blood plasma mixed with buffer two in 1:1. And then, both of them 0.9 mL homogenate added 0.1 mL buffer three, homogenated and putted in the 37°C water bath for 15 min. According to the protocol, buffer four, TMB Substrate and buffer six were fixed in ration, mixed and putted in the 60°C water bath for 10 min.

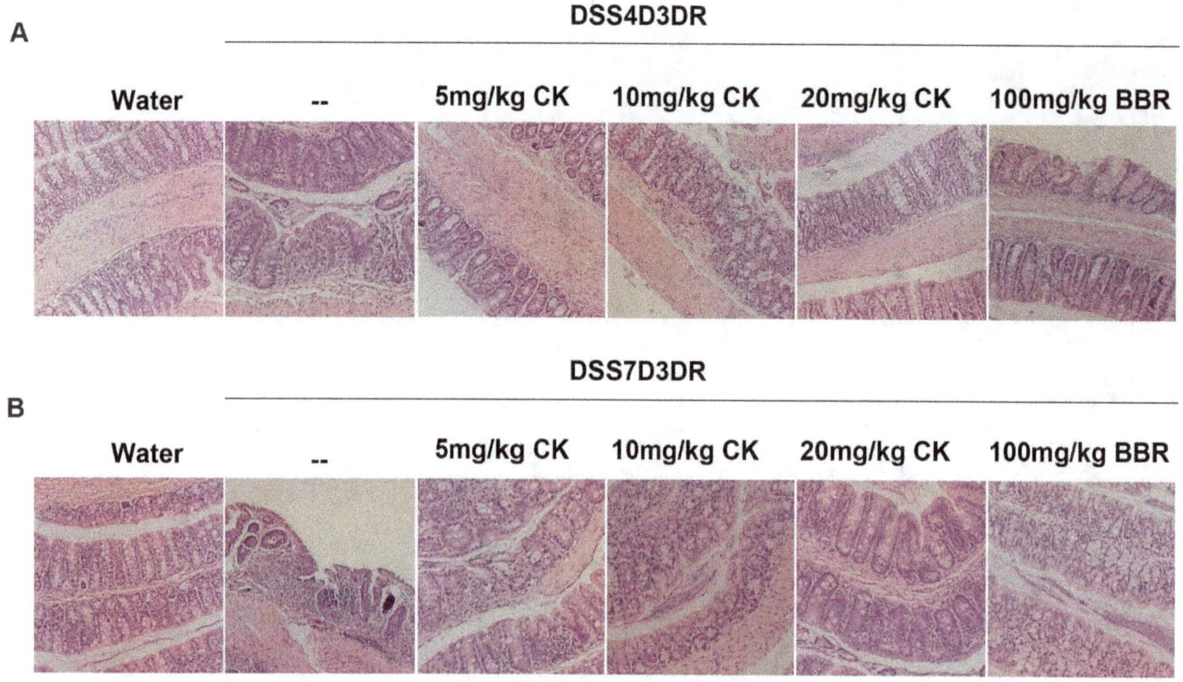

Figure 3. Histology analyze of DSS-induced colitis in mice. (A) Paraffin embedded colon sections were stained with hematoxylin and eosin for light microscopic assessment of epithelial damage of colitis mice, n = 3.

The levels of MPO of colon tissues and blood plasma were be detected in 460 nm absorbance values.

Enzyme-linked Immunosorbent Assay

Weighing the same weight of colon organization, fixed with ice-cold PBS (1:9), homogenated, and centrifugalized (10000 rpm/min, 10 min). The supernatant were reserved. The macrophage RAW 264.7 cells were treated with lipopolysaccharide (LPS) (1 μg/ml) for 10 h in the presence or absence of different dose of CK (10 μM, 20 μM, 50 μM) and BBR (50 μM). After CK or BBR treatment, the supernatants of RAW 264.7 cells were collected and centrifugalized (1000 rpm/min, 5 min). The production of IL-1β, IL-6, TNF-α and IL-10 in colon tissues supernatants, blood serum and RAW 264.7 cell supernatants were determined in duplicate using ELISA kits (R&D System Europe Ltd., UK) as described by the manufacturer.

Cytosolic, Nuclear Protein Isolation

The cytosolic, nuclear protein of colon tissues and RAW 264.7 cells fractions were isolated according to our previously reported procedure [13,14]. Briefly, tissues and cells were scraped in ice-cold homogenization buffer. And then re-suspended in 5 volumes of ice-cold extract buffer A and were homogenized. The homogenates were putted in ice for 15 min, and then added buffer B and centrifuged at 16000 g for 5 min to obtain the cytoplasm pellets. The supernatants were further fixed buffer C and putted in ice for 40 min. The supernatants centrifuged at 160000 g for 1 h to collect the supernatants (the nuclear fraction).

Western Blotting Analysis

Western blotting was performed as in our previous publications [13,14]. Protein assay kit for protein quantity analysis was purchased from Bio-Rad (Hercules, CA). The enhanced chemiluminescence (ECL) detection system was purchased from Arlington Heights, IL. IamgeJ2X software was used to analyze the relative density of each band.

Statistical Analysis

All values are expressed as the means ± S.D. for at least three separate determinations for each group. Statistical significance for multiple comparisons in each study was determined by one-way ANOVA followed by Newman-Keuls analysis using Prism 5.0 (GraphPad Software). Statistical analysis was performed by Student's t-test.

Results

Anti-inflammatory Effects of CK in DSS-induced Colitis in Mice

The DSS mouse model of acute colitis is well-characterized by increased epithelial injury in previous work [2–5], and it has been proved that BBR has influence on promoting the recovery of DSS-treated colitis [1]. To confirm the efficiency of anti-inflammatory effects of CK and explore its functional mechanism, mice were treated with DSS for 4 days to induce mild colitis, and then CK was administered *via* intraperitoneal injection for the following 3 days recovery (Fig. 1B, upper panel). To induced severe colitis, mice were treated with DSS for 7 days, and CK was given to mice for the following 3 days recovery periods (Fig. 1B, lower panel). The mice which were just given water were used as control. In the mild colitis group, the mice body weight reached 96.08±5.41% of their original body weight at the average (p<0.05), but the CK or BBR treatment groups have no statistical significance (Fig. 1C). However, in the severe colitis group, the body weight began to lose after 5 days until the day end of the DSS treatment. When given CK or BBR, the body weight began to recover from day 8 to day 10. CK (20 mg/kg) and BBR (100 mg/kg) significantly improved body weight recovery from day 8 to day 10 (Fig. 1D). Compared

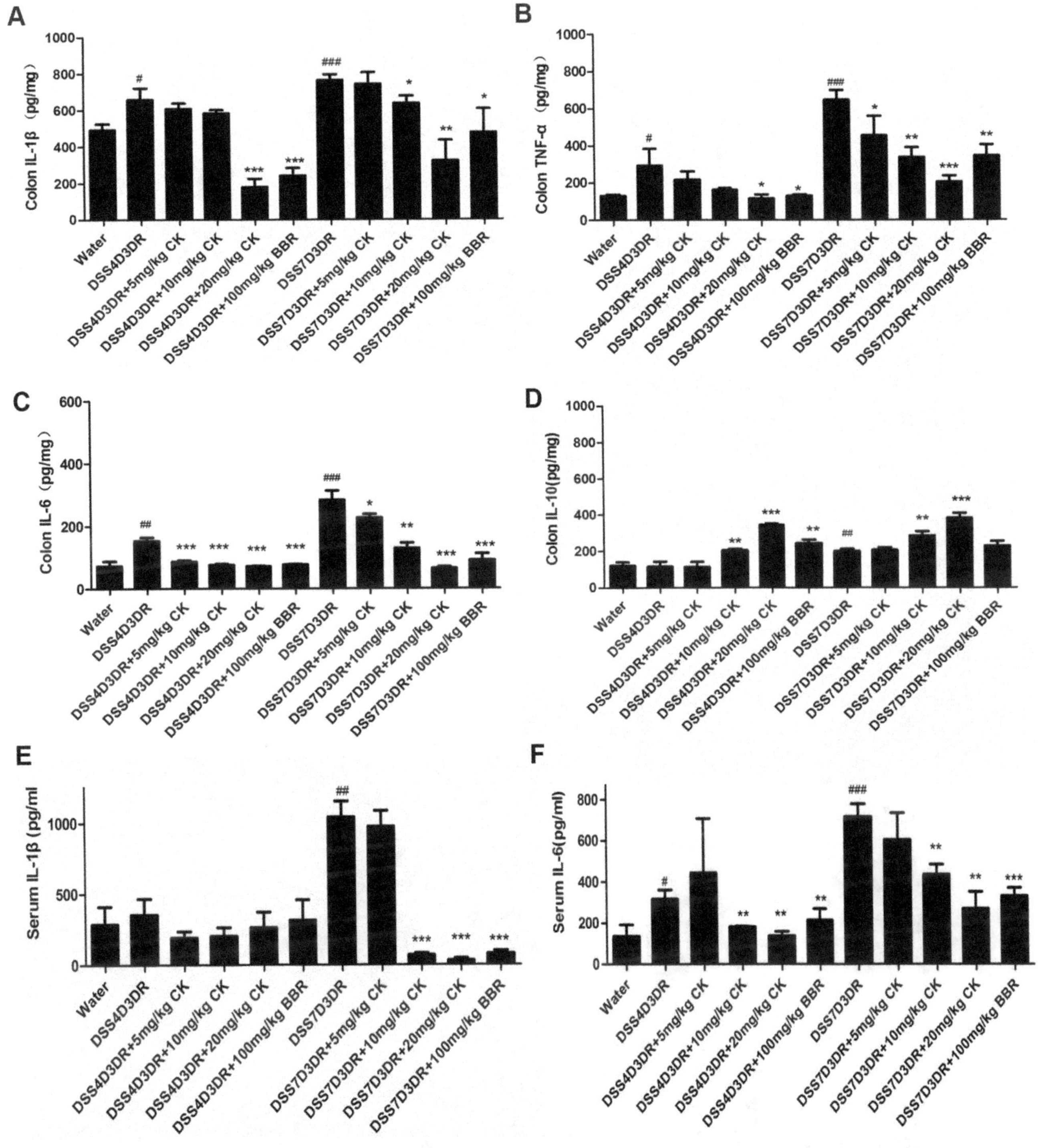

Figure 4. CK reduces production of inflammatory cytokines in DSS-induced colitis in mice. The colon tissues and mice serum were collected as the mean shows in method and materials. Before it performed, the tissues were fixed with ice-cold PBS in 1:9 rations, homogenated, and centrifugalized. The supernatants were collected and IL-1β, TNF-α, IL-6 and IL-10 expressions were measured by ELISA (n = 3). The results were shown in (A), (B), (C) and (D), respectively. (E) and (F) The mice serum is detected the production of IL-1β, IL-6 directly by ELISA (n = 3). # $p<0.05$, ## $p<0.01$, ### $p<0.01$ compared with the control group. *p compared with DSS4D3DR or DSS7D3DR group. *$p<0.05$, **$p<0.01$, ***$p<0.01$.

the average weight to the original, the severe colitis group weight was 90.65±10.16% ($p<0.01$). Meanwhile, the 20 mg/kg CK group was 95.45±7.63% and the BBR group was 94.94±8.39% of their original body weight at the average (Fig. 1D). Obviously, high concentrations of CK and BBR have significant effects on alleviating the DSS-induced colitis mice weight loss.

Moreover, shortening of the colon length is also a marker for colitis. Compared with control group and two colitis models, the colon length of the light colitis group was 3.30±0.53 cm shorter at

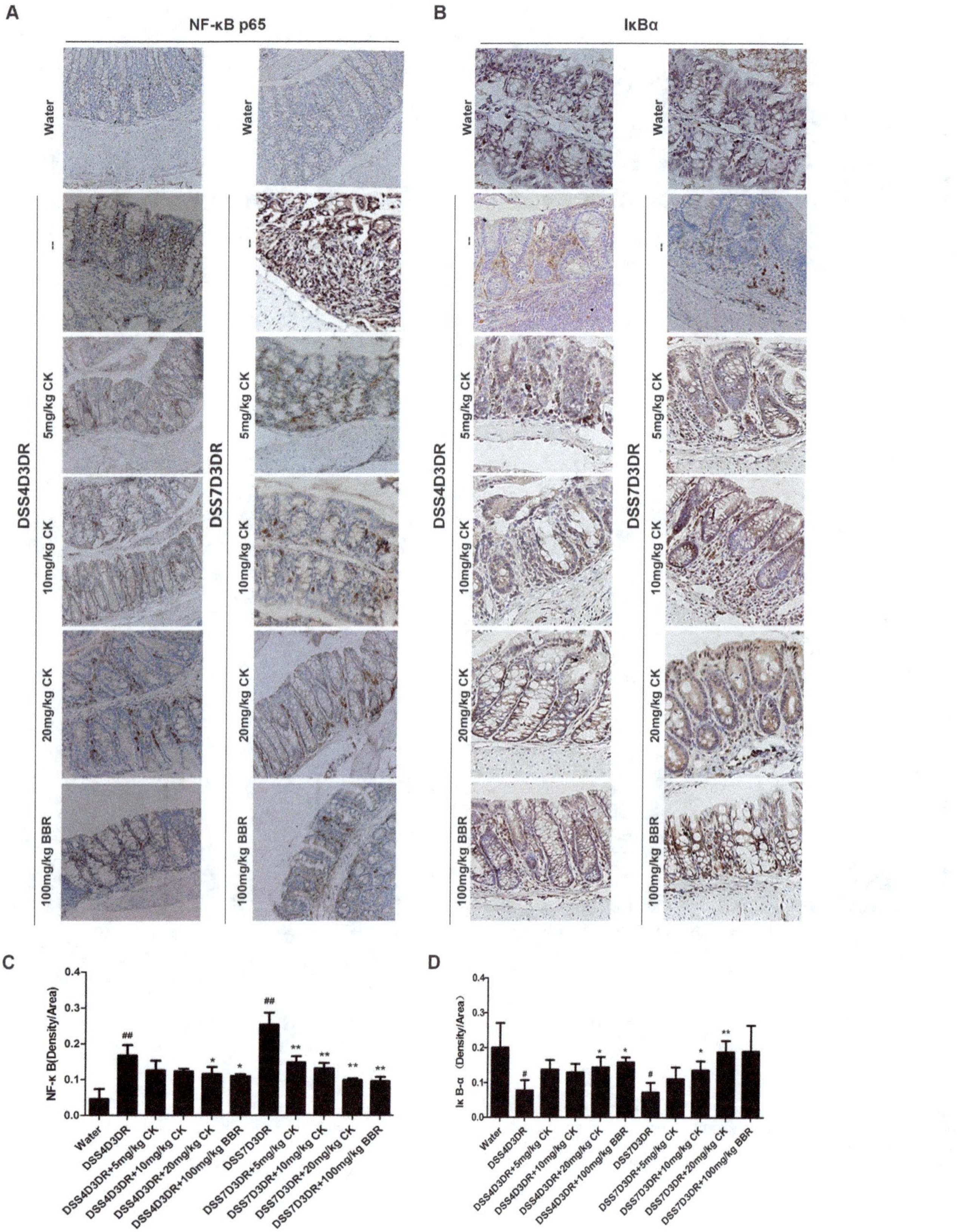

Figure 5. CK inhibits the NF-κB activation in DSS-induced colitis in mice. Representative images of IHC staining of NF-κB (p65) and IκB-α in mild colitis and severe colitis. (A) The expression of NF-κB (p65). (B) The expression of IκB-α. Software used 20 images. Three animals were analyzed for each type of mice. (C) Quantification of NF-κB (p65) positive density in each group. (D) Quantification of IκB-α positive density in each group (n = 3). # $p<0.05$, ## $p<0.01$ compared with the control group. *p compared with DSS4D3DR or DSS7D3DR group. *$p<0.05$, **$p<0.01$.

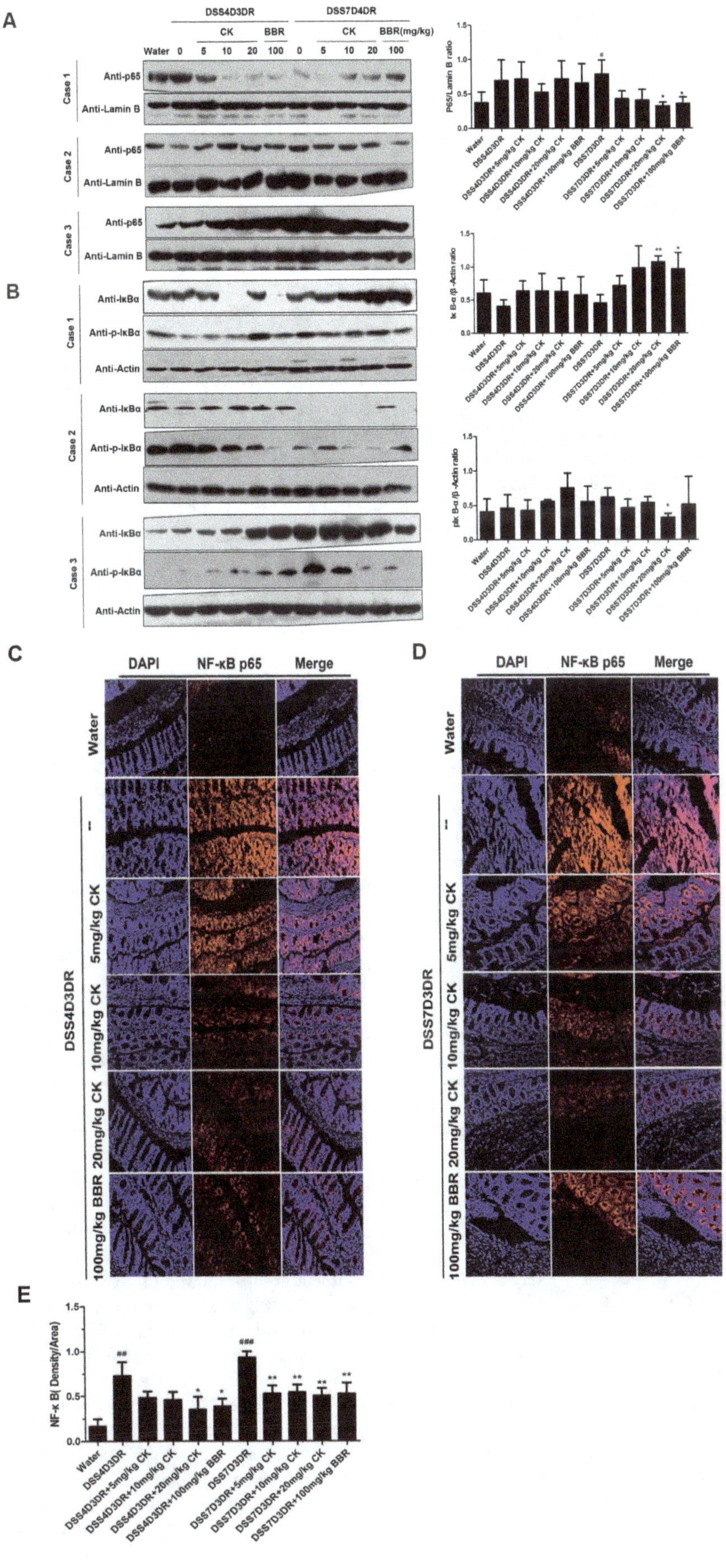
A
B
C
D
E
DSS4D3DR
DSS7D4DR
CK
BBR
BBR(mg/kg)
Water
Case 1
Case 2
Case 3
Anti-p65
Anti-Lamin B
Anti-IκBα
Anti-p-IκBα
Anti-Actin
DAPI
NF-κB p65
Merge
5mg/kg CK
10mg/kg CK
20mg/kg CK
100mg/kg BBR
DSS7D3DR
NF-κ B(Density/Area)

Figure 6. CK inhibits the NF-κB signaling activation in DSS-induced colitis mice. (A) Western blotting analysis of p65 expression in nucleus in different doses of CK and BBR mice group. Three animals were analyzed for each type of mice As shown in the left panel. In the right panel, the relative density of the activated nucleus p65 band was compared with the lamin B band in each group. (B) Analysis of IκB-α and p-IκBα in mild colitis and severe colitis mice tissues cytoplasm protein. In the right panel, the relative density of IκB-α and p-IκBα bands were compared with the β-actin band in each group. (C) and (D) Paraffin-embedded colon tissues sections of mild colitis group and severe colitis group were used to determine p65 translocated to the nucleus by immunofluorescence. (E) Quantification of NF-κB (p65) positive density in each group under 20X image. ## $p<0.01$, ### $p<0.01$ compared with the control group. *p compared with DSS4D3DR or DSS7D3DR group. $p<0.05$, ** $p<0.01$.

the average (Fig. 1E, 1G, $p<0.001$) and the severe one was about 4.53±0.48 cm shorter at the average (Fig. 1F, 1G, $p<0.001$) either. Strikingly, CK and BBR exerted preventive effects on the colon lengh of both mild colitis mice and sever colitis mice.

Furthermore, DSS induces neutrophil infiltration in the colon leading to increasing colonic MPO activity, which is treated as another inflammatory marker for colitis. In mild colitis mice groups, after 20 mg/kg CK and 100 mg/kg BBR treatment, MPO activity in the colon was reduced by 401±41.29 mU/g ($p<0.01$) and 235±76.37 mU/g ($p<0.05$) (Fig. 2A) compared to the model group. Meanwhile, 20 mg/kg CK and 100 mg/kg BBR treatment reduced the MPO by 705.3±11.27 mU/g ($p<0.001$) and 558.3±30.71 mU/g ($p<0.001$) in severe colitis mice compared to the model group, respectively (Fig. 2A). We also found that the reducing tendency of MPO after CK and BBR treatment in colitis mice plasma was the same as the colon MPO activity (Fig. 2B). Above results indicated that DSS-treated mice demonstrated colon injury and acute colitis (mild colitis and sever colitis), including body weight loss, colon length shorten and MPO activity, all of which could be reduced by CK and BBR.

Histology of DSS-induced Colitis in Mice

DSS-induced mice emerge massive colon ulceration, crypt damage, and severe inflammation [4,5]. These abnormalities were reduced by treatment with BBR which we have authenticated in previous work [10–12]. In order to confirm more possible functional mechanisms of CK, we then did the H&E staining in paraffin-embedded colon tissues sections (n = 3, Fig. 3). DSS treatment caused no significant observable macroscopic changes in colonic tissue architecture between the experimental groups, including the untreated mice. However, DSS treatment tended to accelerate initial damage to the mucosa, characterized by the loss of goblet cells and the occurrence of a more diffuse crypt architecture compared to the colon of healthy mice in H&E staining sections (Fig. 3A, 3B). Additionally, the accumulation of neutrophils infiltrating the lamina propria could be observed more frequently in colonic slices of DSS-treated mice in both mild colitis mice and severe colitis groups (Fig. 3A, 3B). When treated with different concentrations of CK and BBR, the severity of inflammation seemed to be much lower (Fig. 3A, 3B). These data suggest that CK and BBR exerted therapeutic effects on both mild and severe colitis associated with intestinal epithelial cell injury repairmen, particularly the high concentration of CK.

CK Reduced Pro-inflammatory Cytokines Production in DSS-treated Mice

The biological activities of CK include anti-metastatic, anti-carcinogenic, and anti-allergic effects, but its role in DSS-induced inflammatory signaling is poorly understood [20–24]. To examine the function of CK on treating colitis, the production of cytokines in colon tissues and serum were detected. In the mild colitis group, the expression of pro-inflammatory cytokines TNF-α, IL-6, IL-1β were increased to about 1.5 folds (Fig. 4A, 4B, 4C, $p<0.05$), and in the severe colitis group IL-6, TNF-α, IL-1β expression were increased to about 3, 2, and 1.5 folds (Fig. 4A, 4B, 4C) compared to the water group. After the treatment of CK, it was obvious that CK inhibited the DSS-induced expression ofpro-inflammatory cytokines and increased anti-inflammatory cytokine (IL-10) production (Fig. 4D). Investigation of the production of IL-1β and IL-6 in colitis mice serum confirmed our results. 7-day DSS treatment group increased the expression of IL-1β about 5 folds ($p<0.01$) compared to the water group (Fig. 4E) and then the 10 mg/kg, 20 mg/kg CK and 100 mg/kg BBR treatment groups decreased the IL-1β production all about 10 folds ($p<0.001$) (Fig. 4E). But the 4-day DSS treatment and 3-day recovery group didn't have significant results. The mild colitis group increased the expression of IL-6 about 2 folds (Fig. 4F, $p<0.05$) and the severe group increased about 5 folds (Fig. 4F, $p<0.01$) compared to the water group. CK can also down-regulated the IL-6 secretion in mice serum. Obviously, the serum levels of IL-1β and IL-6 were significantly suppressed in mice after administration of CK (Fig. 4E, 4F). Together, our findings suggest that CK, similar to BBR, suppressed pro-inflammatory cytokines production in DSS-induced mild and severe colitis in both mice tissues and blood.

CK Inhibited the NF-κB Pathway in DSS-induced Colitis in Mice

The transcription factor NF-κB is a central mediator in inflammation and several other cellular responses [12,25]. NF-κB is translocated to the nucleus by phosphorylation of IκB and subsequent degradation of IκB subunit. BBR can inhibit the activation of the NF-κB pathway in DSS-induced mice [1,26]. To reveal the anti-inflammatory mechanisms of CK on treating colitis in mice, IHC analysis showed that nuclear p65 was significantly reduced in CK and BBR treatment groups compared to control groups (Fig. 5A). Quantification of staining density in multiple samples indicated that in the 4-day DSS treatment group and 7-day water group, nuclear p65 increased 3 folds and 5 folds respectively, compared with the water group (Fig. 5C, $p<0.01$, n = 6). Yet, after administered CK and BBR for the following three recovery days, the nuclear p65 enormously decreased (Fig. 5C, n = 6). Nevertheless, 20 mg/kg CK on 4-day DSS treatment groups reduced the nuclear p65 by 2 folds (Fig. 5C, $p<0.05$, n = 6). We also examined the IκB-α expression in colon tissues and the results showed that IκB-α expression would be much higher in the CK and BBR treatment groups (Fig. 5B, n = 6). Obviously, the mild colitis groups and sever colitis groups presented the same tendency. Quantification of staining density of IκB-α, both in 4-day and 7-day DSS treatment groups, showed that CK and BBR have substantially facilitated the IκB-α expression (Fig. 5D, n = 6). Taken together, with the observation of nuclear p65 activation and IκB-α degradation, these results indicated that NF-κB signaling pathway was inhibited by CK and BBR.

Western blotting analysis was used to further confirm our results. Three colon tissues samples from each group and three separate tests were done. The expression of p65 was shown in figure 6A (left panel). The relative density of the activated nuclear p65 compared with Lamin B in each group was shown in figure 6A right panel. Strikingly, CK treatment caused a dose-dependent decrease in p65 expression in colon tissues. The 20 mg/kg CK

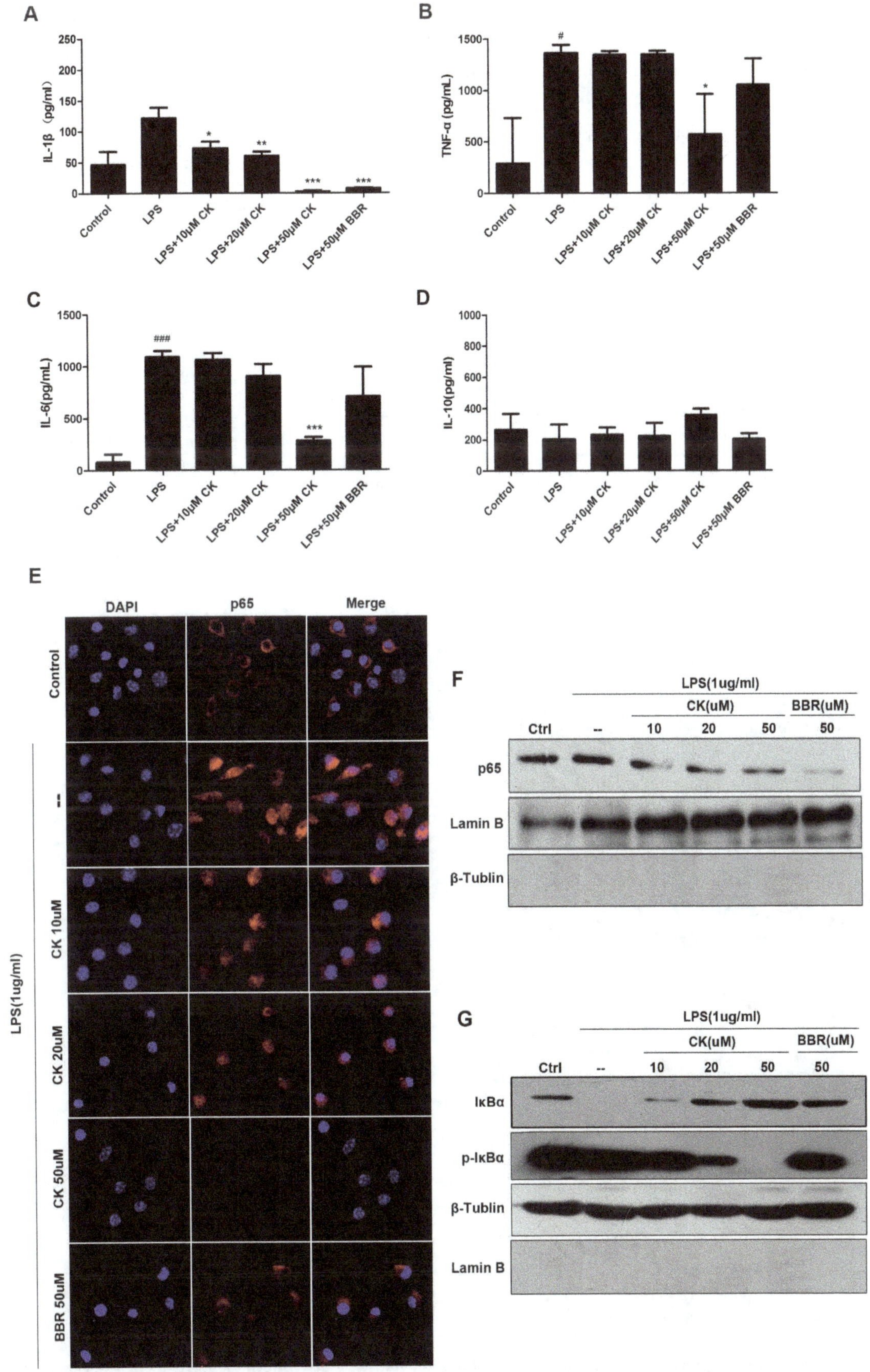

Figure 7. CK inhibits the NF-κB signaling activation in macrophage RAW 264.7 cells. The RAW 264.7 Cells were stimulated with lipopolysaccharide (LPS) (1 μg/ml) for 10 h in the presence or absence of different dose of CK (10 μM, 20 μM, 50 μM) and BBR (50 μM). The

supernatants were subsequently harvested and measured by ELISA (n = 3). IL-1β, TNF-a, IL-6 and IL-10 expressions were shown in (A), (B), (C), and (D). (E) NF-κB nuclear translocation was detected by immunofluorescence analysis using an antibody for the p65. (F) Western blotting results were shown p65 expression in nuclear fractions. (G) IκB-α and p-IκBα expression in cytosolic fractions. All those have done three separate tests. # $p<0.05$, ### $p<0.01$ compared with the control group. *p compared with DSS4D3DR or DSS7D3DR group. *$p<0.05$, **$p<0.01$, ***$p<0.01$.

group reduced the p65 expression by half (Fig. 6A, right panel, $p<0.05$, n = 3). And BBR could also inhibit p65 access to nucleus (Fig. 6A, right panel, $p<0.05$, n = 3). In addition, in the cytosol, the IκB-α expression increased and p-IκBα decreased after CK and BBR treatment in three independent experiments (Fig. 6A, left panel, n = 3). The relative density of IκB-α and p-IκBα compared with the β-actin in each group was shown in figure 6B right panel. Nevertheless, those results about the protein expression of NF-κB signaling pathway in the whole colon seem not very obvious. According to previous work, colitis signed by intestinal epithelial barrier function damage, and triggered innate immune cells such as macrophages and intestinal epithelia cells secreting cytokines and chemokines, which mostly leading to activate NF-κB pathway and then regulate the inflammatory responses. BBR reduced the colon injury via inhibiting the colon tissues NF-κB pathway activation. So, the notion that the anti-inflammation effects of CK may also regulate the colon tissue NF-κB pathway activation will be more acceptable. However, due to mice individual difference, more samples must be done to verify the statements better.

Paraffin-embedded colon tissues sections were used to determine p65 translocation to the nucleus by immunofluorescence and visualized by fluorescence microcopy (Fig. 6C, 6D). Quantification of fluorescence density was shown in figure 6E. Nucleus p65 expression distinctly reduced after CK and BBR treatment (Fig. 6C, 6D, 6E).

From above, we demonstrated for the first time that CK prevented the progression of DSS-induced colitis mice through inhibiting NF-κB pathway activation, thus leading to preventing p65 translocation to nucleus and IκB-α phosphorylation.

CK Inhibited Activation of NF-κB Pathway in Macrophages

CK and BBR have demonstrated potent anti-inflammation effects in *vivo*. It has been reported that in peritoneal macrophages and RAW264.7 cell lines, BBR can down-regulate NF-κB pathway that mediate pro-inflammatory cytokines production, and contribute to relieve the colitis injury, which suggests that BBR has influence on regulating the innate immune responses. CK, as the active metabolite responsible for the anti-inflammatory effect of ginsenoside, prompted us to investigate its functional mechanismon LPS-induced inflammation *in vitro*. LPS is one of the most potent pro-inflammatory agonists for monocytes and macrophages, and macrophage is one of the functional innate immune cells in inflammatory responses and it regulates innate immune responses by providing cytokine [27–29]. Sustained stimulation with LPS could active NF-κB pathway in RAW 264.7 cells [30]. In this work, RAW 264.7 cells were treated with lipopolysaccharide (LPS) (1 μg/ml) for 10 h in the presence or absence of different dose of CK (10 μM, 20 μM, 50 μM) and BBR (50 μM). The control (cell-only) group was used as a positive control for anti-inflammatory activities. In the LPS exposure group, IL-1β, IL-6, TNF-a productions increased dramatically to 5, 10, 8 folds respectively, compared to the control group. However, CK reduced IL-1β, IL-6 and TNF-a production in a

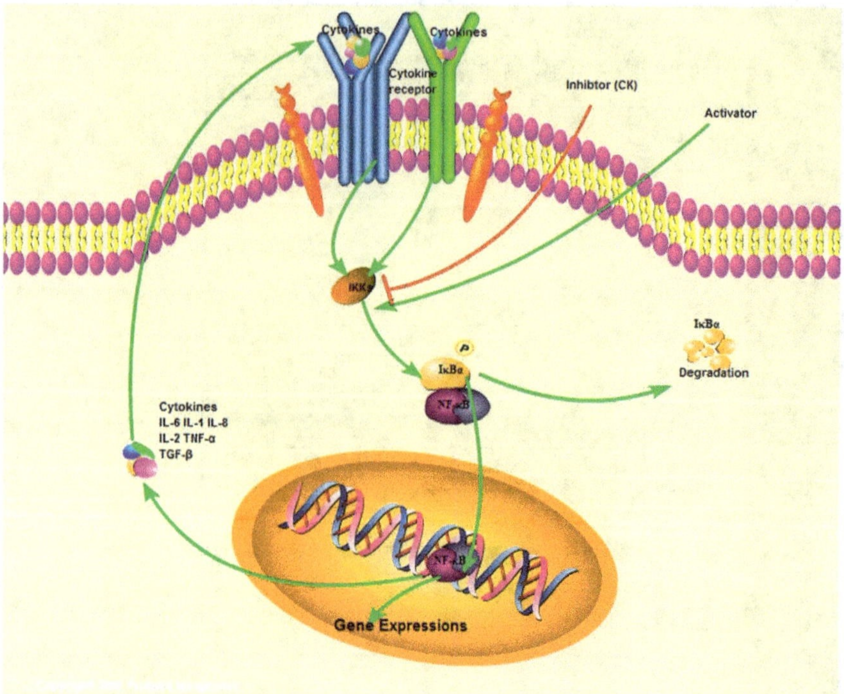

Figure 8. CK prevents inflammatory responses *via* inhibiting NF-κB signaling pathway activation. CK exerts therapy effects on the progression of DSS-induced colitis in mice, and the potential mechanisms may contribute to regulating the innate immune cells such as macrophages activities through modulating NF-κB signaling pathways activation.

dose-dependent manner (Fig. 7A, 7B, 7C). Nevertheless, IL-10 production changed a little (Fig. 7D). BBR (50 μM) also have influence on reducing the pro-inflammation production, expect for IL-10 (Fig. 7A, 7B, 7C, 7D), significantly. In summary, CK and BBR have significant effects on reducing pro-inflammatory cytokines production *in vitro*, and regulating the inflammatory responses in *vivo* via impacting the production of cytokines, which were provided by immune cells, such as macrophages.

According to the previous work, immunofluorescence and western blotting were used to explore the inhibitory effects of CK on inflammation (Fig. 7E, 7F, 7G). The location of nucleus p65 was detected by fluorescence microcopy in RAW 264.7 cells treated with lipopolysaccharide (LPS) (1 μg/ml) for 10 h in the presence or absence of different doses of CK (10, 20, and 50 μM) and BBR (50 μM) It was obvious that CK prevented p65 translocation to nucleus in a concentration-dependent manner. Moreover, western blotting results indicated that CK promoted IκB phosphorylation in a concentration-dependent manner.

Taken together, these data suggest that CK and BBR have influence on reducing LPS-stimulated pro-inflammatory cytokines, increasing anti-inflammatory cytokine expression, contributing to inhibition of the activation of NF-κB pathway, restraining p65 translocated to nucleus, and inhibiting phosphorylation of IκB of macrophage cells, which may serve as mechanism for CK down-regulated inflammatory responses of intestinal disorder *in vivo*.

Discussion

The evaluation of ancient herbal products that have been widely used for many diseases, such as treating diarrhea and bacterial and parasitic infection, may provide insight into developing these herbs into new therapies for other inflammation treatment [1,31]. CK is an intestinal bacterial metabolite of panaxoside, which have been widely reported to exert anti-inflammation and anti-cancer activity [20–26]. *Our studies* and *other previous* work have demonstrated the anti-growth effect of CK in different kinds of tumors cells, such as hepatocellular carcinoma [13]. Although, ginsenoside Rb1 and its metabolites have been confirmed playing an beneficial role in inflammatory responses in TNBS-induced colitis by inhibiting IRAK-1 activation, which contributes to activate IKKβ, linking with NF-κB and MAPK pathways [12]. BBR has been used to treat bacteria associated diarrhea, intestinal parasitic infections, and ocular trachoma infections for several decades [27]. We have proved that BBR induces death in colon tumor cells. Recent work has indicated that BBR promotes recovery of colitis and ameliorate inflammatory responses in DSS-treated mice by promoting colon peritoneal macrophages apoptosis, and decreasing pro-inflammatory production in colonic macrophages and macrophages cell lines [1]. However, the functional mechanisms of CK and BBR on treating those diseases are not clearly known. The purpose of this work was to determine the effects of CK on treatment of the progression of colitis and to provide insight into the potentially functional mechanism.

In the present study, BBR served as a positive agent for treating the DSS-induced colitis mice mode. We showed that CK exerts inhibitory inflammatory effects not only on mild colitis (4-day DSS-induced colitis), but also on severe colitis (7-day DSS-induced colitis), including protection of the weight loss and colon tissues injury, and preservation of of colon length. Furthermore, similar as BBR, CK treatment reduced MPO activity in mice colon and mice plasma in dose-dependent manner. We observed that CK and BBR reduced the production of the pro-inflammatory cytokines, such as IL-1β, IL-6 and TNF-α, but not the anti-inflammatory cytokine, such as IL-10 in colon tissue. In addition, similar results were found in colitis mice serum. *In vitro*, LPS-stimulated macrophage RAW 264.7 cells were treated with BBR and CK and then the supernates cytokines generation was measured. Those results show CK, same as BBR, protected the mice from the colitis injury by increasing the production of the anti-inflammatory cytokines and reducing the pro-inflammatory cytokines in concentration-dependent manners. Based on the cytokines levels that are regulated by CK and BBR, it was possible that they ameliorated colitis through regulating the innate immune system.

As we all known, production of cytokines and chemokines by immune/inflammatory cells that activate transcription factors such as NF-κB in pre-malignant cells to induce genes that stimulate cell proliferation,survival, and growth, as well as angiogenesis, and invasiveness motility [32–35]. In details, NF-κB (p65) is located in cytoplasm and bounds to IκB as an inactive complex [32,33]. The phosphorylation and subsequent degradation of IκB result in separation of the complex, and then NF-κB is activated. The activated NF-κB migrates into the nucleus, and causes the expression of inflammatory cytokines, such as TNF-a, IL-6 and IL-8 [35]. Meanwhile, NF-κB can be activated by inflammatory factors such as IL-1β and TNF-α [35,36]. TNF-α can activate macrophages and initiate immune responses by stimulating secretion of other cytokines [37,38]. IL-1β, mainly synthesized by macrophages, is also an inflammatory cytokine which play important roles in the acute phase response [39,40]. In addition, NF-κB signaling pathway is the downstream pathway of LPS-mediated transduction pathways [29]. As it is been well accepted, in difference forms of inflammation, innate immune cells (including macrophages, neutrophils, mast cells, etc) and adaptive immune cells (T and B lymphocytes) are connected with each other by means of direct contact of cytokines and chemokines, leading to regulating the innate immune responses [40]. Unrestrained reactions may exaggerate inflammatory response and lead to continuous events of injury and tissues damage [41,42].

Our data showed that CK and BBR down-regulated colonic tissues NF-κB signaling pathways in response to the recovery of 4 days DSS-induced and 7 days DSS-induced colitis *in vivo* and inhibited the activation of macrophages NF-κB signaling pathways in LPS-stimulated inflammation *in vitro*. In addition, our data suggest that CK and BBR mediate the progression of the colon disease by regulating innate immune cells, linked with the production of cytokines and chemokines. The potentially singling pathway of this work was shown in figure 8.

In summary, our data indicated that CK exerts effient therapy effects on DSS-induced progression of colitis in mice, and the potential mechanisms for regulating this intestinal inflammation may contribute to regulating the innate immune cells such as macrophages activities through modulating of NF-κB signaling pathways activation that dominate the production of cytokines and chemokines. Since CK has been widely used for treating with many diseases without significant side effects on patients, it has the potential to be developed into a drug for intestinal inflammatory diseases.

Acknowledgments

We thank Hanwei Cao and Yanyan Zhan for their kind comments and support.

Author Contributions

Conceived and designed the experiments: GS JL. Performed the experiments: JL WZ WW SH JY. Analyzed the data: GS JL BZ TH. Wrote the paper: GS JL TH.

References

1. Fang Y, Lihong W, Yan S, Hanwei C, Liping L, et al. (2012) BBR promotes recovery of colitis and inhibits inflammatory responses in colonic macrophages and epithelial cells in DSS-treated mice. Am J Physiol Gastrointest Liver Physiol 302: G504–G514.
2. Sann H, Erichsen J, Hessmann M, Pahl A, Hoffmeyer A (2013) Efficacy of drugs used in the treatment of IBD and combinations thereof in acute DSS-induced colitis in mice. Life Sci 92: 708–718.
3. Mueller K, Blum NM, Mueller AS (2013) Examination of the Anti-Inflammatory, Antioxidant, and Xenobiotic-Inducing Potential of Broccoli Extract and Various Essential Oils during a Mild DSS-Induced Colitis in Rats. ISRN Gastroenterol 2013: 710856.
4. Yoda K, Miyazawa K, Hosoda M, Hiramatsu M, Yan F, et al. (2013) Lactobacillus GG-fermented milk prevents DSS-induced colitis and regulates intestinal epithelial homeostasis through activation of epidermal growth factor receptor. Eur J Nutr.
5. Araki A, Nara H, Rahman M, Onoda T, Li J, et al. (2013) Role of interleukin-21 isoform in dextran sulfate sodium (DSS)-induced colitis. Cytokine 62: 262–271.
6. Rieder F, Karrasch T, Ben-horin S, Schirbel A, Ehehalt R, et al. (2012) Results of the 2nd scientific workshop of the ECCO (III): basic mechanisms of intestinal healing. J Crohns Colitis 6: 373–385.
7. Speca S, Giusti I, Rieder F, Latella G (2012) Cellular and molecular mechanisms of intestinal fibrosis. World J Gastroenterol 18: 3635–3661.
8. Podolsky DK (2002) Inflammatory bowel disease. N Engl J Med 347: 417–429.
9. Blumberg RS (2009) Inflammation in the intestinal tract: pathogenesis and treatment. Dig Dis 27: 455–464.
10. Kim do Y, Park MW, Yuan HD, Lee HJ, Kim SH, et al. (2009) Compound K induces apoptosis via CAMK-IV/AMPK pathways in HT-29 colon cancer cells. J Agric Food Chem 57: 10573–10578.
11. Lee ES, Choi JS, Kim MS, You HJ, Ji GE, et al. (2011) Ginsenoside metabolite compound K differentially antagonizing tumor necrosis factor-alpha-induced monocyte-endothelial trafficking. Chem Biol Interact 194: 13–22.
12. Joh EH, Lee IA, Jung IH, Kim DH (2011) Ginsenoside Rb1 and its metabolite compound K inhibit IRAK-1 activation–the key step of inflammation. Biochem Pharmacol 82: 278–286.
13. Song G, Guo S, Wang W, Hu C, Mao Y, et al. (2010) Intestinal metabolite compound K of ginseng saponin potently attenuates metastatic growth of hepatocellular carcinoma by augmenting apoptosis via a Bid-mediated mitochondrial pathway. J Agric Food Chem 58: 12753–12760.
14. Hu C, Song G, Zhang B, Liu Z, Chen R, et al. (2012) Intestinal metabolite compound K of panaxoside inhibits the growth of gastric carcinoma by augmenting apoptosis via Bid-mediated mitochondrial pathway. J Cell Mol Med 16: 96–106.
15. Zhang Z, Du GJ, Wang CZ, Wen XD, Calway T, et al. (2013) Compound K, a Ginsenoside Metabolite, Inhibits Colon Cancer Growth via Multiple Pathways Including p53-p21 Interactions. Int J Mol Sci 14: 2980–2995.
16. Lee IA, Hyun YJ, Kim DH (2010) Berberine ameliorates TNBS-induced colitis by inhibiting lipid peroxidation, enterobacterial growth and NF-kappaB activation. Eur J Pharmacol 648: 162–170.
17. Jiang Q, Liu P, Wu X, Liu W, Shen X, et al. (2011) Berberine attenuates lipopolysaccharide-induced extracelluar matrix accumulation and inflammation in rat mesangial cells: involvement of NF-kappaB signaling pathway. Mol Cell Endocrinol 331: 34–40.
18. Bae DS, Kim YH, Pan CH, Nho CW, Samdan J, et al. (2012) Protopine reduces the inflammatory activity of lipopolysaccharide-stimulated murine macrophages. BMB Rep 45: 108–113.
19. Ma BL, Yao MK, Zhong J, Ma YM, Gao CL, et al. (2012) Increased systemic exposure to rhizoma coptidis alkaloids in lipopolysaccharide-pretreated rats attributable to enhanced intestinal absorption. Drug Metab Dispos 40: 381–388.
20. Wakabayashi C, Hasegawa H, Murata J, Saiki I (1997) In vivo antimetastatic action of ginseng protopanaxadiol saponins bis based on their intestinal bacterial metabolites after oral administration. Oncol Res 9: 411–417.
21. Hasegawa H, Sung JH, Matsumiya S, Uchiyama M (1996) Main ginseng saponin metabolites formed by intestinal bacteria. Planta Med 62: 453–457.
22. Kim do Y, Yuan HD, Chung IK, Chung SH (2009) Compound K, intestinal metabolite of ginsenoside, attenuates hepatic lipid accumulation via AMPK activation in human hepatoma cells. J Agric Food Chem 57: 1532–1537.
23. Lee BH, Lee SJ, Hur JH, Lee S, Sung JH, et al. (1998) In vitro antigenotoxic activity of novel ginseng saponin metabolites formed by intestinal bacteria. Planta Med 64: 500–503.
24. Hasegawa H, Sung JH, Huh JH (1997) Ginseng intestinal bacterial metabolite IH901 as a new anti-metastatic agent. Arch Pharm Res 20: 539–544.
25. Choo MK, Sakurai H, Kim DH, Saiki I, et al. (2008) A ginseng saponinmetabolite suppresses tumor necrosis factor-alpha-promoted metastasis by suppressing nuclear factor-kappaB signaling inmurine colon cancer cells. Oncol Rep 19: 595–600.
26. Yang CS, Ko SR, Cho BG, Shin DM, Yuk JM, et al. (2008) The ginsenoside metabolite compound K, a novel agonist of glucocorticoid receptor, induces tolerance to endotoxin-induced lethal shock. J Cell Mol Med 12: 1739–1753.
27. Zhou X, Zhang C, Wang X, An B, Zhang P, et al. (2012) Berberine inhibits lipopolysaccharide- and polyethylene particle-induced mouse calvarial osteolysis in vivo. J Surg Res 173: e47–52.
28. Ma BL, Yao MK, Zhong J, Ma YM, Gao CL, et al. (2012) Increased systemic exposure to rhizoma coptidis alkaloids in lipopolysaccharide-pretreated rats attributable to enhanced intestinal absorption. Drug Metab Dispos 40: 381–388.
29. Lee D, Bae J, Kim YK, Gil M, Lee JY, et al. (2013) Inhibitory effects of berberine on lipopolysaccharide-induced inducible nitric oxide synthase and the high-mobility group box 1 release in macrophages. Biochem Biophys Res Commun 431: 506–511.
30. Bae DS, Kim YH, Pan CH, Nho CW, Samdan J, et al. (2012) Protopine reduces the inflammatory activity of lipopolysaccharide-stimulated murine macrophages. BMB Rep 45: 108–113.
31. Kalaiselvi P, Rajashree K, Bharathi Priya L, Padma VV (2013) Cytoprotective effect of epigallocatechin-3-gallate against deoxynivalenol-induced toxicity through anti-oxidative and anti-inflammatory mechanisms in HT-29 cells. Food Chem Toxicol 56: 110–118.
32. Bedirli A, Salman B, Pasaoglu H, Ofluoglu E, Sakrak O (2011) Effects of nuclear factor-kappaB inhibitors on colon anastomotic healing in rats. J Surg Res 171: 355–360.
33. Yan J, Xiang J, Lin Y, Ma J, Zhang J, et al. (2013) Inactivation of BAD by IKK inhibits TNFalpha-induced apoptosis independently of NF-kappaB activation. Cell 152: 304–315.
34. Jo MJ, Lee JR, Cho IJ, Kim YW, Kim SC (2013) Roots of Erigeron annuus Attenuate Acute Inflammation as Mediated with the Inhibition of NF- kappa B-Associated Nitric Oxide and Prostaglandin E2 production. Evid Based Complement Alternat Med 2013: 297427.
35. Grivennikov SI, Greten FR, Karin M (2010) Immunity, Inflammation, and Cancer. Cell 140: 883–899.
36. Aggarwal BB, Vijayalekshmi RV, Sung B (2010) Targeting inflammatory pathways for prevention and therapy of cancer: short-term friend, long-term foe. Clin Cancer Res 15: 425–430.
37. Theiss AL, Simmnons JG, Jobin C, Lund PK (2005) Tumor Necrosis Factor (TNF) a Increases Collagen Accumulation and Proliferation in Intestinal Myofibroblasts via TNF Receptor 2. J Biol Chem 280: 36099–36109.
38. Amasheh M, Fromm A, Krug SM, Amasheh S, Andres S, et al. (2010) TNF-induced and berberine-antagonized tight junction barrier impairment via tyrosine kinase, Akt and NF_B signaling. J Cell Sci 123: 4145–4155.
39. Schirbel A, Fiocchi C (2010) Inflammatory bowel disease: Established and evolving considerations on its etiopathogenesis and therapy. J Dig Dis 11: 266–276.
40. Abaham C, Cho JH (2009) Inflammatory bowel disease. N Engl J Med 361: 2066–2078.
41. Latlla G, Papi C (2012) Crucial steps in the natural history of inflammatory bowel disease. World J Gastroenterol 18: 3790–3799.
42. Clark M, Colombel JF, Feagan BC, Fedorak RN, Hanauer SB, et al. (2006) American gastroenterological association consensus development conference on the use of biologics in the treatment of inflammatory bowel disease, Gastroenterology 133: 312–339.

22

Local and Systemic Immune Mechanisms Underlying the Anti-Colitis Effects of the Dairy Bacterium *Lactobacillus delbrueckii*

Clarissa Santos Rocha[1,3,4], Ana Cristina Gomes-Santos[2], Thais Garcias Moreira[2], Marcela de Azevedo[1], Tessalia Diniz Luerce[1], Mahendra Mariadassou[5], Ana Paula Longaray Delamare[6], Philippe Langella[3,4], Emmanuelle Maguin[3,4], Vasco Azevedo[1], Ana Maria Caetano de Faria[2], Anderson Miyoshi[1¶], Maarten van de Guchte[3,4*¶]

1 Department of General Biology, Instituto de Ciências Biológicas, Universidade Federal de Minas Gerais, Belo Horizonte, Brazil, 2 Department of Biochemistry and Immunology, Instituto de Ciências Biológicas, Universidade Federal de Minas Gerais, Belo Horizonte, Brazil, 3 INRA, UMR1319 Micalis, Jouy-en-Josas, France, 4 AgroParisTech, UMR Micalis, Jouy-en-Josas, France, 5 INRA, Mathématique, Informatique et Génome, UR1077, Jouy-en-Josas, France, 6 Institute of Biotechnology, Universidade de Caxias do Sul, Caxias do Sul, Brazil

Abstract

Several probiotic bacteria have been proposed for treatment or prevention of inflammatory bowel diseases (IBD), showing a protective effect in animal models of experimental colitis and for some of them also in human clinical trials. While most of these probiotic bacteria are isolated from the digestive tract, we recently reported that a *Lactobacillus* strain isolated from cheese, *L. delbrueckii* subsp. *lactis* CNRZ327 (Lb CNRZ327), also possesses anti-inflammatory effects *in vitro* and *in vivo*, demonstrating that common dairy bacteria may be useful in the treatment or prevention of IBD. Here, we studied the mechanisms underlying the protective effects of Lb CNRZ327 *in vivo*, in a mouse dextran sodium sulfate (DSS) colitis model. During colitis, Lb CNRZ327 modulated the production of TGF-β, IL-6, and IL-12 in colonic tissue and of TGF-β and IL-6 in the spleen, and caused an expansion of CD4+Foxp3+ regulatory T cells in the cecal lymph nodes. Moreover, a strong tendency to CD4+Foxp3+ expansion was also observed in the spleen. The results of this study for the first time show that orally administered dairy lactobacilli can not only modulate mucosal but also systemic immune responses and constitute an effective treatment of IBD.

Editor: Markus M. Heimesaat, Charité, Campus Benjamin Franklin, Germany

Funding: This study received financial support from Conselho Nacional de Desenvolvimento Científico e Tecnológico, Brasil (CNPq), Fundação de Amparo a Pesquisa do Estado de Minas Gerais, Brasil (FAPEMIG), Coordenação de Aperfeiçoamento de Pessoal de Nível Superior, Brasil (CAPES), and the EC EST project "LABHEALTH" (Marie Curie Contract MEST-2-CT-2004-514428). The funders had no role in study design, data collection and analysis, decision to publish, or preparation of the manuscript.

Competing Interests: The authors have declared that no competing interests exist.

* E-mail: maarten.vandeguchte@jouy.inra.fr

¶ These authors contributed equally to this work.

Introduction

The gastro intestinal tract (GIT) constitutes the largest surface of contact between the body and the external environment [1], and harbors a diverse population of commensal microorganisms that play an important role in the development and functioning of the immune system [2,3]. Under physiological conditions, the constant exposure to antigens through the gut mucosa leads to local and systemic immunological activities, such as secretory immunoglobulin A (sIgA) production and oral tolerance induction [3,4].

Inflammatory bowel diseases (IBDs), including ulcerative colitis (UC) and Crohn's disease (CD), are characterized by a spontaneous and chronic inflammation of the GIT. Although the causes for IBD remain obscure, there is growing evidence that IBD results from abnormal immune responses to the gut microbiota in individuals with genetic predisposition. The state of tolerance to the native microbiota is disturbed by the presence of a deregulated effector T cell population that reacts to the normal microbiota or, alternatively, by the presence of a defective Treg (regulatory T-cell) population that does not properly modulate the effector T cell responses [5,6].

Patients with IBD present an abnormal luminal microbiota and it has been suggested that the lack of bacteria with anti-inflammatory properties observed in the dysbiosis accompanying IBD could be a key factor in the persistence of inflammation [7,8]. In this context, the administration of probiotics may balance the indigenous microbiota and several have been proposed for IBD treatment, showing a protective effect in animal models of experimental colitis and for some of them also in human clinical trials [9,10]. Although the mechanisms underlying the protective effects of probiotics in IBD remain largely unknown, some of them have been partially characterized. These include the enhancement of the intestinal barrier function [11], the secretion of antimicrobial compounds [12], and the modulation of intestinal epithelial and mucosal immune cell responses [13]. Several probiotics have been reported to exert anti-inflammatory effects by the modulation of innate and adaptive immune responses. It has been shown that they can modulate the balance between Th1, Th2, Th17 and Treg cells, down-regulate the production of pro-inflammatory cytokines and stimulate anti-inflammatory cytokine production [14,15].

We recently reported that a dairy *Lactobacillus* isolated from cheese, *Lactobacillus delbrueckii* subsp. *lactis* CNRZ327 (Lb CNRZ327) inhibits TNF-α-induced NF-κB activation in intestinal epithelial cells, *in vitro*, by reducing IκB phosphorylation [16]. The nuclear factor κB is a key transcription factor in the establishment of an inflammatory response and its inhibition has been proposed as an important therapeutic target for IBD [17]. The same *Lactobacillus* strain also attenuated the symptoms of DSS induced colitis in mice [16]. Here, we examine the immune modulation mechanisms underlying its protective effect *in vivo*.

Materials and Methods

Ethics statement

Conventional female C57BL/6 mice (Federal University of Minas Gerais, Brazil), 10 to 12 weeks of age, were kept in an environmentally controlled room (21°C, 55% RH) with a 12-h light-dark cycle in the conventional experimental animal facility of Laboratório de Imunobiologia, Instituto de Ciências Biológicas, Universidade Federal de Minas Gerais, Belo Horizonte, Brasil. Mouse chow and water were administered *ad libidum*. At the end of the experiments, mice were sacrificed by cervical dislocation. This study was approved by the local Ethical Committee for Animal Experimentation (CETEA - UFMG, CETEA # 114/2010).

Bacterial strain

Lactobacillus delbrueckii subsp. *lactis* CNRZ327 (Lb CNRZ327) from the INRA collection was grown at 42°C under microaerobic conditions in MRS broth (Difco) or on the same medium solidified with 2% agar.

DSS-induced colitis

Experiments were performed several times with 5 to 10 mice per group in each experiment (see Figure legends for details on the number of repetitions for each parameter measured). After acclimatization, colonic inflammation was induced by the administration of a 2% (w/v) DSS (Dextran Sodium Sulphate; 40 kDa, ICN n° 160110) aqueous solution as the only source of drinking water for 7 days. All mice were sacrificed at day 8. Liquid consumption was monitored and all mice groups consumed similar volumes of DSS solution daily. Lb CNRZ327 was administered intragastrically from the day before the beginning of the DSS treatment, and daily until day 7. For this purpose, daily cultures of Lb CNRZ327 ($OD_{600} = 1$) were prepared in MRS medium (Difco). Cultures were centrifuged and collected cells were washed with 0.9% NaCl and resuspended in phosphate buffered saline (PBS; NaCl 8 g/L, KCl 0.2 g/L, NaH_2PO_4 1.44 g/L, K_2HPO_4 0.24 g/L, pH 7.4) to obtain a final concentration of 2.5×10^{10} colony forming units (CFU) per mL. Each mouse received 0.2 mL of bacterial suspension by intragastric administration (5×10^9 CFU/mouse/day). Negative control mice, called PBS group, received PBS intragastrically, and no DSS was added to their drinking water. Positive control mice (DSS group) received PBS intragastrically, and DSS was added to their drinking water. Animals from the experimental group received Lb CNRZ327 intragastically and DSS was added to their drinking water (327+DSS group).

Macroscopic analysis

Body weight was assessed at the start of the experiment and daily until the end of the experiment (day 8). Weight change is expressed as percentage change in weight compared with the starting weight. The disease activity index (DAI) was obtained as described by Murthy *et al.* [18] by scoring three major clinical signs: weight loss, diarrhea, and rectal bleeding.

Histological analysis

The colon was dissected free of fat and mesentery tissue, opened and cleaned with PBS. For histological inflammation scoring, sections of paraffin embedded descendent colon tissue were stained with haematoxylin and eosin, and observed under the microscope. Histological scoring was based on a semiquantitative scoring system described by McCafferty *et al.* [19] in which the following features were graded: extent of destruction of normal mucosal architecture (0, normal; 1, 2, and 3, mild, moderate, and extensive damage, respectively), presence and degree of cellular infiltration (0, normal; 1, 2, and 3, mild, moderate, and transmural infiltration, respectively), extent of muscle thickening (0, normal; 1, 2, and 3, mild, moderate, and extensive thickening, respectively), presence or absence of crypt abscesses (0, absent or 1, present), and presence or absence of goblet cell depletion (0, absent or 1, present). Mice were scored blindly by an expert.

Measurement of colon and spleen cytokines

Colon or spleen samples were weighed and homogenized in PBS containing 0.05% Tween-20, 0.1 mM phenylmethylsulphonyl fluoride, 0.1 mM benzethonium chloride, 10 mM EDTA and 20 KIU Aprotinin A using a tissue homogenizer (100 mg tissue/ml buffer). Suspensions were centrifuged at 12.000× g for 20 min at 4°C and the supernatants were transferred to microtubes and stored at −80°C until analysis. Concentrations of IL-4, IL-6, IL-10, IL-12, IL-17 and TGF-β were measured by enzyme-linked immunosorbent assay (ELISA) as described by Maron *et al.* [20]. Briefly, supernatants were added to microtitre plates (Nunc), previously coated with purified monoclonal antibodies reactive to IL-4, IL-6, IL-10, IL-12, IL-17 and TGF-β (BD Bioscience). Standards and samples were added and incubated overnight at 4°C. Biotinylated monoclonal antibodies against cytokines were added and incubated for 1 h at room temperature, after which peroxidase-labelled streptavidin (Sigma) was added. A color reaction was developed at room temperature with 100 uL/well of orthophenylenediamine (1 mg/ml) and 0.04% H_2O_2 substrate in sodium citrate buffer. The reaction was terminated by the addition of 20 μL/well of 2 N H_2SO_4. Absorbance was measured at 492 nm by an ELISA reader (Bio-Rad Model 450 Microplate Reader). Results are presented as a percentage of the values obtained for the negative control group which received the value of 100.

Measurement of secreted IgA (sIgA)

Fecal samples were weighed and homogenized in PBS (100 mg feces/ml buffer). The suspensions were centrifuged at 12.000 g for 20 min at 4°C, and the levels of sIgA in the supernatant were determined by ELISA as previously described [20].

Analysis of cell subsets by flow cytometry

Briefly, 1×10^6 cells isolated from spleen or cecal lymph nodes were resuspended in PBS containing 0.2% BSA (Bovine Serum Albumin) and 0.1% NaN_3 (PBS-BSA-NaN_3, pH 7.4). For surface antigen detection, the cells were labeled with monoclonal antibodies (FITC-conjugated anti-mouse CD4 and Cy5-conjugated anti-mouse CD69) for 30 min at 4°C. For intracellular staining, cells were fixed and permeabilized with Fixation/Permeabilization working solution (eBioscience) for one hour on ice and subsequently incubated with PE-conjugated anti-mouse Foxp3 for 30 min at 4°C. The cells were then washed in PBS-BSA-NaN_3 and centrifuged at 1200× g for 2 min at 4°C. The supernatant was discarded and the cells resuspended in 200 µL of the same buffer containing 1% paraformaldehyde. Cells were acquired using a FACSCan (BECTON & DICKINSON) and data were analyzed by FlowJo (TREESTAR). At least 30,000 events were counted for each sample. Results are presented as a percentage of the negative control group which received the value of 100.

Statistical analysis

Data were analyzed in accordance with an unbalanced factorial experimental design, as all parameters (e.g. cytokine-levels) were measured in all combinations of tissue and treatment but with unequal sample sizes and not always during the same experiment. The effect of a treatment was examined independently for each parameter within each tissue, when applicable. This led to a total of 20 analyses (2 tissues×6 cytokine levels, 2 tissues×2 cell counts, and weight, DAI, IgA and histological score not related to tissue). Cytokine levels and cell counts showed considerable scale variations between experiments, and were therefore expressed as a percentage of the average level or count in the negative control (PBS) in the same experiment. This type of normalization was not necessary for the parameters weight, DAI, IgA and histological score. For all parameters, a clear (additive) experiment effect was observed which was modeled as a random effect in downstream analyses. To assess the effect of treatment on each parameter, linear mixed models were used as implemented in the lmer function of the R lme4 package [21]. Treatment was used as a fixed effect, Experiment as a random effect, and an interaction [Treatment×Experiment] was added to the model when found significant ($p<0.05$). The overall effect of the treatment was then assessed with a likelihood ratio test. In case of a significant difference, a post-hoc analysis using Tukey's HSD test was performed to detect significantly different pairs of treatments. All data are expressed as mean ± standard error of the mean (SEM), which are computed under the abovementioned linear mixed model framework. They are the analogs of standard mean and SEM, taking the grouping of mice in independent experiments into account.

The possible existence of correlations between cytokine levels and cell counts in different tissues was analyzed where the experimental data allowed so. Because of the incomplete design, only 16 such correlations (2 tissues×2 cell counts×4 cytokine levels) out of the 24 theoretical ones could be computed. Although the factor "Experiment" still had the potential to be a confounding factor in this analysis, visual inspection confirmed by linear mixed modeling did not show any Experiment effect. Therefore, only simple correlations were computed.

Results

L. delbrueckii shows anti-inflammatory properties in DSS-induced colitis in C57BL/6 mice

DSS administration in the drinking water induces an acute inflammation in the gut with symptoms resembling those of human UC [22]. The impact of Lb CNRZ327 on DSS-induced colitis in mice was evaluated through the analysis of the major clinical signs (weight loss, diarrhea, and rectal bleeding), yielding a combined DAI (disease activity index) score, and colon histology, in comparison with mice that received no bacteria (DSS group). All parameters were analyzed at day 8, after the last administration of DSS in the drinking water. In three out of 4 experiments, no difference was observed in weight change over the course of the experiment between the DSS and PBS group, despite clear signs of inflammation (diarrhea and rectal bleeding) in the former (data not shown). In the fourth experiment, PBS-treated mice gained weight (~1.6%) by the end of the experiment while DSS exposure severely affected the weight of the mice, resulting in a weight loss of about 19%. Administration of Lb CNRZ327 significantly reduced weight loss to about 3% at the end of this experiment (Fig. 1A). Figure 1B shows the DAI at the end of the experiment. The DSS-treated mice without bacteria obtained a score of 6.5 whereas a significantly reduced score of 3.4 was observed in Lb CNRZ327-treated mice. Microscopic examination showed that control mice without DSS presented a normal colon histology (Fig. 2A) while DSS exposure provoked the loss of mucosal architecture with ulcerations, transmural immune cell infiltration through the mucosa and submucosa, edema, goblet cell depletion and increased thickness of the intestinal mucosa and submucosa (Fig. 2B). The administration of Lb CNRZ327 almost abrogated these intestinal changes (Fig. 2C). Colonic tissue damage was given a score taking into account the extent of destruction of the normal mucosal architecture, the presence and degree of cellular infiltration, the extent of muscle thickening, the presence or absence of crypt abscesses and the presence or absence of goblet cell depletion. The DSS-treated group without bacteria obtained a score of 8.9 which was significantly reduced to 5 in Lb CNRZ327-treated mice (Fig. 2D).

L. delbrueckii tends to increase the level of secretory IgA (sIgA)

An increasing number of probiotic strains have been shown to increase IgA secretion, which is important to selectively exclude the entrance of pathogenic agents [23,24]. We therefore analyzed the impact of Lb. CNRZ327 on the sIgA levels in the feces of DSS-treated mice. As shown in Fig. 3, the level of IgA in DSS-exposed mice did not significantly differ from the levels found in the PBS group. The administration of DSS and Lb CNRZ327 increased the s-IgA level to a level that was significantly higher

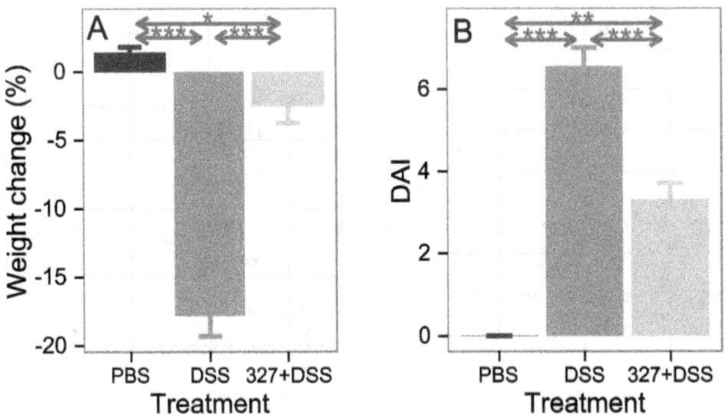

Figure 1. Effect of Lb CNRZ327 on body weight and DAI in DSS-induced colitis. A. Body weight change from day 1 to day 8. Each bar represents the average body weight change ± SEM of the 5 mice in the group (one experiment, see text for further details) as a percentage of their initial weights. **B.** Disease activity index (DAI) on day 8. Bars represent the mean ± SEM calculated across three independent experiments, with 5 to 10 mice per group in each experiment (combined sample sizes: 17 to 20 mice per treatment). * = $p<0.05$; ** = $p<0.01$; *** = $p<0.001$.

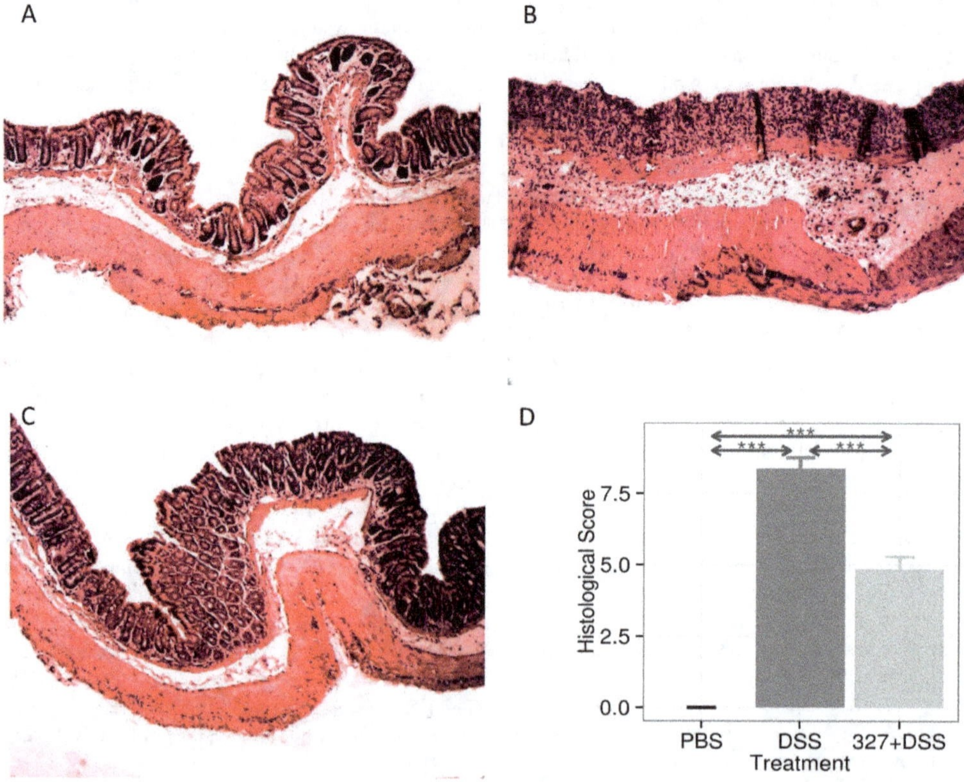

Figure 2. Colon histology after DSS-induced colitis. **A**. Descending colon of the negative control group (without bacteria or DSS). **B**. Descending colon of the positive group control (only DSS). **C**. Descending colon of the experimental group (DSS plus Lb CNRZ327). A, B, and C each show representative results from three independent experiments. **D**. Histological score of the groups described above. Bars represent the mean ± SEM calculated across three independent experiments, with 4 or 5 mice per group in each experiment (combined sample sizes: 13 to 14 mice per treatment). *** = p<0.001.

than in the PBS group, although the difference with the DSS group was not significant.

L. delbrueckii modulates the production of cytokines and T-cell differentiation in colonic tissue

In order to determine if Lb CNRZ327 can modulate DSS-induced cytokines, we measured the levels of TGF-β, IL-4, IL-6, IL-10, IL-12, and IL-17 in colonic tissue. The exposure of C57BL/6 mice to 2% DSS led to significant 1.5, 2.7, 2.4, and 1.5-fold increases in colonic TGF-β, IL-4, IL-6, and IL-12 levels, respectively. The administration of Lb CNRZ327 diminished the production of TGF-β, IL-6 and IL-12 to levels that are not significantly different from those measured in the PBS control group, while the amounts of IL-4 were not significantly affected (Fig. 4, upper panel). Lb CNRZ327 did not affect the decrease in colonic levels of IL-10 and IL-17 induced by the administration of DSS (Fig. 4).

As patients with IBD present a disrupted balance between effector and regulatory T cells [5,6], we analyzed the effect of DSS and Lb CNRZ327 administration on the frequencies of T-cell subtypes in cecal lymph nodes (CLN). Neither DSS nor the combination of DSS and Lb CNRZ327 significantly affected the frequency of T cells expressing the early activation marker CD69 in CLN (Fig. 5, upper panel). While T cells with a regulatory phenotype ($CD4^+$ $Foxp3^+$) were less frequent after DSS treatment (Fig. 5), Lb CNRZ327 restored the levels of $Foxp3^+$ cells within the $CD4^+$ compartment in the CLN of DSS-treated mice to those found in the control group (Fig. 5).

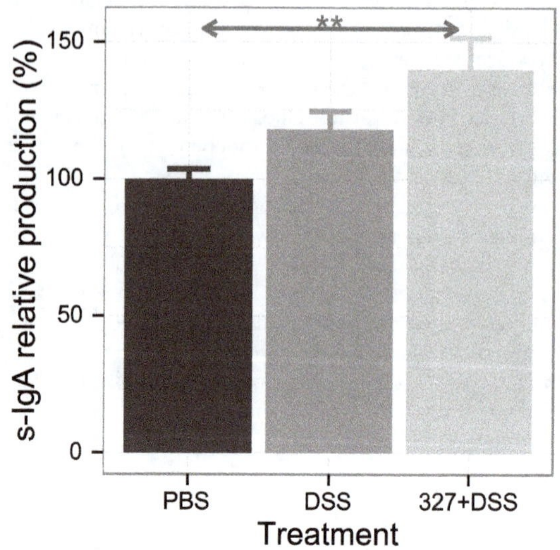

Figure 3. Secretory IgA levels after DSS-induced colitis. Feces were collected and total sIgA was measured by ELISA. PBS, control without bacteria or DSS; DSS, DSS only, without bacteria; 327+DSS, DSS plus Lb CNRZ327. 100 (the average amount observed in the PBS control group) corresponds to the range of 61.5 to 126 pg/mL. Bars represent the mean ± SEM calculated across three independent experiments, with 3 to 10 mice per group in each experiment (combined sample sizes: 15 to 24 mice per treatment). ** = p<0.01.

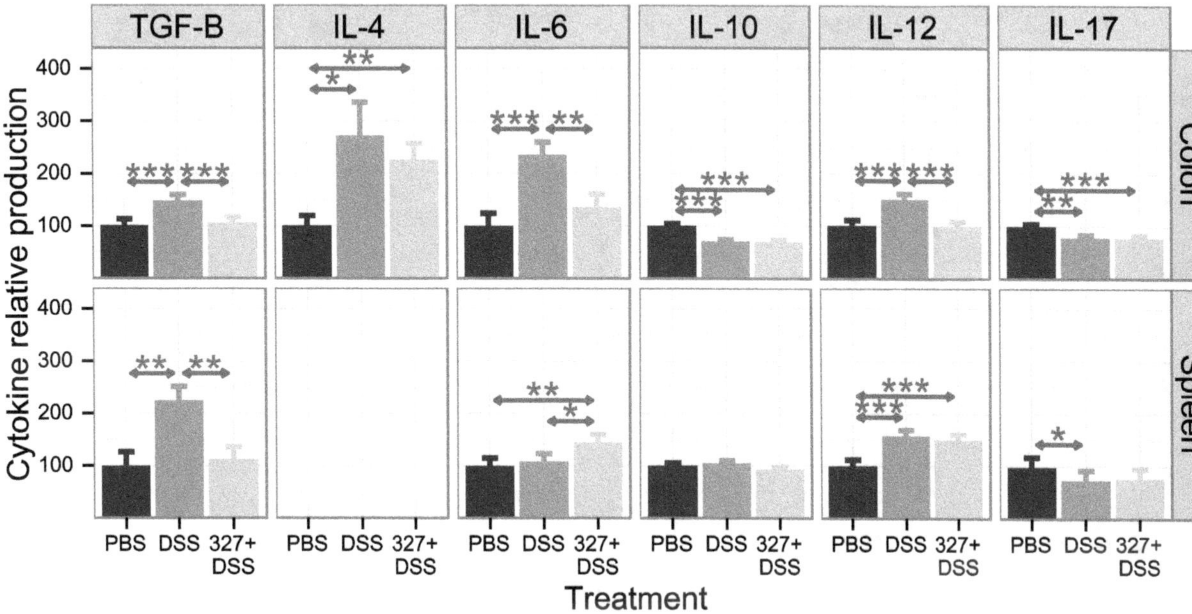

Figure 4. Cytokine production in colonic tissue and spleen after DSS-induced colitis. Cytokine concentrations in homogenized tissues are presented as a percentage of the amount observed in the PBS control group (range from different experiments given in parentheses for each cytokine) which received the value of 100. Upper panel, colon: TGF-β (100 = 69 to 131.4 pg/mL), IL-4 (100 = 70.8 to 161.2 pg/mL), IL-6 (100 = 63.2 to 159.2 pg/mL), IL-10 (100 = 72.8 to 146.2 pg/mL), IL-12 (100 = 71.4 to 168.8 pg/mL), IL-17 (100 = 83.3 to 143.4 pg/mL). Lower panel, spleen: TGF-β (100 = 80.7 to 169.7 pg/mL), IL-6 (100 = 80.1 to 134 pg/mL), IL-10 (100 = 73.1 to 143.2 pg/mL), IL-12 (100 = 53.1 to 123 pg/mL), IL-17 (100 = 68.3 to 136.2 pg/mL). PBS, control without bacteria or DSS; DSS, DSS only, without bacteria; 327+DSS, DSS plus Lb CNRZ327.Bars represent the mean ± SEM calculated across two to six independent experiments, with 2 to 10 mice per group in each experiment (combined sample sizes: 9 to 33 mice per treatment (colon) and 5 to 12 mice per treatment (spleen)). * = $p<0.05$; ** = $p<0.01$; *** = $p<0.001$.

Systemic effects of *L. delbrueckii*

In order to see if the effects of the oral administration of *L. delbrueckii* were restricted to the gut and associated tissues or more widespread, we measured TGF-β, IL-6, IL-10, IL-12, and IL-17 in the spleen of the mice. DSS exposure increased the levels of splenic TGF-β and IL-12 (Fig. 4, lower pannel). Lb CNRZ327 abolished the increase in TGF-β, but did not affect IL-12 levels. The secretion of splenic IL-17 was reduced by DSS, and Lb CNRZ327-treatment did not restore the production of this cytokine (Fig. 4). The production of splenic IL-6 was not affected by DSS, but slightly enhanced in the presence of DSS and Lb CNRZ327, and IL-10 was not affected by either DSS or DSS and Lb CNRZ327 (Fig. 4).

Regarding T-cell differentiation, neither DSS nor the combination of DSS and Lb CNRZ327 significantly affected the frequency of T cells expressing the early activation marker CD69 in the spleen (Fig. 5, lower panel). However, while DSS-treatment resulted in an important reduction in the frequency of T cells with a regulatory phenotype ($CD4^+Foxp3^+$) in the spleen (Fig. 5), we observed a strong tendency of augmentation of this cell-type after treatment with Lb CNRZ327 (Fig. 5). This tendency reflects the changes observed in the colon, and is further supported by the strong correlation that can be observed between the frequencies of $CD4^+Foxp3^+$ cells in the spleen and in the colon (Fig. 6).

Together, these results clearly demonstrate that the immune-modulation effects of *L. delbrueckii* go beyond a local effect in gut-associated tissues.

Discussion

The aim of this study was to characterize the mechanisms involved in the anti-inflammatory effects of Lb CNRZ327 in DSS-induced colitis in mice. We induced colitis in C56BL/6 mice by adding 2% (w/v) DSS in the drinking water for 7 consecutive days. At this concentration, DSS triggered a strong colonic inflammation accompanied by diarrhea and rectal bleeding. No mortality was observed. The administration of Lb CNRZ327 significantly attenuated diarrhea and rectal bleeding. In only one out of 4 independent experiments, weight loss was observed in the DSS group compared with the negative control group, and Lb CNRZ327 significantly reduced this weight loss. In other experiments we observed no weight loss after DSS exposure. Variability of this parameter after DSS treatment has been reported earlier [25]. At the histological level, the administration of Lb CNRZ327 strongly diminished the tissue damage induced by DSS, demonstrating its anti-inflammatory effects.

We previously reported that Lb CNRZ327 attenuates DSS-induced colitis in BALB/c mice [16]. In the present study, we observed an even stronger anti-colitis effect of Lb CNRZ327 in C56BL/6 mice. Although a direct comparison is precluded as we did not perform experiments using C56BL/6 and BALB/c mice in parallel in the same laboratory, the difference may be explained by the fact that these mice strains differ in their response to DSS due to their different genetic background [26].

The administration of Lb CNRZ327 tended to increase the level of gut secretory IgA (sIgA), although the difference with the DSS group was not statistically significant. Several other studies reported that the consumption of probiotics was associated with increased sIgA levels [23,24] which could reinforce the gut barrier and limit the penetration of bacteria (commensal and pathogenic)

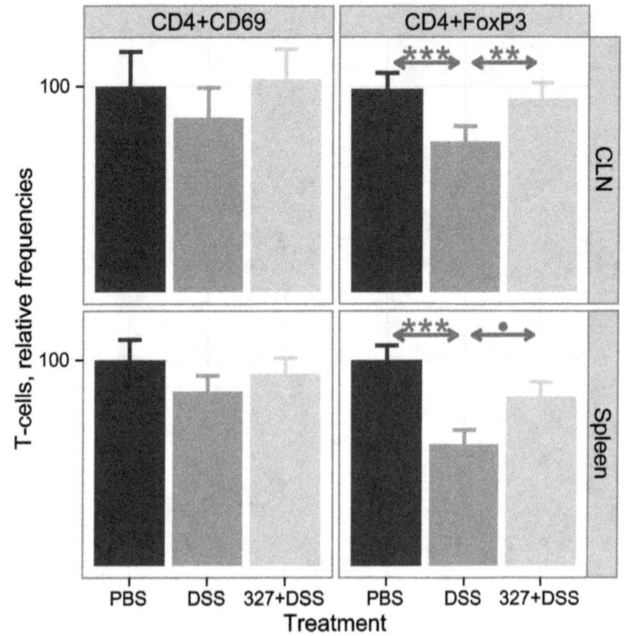

Figure 5. T lymphocyte profiles in cecal lymph nodes and spleen after DSS-induced colitis. T cells were isolated from cecal lymph nodes (CLN, upper panel) and spleen (lower panel) at the end of the experiment, and the frequencies of $CD4^{+}CD69^{+}$ and $CD4^{+}Foxp3^{+}$ T cells, as percentage of CD4+ T cells, were assessed by flow cytometry. T-cell frequencies are presented relative to the average frequency observed in the PBS control group (range from different experiments given in parentheses for each T cell type) which received the value of 100. Upper panel, CLN: CD4+CD69+ (100 = 2.7 to 3.54), CD4+FoxP3+ (100 = 3.41 to 5.41). Lower panel, spleen: CD4+CD69+ (100 = 4.5 to 4.51), CD4+FoxP3+ (100 = 1.59 to 4.02). PBS, control without bacteria or DSS; DSS, DSS only, without bacteria; 327+DSS, DSS plus Lb CNRZ327. For $CD4^{+}CD69^{+}$ T cells, bars represent the mean ± SEM of one experiment, with 2 or 3 mice in the PBS control groups and 5 mice in each of the other groups. For $CD4^{+}$FoxP3+ T cells, bars represent the mean ± SEM calculated across two independent experiments, with 3 to 5 mice per group in each experiment (combined sample sizes: 8 to 10 mice per treatment (colon) and 8 mice per treatment (spleen)). ** = $p<0.01$; *** = $p<0.001$; • = $p = 0.053$.

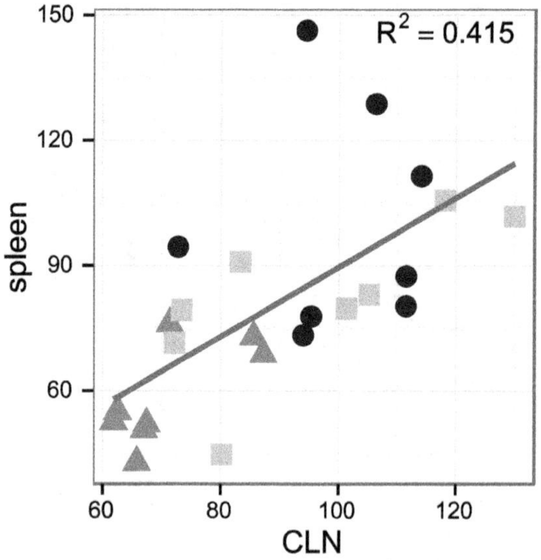

Figure 6. Correlation between relative frequencies of CD4+FoxP3 T cells in CLN and spleen. Each point represents one mouse, placed as a function of relative CD4+FoxP3 T cell frequencies in CLN and spleen (cf legend to Fig. 5). Black dots, PBS (control without bacteria or DSS); grey triangles, DSS (DSS only, without bacteria); light grey squares, 327+DSS (DSS plus Lb CNRZ327). The grey line describes the linear relationship between the frequencies of $CD4^{+}Foxp3^{+}$ cells in the spleen and in the colon ($R^2 = 0.415$).

into host tissues (reviewed in [27]). This is particularly relevant in the DSS model of colitis as DSS is directly toxic to gut epithelial cells and affects the integrity of the epithelial barrier [28,29]. The mechanisms by which Lb CNRZ327 affects sIgA production remain to be elucidated.

Since cytokines are major mediators of inflammation and regulatory activity in the gut mucosa, we analyzed the ability of Lb CNRZ327 to modulate the production of cytokines in colonic tissue of the mice. TGF-β, IL-4, IL-6 and IL-12 were found to be significantly increased in the colonic tissue of DSS-treated mice when compared with the negative control. Lb CNRZ327 decreased the production of TGF-β, IL-6 and IL-12 to reach a level similar to that in the negative control. TGF-β1 is an abundant cytokine in the intestinal mucosa where it has immunosuppressive as well as pro-inflammatory properties. TGF-β1 can inhibit T cell proliferation, macrophage activity and secretion of several pro-inflammatory cytokines. Secretion of this cytokine can be triggered in regulatory T cells and epithelial gut cells as a protective mechanism to control tissue damage and overt inflammation. On the other hand, in combination with the pro-inflammatory cytokine IL-6, TGF-β can induce differentiation of Th17 cells, a T cell subset with a prominent pathogenic role in inflammatory bowel diseases [30]. Therefore, elevated levels of local TGF-β1 and IL-6 in colitis can be correlated with inflammatory events, fibrosis and structuring of the disease [31]. IL-12 is a pro-inflammatory cytokine that plays a pivotal role in the differentiation of Th1 cells and is upregulated in patients with IBD, especially those with CD [32,33], while IL-4 is critical in generating CD4+ Th2 effector cells [34]. Interestingly, Mannon *et al.* [35] demonstrated that treatment with a monoclonal antibody against IL-12 induces remission in patients with active CD. Therefore, the reduced levels of TGF-β, IL-6 and IL-12 at the peak of colonic inflammation in mice treated with Lb CNRZ327 may be an indicator and explaining factor of the lower degree of inflammation in these mice.

The modulation of pro- and anti-inflammatory cytokines is an important mechanism underlying the effects of several probiotics although the actual cytokines affected may differ. While for *Lactobacillus casei* DN-114 001, for example, an increase in IL-10 seems to explain the observed anti-inflammatory effect [36], here a different mechanism appears to be involved. We observed clear anti-inflammatory effects, but no changes in colonic tissue IL-10 levels. Other studies have shown that several other lactic acid bacteria are, like *L. delbrueckii*, able to reduce the production of the pro-inflammatory cytokine IL-6 in the inflamed colon of mice [37–39].

In addition to cytokine levels in colonic tissue, DSS and Lb CNRZ327 affected cytokine levels in the spleen. TGF-β was increased in the spleen of DSS treated mice and, as observed in the colonic tissue, Lb CNRZ327 restored TGF-β levels to those found in the non-inflamed mice, demonstrating the ability of Lb CNRZ327 to modulate not only local but also systemic immune responses. No significant differences between mice treated with DSS or DSS and Lb CNRZ327 were found for the other splenic cytokines measured, except for IL-6 which was increased by ~34% after administration of the bacterium, at a difference with the colon where Lb CNRZ327 caused a reduction of this cytokine.

However, the latter difference should be regarded in the light of the DSS-mediated strong induction of IL-6 in the colon, which is nearly annulled by Lb CNRZ327, and the absence of IL-6 induction by DSS in the spleen. Lb CNRZ327 thus appears to correct the large change in IL-6 brought about by DSS treatment in the colon, while inducing a small raise of IL-6 in both the spleen and colon when compared to the PBS control.

Few studies have addressed the systemic immune responses triggered by orally administered bacteria. The consumption of *Lactobacillus fermentum* CECT5713 was reported to enhance the production of Th1 cytokines (especially IL-12) in the spleen of healthy mice while *Lactobacillus salivarius* induced IL-10 production [40]. Lavasani *et al.* [41] demonstrated that the oral administration of three strains of *lactobacilli* (*Lactobacillus paracasei* DSM 13434, *L. plantarum* DSM 15312 and *L. plantarum* DSM15323) prevented the signs of multiple sclerosis, a T cell mediated inflammatory autoimmune disease affecting the central nervous system, in mice, and that effect correlated with the attenuation of pro-inflammatory Th1 and Th17 cytokines followed by IL-10 induction in the mesenteric lymph nodes (MLN), spleen and blood.

In addition to the effects of Lb CNRZ327 on cytokine production, we evaluated two cellular parameters. CD4+ T cells expressing the Foxp3 transcription factor constitute a classical subset of regulatory T cells (Tregs) that play a crucial role in preventing the development and activity of inflammatory effector T cells. Natural CD4+Foxp3+ are generated in the thymus as key elements to regulate autoimmune reactivity in the body [42]. CD4+Foxp3+ T cells can also be generated in peripheral lymphoid sites and the gut associated lymphoid tissue is especially prone to induce the differentiation of these cells [42]. These cells were shown to be important players in the homeostasis of the gut mucosa [43], and individuals with IBD present altered frequencies of these cells [44,45]. Our results show that DSS exposure leads to a decrease in the frequency of CD4+Foxp3+ T cells in the CLN and that Lb CNRZ327 is able to restore the frequency to a level similar to that in the negative control. Lb CNRZ327 did not affect the frequency of T cells expressing the activation marker CD69+, demonstrating that this strain is not able to activate CD4+ lymphocytes, thus confirming that Lb CNRZ327 does not induce inflammatory responses.

These results are reminiscent of those obtained with several probiotics, that attenuated colitis symptoms through the local expansion of different Tregs subtypes. The anti-colitis effect of *L. salivarius* 33 was correlated with the expansion of CD4+Foxp3+ T cells in the MLN [46] while VSL#3 increased the population of Tregs bearing surface TGF-beta in the form of latency-associated protein (LAP) (LAP+ T cells) in the lamina propria [14].

Here, in addition we observed a strong tendency of restoration of CD4+Foxp3+ regulatory T cells in the spleen of mice treated with DSS and Lb CNRZ327, as compared to mice treated with DSS alone, highlighting the systemic improvement of inflammation parameters by Lb CNRZ327. Expansion of regulatory T cells in the spleen had earlier been reported after treatment with *Lactobacillus plantarum*, but only in healthy mice (i.e. without induction of colitis) [47].

In conclusion, we confirmed the anti-inflammatory effect of the dairy *Lactobacillus delbrueckii* strain Lb CNRZ327 in DSS-induced colitis in mice, and showed some of the mechanisms underlying its probiotic effects, at the local and systemic level. For the cytokines and cellular parameters where Lb CNRZ327 has an effect, the bacteria tend to correct the changes brought about by the DSS treatment. To our knowledge, this is the first demonstration of systemic immune modulation effects exerted by a dairy *Lactobacillus* strain.

Acknowledgments

We are thankful to Ilda Marçal de Souza for her excellent work taking care of the mice facilities.

Author Contributions

Conceived and designed the experiments: AMCdF CSR MvdG AM PL EM VA. Performed the experiments: CSR ACGS TGM MdA TDL. Analyzed the data: CSR AMCdF MM MvdG APLD AM. Wrote the paper: CSR MvdG.

References

1. Neish AS (2009) Microbes in gastrointestinal health and disease. Gastroenterology 136: 65–80.
2. Hooper LV, Macpherson AJ (2010) Immune adaptations that maintain homeostasis with the intestinal microbiota. Nature reviews Immunology 10: 159–169.
3. Kamada N, Seo SU, Chen GY, Nunez G (2013) Role of the gut microbiota in immunity and inflammatory disease. Nature reviews Immunology 13: 321–335.
4. Faria AM, Weiner HL (2005) Oral tolerance. Immunological reviews 206: 232–259.
5. Strober W, Fuss I, Mannon P (2007) The fundamental basis of inflammatory bowel disease. J Clin Invest 117: 514–521.
6. Bouma G, Strober W (2003) The immunological and genetic basis of inflammatory bowel disease. Nat Rev Immunol 3: 521–533.
7. Sokol H, Pigneur B, Watterlot L, Lakhdari O, Bermudez-Humaran LG, et al. (2008) Faecalibacterium prausnitzii is an anti-inflammatory commensal bacterium identified by gut microbiota analysis of Crohn disease patients. Proc Natl Acad Sci U S A 105: 16731–16736.
8. Sokol H, Seksik P, Furet JP, Firmesse O, Nion-Larmurier I, et al. (2009) Low counts of Faecalibacterium prausnitzii in colitis microbiota. Inflamm Bowel Dis 15: 1183–1189.
9. Mileti E, Matteoli G, Iliev ID, Rescigno M (2009) Comparison of the immunomodulatory properties of three probiotic strains of Lactobacilli using complex culture systems: prediction for in vivo efficacy. PloS one 4: e7056.
10. Meijer BJ, Dieleman LA (2011) Probiotics in the treatment of human inflammatory bowel diseases: update 2011. Journal of clinical gastroenterology 45 Suppl: S139–144.
11. Ohland CL, Macnaughton WK (2010) Probiotic bacteria and intestinal epithelial barrier function. American journal of physiology Gastrointestinal and liver physiology 298: G807–819.
12. Lievin V, Peiffer I, Hudault S, Rochat F, Brassart D, et al. (2000) Bifidobacterium strains from resident infant human gastrointestinal microflora exert antimicrobial activity. Gut 47: 646–652.
13. de Moreno de Leblanc A, Del Carmen S, Zurita-Turk M, Santos Rocha C, van de Guchte M, et al. (2011) Importance of IL-10 modulation by probiotic microorganisms in gastrointestinal inflammatory diseases. ISRN gastroenterology 2011: 892971.
14. Di Giacinto C, Marinaro M, Sanchez M, Strober W, Boirivant M (2005) Probiotics ameliorate recurrent Th1-mediated murine colitis by inducing IL-10 and IL-10-dependent TGF-beta-bearing regulatory cells. J Immunol 174: 3237–3246.
15. Round JL, Mazmanian SK (2010) Inducible Foxp3+ regulatory T-cell development by a commensal bacterium of the intestinal microbiota. Proc Natl Acad Sci U S A 107: 12204–12209.
16. Santos Rocha C, Lakhdari O, Blottiere HM, Blugeon S, Sokol H, et al. (2012) Anti-inflammatory properties of dairy lactobacilli. Inflamm Bowel Dis 18: 657–666.
17. Jobin C, Sartor RB (2000) The I kappa B/NF-kappa B system: a key determinant of mucosalinflammation and protection. American journal of physiology Cell physiology 278: C451–462.
18. Murthy SN, Cooper HS, Shim H, Shah RS, Ibrahim SA, et al. (1993) Treatment of dextran sulfate sodium-induced murine colitis by intracolonic cyclosporin. Dig Dis Sci 38: 1722–1734.
19. McCafferty DM, Sihota E, Muscara M, Wallace JL, Sharkey KA, et al. (2000) Spontaneously developing chronic colitis in IL-10/iNOS double-deficient mice. Am J Physiol Gastrointest Liver Physiol 279: G90–99.
20. Maron R, Hancock WW, Slavin A, Hattori M, Kuchroo V, et al. (1999) Genetic susceptibility or resistance to autoimmune encephalomyelitis in MHC congenic mice is associated with differential production of pro- and anti-inflammatory cytokines. Int Immunol 11: 1573–1580.

21. Pinheiro J, Bates D (2000) Mixed-effects models in S and S-PLUS. Berlin: Springer.
22. Solomon L, Mansor S, Mallon P, Donnelly E, Hoper M, et al. (2010) The dextran sulphate sodium (DSS) model of colitis: an overview. Comp Clin Pathol 19: 235–239.
23. O'Sullivan DJ (2001) Screening of intestinal microflora for effective probiotic bacteria. J Agric Food Chem 49: 1751–1760.
24. Malin M, Suomalainen H, Saxelin M, Isolauri E (1996) Promotion of IgA immune response in patients with Crohn's disease by oral bacteriotherapy with Lactobacillus GG. Ann Nutr Metab 40: 137–145.
25. Hamilton MJ, Sinnamon MJ, Lyng GD, Glickman JN, Wang X, et al. (2011) Essential role for mast cell tryptase in acute experimental colitis. Proc Natl Acad Sci U S A 108: 290–295.
26. Melgar S, Karlsson A, Michaelsson E (2005) Acute colitis induced by dextran sulfate sodium progresses to chronicity in C57BL/6 but not in BALB/c mice: correlation between symptoms and inflammation. Am J Physiol Gastrointest Liver Physiol 288: G1328–1338.
27. Thomas CM, Versalovic J (2010) Probiotics-host communication: Modulation of signaling pathways in the intestine. Gut microbes 1: 148–163.
28. Okayasu I, Hatakeyama S, Yamada M, Ohkusa T, Inagaki Y, et al. (1990) A novel method in the induction of reliable experimental acute and chronic ulcerative colitis in mice. Gastroenterology 98: 694–702.
29. Laroui H, Ingersoll SA, Liu HC, Baker MT, Ayyadurai S, et al. (2012) Dextran sodium sulfate (DSS) induces colitis in mice by forming nano-lipocomplexes with medium-chain-length fatty acids in the colon. PloS one 7: e32084.
30. Letterio JJ, Roberts AB (1998) Regulation of immune responses by TGF-beta. Annu Rev Immunol 16: 137–161.
31. Fichtner-Feigl S, Fuss IJ, Young CA, Watanabe T, Geissler EK, et al. (2007) Induction of IL-13 triggers TGF-beta1-dependent tissue fibrosis in chronic 2,4,6-trinitrobenzene sulfonic acid colitis. J Immunol 178: 5859–5870.
32. Pallone F, Monteleone G (1998) Interleukin 12 and Th1 responses in inflammatory bowel disease. Gut 43: 735–736.
33. Brand S (2009) Crohn's disease: Th1, Th17 or both? The change of a paradigm: new immunological and genetic insights implicate Th17 cells in the pathogenesis of Crohn's disease. Gut 58: 1152–1167.
34. Swain SL, Weinberg AD, English M, Huston G (1990) IL-4 directs the development of Th2-like helper effectors. Journal of immunology 145: 3796–3806.
35. Mannon PJ, Fuss IJ, Mayer L, Elson CO, Sandborn WJ, et al. (2004) Anti-interleukin-12 antibody for active Crohn's disease. The New England journal of medicine 351: 2069–2079.
36. Chung YW, Choi JH, Oh TY, Eun CS, Han DS (2008) Lactobacillus casei prevents the development of dextran sulphate sodium-induced colitis in Toll-like receptor 4 mutant mice. Clin Exp Immunol 151: 182–189.
37. Philippe D, Heupel E, Blum-Sperisen S, Riedel CU (2011) Treatment with Bifidobacterium bifidum 17 partially protects mice from Th1-driven inflammation in a chemically induced model of colitis. International journal of food microbiology 149: 45–49.
38. Kim SW, Kim HM, Yang KM, Kim SA, Kim SK, et al. (2010) Bifidobacterium lactis inhibits NF-kappaB in intestinal epithelial cells and prevents acute colitis and colitis-associated colon cancer in mice. Inflamm Bowel Dis 16: 1514–1525.
39. Nishitani Y, Tanoue T, Yamada K, Ishida T, Yoshida M, et al. (2009) Lactococcus lactis subsp. cremoris FC alleviates symptoms of colitis induced by dextran sulfate sodium in mice. International immunopharmacology 9: 1444–1451.
40. Diaz-Ropero MP, Martin R, Sierra S, Lara-Villoslada F, Rodriguez JM, et al. (2007) Two Lactobacillus strains, isolated from breast milk, differently modulate the immune response. Journal of applied microbiology 102: 337–343.
41. Lavasani S, Dzhambazov B, Nouri M, Fak F, Buske S, et al. (2010) A novel probiotic mixture exerts a therapeutic effect on experimental autoimmune encephalomyelitis mediated by IL-10 producing regulatory T cells. PloS one 5: e9009.
42. Curotto de Lafaille MA, Lafaille JJ (2009) Natural and adaptive foxp3+ regulatory T cells: more of the same or a division of labor? Immunity 30: 626–635.
43. Fontenot JD, Gavin MA, Rudensky AY (2003) Foxp3 programs the development and function of CD4+CD25+ regulatory T cells. Nat Immunol 4: 330–336.
44. Makita S, Kanai T, Oshima S, Uraushihara K, Totsuka T, et al. (2004) CD4+CD25bright T cells in human intestinal lamina propria as regulatory cells. J Immunol 173: 3119–3130.
45. Maul J, Loddenkemper C, Mundt P, Berg E, Giese T, et al. (2005) Peripheral and intestinal regulatory CD4+ CD25(high) T cells in inflammatory bowel disease. Gastroenterology 128: 1868–1878.
46. Macho Fernandez E, Valenti V, Rockel C, Hermann C, Pot B, et al. (2011) Anti-inflammatory capacity of selected lactobacilli in experimental colitis is driven by NOD2-mediated recognition of a specific peptidoglycan-derived muropeptide. Gut 60: 1050–1059.
47. Smelt MJ, de Haan BJ, Bron PA, van Swam I, Meijerink M, et al. (2012) L. plantarum, L. salivarius, and L. lactis attenuate Th2 responses and increase Treg frequencies in healthy mice in a strain dependent manner. PLoS One 7: e47244.

Permissions

All chapters in this book were first published in PLOS ONE, by The Public Library of Science; hereby published with permission under the Creative Commons Attribution License or equivalent. Every chapter published in this book has been scrutinized by our experts. Their significance has been extensively debated. The topics covered herein carry significant findings which will fuel the growth of the discipline. They may even be implemented as practical applications or may be referred to as a beginning point for another development.

The contributors of this book come from diverse backgrounds, making this book a truly international effort. This book will bring forth new frontiers with its revolutionizing research information and detailed analysis of the nascent developments around the world.

We would like to thank all the contributing authors for lending their expertise to make the book truly unique. They have played a crucial role in the development of this book. Without their invaluable contributions this book wouldn't have been possible. They have made vital efforts to compile up to date information on the varied aspects of this subject to make this book a valuable addition to the collection of many professionals and students.

This book was conceptualized with the vision of imparting up-to-date information and advanced data in this field. To ensure the same, a matchless editorial board was set up. Every individual on the board went through rigorous rounds of assessment to prove their worth. After which they invested a large part of their time researching and compiling the most relevant data for our readers.

The editorial board has been involved in producing this book since its inception. They have spent rigorous hours researching and exploring the diverse topics which have resulted in the successful publishing of this book. They have passed on their knowledge of decades through this book. To expedite this challenging task, the publisher supported the team at every step. A small team of assistant editors was also appointed to further simplify the editing procedure and attain best results for the readers.

Apart from the editorial board, the designing team has also invested a significant amount of their time in understanding the subject and creating the most relevant covers. They scrutinized every image to scout for the most suitable representation of the subject and create an appropriate cover for the book.

The publishing team has been an ardent support to the editorial, designing and production team. Their endless efforts to recruit the best for this project, has resulted in the accomplishment of this book. They are a veteran in the field of academics and their pool of knowledge is as vast as their experience in printing. Their expertise and guidance has proved useful at every step. Their uncompromising quality standards have made this book an exceptional effort. Their encouragement from time to time has been an inspiration for everyone.

The publisher and the editorial board hope that this book will prove to be a valuable piece of knowledge for researchers, students, practitioners and scholars across the globe.

List of Contributors

Kyoko Oh-oka and Kayoko Ishimaru
Department of Immunology, University of Yamanashi Faculty of Medicine, Yamanashi, Japan,

Hiroshi Kono
The First Department of Surgery, University of Yamanashi Faculty of Medicine, Yamanashi, Japan

Kunio Miyake and Takeo Kubota
Department of Epigenetic Medicine, University of Yamanashi Faculty of Medicine, Yamanashi, Japan

Hideoki Ogawa and Ko Okumura
Atopy Research Center, Juntendo University School of Medicine, Tokyo, Japan

Shigenobu Shibata
Department of Physiology and Pharmacology, School of Advanced Science and Engineering, Waseda University, Tokyo, Japan

Atsuhito Nakao
Department of Immunology, University of Yamanashi Faculty of Medicine, Yamanashi, Japan Atopy Research Center, Juntendo University School of Medicine, Tokyo, Japan

Rita Aldini
Ospedale Policlinico S.Orsola and Dipartimento di Scienza dei Metalli, Elettrochimica e Tecniche Chimiche, Universita degli Stu di Bologna, Bologna, Italy

Roberta Budriesi, Matteo Micucci, Pierfranco Ioan and Alberto Chiarini
Dipartimento di Scienze Farmaceutiche, Universita degli Studi di Bologna, Bologna, Italy

Giulia Roda, Alessandro Sartini, Elena Guidetti, Margherita Marocchi, Monica Cevenini, Marco Montagnani and Giuseppe Mazzella
Dipartimento di Medicina Clinica, Universita degli Studi di Bologna, Ospedale Policlinico S. Orsola, Bologna, Italy

Antonia D'Errico-Grigioni and Francesca Rosini
Dipartimento di Medicina Interna, dell'Invecchiamento e Malattie Nefrologiche, Universita degli Studi di Bologna; Ospedale Policlinico S. Orsola, Bologna, Italy

Corinne Schaer, Stefanie Hiltbrunner, Bettina Ernst and Manfred Kopf
Molecular Biomedicine, Institute of Integrative Biology, Swiss Federal Institute of Technology, Zurich, Switzerland

Christoph Mueller
Institute of Pathology, University of Bern, Bern, Switzerland

Michael Kurrer
Institute of Pathology, Cantonal Hospital Aarau, Aarau, Switzerland

Nicola L. Harris
Swiss Vaccine Research Institute and Global Health Institute, Ecole Polytechnique Fédérale, Lausanne, Switzerland

Zuzana Zakostelska, Miloslav Kverka, Klara Klimesova, Pavel Rossmann, Michaela Hornova and Helena Tlaskalova- Hogenova
Institute of Microbiology, Academy of Sciences of the Czech Republic, Prague, Czech Republic

Dagmar Srutkova and Tomas Hudcovic
Institute of Microbiology, Academy of Sciences of the Czech Republic, Novy Hradek, Czech Republic

Jakub Mrazek and Jan Kopecny
Institute of Animal Physiology and Genetics, Academy of Sciences of the Czech Republic, Prague, Czech Republic

Jakub Ridl
Institute of Molecular Genetics, Academy of Sciences of the Czech Republic, Prague, Czech Republic

Hamed Laroui, Mark T. Baker, Saravanan Ayyadurai and Moiz A. Charania
Department of Biology, Center Diagnostics and Therapeutics, Georgia State University, Atlanta, Georgia, United States of America

Famina Laroui
Veterans Affairs Medical Center, Decatur, Georgia, United States of America

Yutao Yan, Didier Merlin and Sarah A. Ingersoll
Department of Biology, Center Diagnostics and Therapeutics, Georgia State University, Atlanta, Georgia, United States of America
Veterans Affairs Medical Center, Decatur, Georgia, United States of America

Shanthi V. Sitaraman
Department of Medicine, Division of Digestive Diseases, Emory University, Atlanta, Georgia, United States of America

Hong Chun Liu
Department of Medicine, Division of Digestive Diseases, Emory University, Atlanta, Georgia, United States of America
Department of Gastroenterology, Zhongshan Hospital, Fudan University, Shanghai, China

Serge Hardy and Noriko Uetani
Rosalind and Morris Goodman Cancer Centre, McGill University, Montreal, Canada

Syed-Wajahat Hassan
Rosalind and Morris Goodman Cancer Centre, McGill University, Montreal, Canada Department of Medicine, Division of Experimental Medicine, McGill University, Montreal, Canada

Karen M. Doody
Rosalind and Morris Goodman Cancer Centre, McGill University, Montreal, Canada
Department of Biochemistry, McGill University, Montreal, Canada

Michel L. Tremblay
Rosalind and Morris Goodman Cancer Centre, McGill University, Montreal, Canada
Department of Medicine, Division of Experimental Medicine, McGill University, Montreal, Canada
Department of Biochemistry, McGill University, Montreal, Canada

Denis Cournoyer
Rosalind and Morris Goodman Cancer Centre, McGill University, Montreal, Canada
Department of Medicine, Division of Experimental Medicine, McGill University, Montreal, Canada
Department of Oncology, McGill University, Montreal, Canada

Ke Wang
Department of Immunology, School of Basic Medical Sciences, Central South University, Changsha, P. R. China
Department of Immunology, Institute of Basic Medical Sciences, Beijing, P. R. China

Gencheng Han, Yi Wang, Renxi Wang, He Xiao, Xinying Li, Yan Li, Guojiang Chen, Chunmei Hou and Beifen Shen
Department of Immunology, Institute of Basic Medical Sciences, Beijing, P. R. China

Yan Dou
Department of Gastroenterology, General Hospital of PLA, Beijing, P. R. China

Guijun Liu and Yanchun Shi
Center of Molecular Biology, Inner Mongolia Medical College, Hohhot, P. R. China

Renfeng Guo
InflaRx GmbH, Jena, Germany

Johan Gottfries
Department of Chemistry, University of Gothenburg, Gothenburg, Sweden

Silvia Melgar
Alimentary Pharmabiotic Centre, University College Cork, National University of Ireland, Cork, Ireland

Erik Michaëlsson
Department of Bioscience, Cardiovascular and Gastrointestinal IMED, AstraZeneca R&D Mölndal, Mölndal, Sweden

Helmut Neumann, Claudia Günther, Martin Grauer, Nadine Wittkopf, Jonas Mudter, Raja Atreya, Christoph Becker and Markus F. Neurath
Department of Medicine I, University of Erlangen-Nuremberg, Erlangen, Germany

Michael Vieth
Institute of Pathology, Klinikum Bayreuth, Bayreuth, Germany

Christoph Schoerner
Institute of Microbiology, Immunology and Hygiene, University of Erlangen-Nuremberg, Erlangen, Germany

Hiroshi Yukitake, Haruhide Kimura, Hirobumi Suzuki, Yasukazu Tajima, Yoshimi Sato, Toshihiro Imaeda and Masayuki Takizawa
Pharmaceutical Research Division, Takeda Pharmaceutical Company Limited, Fujisawa, Japan

Masahiro Kajino
Chemistry, Manufacturing and Controls, Takeda Pharmaceutical Company Limited, Osaka, Japan

Jana Hemmerling, Katharina Heller, Gabriele Hörmannsperger, Monika Bazanella, Thomas Clavel and Dirk Haller
Chair of Nutrition and Immunology, Technische Universität München, Freising- Weihenstephan, Bavaria, Germany
ZIEL - Research Center for Nutrition and Food Sciences, Freising-Weihenstephan, Bavaria, Germany

George Kollias
Biomedical Sciences Research Centre, Institute for Immunology, Alexander Fleming, Vari, Athens, Greece

Ramzi Fattouh, Cong-Hui Guo, Grace Y. Lam and Melanie G. Gareau
Cell Biology Program, Hospital for Sick Children, Toronto, Ontario, Canada

Bo-Yee Ngan
Department of Pathology, Hospital for Sick Children, Toronto, Ontario, Canada

Michael Glogauer
Faculty of Dentistry, University of Toronto, Toronto, Ontario, Canada

Aleixo M. Muise
Cell Biology Program, Hospital for Sick Children, Toronto, Ontario, Canada
Division of Gastroenterology, Hepatology, and Nutrition, Department of Pediatrics, Hospital for Sick Children, University of Toronto, Toronto, Ontario, Canada
Institute of Medical Science, University of Toronto, Toronto, Ontario, Canada
Sickkids IBD Centre, Hospital for Sick Children, Toronto, Ontario, Canada

John H. Brumell
Cell Biology Program, Hospital for Sick Children, Toronto, Ontario, Canada
Institute of Medical Science, University of Toronto, Toronto, Ontario, Canada
Sickkids IBD Centre, Hospital for Sick Children, Toronto, Ontario, Canada
Department of Molecular Genetics, University of Toronto, Toronto, Ontario, Canada

Toshinori Ito
Departments of Complementary and Alternative Medicine, Graduate School of Medicine, Osaka University, Osaka, Japan

Yasuaki Sanada
Departments of Complementary and Alternative Medicine, Graduate School of Medicine, Osaka University, Osaka, Japan
Department of Hospital Pharmacy Education, Graduate School of Pharmaceutical Science, Osaka University, Osaka, Japan

Etsuko Uejima
Department of Hospital Pharmacy Education, Graduate School of Pharmaceutical Science, Osaka University, Osaka, Japan

Tsunekazu Mizushima, Yasuyuki Kai and Junichi Nishimura
Department of Surgery, Gastroenterological Surgery, Graduate School of Medicine, Osaka University, Osaka, Japan

Hiroshi Hagiya and Haruto Kurata
Minase Research Institute, Ono Pharmaceutical Co., Ltd, Osaka, Japan

Hirotaka Mizuno
Tsukuba Research Institute, Ono Pharmaceutical Co., Ltd, Ibaraki, Japan

Steven R. Tannenbaum and Yu Zeng
Biological Engineering Department, Massachusetts Institute of Technology, Cambridge, Massachusetts, United States of America

David B. Schauer
Biological Engineering Department, Massachusetts Institute of Technology, Cambridge, Massachusetts, United States of America
Division of Comparative Medicine,Massachusetts Institute of Technology, Cambridge, Massachusetts, United States of America

Nicola Parry
Division of Comparative Medicine,Massachusetts Institute of Technology, Cambridge, Massachusetts, United States of America

Megan E. McBee
Biological Engineering Department, Massachusetts Institute of Technology, Cambridge, Massachusetts, United States of America
Department of Pathology, The University of Chicago, Chicago, Illinois, United States of America

Cathryn R. Nagler
Department of Pathology, The University of Chicago, Chicago, Illinois, United States of America

Laura Goeser and Ting-Jia Fan
Center for Gastrointestinal Biology and Disease, University of North Carolina at Chapel Hill, Chapel Hill, North Carolina, United States of America

Jonathan J. Hansen
Center for Gastrointestinal Biology and Disease, University of North Carolina at Chapel Hill, Chapel Hill, North Carolina, United States of America
Department of Medicine, Division of Gastroenterology and Hepatology, University of North Carolina at Chapel Hill, Chapel Hill, North Carolina, United States of America

Yong Huang and Eugene B. Chang
Department of Medicine, Section of Gastroenterology, University of Chicago Medical Center, Chicago, Illinois, United States of America

Daniel A. Peterson
Department of Pathology, Johns Hopkins University School of Medicine, Baltimore, Maryland, United States of America

R. Balfour Sartor
Center for Gastrointestinal Biology and Disease, University of North Carolina at Chapel Hill, Chapel Hill, North Carolina, United States of America
Department of Medicine, Division of Gastroenterology and Hepatology, University of North Carolina at Chapel Hill, Chapel Hill, North Carolina, United States of America
Department of Microbiology and Immunology, University of North Carolina at Chapel Hill, Chapel Hill, North Carolina, United States of America

Marc-Andre Wurbel, Peter Dwyer and Edda Fiebiger
Division of Gastroenterology and Nutrition, Children's Hospital Boston, and Department of Pediatrics, Harvard Medical School, Boston, Massachusetts, United States of America

Maria G. McIntire
Department of Pathology, Harvard Medical School, Brigham and Women's Hospital, Boston, Massachusetts, United States of America

Yuan-Chin Hsiung and Sung-Ling Yeh
School of Nutrition and Health Sciences, Taipei Medical University, Taipei, Taiwan

Jun-Jen Liu
School of Medical Laboratory Science and Biotechnology, Taipei Medical University, Taipei, Taiwan

Yu-Chen Hou
Department of Surgery, National Taiwan University Hospital, Taipei, Taiwan

Chiu-Li Yeh
Department of Food and Nutrition, Chinese Culture University, Taipei, Taiwan

Yeonsoo Joe, Md. Jamal Uddin, Hyo Jeong Kim, Yingqing Chen, Nal Ae Yoon, Jeong Woo Park and Hun Taeg Chung
Department of Biological Sciences, University of Ulsan, Ulsan, Korea

Min Zheng
Department of Biological Sciences, University of Ulsan, Ulsan, Korea
Department of Thoracic and Cardiovascular Surgery, Affiliated Hospital of Yanbian University, Yanji, China

Gyeong Jae Cho
Department of Anatomy, School of Medicine and Institute of Health Sciences, Gyeongsang National University, Jinju, Korea

Christoph Thelemann, Remzi Onur Eren, Manuel Coutaz, Muriel Rosa, Anais Duval, Christine Lavanchy, Vanessa Mack and Hans Acha-Orbea
Department of Biochemistry, University of Lausanne, Epalinges, Switzerland

Jennifer Brasseit and Christoph Mueller
Institute of Pathology, University of Bern, Bern, Switzerland

Hanifa Bouzourene
Unilabs Pathologie Suisse Romande, Epalinges, Switzerland

Walter Reith
Department of Pathology and Immunology, University of Geneva, Geneva, Switzerland

Saravanan Ayyadurai, Moiz A. Charania, Bo Xiao and Yuchen Zhang
Department of Biology and Chemistry, Center for Diagnostics and Therapeutics, Georgia State University, Atlanta, Georgia, United States of America

Emilie Viennois and Didier Merlin
Department of Biology and Chemistry, Center for Diagnostics and Therapeutics, Georgia State University, Atlanta, Georgia, United States of America
Veterans Affairs Medical Center, Decatur, Georgia, United States of America

Juan Li, Wei Zhong, Weiwei Wang, Shaoping Hu, Jiahui Yuan, Tianhui Hu and Gang Song
Cancer Research Center, Medical College of Xiamen University, Xiamen, China

Bing Zhang
Department of Basic Medicine, Medical College of Xiamen University, Xiamen, China

Marcela de Azevedo, Tessalia Diniz Luerce, Vasco Azevedo and Anderson Miyoshi
Department of General Biology, Instituto de Ciências Biológicas, Universidade Federal de Minas Gerais, Belo Horizonte, Brazil

Ana Cristina Gomes-Santos, Ana Maria Caetano de Faria and Thais Garcias Moreira
Department of Biochemistry and Immunology, Instituto de Ciências Biológicas, Universidade Federal de Minas Gerais, Belo Horizonte, Brazil

Philippe Langella, Emmanuelle Maguin and Maarten van de Guchte
INRA, UMR1319 Micalis, Jouy-en-Josas, France
AgroParisTech, UMR Micalis, Jouy-en-Josas, France

Clarissa Santos Rocha
Department of General Biology, Instituto de Ciências Biológicas, Universidade Federal de Minas Gerais, Belo Horizonte, Brazil INRA, UMR1319 Micalis, Jouy-en-Josas, France, AgroParisTech, UMR Micalis, Jouy-en-Josas, France

Mahendra Mariadassou
INRA, Mathématique, Informatique et Génome, UR1077, Jouy-en-Josas, France

Ana Paula Longaray Delamare
Institute of Biotechnology, Universidade de Caxias do Sul, Caxias do Sul, Brazil

Index